Foundations for Community Health Workers

Tim Berthold

Jeni Miller

Alma Avila-Esparza

EDITORS

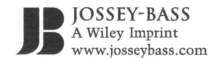

JOSSEY-BASS
A Wiley Imprint
www.josseybass.com

Published by Jossey-Bass
A Wiley Imprint
989 Market Street, San Francisco, CA 94103–1741—www.josseybass.com

Readers should be aware that Internet Web sites offered as citations and/or sources for further information may have changed or disappeared between the time this was written and when it is read.

Limit of Liability/Disclaimer of Warranty: While the publisher and author have used their best efforts in preparing this book, they make no representations or warranties with respect to the accuracy or completeness of the contents of this book and specifically disclaim any implied warranties of merchantability or fitness for a particular purpose. No warranty may be created or extended by sales representatives or written sales materials. The advice and strategies contained herein may not be suitable for your situation. You should consult with a professional where appropriate. Neither the publisher nor author shall be liable for any loss of profit or any other commercial damages, including but not limited to special, incidental, consequential, or other damages.

Jossey-Bass books and products are available through most bookstores. To contact Jossey-Bass directly call our Customer Care Department within the U.S. at 800–956–7739, outside the U.S. at 317–572–3986, or fax 317–572–4002.

Jossey-Bass also publishes its books in a variety of electronic formats. Some content that appears in print may not be available in electronic books.

Library of Congress Cataloging-in-Publication Data
Foundations for community health workers / Tim Berthold, Jennifer Miller, alma Avila-Esparza, editors.
      p.   cm.
Includes index.
ISBN 978-0-470-17997-0 (pbk.)
      1. Community health aides. 2. Community health services. I. Berthold, Tim. II. Miller, Jennifer, 1963-
III. Avila-Esparza, Alma.
RA427.F66   2009
362.12—dc22
                                                                                    2009021665

Printed in the United States of America
PB Printing   10 9 8 7 6 5 4

CONTENTS

INTRODUCTION

This book is based on the curriculum developed for the Community Health Worker Certificate Program established at the City College of San Francisco (CCSF) in 1992 (www.ccsf.edu/hlth). The certificate program was developed through Community Health Works, a partnership between CCSF and San Francisco State University (SFSU), based on research on the roles and core competencies of community health workers (CHWs) undertaken by Mary Beth Love and colleagues (www.communityhealthworks.org).

When we started the CHW Certificate Program, we were unable to locate an existing curriculum that addressed these core roles and competencies. Over the past fifteen years, faculty at CCSF have collaborated with students, internship preceptors, working CHWs, and their employers to develop, evaluate, and revise a curriculum that is responsive to the field of public health and the emerging roles of CHWs. Over time, the idea emerged to write a textbook that could be used in our classrooms. This book is for CHWs in training. In the future, we hope to develop a companion resource to guide those who facilitate these trainings.

The book is divided into three parts. Part One provides information about the broad context that informs the work of CHWs, including an introduction to the role and history of CHWs, the discipline of public health, health inequalities, globalization, the U.S. health care system, the public policy process, and working effectively across cultures in an increasingly diverse society. Part Two addresses professional skills and the competencies that CHWs use when working with individual clients: conducting initial client interviews, client-centered counseling, case management, and home visiting. Part Two also addresses concepts of ethics, scope of practice and skills for stress management, conflict resolution, and working in a professional environment. Part Three addresses competencies that CHWs use when working at the group and community levels, including how to conduct a health outreach and a community diagnosis, how to facilitate educational trainings, support groups, and community organizing and advocacy efforts.

One book cannot possibly address all the knowledge and skills required of CHWs. Our intention is to provide an introduction to the competencies most commonly required of CHWs. We acknowledge that the topics addressed in each chapter could form the basis of its own book. We ask you to keep this in mind, and to remember that the process of becoming a CHW is ongoing. Your knowledge and skills will be influenced by a wide variety of factors, including your training, on-the-job experience, guidance and support from experienced CHWs, supervisors, and other colleagues. Your life experience, cultural identity, and personality also contribute to your work as a CHW. Most important, you will learn from the clients and communities you work with.

Guiding principles that inform this book include a commitment to social justice, cultural humility, and client- and community-centered practice that respects the experience, wisdom, and autonomy of those we work with. The book is also inspired by the ideas of popular education and the works of Paolo Freire, who believed that education should be a process of political awakening and liberation.

This book was created in collaboration with many people. Some contributors have experience working as CHWs. Some have experience teaching CHWs in the classroom or community-based setting. Some have experience working in public health in other ways, and others have experience conducting research and advocating with and on behalf of CHWs. *All* of us have had the privilege of knowing and working with CHWs. We have witnessed the passion, commitment, skills, and creativity that CHWs bring to their work. Because the contributors have different life and professional experiences, we bring different writing styles and different opinions to this book. These differences echo those that exist in the field of public health and among CHWs.

CHWs contributed to this book in a variety of ways. Some chapters were written by CHWs or former CHWs. We recruited four working CHWs who graduated from the CCSF Program—Ramona Benson, Lee Jackson, Phuong An Doan-Billings, and Alvaro Morales— to participate in qualitative interviews about their work. They also participated in a Photovoice project, taking photographs to document their communities and the work they do. Their quotes and photos appear throughout the book (please note that the CHWs spoke with clients at length before obtaining informed consent to take their photographs). A detailed introduction to each of these four CHWs is included in Chapter One. In addition, nationally recognized and respected CHWs have shared their thoughts or experiences on crucial topics covered in the book, such as the history of the field and the role of CHWs.

The editors and most of the contributors to this book are based in the San Francisco Bay Area. For these reasons, the photos and stories are not representative of the full range of diversity of CHWs or their work throughout the United States and the world. We are confident, however, that the knowledge and skills presented in this book are relevant to all CHWs, regardless of the communities they work with and the health issues they address.

We have written this book for CHWs and for the agencies and institutions who train CHWs. We understand that CHWs are trained in a variety of ways: by the agencies they work or volunteer for, by participating in workshops or training institutes in the community, and in college settings. While this book is based on our experience training CHWs at a community college, we support programs that provide high-quality training of CHWs in any setting. We are opposed to policy efforts that would require college-based training of CHWs or certification of CHWs that would discriminate against any community, such as communities who do not speak English, English Language Learners, undocumented residents, or formerly incarcerated communities. We address these issues in greater detail in Chapters One and Two of the book.

This book is rooted in a deep hope for a world characterized by social justice and equal access to the basic resources—including education, employment, food, housing, safety, health care, and human rights—that everyone needs in order to be healthy. CHWs play a vital role in helping to create such a world. They partner with clients and communities and support them to take action to transform this hope into a reality.

We welcome your responses to this book and your suggestions for how to improve it, should we have that opportunity. Your comments may be sent to us at

The CHW Program
Health Education Department
City College of San Francisco
50 Phelan Avenue, C363
San Francisco, CA 94112

ACKNOWLEDGMENTS

This book would not have been possible without the leadership of Mary Beth Love and Vicki Legion. Mary Beth is the chair of the Health Education Department at San Francisco State University (SFSU) and founder of Community Health Works, a unique and enduring partnership between the Health Education Departments at SFSU and City College of San Francisco (CCSF) (www.communityhealthworks.org). This partnership established the CHW Certificate Program at CCSF. Vicki Legion served as the first coordinator and created the model CHW program that serves as the basis for this book.

We thank the faculty who have taught in the CHW Certificate Program and collaborated with students and community-based organizations to develop the curriculum that informs this book, including Alma Avila-Esparza, Susanna Hennessy-Lavery, Melissa Jones, Obiel Leyva, Joani Marinoff, Marcellina Ogbu, Abby Rincon, and Darouny Somsanith.

Cindy Tsai helped to establish the CCSF CHW Certificate Program and was instrumental in creating the vision for this book. Len Finocchio proposed doing a Photovoice project to document the work of CHWs for use in the book. He trained and supervised five graduates of the CHW program to take photographs of their communities and their work. These photographs, along with others taken by Len and Cindy Tsai, are used throughout the book.

Regina Rowland served as our creative director and developed the graphic design for this book. We owe a deep debt of gratitude to Mickey Ellinger, who conducted qualitative interviews with CHWs, cowrote several chapters of the book, and served as an editor for many others. Maia Russell provided a steady hand and endless patience in her role as administrative coordinator of the book project. We also acknowledge the leadership and support provided by several CCSF colleagues: Carol Cheng, administrative coordinator of the Health Education Department; Linda Squires-Grohe, dean of the School of Health and Physical Education; Janey Skinner, program director for the Interior Bay Area Regional Health Occupations Resource Center; and Bob Gabriner, vice chancellor of institutional advancement.

We wish to thank all CHWs who contributed to the book through their interviews and photographs, including Veronica Aburto, Kathleen Banks, Ramona Benson, Esther Chavez, Phuong An Doan-Billings, Durrell Fox, Thomas Ganger, Lee Jackson, Sergio Matos, Alvaro Morales, David Pheng, Kent Rodriguez, Romelia Rodriguez, LaTonya Rogers, Somnang Sin, Letida Sot, Jason Stanford, and Manith Thaing.

A number of reviewers provided critical feedback on key book chapters, including Nell Bronstein, Durrell Fox, Vicki Legion, Sergio Matos, Carl Rush, Janey Skinner, Jill Tregor, and the Steering Committee of the American Association of CHWs (AACHW).

We also acknowledge those who provided grants and donations to support the development of this book: Kaiser Permanente, Northern California Community Benefits, and Eastman Kodak. This book would not have been possible without our previous work on the *Yes We Can Manual*, a curriculum for training clinical care teams—including CHWs—to manage childhood asthma. The *Yes We Can Manual* was funded by the California Endowment and Kaiser Permanente and was supported by the Pediatric Asthma Clinic at San Francisco General Hospital, University of California, San Francisco, and the San Francisco Department of Public Health, Primary Care Division.

Most important, this book acknowledges and is dedicated to community health workers past, present, and future.

CONTRIBUTORS

Alma Avila-Esparza, MPH Alma Avila-Esparza is the coordinator for the community health worker (CHW) program at the City College of San Francisco. Alma has a master's degree in public health and has been involved with community health worker programs and *promotora* programs for more than fifteen years.

Tim Berthold, MPH Tim Berthold is chair of the Health Education Department at the City College of San Francisco. He has twenty years' experience working with diverse communities to train community health and human rights workers.

Philip Colgan, PhD Philip Colgan is a psychologist in private practice in San Francisco, specializing in the treatment of attachment disorders in close relationships, including problems with addiction, communication, and sexuality. He teaches at the City College of San Francisco and at Diablo Valley College in Pleasant Hill, California.

Mickey Ellinger, PhD Mickey Ellinger interviewed community health workers and wrote early drafts of some chapters of the textbook. She was part of the team that produced Community Health Works' *Asthma Toolkit—Managing Children's Asthma*.

Len Finocchio, DrPH Len Finocchio is a senior program officer at the California HealthCare Foundation. He also teaches courses on the health care system and health policy at San Francisco State University and the City College of San Francisco.

Edith Guillén-Núñez, JD, MS, LMFT Edith Guillén-Núñez is an educator, attorney, and licensed marriage family therapist. She is a faculty member in the Health Education Department at the City College of San Francisco. Her therapy practice focuses on working with families and children in the areas of family violence, trauma, and substance abuse. She specializes in family law and consults in the area of ethical and legal issues to mental health agencies.

Susana Hennessey Lavery, MPH Susana Hennessey Lavery is a health educator with the San Francisco Department of Public Health, Tobacco Free Project, where she works on food systems and food security, community health worker, and popular education projects. For thirteen years she worked as a community health educator and coordinated the Casa CHE program at La Clínica de la Raza in Oakland, California.

Mele Lau-Smith, MPH Mele Lau-Smith is the health program coordinator with the San Francisco Department of Public, Tobacco Free Project. She is involved in the development and implementation of the comprehensive tobacco control plan for San Francisco.

This includes training, contract management, and development of advocacy and community capacity-building projects, as well as providing resources to the groups working to address the global impact of tobacco.

Joani Marinoff, MPH   Joani Marinoff is the coordinator of HIV/STI Prevention Studies in the Health Education Department at City College of San Francisco. She has more than thirty-five years of experience in health care and education, participatory learning, and organizing strategies for addressing health disparities through reflection and community action. She is also a longtime meditator and teaches restorative yoga.

Jeni Miller, PhD   Jeni Miller is communications manager and codirector of Partnership for the Public's Health, a project of the Public Health Institute. In this role, she assists people and institutions work together to make their communities healthier places to live, with access to fresh foods, places to play and be active, and places where people have a voice in shaping their own neighborhoods, schools, and communities.

Sal Núñez, PhD, LMFT   Sal Núñez is a full-time instructor and program coordinator at the Health Education Department of the City College of San Francisco. He practices as a clinical psychologist, consultant, and researcher and is interested in pediatric health, indigenous medicine, neuropsychology, clinical biofeedback, chemical dependence, and therapeutic/healing drumming as a treatment modality.

Rhonella C. Owens, MEd, PhD   Rhonella C. Owens has a B.S. in both business education and general business, an M.Ed. in counseling, and a Ph.D. in psychology (emphasis in integrating traditional Western psychology with Eastern traditions of personality). She has been a counselor and instructor at the City College of San Francisco for twenty-two years. Rhonella is also the author of *The Journey of Your Life* (life coaching workbook) and *Turn Your Dreams into Reality* (goal setting and achievement).

Abby M. Rincón, MPH   Abby M. Rincón is director of diversity at U.C. Berkeley's School of Public Health, is a part-time faculty member at the City College of San Francisco, and has been teaching in the Community Health Worker program since 2002. She has been in the field of public health for more than twenty-five years and has developed health education programs for migrant farmer workers in a rural community, served as the director of health promotion for the University Health Services at U.C. Berkeley, and participated in creating a primary care counselor program in Zimbabwe focusing on HIV/AIDS.

E. Lee Rosenthal, PhD, MS, MPH   E. Lee Rosenthal is an assistant professor in the Department of Health Promotion at the University of Texas at El Paso. She directed the Annie E. Casey Foundation-funded National Community Health Advisor Study (University of Arizona, 1998) and is a coinvestigator on a study entitled "Can *Promotores* Change Clinical Outcomes for Chronic Disease?" funded by the National Institutes of Health National Center on Minority Health and Health Disparities. She is also codirector of the Community Health Worker National Education Collaborative funded by the U.S. Department of Education.

Darouny Somsanith, MPH   Darouny Somsanith is currently an instructor at the City College of San Francisco within the Health Education Department. Along with teaching, she coordinates a program to bring work-based training and education to frontline staff at a local social service agency.

Amber Straus, MEd   Amber Straus teaches academic literacy at the City College of San Francisco. She loves working with and learning from students. Amber sees education as a vital tool for ending cycles of oppression and creating social justice.

Jill Tregor, MPH   Jill Tregor is the program director for the Regional Health Occupations Resource Center at the City College of San Francisco. Over the course of her career, Jill has developed and led training and education sessions for law enforcement, teachers, court staff, and students from kindergarten through college, on topics ranging from hate crime awareness and prevention and cultural awareness to providing assistance to survivors of domestic violence.

Sharon Turner, MPH   Sharon Turner has worked at CCSF in a variety of capacities since 2004. She has worked for the Drug and Alcohol Studies Department; taught general health education classes, women's health, and CPR/First Aid; and developed and taught a class on global health based on her international experience in Uganda.

Darlene Weide, MPH, MSW   Darlene Weide is a faculty member in the Health Education Department at the City College of San Francisco and the executive director of Community Boards, the nation's longest-running community-based dispute resolution organization.

Craig Wenzl, BA   Craig Wenzl is associate director of drug and alcohol studies at the City College of San Francisco. Prior to City College, Craig worked for ten years as the director of programs at the Monterey County AIDS Project (MCAP) in Seaside and Salinas, California. In addition to program coordinating, Craig also worked as a community health outreach worker, HIV testing counselor, and group facilitator, with a focus on sexual risk and substance use.

Ellen Wu, MPH   Ellen Wu is the executive director of the California Pan-Ethnic Health Network (CPEHN), a statewide network of multicultural health organizations working together to ensure that all Californians have access to quality health care and can live healthy lives. Ellen has worked with a culturally diverse low-income and uninsured population since 1996, and prior to CPEHN, she was the director of health education and cultural/linguistic services at the Alameda Alliance for Health.

PART 1

The Changing World of the Community Health Worker

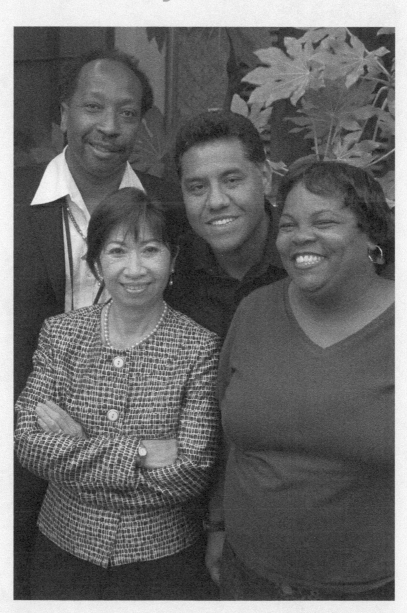

1

The Role of CHWs

Darouny Somsanith

I was homeless, living in a shelter with my daughter. There was a nurse practitioner who provided prenatal care at the shelter two days a week. When a pregnant woman came in, sometimes they came in the middle of the night, so I would give them a short presentation about the prenatal services at the shelter, and tell them when the nurse practitioner lady was coming in.

I didn't know why I was doing it, I just was doing it. I got housing after three months of being at the shelter. While I was there, I was interacting with the nurse practitioner. And when I got ready to move into my housing, she asked me did I want to become a community health worker for her. I'm like, "Sure, but what is a community health worker?" I was the second CHW with her organization. She had just started this organization called the Homeless Prenatal Program, and she and a part-time social worker took me on the streets to show me what a CHW does. I learned the ropes and I used my life experience, and the part-time social worker showed me what to do in the community, and then I just took off from there. That's how I became a CHW.

—*Ramona Benson, Community Health Worker*
Black Infant Health Program, Berkeley, California

INTRODUCTION

This chapter introduces you to the key roles and skills of community health workers (CHWs) and addresses common qualities and values of successful CHWs. It will introduce you to the four CHWs pictured in the photograph at the beginning of this chapter. They are each graduates of the CHW Certificate Program at City College of San Francisco, on which this book is based. Their quotes and photographs appear throughout the book, providing examples of the work they do to promote community health.

You may already possess some of the qualities, knowledge, and skills common among CHWs. Are you a trusted member of your community? Have you ever assisted a family member or friend to obtain health care services? Are there things harming your community's health that you feel passionate about changing? Have you participated in efforts to advocate for social change? Do you hope that, in your work, you can work with your community members to become healthy, strong, and in charge of their lives? If you answered yes to any of these questions, you have some of the characteristics of a successful CHW.

WHAT YOU WILL LEARN

By studying the information in this chapter, you will be able to:

- ✪ Describe CHWs and what they do
- ✪ Identify where CHWs work, the populations they work with, and the health issues they address
- ✪ Explain the core roles that CHWs play in the health and social services fields
- ✪ Discuss the core skills necessary to become an effective CHW
- ✪ Describe personal qualities and values that are common among successful CHWs

WORDS TO KNOW

Mortality	Social Justice	Competencies
Credentialing	Advocate (noun)	
Advocate (verb)	Health Inequalities	

1.1 WHO ARE CHWs AND WHAT DO THEY DO?

CHWs generally come from the communities they serve and are therefore uniquely prepared to provide culturally and linguistically appropriate services (Love and others, 1997). They work with diverse communities who are most at risk of illness, disability, and death. CHWs provide a wide range of services, including outreach, home visits, health education, and client-centered counseling and case management. They support clients in accessing high-quality health and social services programs. They facilitate support groups and workshops and support communities to organize and **advocate** (to actively speak up and support a client, community, or policy change) for social change that promotes their health and welfare. CHWs also work with health care and social services agencies to enhance their capacity to provide culturally sensitive services that truly respect the diverse identities, strengths, and needs of the clients and communities they serve. As a result of the work of CHWs, clients and communities learn new information and skills, increase their confidence, and enhance their ability to successfully advocate for themselves. Most important, the work that CHWs do reduces persistent **health inequalities** or differences in the rates of illness, disability, and death (or **mortality**) among different communities (Ro and others, 2003).

The U.S. Bureau of Labor Statistic's *Occupational Outlook Handbook* (2009) projected "social and human service assistants" (the category that until recently included CHWs) to be one of the fastest growing occupations for the years 2000 to 2010. Increasingly, health departments, community-based organizations, hospitals and clinics, foundations, and researchers recognize the important contributions of CHWs to promoting the health of low-income and at-risk communities.

CHWs work under a wide range of professional titles. Some of the most popular include:

Case manager/Case worker
Community health advocate
Community health outreach worker
Community liaison
Community organizer
Community outreach worker
Enrollment specialist
Health ambassador
Health educator
Health worker
Patient navigator
Peer counselor
Peer educator
Promotor/a
Public health aide

Can you think of other titles that CHWs go by?

Because CHWs work under many different job titles and perform a wide variety of duties, it has been difficult to determine how many people are working in the field in the United States and what types of jobs they hold. A study of the CHW field was completed in 2007 by the U.S. Department of Health and Human Services and the University of Texas in San Antonio. The study was called the Community Health Worker National Workforce Study (CHWNWS, 2007) and to date is the most accurate national estimate of the workforce. The following are highlights of the study's findings:

OVERALL NUMBER, GENDER, AND ETHNICITY

- In 2000, there were approximately 86,000 CHWs working in the United States. California (9,000) and New York (8,000) had the most CHWs.
- The majority of CHWs were female (82 percent) between the ages of 30 and 50. One-fourth of the workforce was younger than 30 and one-fourth was older than 50 years old.
- CHWs were Hispanic (35 percent) or Non-Hispanic Whites (39 percent); African Americans made up 15.5 percent of the workforce, followed by Native Americans (5 percent), and Asian and Pacific Islanders (4.6 percent).

EDUCATION AND WAGES

- Thirty-five percent of CHWs had high school diplomas, 20 percent had completed some type of college, and 31 percent had at least a four-year college degree. When comparing volunteers and paid CHWs, the volunteers tended to have less than a high school diploma, while paid workers were more likely to have completed some college.
- The majority of experienced CHWs (70 percent) received an hourly wage of $13 or more, and about half received $15 or more.

POPULATIONS SERVED

CHWs provided services to all racial and ethnic communities: Hispanic/Latino (78 percent), Black/African American (68 percent), and Non-Hispanic White (64 percent). One-third of CHWs surveyed reported services to Asian/Pacific Islander (34 percent) and American Indian/Alaska Natives (32 percent).

The majority of the clients served were females and adults ages 18 to 49.

Other populations served included the uninsured (71 percent), immigrants (49 percent), homeless individuals (41 percent), isolated rural and migrant workers (31 percent each), and colonial or community residents (9 percent).

Programs serving immigrants, migrant workers, and the uninsured were more likely to have volunteer CHWs.

CHWs work primarily with low-income communities. They work with children, youth and their families, adults and seniors, men and women, and people of all sexual orientations and gender identities.

HEALTH ISSUES AND ACTIVITIES

- The top health areas that CHWs were found to work in were women's health and nutrition, child health and pregnancy/prenatal care, immunizations, and sexual behaviors.
- The most common specific illnesses CHWs were working to address included HIV/AIDS (39 percent), diabetes (38 percent), high blood pressure (31 percent), cancer (27 percent), cardiovascular diseases (26 percent), and heart disease (23 percent).

○ Specific work activities included culturally appropriate health promotion and education (82 percent), assistance in accessing medical and nonmedical services and programs (84 percent and 72 percent, respectively), translating (36 percent), interpreting (34 percent), counseling (31 percent), mentoring (21 percent), social support (46 percent), and transportation (36 percent).

○ Related to the work activities listed, specific CHWs duties included case management, risk identification, patient navigation, and providing direct services such as blood pressure screening.

Because most CHWs work within the field of public health (see Chapter Three), they address the widest range of health issues, including issues such as homelessness, violence, environmental health, mental health recovery, and civil and human rights issues.

CHWs work directly with individual clients and families, with groups, and at the community level. They provide health education and case management services, facilitate support groups and educational workshops or trainings, and support communities to organize and advocate for social change and social justice.

MODELS OF CARE

The study further identified five "models of care" that incorporated CHWs within them:

1. *Member of a care delivery team:* CHWs work with other providers (for example, doctors, nurses, social worker) to care for individual patients.

2. *Navigator:* CHWs are called upon to use their extensive knowledge of the complex health care system to assist individuals and patients in accessing the services they need and gain greater confidence in interacting with their providers.

3. *Screening and health education provider:* CHWs administer basic health screening (for example, pregnancy tests, blood pressure checks, and rapid HIV antibody tests) and provide prevention education on basic health topics.

4. *Outreach/enrolling/informing agent:* CHWs go into the community to reach and inform individuals and families about the services that they qualify for and encourage them to enroll in the programs.

5. *Organizer:* CHWs work with other community members to advocate for change on a specific issue or cause. Often their work aids community members to become stronger advocates for themselves.

? *When did you first become aware of CHWs?*

? *Are there CHWs working in your community?*

? *Can you think of other populations that CHWs work with? Other health issues that they address or other work activities that they do?*

The term *community health worker* describes both community volunteers who work informally to improve their community's health and those who are paid for providing these services. Regardless of their compensation, they are referred to as "frontline" health and social service workers and are often a community member's first contact with a health or social service agency. CHWs typically spend a lot of time in the community, developing trust and learning about key resources, challenges, and needs. This knowledge guides CHWs in providing assistance and support in a way that is culturally appropriate to community members.

Community health work grew out of compassion and the desire to assist those in need. This motivation propels CHWs to work for equality and **social justice** or equal access to essential health resources such as housing, food, education, employment, health care, and civil rights. Some CHWs take on this work because they have experienced discrimination and poverty and can relate to the situations of those they are working with. Others simply see a need and want to change the inequalities that exist in their communities. Regardless of how the CHW comes to the work, every CHW is an **advocate**— someone who speaks up for a cause or policy or on someone else's behalf—working to promote the health, and the conditions that support the health, of local communities.

ESTHER CHAVEZ: The reason I got into community health work was because of the immediate need in my community. There was a lack of education among youth with regard to safe sex and sexually transmitted diseases. It didn't seem to be an important topic for the other community-based organization and the need was great. So my colleague and I started an organization that provided sex education and peer support around health issues for youth in our community.

CHWs are working throughout the world, on every continent and in every country, including China's barefoot doctors, Latin American *promotoras de salud*, Bangladesh Rural Advancement Committee (BRAC) outreach workers in Bangladesh, *accompagnateurs* in Haiti, doulas in the United States, and community health representatives in Alaska and the southwestern United States. Wherever they work, their roles, duties, and even titles are flexible; they adapt to the needs of the communities they serve. This responsiveness to the needs of the communities and clients they work with is what makes CHWs so important to the health of populations throughout the world.

In October 2007, a peer-reviewed journal published by the Public Library of Science asked renowned public health leaders this question: "Which single intervention would do the most to improve the health of those living on less than \$1 per day?" Dr. Paul Farmer, founding director, Partners in Health and Presley Professor of Medical Anthropology, Harvard Medical School, Boston, provided the following answer:

> *Hire community health workers to serve them* [emphasis added]. In my experience in the rural reaches of Africa and Haiti, and among the urban poor too, the problem with so many funded health programs is that they never go the extra mile: resources (money, people, plans, services) get hung up in cities and towns. If we train village health workers, and make sure they're compensated, then the resources intended for the world's poorest—from vaccines, to bed nets, to prenatal care, and to care for chronic diseases like AIDS and tuberculosis—would reach the intended beneficiaries. Training and paying village health workers also creates jobs among the very poorest. (Yamey, 2007)

1.2 CHWs AND PUBLIC HEALTH

CHWs usually work within the field of public health (see Chapter Three). Unlike medicine, public health works to promote the health of entire communities and populations

Public health understands the primary causes of illness and health to be whether or not people have equal access to basic resources and rights, including food, housing, education, employment with safe working conditions and a living wage, transportation, clean air and water, and civil rights. Collectively, these are called the "social determinants of health." The field of public health not only provides services designed to prevent illness and increase access to quality health care, it also seeks to influence the social determinants of health by advocating for policies that increase access to basic resources and rights for all people.

> As we continue to uncover the inequities that limit access to social, economic, political, and environmental well-being, the foundation and history of community health workers as advocates for social justice becomes increasingly relevant. (Perez and Martinez, 2008)

1.3 ROLES AND COMPETENCIES OF CHWs

The roles of CHWs keep evolving to respond to changes in the field of public health and to ensure that communities are provided with culturally and linguistically appropriate services. As the field develops, and more research about CHWs is undertaken, the primary roles and skills of CHWs become more defined. These definitions are used to guide CHW training programs and to advocate for increased respect and funding for CHWs.

However, as the CHW field develops, it also experiences inevitable growing pains and tensions. Some people are worried that "professionalization" of the field may be used to restrict the roles that CHWs play. For example, some people are hesitant to have the scope of practice for CHWs defined. A *scope of practice* refers to the range of services and duties that a category of worker, such as CHWs, is competent to provide. While many CHWs express mixed feelings about how far the field should be formalized, all agree that the work they do deserves more recognition from government and other professionals, and increased funding.

A stepping-stone toward national recognition is to be officially classified by the U.S. Department of Labor, Bureau of Labor Statistics. In 2007, CHWs in the American Public Health Association (APHA) submitted the following description of the CHW field to the U.S. Department of Labor to formally classify the profession:

> A Community Health Worker (CHW) is a frontline public health worker who is a trusted member of and/or has an unusually close understanding of the community served. This trusting relationship enables the CHW to serve as a liaison/link/intermediary between health and social services and the community, to facilitate access to services and improve the quality and cultural competence of service delivery. A CHW also builds individual and community capacity by increasing health knowledge and self-sufficiency through a range of activities such as outreach, community education, informal counseling, social support and advocacy.

In March of 2009, the Department of Labor approved a separate occupational category and new definition—21-1094—for CHWs (U.S. Bureau of Labor Statistics, 2009). At the time of publication, the DOL is still accepting public comments, and the final definition for CHWs has not yet been released.

? *What do you think of this definition of the CHW field?*

While CHWs within the APHA submitted the classification, another study aided in defining and clarifying the roles and skill sets of CHWs. This study by the University of Arizona looked at the duties of working CHWs (under various titles) (Rosenthal and others, 1998).

WHAT ARE "CORE ROLES AND COMPETENCIES"?

Core roles are the major functions a person commonly performs on the job. For example, the core roles of a farmer include clearing fields, planting, and harvesting crops. The core roles of CHWs include providing outreach, health education, client-centered counseling, case management, community organizing, and advocacy. Core competencies are the knowledge and skills a person needs in order to do his or her job well. Again, a farmer must be able to operate equipment, assess timing for planting, and prepare the soil. Core competencies for CHWs include knowledge of public health, behavior change, ethics, and community resources and the ability to provide health information, facilitate groups, resolve conflicts, and conduct an initial client interview or assessment. CHW educational programs seek to strengthen CHW competencies or skills.

While the study took care not to overclassify or narrow CHW functions, it did group similar roles and skills to identify common duties that most or all CHWs performed, and the key skill sets that are necessary to be a good CHW. Identifying these **competencies** or key knowledge and skills (see feature) allows trainers and employers to better support current and new CHWs in their work. All in all, the study identified seven core roles and eight core competencies for a CHW.

CORE CHW ROLES

1. Cultural mediation between communities and the health and social services systems

Intimate knowledge of the communities they work with permits CHWs to serve as cultural brokers between their clients and health and social services systems. By being a bridge that links community members to essential services, CHWs ensure that the clients receive culturally appropriate quality care.

LETIDA SOT: As a CHW, I work regularly with doctors to assist them to communicate with our Cambodian patients. Because the Cambodian community is so small, sometimes patients have to wait many hours to speak to someone at a clinic who can understand them. By me working at the clinic, the patient doesn't get lost in the system—they can easily come to me for what they need. Besides not understanding English, some of our patients don't read or write well and have a hard time understanding their medications. One of the patients I worked with suffered from hypertension, diabetes, and heart disease. She thought that she needed to finish one type of medicine first before she can start on another, even though sometimes she needed to take fifteen different medications a month. Because of this, her diabetes was out of control and the doctor asked me to aid in the arrangement of her daily medication schedule. When I explained to her that she could take the medications simultaneously, she was shocked because she had been doing what she thought was right for ten years.

2. Informal counseling and social support

CHWs provide client-centered counseling and support to assist clients to live healthier and better lives. A CHW may provide information about healthy behaviors, such as smoking cessation, healthy eating habits, and family planning, and may use techniques such as motivational interviewing (see Chapter Ten) to support clients in reducing health-related risk behaviors.

TINA DIEP: Smoking within the Asian community, especially with men, is very integrated into the cultures. Many men know about some of the health hazards of smoking for themselves but don't really know about secondhand smoke or the other health impacts of smoking on their families. Because it is so hard for them to quit, the doctors refer them to me to get smoking cessation counseling. Of course not everyone is ready to quit or even wants to quit, but for those who are, I assist them in creating a plan to reduce or stop smoking, give them some education on the harmful effects of cigarettes, and just provide support and encouragement. In every session, I talk with them about their smoking experience and explore their ambivalence to quitting. Sometimes just talking will get those who were not ready to quit at least thinking about the possibility of it, and this can lead to another appointment and another opportunity to make a plan to quit.

3. Providing direct services and referrals

Some CHWs provide direct care to clients through the services they are trained and qualified to provide, such as reproductive health counseling or HIV-antibody test counseling. They may also provide case management services or otherwise link clients to services by knowing what services exist and referring clients appropriately.

SOMNANG SIN: When I can't provide the services for a patient, I refer them to services at another program or agency. It is important as a CHW to know what resources are available in the community. Part of my job is to make sure the patient gets the right care—I'll walk them to their appointment or to another agency if the patient needs me to.

4. Providing culturally appropriate health education

Because CHWs usually come from the communities they serve, they are familiar with the cultures of the clients they work with (for example, language, values, customs, sexual orientation, and so on) and are better prepared to provide health information in ways that the community will understand and accept.

DAVID PHENG: I am a CHW at a clinic in Oakland [California]. I see and give presentations to patients who are young adults ages fourteen to twenty. I find that during my presentations, I have to ditch lecture-based teaching and make it as entertaining as possible. But the entertainment is also speaking to the youth and relating to their everyday experiences—not from a textbook but from the radio, Internet, music, and the everyday words they use. Being culturally appropriate isn't just knowing their language but relating to them as youth, not talking down to them, and respecting their space so they feel comfortable and willing to ask questions. I find the more the youth laugh, the more they pick up on ideas and information that deal with safer sex practices and access to clinical services.

5. Advocating for individual and community needs

CHWs speak out with and on behalf of the clients and communities they work with. They advocate—with the community whenever possible—to make sure that clients are treated respectfully and given access to the basic resources that they need in order to live healthy lives.

JINYOUNG CHUN: For a couple of years now, I've taken my clients to Sacramento [California] for Immigrant Day. I think it is important that they understand how our government works and that they can have a chance to talk directly to their legislators. The clients also get to see and connect with community members from other cultures that are there for the same cause. They see that they are not alone and that people can come together and make a difference. At the legislative meetings, the clients talk about issues that impact their lives and their community while I interpret. We do a lot of preparation together before the day so they understand the process and decide what they want to say. After the meeting, they feel so empowered and heard! Many of the clients I work with now also attend and speak at local Board of Supervisor's meetings, as well as other community events on issues that they are passionate about.

6. Assuring people get the services they need

A CHW often is the first person many clients interact with. It is the job of the CHW to ensure that these clients get the services they need.

DAVID PHENG: We are usually the first ones to receive questions—and complaints— from the patients. It's fun but challenging work, because the routine is never the same. Once patients come in, I find out what services they need and assist them to get these services. I try to empower the patients to seek the services themselves, but if they need it, I'll assist in guiding them through the clinical side of checking in, seeing a doctor and offering additional resources. I see what else they might need and try to find an organization in the community that can assist them, like with food or legal issues.

7. Building individual and community capacity

CHWs support clients and community members to develop the skills and the confidence to promote and advocate for their own health and well-being.

ALVARO MORALES: One of the most important ways that I know that I am doing a good job is when my clients no longer need me, or need me as much. Everything I do is based on supporting the client not to be dependent on me any more. I want to support them to take charge of their own health, to negotiate healthy relationships, to navigate the health care system, to communicate with health care providers to get the treatment they want and deserve. And sometimes I get to work with communities and to support them to speak out for policy changes. Instead of me testifying before the Board of Supervisors (City Council) on behalf of the communities I work with, I want to support them to testify and speak out for themselves. They are the experts about what they need and want, and their voices are the voices that need to be heard.

David Pheng counseling youth at a health center.

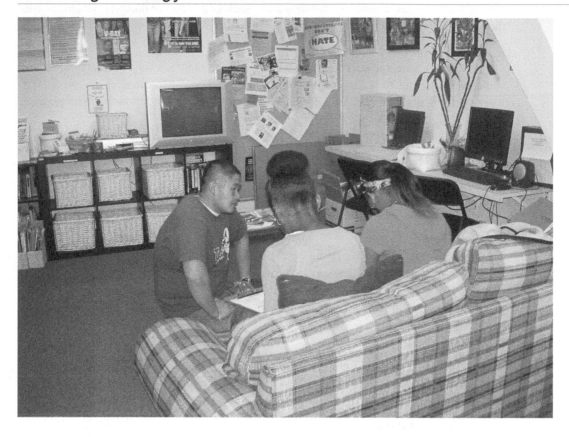

? *Have you ever taken on any of these CHWs' roles?*

? *What were some of the challenges that you faced in perform-ing the role?*

? *Can you think of other roles that a CHW might play?*

Besides sharing common roles, CHWs also share common knowledge and skills.

EIGHT CORE COMPETENCIES FOR CHWs

1. Communication skills

CHWs must be good listeners in order to learn about their clients' experiences, behaviors, strengths and needs, and to provide health information and client-centered counseling. They must also develop skills to communicate in situations of conflict or stress. Group communica-tions skills become important for leading group health education or community advocacy.

2. Interpersonal skills

CHWs work with diverse groups of people and must be able to develop positive relationships with clients, community members, supervisors, nurses, social workers, and policymakers.

3. Knowledge base about the community, health issues, and available services

CHWs often support community members to gain access to local resources. In order to do this effectively, they must spend time getting to know the communities they work with and the range of health and related services that may be available to clients. CHWs must also be knowledgeable about the health issues—such as diabetes or domestic violence—that they address day to day.

4. Service coordination skills

The health care and social service systems are complex, not very well integrated, and sometimes difficult to access. CHWs sometimes work as case managers and frequently work with clients to access available services and to create and follow realistic plans to improve their health, despite the complexity of the systems.

5. Capacity-building skills

CHWs do not want clients and communities to become dependent upon them or other service providers. They teach and support clients and communities to develop new skills and confidence to promote their own health, including, for example, communication skills, risk reduction behaviors, and community organizing and advocacy skills.

6. Advocacy skills

CHWs sometimes speak up on behalf of their clients and their communities within their own agencies, with other service providers, and to support changes in public policies. More important, CHWs support clients and communities in raising their own voices to create meaningful changes—including changes in public policies—that influence their health and well-being.

7. Teaching skills

CHWs educate clients about how to prevent and manage health conditions. CHWs teach about healthy behaviors and support clients in developing healthier habits. They also teach community members how to advocate for social change.

8. Organizational skills

CHWs support individuals, families, and communities in getting the services they need. The work is demanding, with many things to keep track of, not only for oneself but also for one's clients. Being organized is critical to ensure that CHWs are able to properly follow up with clients and accurately document data for their employers.

? *What other skills are important for CHWs to have?*

? *Do you already have some of the skills identified?*

? *Which skills do you want to learn or improve?*

1.4 PERSONAL QUALITIES AND VALUES OF CHWs

All of us bring unique life experiences to our work. These experiences, along with our individual personalities, shape our value systems and how we see the world around us. The work of a CHW depends heavily on building positive interpersonal relationships with people of diverse backgrounds and identities. Without the capacity to build relationships based on trust, CHWs cannot do their job effectively. The qualities that enable this capacity can be strengthened through practice and self-reflection. We highlight several desirable personal qualities and values in Table 1.1, adapted from work of the International Training and Education Center on HIV in Zimbabwe (I-TECH, 2004).

With these qualities and values, CHWs inspire confidence and trust and build positive professional relationships with those whom they work with.

Table 1.1.   Personal Characteristics of Successful CHWs.

Personal Characteristics	Definitions
1. Interpersonal warmth	The ability to listen, care, and respond to clients and communities with compassion and kindness
2. Trustworthiness	Being honest, allowing others to confide in you, maintaining confidentiality, and upholding professional ethics
3. Open-mindedness	The willingness to embrace others' differences, including their flaws, and be nonjudgmental in your interactions with them
4. Objectivity	Striving to work with and view clients and their circumstances without the influence of personal prejudice or bias
5. Sensitivity	To be aware of and truly respect the experience, culture, feelings, and opinions of others
6. Competence	Developing the knowledge and skills required to provide quality services to all the clients and communities you work with
7. Commitment to social justice	The commitment and heart to fight injustice and to advocate for social changes that promote the health and well-being of clients and communities
8. Good psychological health	Having the mental and emotional capacity to perform your work professionally, without doing harm to clients, colleagues, or yourself
9. Self-awareness and understanding	Being willing and able to reflect upon and analyze your own experiences, biases, and prejudices, to ensure that they do not negatively affect your interactions with clients and colleagues

? *What other personal qualities and values should CHWs have?*

? *What personal qualities and values do you bring to this work?*

? *What qualities do you want to build and enhance?*

Characteristic number 9 has special importance: self-awareness serves as a foundation that assists CHWs to cultivate other key qualities and skills. Developing awareness of our own personal biases aids in ensuring that we do not harm a client or the community by judging them according to our own experiences, values, and beliefs. This is an ethical obligation for all CHWs and is essential for two key principles of CHW practice: client- and community-centered practice and cultural humility.

Throughout this book you will find questions directed to you as a person who is training to become a CHW or to enhance your CHW skills. Some of the questions invite you to take time to reflect and to cultivate self-awareness. The questions also invite you to bring your own experience, insights, ideas, and wisdom into the conversation. Your life experience, whatever it may be, is an important foundation for the work you will do as a CHW.

The challenges of developing self-awareness and using it to inform your work as a CHW is a theme that runs throughout this book. It is addressed in Chapters Seven and Eight.

1.5 EMERGING ROLE IN THE MANAGEMENT OF CHRONIC CONDITIONS

As CHWs become more recognized and respected, their role within the health and social services field is expanding, especially in the area of primary care and chronic disease management.

CHRONIC DISEASE: THE DOMINANT TYPE OF ILLNESS IN THE UNITED STATES

Today, chronic diseases—such as cardiovascular disease (primarily heart disease and stroke), cancer, and diabetes—are the most common, costly, and preventable of all health problems in the United States. Data from the Centers for Disease Control (CDC) show that:

- More than 90 million Americans live with chronic illnesses.
- Seven of every ten Americans who die each year, or more than 1.7 million people, die of a chronic disease. Chronic diseases account for 70 percent of all deaths in the United States.
- The costs of medical care for people with chronic diseases account for more than 75 percent of the nation's $1.4 trillion medical care costs.
- Chronic diseases account for one-third of the years of potential life lost before age sixty-five. The prolonged illness and disability from chronic diseases such as diabetes and arthritis result in extended pain and suffering and decreased quality of life for millions of Americans.

CHWs WITHIN THE HEALTH CARE DELIVERY TEAM

Many clinics and hospitals now employ CHWs as members of a care delivery team for patients with chronic diseases. CHWs may work with doctors, nurses, and other providers. The care delivery team may combine social support (provided by CHWs) and clinical care (provided by doctors and nurses) to assist patients to more effectively manage and control their illnesses (Legion and others, 2006). Within this model, CHWs are trained to educate, counsel, and work with patients to improve their health through one-on-one and group sessions. CHWs may also provide home visits. Some of the chronic conditions that CHWs address in their work include diabetes, high blood pressure, HIV/AIDS, and smoking cessation.

Dr. Thomas Bodenheimer, a clinical professor within the Department of Family and Community Medicine at the University of California, San Francisco, advocates including CHWs as part of a "Team Care Model." Including CHWs as part of the team, he argues, and changing the dynamic of a primary care visits, will not only make better use of limited health care resources, but will also improve care. The three main goals of the Team Care Model (Bodenheimer, 2006) and the CHWs roles within each goal are to:

1. Improve quality, access, and patient centeredness
   - CHWs speak the languages of their patients and can connect them to culturally appropriate health and social services resources. By being a cultural bridge between their community and the service providers, CHWs ensure that clients receive better care.
   - Increasing access to quality health and social services improves health outcomes and reduces health inequalities.

2. Reduce health care costs for high-cost patients
   - CHWs provide clients with the health education, social support, and follow-up required to manage their chronic health conditions. Successful self-management of the condition will mean fewer complications, thereby decreasing the chances of a patient ending up in the emergency room, where care is more expensive.
   - The contributions of CHWs free nurses and other clinicians to invest their time caring for patients requiring urgent attention.
3. Change primary care from a doctor game to a team game
   - A clinical team model that features the role of CHWs expands the capacity of clinics and hospitals to see more patients.
   - While doctors still supervise the overall care of the patient, employing CHWs within a primary care setting will increase opportunities for patient education and prevention.

Including CHWs within a team model for clinical care will improve the quality of care for patients, improve the health of the community, decrease health inequalities, and ensure that health care services are used appropriately, which in turn will aid in reducing health care costs. As our society grows and diversifies, and as poorly treated chronic conditions become an increasing strain on the health care system, employing CHWs is a cost effective and culturally appropriate solution.

1.6 PROFESSIONALIZING THE WORK

The CHW field is growing and transforming. You will learn more about this in Chapter Two. There are disagreements among CHWs, CHW supporters, researchers, educators, employers, and other health professions about how best to professionalize the field. Some people advocate for **credentialing** (CHWs would need certification from an educational institution, professional association, or employer in order to work—see Chapter Two for more details) and greater integration into the health care field. Others worry that CHWs may lose their connection to the community and their commitment to social justice. Everyone, however, seems to agree that the field deserves greater recognition, respect, and funding.

Strategies that are being used to advance the CHW field include:

- Conducting research about the field to further clarify what CHWs do and how effective they are
- Founding national and regional CHW organizations as a way for CHWs to have a collective voice on their own behalf, as well as on behalf of the communities they serve
- Identifying appropriate ways to credential or certify the work of CHWs
- Developing training programs and materials that teach the core competencies required for success as a CHWs
- Advocating for policy changes that will result in more stable funding for CHWs

The tension between working as part of the health care and social service industries and working to foster client and community independence is an ongoing challenge for CHWs.

? *What do you see as the key opportunities and challenges for CHWs, and for the communities they serve, as the field becomes more professionalized?*

AN INHERENT TENSION

Sergio Matos, longtime CHW and current (2009) Chair of the CHW Special Primary Interest Group of the American Public Health Association, discusses issues that arise as the role of CHWs within the health and social services systems expands.

"There is tension between our community's needs and desires, and the programs that pay CHWs—they often have conflicting goals and objectives. There is a big risk that CHWs will just get co-opted by the service industry. It's attractive—it provides salaries, it provides benefits, it provides a lot of stuff. But it betrays much of our tradition and history.

"Our society has become a service economy and in order to keep it going you need clients to sell your service to. We often don't even think about it, but we continuously label people in a way that oppresses them so that they are dependent on our services. So, for example, people are no longer people but they're diabetics, or they are handicapped or disabled, they're homeless, they're poverty stricken, or underprivileged. All these labels that we put on people—and once we get you to accept that label we say, 'Oh, but fear not, we have a service for you!'

"The work of CHWs is directly opposed to that—directly and fundamentally opposed to that. A CHW is successful when the person they work with no longer needs us. That's our true measure of success—when we've helped somebody develop self-sufficiency and independence so that they no longer need us or our services."

1.7   INTRODUCING FOUR CHWs

Throughout this book, you will find quotes from CHWs who have firsthand knowledge, experience, and information to share. Quotes and photographs from four CHWs appear most frequently throughout the entire book. The CHWs are **Ramona Benson**, **Phuong An Doan-Billings**, **Lee Jackson**, and **Alvaro Morales**. They each graduated from the CHW Certificate Program at City College of San Francisco and contributed to the development of this book by participating in extensive interviews and taking photographs that represent their work. In this section, each of them is introduced. Through the rest of the book, you'll see an icon of a CHW badge every time we include a quote from a CHW.

RAMONA BENSON: Ramona Benson journeyed from being a client at a San Francisco homeless shelter to becoming a CHW with the Homeless Prenatal Program in San Francisco in 1990. She completed her CHW certificate from City College of San Francisco in 1994 and trained CHWs at the Homeless Prenatal Program until 2000. She was the supervisor of supportive services at San Francisco's Tenderloin Housing Clinic from 2000 to 2001, when she became the CHW at the Black Infant Health Program in Berkeley, California. She is currently completing an A.A. degree. Ramona says:

You have to have a variety of skills to be effective as a CHW. There are gonna be some long hours that you're not gonna get paid for. You gotta be committed and passionate and you gotta be a team player: we can't do it all by ourselves. My reward is seeing my community become healthy, becoming empowered. That's how I measure my success, by watching those who I've worked with overcome barriers. They may have had ten barriers and they overcame two of 'em—but that's success, for me.

From top clockwise, Lee Jackson, Alvaro Morales, Ramona Benson, and Phuong An Doan-Billings.

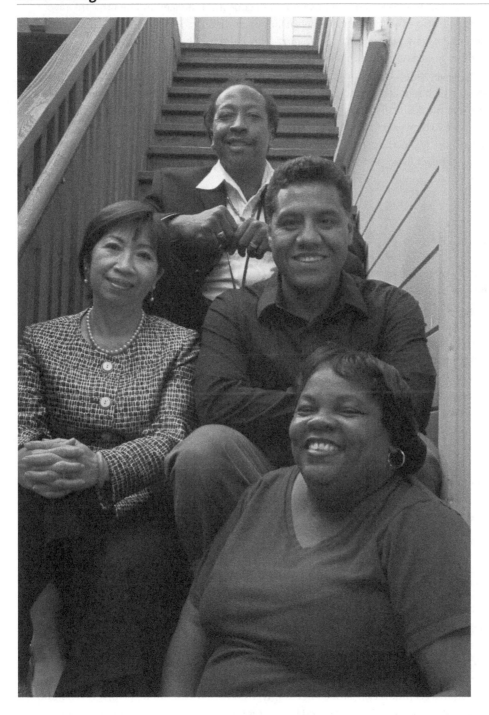

PHUONG AN DOAN-BILLINGS: Born in Vietnam, Phuong An Doan-Billings holds a B.A. degree in English from Saigon University (1979). She taught French and English in Vietnam until she came to the United States in 1990. She started working for Asian Health Services (AHS) in Oakland in 1992 as a health care interpreter and CHW.

(Continued)

In 2006, Phuong An started to supervise the AHS Community Liaison Unit, which reaches out to Asian communities for health education services and health care advocacy. She also contributes her in-depth language skills to the AHS Language Culture Access Program, which provides training for hundreds of health care interpreters in the Bay Area. Sharing her philosophy about work, Phuong An says:

I never forget the desire of learning I used to see in the eyes of the poor students in a remote high school of my home country where I was a teacher at the age of twenty-three. I believe the desire of learning is rooted in everyone. Working with community people for the past sixteen years, for me, is just the continuation of the teaching work I have done in the past. My job has always been to encourage people to learn to better yourself and other people's lives spiritually, psychologically, mentally, and physically). I love teaching.

 LEE JACKSON :   Lee Jackson has certificates from City College of San Francisco in Drug and Alcohol Studies, HIV/STI Outreach, Case Management and Group Facilitation; he completed the CHW certificate in 2004. Originally from Texas, Lee moved to Los Angeles in 1979 and San Francisco in 1987. He has worked as a CHW at several non-profits including the South Beach Resource Center, Walden House, and PlaneTree, and currently works for San Francisco Department of Public Health's Early Intervention Program at Southeast Health Center. Lee works with clients who are HIV positive, multiply diagnosed, or struggling with substance abuse. Lee is working to complete an A.A. degree. Lee says:

As a CHW, you have to work from the heart and give your call to do what's best for your client. Some of my clients are really sick and I go wherever I have to find them. I visit them on the streets and in their apartments, in detox and residential drug recovery programs, in jail and at the General Hospital. I even accompany them to court when they have legal problems. In this work, you have to learn how to take care of yourself to. I'm really into jazz, so I listen to music a lot. And my faith keeps me going, and my community at church.

 ALVARO MORALES: I am originally from Guatemala, where I got an accounting degree. I started out working here in the United States as a cook for a big hotel in San Francisco. But that isn't what I wanted to do. I started volunteering for an AIDS hotline, answering questions, talking to people over the phone. Someone told me about the CHW training program at City College. I started the program, and for my internship I went to a community health center and worked with their outreach worker. We went out on the streets, to the parks, and to different agencies, talking to people about HIV, passing out condoms, telling people about the health center, and about how to get tested for HIV. It was a great training because I learned to work with all kinds of people, to talk with people about all kinds of topics, including things like relationships and sex and drug use and to work in both Spanish and English. When the outreach worker quit, they offered me the job.

Then I started doing HIV antibody test counseling at the clinic. It was a great chance to learn how to do client-centered counseling, how to assist people to reduce their risks for HIV, and how to work with people that were HIV positive to stay healthy. I listened a lot, and provided emotional support and a safe place for people to talk about things that are private, or that they were scared of. I had great supervisors who really taught me a lot about this work.

Since then, I worked all around the [San Francisco] Bay Area. I managed a mobile HIV testing project for a local health department. I did Healthy Families (SCHIP) outreach and enrollment, assisting low-income families in getting health insurance and primary health care for their children. I worked at a drop-in center for the homeless. And now I'm back in the Mission, where I started out fourteen years ago. I work for the San Francisco Department of Public Health, doing environmental health work for day laborers and restaurant workers.

I have benefited from every experience working as a CHW and everyone I ever worked with. I think, as a CHW, you learn a lot from your colleagues, but you learn the most from your clients. I try to keep them in mind, to remember the things they have taught me, and to put that to use in the work I am doing today. But I also know that I don't know it all. I'm a person who likes to keep learning. Not just for my job, but for myself too, and my family.

About ten years after I finished the CHW certificate at City College, I went back to school. In December 2007, I completed my B.A. in Humanities with an emphasis on Social Change and Activism. In September 2008, I started a master's degree program in public health at San Francisco State University. It's a sacrifice, because I have a young son and daughter, but I want to keep learning, and I want my family to be proud of me. There is so much more that I want to do in public health.

CHAPTER REVIEW

1. Which communities or populations do CHWs most commonly work with?
2. Which health issues do CHWs most commonly address in their work?
3. Provide new examples of how CHWs may fulfill each of their seven core roles.
4. Which of these core roles are you most comfortable fulfilling? Which do you know the least about?
5. Explain the eight core competencies of CHWs, and provide an example of each. Have you had the opportunity to develop and practice any of these skills? Which of these skills are you currently least prepared to put into practice?
6. Describe personal qualities that are common among successful CHWs. Which of these qualities will you bring to the work? What additional qualities and values will you bring?
7. As the profession grows, what are some of the challenges you see CHWs encountering?

REFERENCES

Bodenheimer, T. 2006. Improving Primary Care: The Team Care Model. Draft manuscript. San Francisco.

Legion, V., Love, M. B., Miller, J., and Malik, S. 2006. *Overcoming Chronic Under-Funding for Chronic Conditions. Sustainable Reimbursement for Children's Asthma Care Management: Practical Tools.* San Francisco: Community Health Works: A Partnership of San Francisco State University and City College of San Francisco.

Love, M. B., Gardner, K., and Legion, V. 1997. Community Health Workers: Who They Are and What They Do. *Health Education Behavior* 24: 510–522.

Perez, L. M., and Martinez, J. 2008. Community Health Workers: Social Justice and Policy Advocates for Community Health and Well-Being. *American Journal of Public Health* 98: 11–14.

Ro, M., Treadwell, H. M., and Northridge, M. 2003. *Community Health Workers and Community Voices: Promoting Good Health.* A Community Voices Publication. Atlanta: National Center for Primary Care at Morehouse School of Medicine.

Rosenthal, E. L., Wiggins, N., Brownstein, J. N., and others. (Eds.). 1998. *The Final Report of the National Community Health Advisor Study: Weaving the Future.* Tucson: University of Arizona, Mel and Enid Zuckerman College of Public Health, pp. 11–17.

U.S. Bureau of Labor Statistics. 2008. *Occupational Outlook Handbook, 2008–09 Edition.* Washington, DC:

U.S. Bureau of Labor Statistics Office of Occupational Statistics and Employment Projects. Accessed on April 12, 2009: www.bls.gov/OCO/

U.S. Bureau of Labor Statistics. Standard Occupational Classification. Responses to Comments on 2010 SOC. Multiple Dockets. Accessed on January 21, 2009: www.bls.gov/soc/soc2010responses.htm.International Training and Education Center on HIV (I-TECH) and the Zimbabwe Ministry of Health. 2004. Integrated Counseling for HIV and AIDS Prevention and Care: Primary Care Counselor Training: Trainer's Guide. Unpublished. Seattle and San Francisco: I-TECH.

Yamey, G., on behalf of interviewees. 2007. *Which Single Intervention Would Most Improve the Health of Those Living on Less Than $1 Per Day.* Public Library of Science Medicine. Accessed on April 12, 2009: http://medicine.plosjournals.org.

ADDITIONAL RESOURCES

American Public Health Association (APHA). Special Primary Interest Group. Member Groups and State Affiliates. Community Health Workers. Accessed on April 12, 2009: www.apha.org.

Center for Sustainable Health Outreach. The University of Southern Mississippi and Harrison Institute for Public Law of Georgetown University Law Center. Accessed on April 12, 2009: www.usm.edu.

Centers for Disease Control and Prevention. Department of Health and Human Services. Chronic Disease Prevention. Chronic Disease Overview. Accessed on April 12, 2009: www.cdc.gov.

City College of San Francisco. Health Education and Community Health Sciences Department. Community

Health Worker Certificate Program. Accessed on April 12, 2009: www.ccsf.edu.

Community Health Workers National Workforce Study. U.S. Department of Health and Human Services. Health Resources and Services Administration. Accessed on April 12, 2009: http://bhpr.hrsa.gov.

Community Health Works. A Partnership of San Francisco State University and City College of San Francisco. Accessed on April 12, 2009: http://communityhealthworks.org/.

National Community Health Advisor Study. University of Arizona Rural Health Office. Accessed on April 12, 2009: www.rho.arizona.edu.

2

The Evolution of the CHW Field in the United States

THE SHOULDERS WE STAND ON

E. Lee Rosenthal

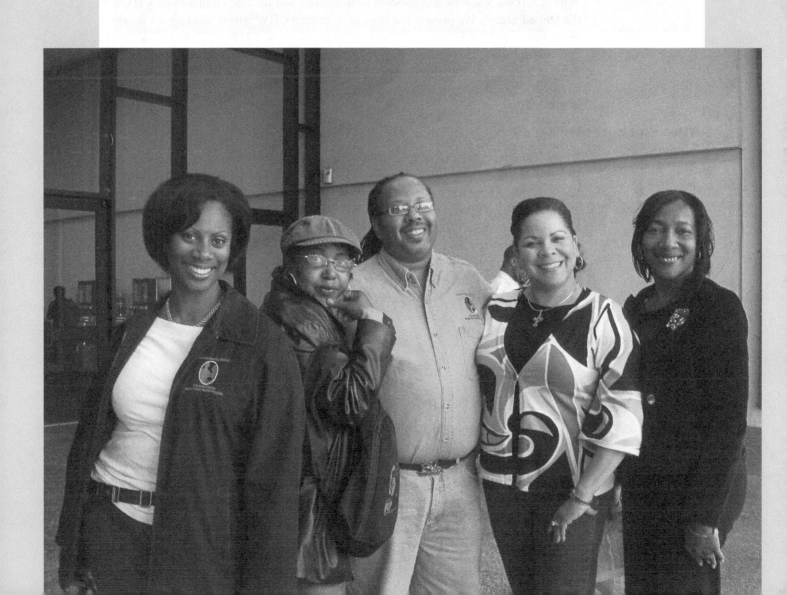

A great river always begins somewhere. Often it starts as a tiny spring bubbling up from a crack in the soil, just like the little stream in my family's land (in Ihithe), which starts where the roots of the fig tree broke though the rocks beneath the ground. But for the stream to grow into a river, it must meet other tributaries and join them as it heads for a lake or the sea . . .

—*Wangari Maathai, Unbowed (2007)*

INTRODUCTION

There are many CHWs throughout the United States and the world. In the United States, we see natural aid-giving networks that may include CHWs in all communities. However, formal CHW programs, with both paid and volunteer CHWs, are not found in all the communities that could benefit from them. CHWs are a rising force for improving the health of community members. They are being recognized for their important contributions to reducing health inequalities by assisting people to access health care and improve health status.

The focus of this chapter is the journey of the CHW profession. We address ongoing efforts to define CHWs and the range of their scope of practice. We briefly explore CHWs' roots in international communities and the known history of CHWs in the United States. We present the story of a veteran CHW whose work spans many of those years, and we look at various trends that affect the CHW field, including developments in evaluation and research; education and capacity building; credentialing; funding; polices aimed at sustaining CHW programs; and CHW local and national network building.

WHAT YOU WILL LEARN

By studying the material presented in this chapter, you will be able to:

✪ Describe the presence and importance of both formal and informal CHWs in promoting healthy individuals and communities in the United States and internationally
✪ Discuss the role that CHWs have played in advocating for greater recognition and respect for their field
✪ Identify and discuss major trends and debates in the development of the CHW field in the United States
✪ Consider what place you want to have in the CHW field

WORDS TO KNOW

Capacity Building   Curriculum

The history of the CHW field in the United States includes the contributions of many individuals and organizations working together to establish new ways of promoting the health of our most vulnerable communities. CHWs and their allies understand how CHWs support families and communities to empower themselves and claim greater control over their own lives and health. Following is a brief summary of the history of the CHW field, without the space to share all the important stories and contributions. If you have been a part of the field, take a moment to ask yourself, "Where have I made my contributions?" If you are new to CHW work, then ask yourself, "Where will I fit into this history?" Think about your role in assisting people to make communities healthier. You already have, or one day will have, an important story to tell about your contributions as a CHW.

A NOTE ON WRITING DOWN HISTORIES

Sometimes, when people met my mother, she would tell them about her life and the work she did, and they would say, "You should write down your story." And she would say, "I am too busy living my life and doing my work to stop and write it down." Just because something is published in a book or article does not mean that it the only story or the best story. Research can only tell us about what has been documented in some way, especially the literature published in scientific journals. That literature is a valuable source of history. Yet our experiences are also valuable sources of information. As someone who has played a role in the CHW field for a number of years, I have been honored to contribute to its history. I am pleased to have a chance to share some of what I have witnessed and learned. I also understand that, even with the literature to help me, I am only able to shed light on a small piece of the much bigger and richer CHW story.

—E. Lee Rosenthal

2.1 NEIGHBOR ASSISTING NEIGHBOR

The history of CHWs began when neighbors first aided each other to take care of their health. Over time, this *natural* aid giving grew to include more formal approaches to CHW work. The many programs we see today include both paid CHWs and volunteer "lay" aid programs and networks. The informal assistance-giving tradition still continues.

WHAT IS A "NATURAL" ASSISTANCE SYSTEM?

A natural assistance system is a naturally occurring community network through which family, friends, neighbors, and others connected by shared experience watch out for one another and reach out with assistance on a regular basis, as well as in times of natural and human-made disasters. *Who are the natural aid-givers in your community?*

2.2 CHW NAMES AND DEFINITIONS

MANY NAMES FOR CHWs

As the CHW field has evolved, no one definition for a CHW has been adopted. In this book we use the term *community health worker* to include the volunteer and paid health practitioners known nationally and internationally by many different names or titles. The National Community Health Advisor Study (NHCHAS) identified more than sixty-six titles for CHWs, including lay health advocate, *promotor,* outreach educator, Community Health Representative, peer health promoter, and of course, CHW (Rosenthal and others, 1998). This last term, used by the World Health Organization, is the one most used in international settings.

During a series of meetings in the mid '90s of diverse leaders in the CHW movement in the United States, it was decided that we needed a unifying, umbrella term for the over sixty titles CHWs fall under. CHW was the agreed-upon, common, unifying term to help progress the movement for sustainability of our CHW workforce, especially to help inform policy development.

— Durrell Fox, CHW, cochair, American Association of CHWs, 2008

IDENTIFYING CHW ROLES AND QUALITIES

There is no consensus or broad agreement about the core roles (related to CHW activities) and qualities of a CHW. Nevertheless, common elements have been identified across many CHW job descriptions, including the roles described in Chapter One. Beyond the core roles, there is general agreement in the field that CHWs must be connected to the community they serve in unique ways, through geographic, social, or cultural identities or relationships. These connections provide CHWs with unique personal understanding of the needs and strengths of the communities with whom they work.

2.3 THE INTERNATIONAL ROOTS OF CHWs

CHWs THROUGHOUT HISTORY AND AROUND THE WORLD

As a CHW you are part of a worldwide community with historical roots that go back hundreds of years. In this section of the chapter, I explain three of the historical roots that produced CHW programs outside the United States.

In nearly all human communities, people have been recognized for their skill in preserving and restoring health. These informal healers have gone by many names: *curanderos*, shamans, elders, and *sobadores,* among others. At a certain point in history, these informal healers began to be differentiated from the more formal healers who practiced health care as a profession. But in many places around the world, especially in rural areas, there were not enough formal healers to go around, and community members were trained to fill the gap. For example, in seventeenth-century Russia, laypeople called *feldshers* were trained for one year so that they could care for the health of civilians and soldiers. *Feldshers* are still part of the health care system in many parts of the Russian-speaking world. Three centuries later, Chinese leader Mao Tse-Tung promised that he would increase access to health care in the rural areas. Initially, he sent doctors from the cities to serve rural communities. But the urban doctors didn't want to stay, so the Chinese government began to train villagers to treat common illnesses, promote sanitation, and give immunizations. They were called "barefoot doctors" because many were so poor they could not afford shoes. Similarly, in the 1960s and 1970s, newly independent Tanzania in East Africa and Zimbabwe in southern Africa developed programs of community health promoters. People with some formal education were trained for a relatively brief time—six months was common—to improve access to health services. These early programs were staffed by locally supported volunteers or, in the case of China, as part of the revolutionary division of labor.

Another important factor that led to the creation of CHW programs was the desire to create more just and equitable societies. In many colonial societies, and among colonized communities of color in the United States, health care and education had been systematically denied in order to keep people under control.

DEFINING CHWs

Because CHWs work in so many communities, under a wide variety of titles, and provide such a wide variety of services, the field and the occupation have not been well defined. As part of a movement for greater recognition and respect for the work that CHWs do, several groups have been advocating for a formal definition of CHW. In the early 2000s, a newly formed Policy Committee for the American Public Health Association CHW Special Primary Interest Group (APHA CHW SPIG) took the lead in developing such a definition. As a part of this effort, the Center for Sustainable Health Outreach (CSHO) collected definitions from hundreds of CHWs and CHW networks across the United States and from other sources.

In 2006, the APHA CHW SPIG submitted a definition of CHWs (see Chapter One) to the U.S. Department of Labor and Statistics (DOL) for consideration. Other groups have also submitted definitions for consideration. In March of 2009, the U.S. Department of Labor approved a separate occupational category—21-1094—for CHWs (U.S. Bureau of Labor Statistics, 2009). At the time of this writing, the DOL is still accepting public comments on the new CHW occupational category, and the final definition for CHWs has not yet been released.

Popular movements for social justice throughout the world influenced or supported the development of CHW programs. For example, CHWs or *promotores de salud* throughout Latin America became active in promoting the health of poor communities, often supporting these communities to organize and advocate for greater access to basic rights and resources. In many parts of Latin America, such as El Salvador, CHWs were targeted for intimidation, violence, and death by right-wing governments and affiliated paramilitary groups and death squads simply because they worked with and on behalf of poor communities or were associated with organizations, including the Catholic Church, that had been labeled "subversive."

The final root of CHW programs outside the United States is the effort to provide primary health care for all. In 1978, at a conference in Alma Ata, Russia, the World Health Organization (WHO) adopted the concept of primary health care (PHC) as its main strategy for achieving "health for all by the year 2000." An important part of this strategy was "community participation in health," which meant involving community members to identify health problems and participate in their solution. The WHO said that "village health workers" (VHWs) were the best strategy for achieving community participation in health. This formal recognition and support led in the 1970s and 1980s to large-scale government-sponsored CHW programs in developing countries such as Indonesia, Costa Rica, and Colombia.

A variety of historical situations have produced CHW programs in many parts of the world. However, none of these programs could have been created if community members were not motivated to aid other community members achieve more control over their lives and their health. This is, in the final analysis, the most important root of CHW programs.

Additional information from Noelle Wiggins about the international roots of CHWs, including a participatory Radio Play, has been posted on the Web site of the CCSF Health Education Department (www.ccsf.edu).

Source: Noelle Wiggins, MSPH, founder and manager, Community Capacitacion Center, Multnomah County Health Department, Oregon.

2.4 CHWs IN THE UNITED STATES

In many cultures, there are traditional healing systems that were developed before Western medicine and many now exist along with it. In the United States, these systems take many forms. In American Indian communities, traditional healers such as medicine men were and are an important part of health networks (Mohatt and Eagle Elk, 2000). In Latino communities, *curanderos* assist in promoting health in the community. In addition to these more formal healing practitioners, there have been natural or "lay" aides. *Promotores* are found in communities throughout the United States (Ramos, Hernandez, Freirre-Pinto, Ortiz, and Somerville, 2006; Gonzalez and Ortiz, 2004). Church groups often lead CHW projects to promote health and address other issues in their communities. There have also been many projects based in communities and led by community members who work to change conditions that harm their health. In all communities, natural volunteers play an important role in supporting the health of community members.

Public health and other health professionals reach out to these natural networks (Eng and Young, 1992) to address health related issues, often those prioritized by community members themselves. Health professionals often hire CHWs into programs based within public health departments, hospitals, or other institutions. Other CHWs contribute on a volunteer basis. In these cases, programs often provide incentives such as educational credits or modest financial stipends to CHWs to support their participation. Estimates are that approximately one-third of formal CHW programs are volunteer based, while the rest are paid CHW programs (Rosenthal and others, 1998; Human Resources and Services Administration [HRSA], 2007).

Generally, health professions, like other professions, have achieved recognition through a process of defining themselves and assisting others understand what members of the profession do to improve health. At times, health professionals have faced conflicts with other professions and have had to struggle for respect and legitimacy. This has been true for nurses, midwives, physicians, and acupuncturists, as well as CHWs. CHWs are actively organizing on local, state, and national levels to ensure that their knowledge, skills, and contributions are valued, respected, and integrated into health and public health systems.

CHWs' FORMAL HISTORY IN THE UNITED STATES: 1950–2000

The documented history of CHWs begins in the late 1950s to early 1960s.

In the 1950s, the first documented volunteer and paid CHW programs were established in the United States (Hoff, 1969; Giblin, 1989; Meister, Warrick, de Zapien, and Wood, 1992; Gould and Lomax, 1993). During this period, programs started in Native American communities in the West and among migrant farm workers in the southeastern United States. Strong CHW programs still serve these communities today.

In the 1960s and 1970s, new CHW programs were developed throughout U.S. rural and urban communities. CHW programs addressed important public health issues, and at the same time they were often credited with creating valuable employment opportunities for low-income women and families who had difficulty entering the paid workforce (Domke and Coffey, 1966). The Office of Economic Opportunity invested in CHWs in numerous urban areas (Meister, 1997). CHWs and other community-based workers were seen as critical to the reorganization of the human services system (Pearl and Reissman, 1965). CHWs were recognized for their connection to the community and their unique insight into the individuals they served (Withorn, 1984).

The Federal Migrant Act of 1962 required federally qualified migrant clinics to conduct outreach in migrant labor camps. CHWs were hired to provide this outreach, a move that established many CHW programs. This outreach built on the *promotor(a)* tradition common in Mexico and Latin America, where many farm workers were raised or have family ties (Mahler, 1978).

In many states, CHWs were an important part of the Community Health Center (CHC) movement. Today, many CHCs integrate CHWs into their health promotion and related programs.

In the 1950s and 1960s, opportunities for paid and volunteer CHWs and *promotores* increased and were hailed as contributing to the reorganization of health and human services delivery systems (Pynoos, Hade-Kaplan, and Fleisher, 1984; Service and Salber, 1977). In the 1960s, CHWs were paid to work in a variety of health projects and programs (Hoff, 1969; Wilkinson, 1992; Potts and Miller, 1964). In this era, groups like the Black Panther Party and the Young Lords advocated for the government to provide free health care, including prevention services, and accessible services to treat drug addiction for African American, Latino, and all oppressed peoples. Though their more controversial activities received public attention, the Black Panthers also created free breakfast programs for school children and free medical clinics for their communities (Brand and Burt, 2006; Black Panther Party Research Project, 2009).

The largest and perhaps the oldest CHW program in the United States also got its start in the late 1960s in Native American communities (Satterfield and Burd, 2002). The Community Health Representative (CHR) program was created in 1968 by Indian Health Services in collaboration with American Indian tribes (Indian Health Service, 2006). The CHR program is still strong today, with more 1,500 CHRs serving in more than 250 tribes throughout the United States. CHRs address maternal and child health issues, diabetes management, and other chronic disease management. They also assist families with transportation to health care providers.

In the 1970s, Service and Salber (1977) started to use the term "lay health advisors" (LHAs) and called attention to the important community roles of LHAs, such as health promotion, social support, mediation (helping two sides reach an agreement), and community empowerment (Salber, 1979).

In the 1980s, funding for job creation programs slowed, and the number of paid CHWs participating in forums such as the American Public Health Association declined. At the same time, a number of CHW programs expanded their roles. Programs for migrants grew with funding from private and government sources (Harlan, Eng, and Watkins, 1992; Meister, Warrick, de Zapien, and Wood, 1992; Booker, Grube-Robinson, Kay, Najjera, and Stewart, 2004). The number of CHWs making home visits to aid mothers and infants increased (Poland, Giblin, Waller, and Hankin, 1992; Julnes, Konefal, Pindur, and Kim, 1994; McFarlane and Fehir, 1994; Larson, McGuire, Watkins, and Mountain, 1992). The federal Healthy Start program began to rely on outreach workers to address infant mortality issues and inequalities in infant mortality, especially in cities that were addressing the needs of African Americans mothers and infants. CHWs also started supporting community members at risk for chronic conditions or diseases (for example, high blood pressure, cancer, diabetes) to maintain better control, keep appointments with and talk to their doctors, check their blood pressure and blood sugar levels, and know the signs of serious illness (Brownstein, Bone, and Dennison, 2005; Norris, Chowdhury, and Van Le, 2006; Brandeis University, 2003).

In the 1980s, the AIDS epidemic motivated activists to organize and advocate for civil rights protections and investment in community health outreach, education and testing programs, research into treatments, and access to quality health care. Perhaps the best-known activist organization was the AIDS Coalition to Unleash Power (ACT UP), founded in 1987. ACT UP built on the protest traditions that came out of the civil rights movement and opposition to the Vietnam War (Klitzman, 1997). Activists were successful in building strategic alliances with health and public health professionals, in drawing public attention to HIV/AIDS, in advocating for changes to public policies and the creation of new public health programs and research on treatments for HIV disease. As a result, local health departments and community-based organizations began to hire CHWs to conduct outreach and provide client-centered education, counseling, and HIV antibody testing services. CHWs conducted home and hospital visits, facilitated support groups, trained physicians and other providers in providing culturally competent care, initiated syringe exchange programs, and much more. With the development of the AIDS epidemic in the United States "a disease [became] the basis of a political movement" (Klitzman, 1997). The success of CHWs in aiding to address the HIV epidemic in turn influenced the development of the CHW field.

In the 1990s, CHWs gained increased recognition for their important contributions to health and job creation (Witmer, Seifer, Finocchio, Leslie, and O'Neil, 1995; Rosenthal and others, 1998). Jobs creation was pushed by Welfare Reform, which brought with it renewed federal attention and resources. Welfare-to-work programs explored CHW jobs as an important option for individuals newly entering or reentering the paid workforce. CHW program coordinators reminded all involved of the importance of looking for individuals who were already known to be natural aides in their communities when recruiting CHWs (Aguirre and Palacio-Waters, 1997). At the same time, public and private grant funding for CHW programs continued to grow, focusing on assisting individuals in managing health conditions such as HIV disease, diabetes, and asthma (Norris and others, 2006).

In the 1990s and beyond, people began to learn more about the work of CHWs. Workforce studies, articles, and reports about CHWs became more common (Love and others, 2004; Proulx, 2000a). Local, state, and national networks and conferences began bringing CHW together.

2.5 INTERVIEW WITH CHW YVONNE LACEY

FROM THE FRONT DOOR TO THE HEAD OF THE TABLE: 1970–2007

Yvonne Lacey retired as coordinator of the City of Berkeley, California, Black Infant Health Program in 2007, after more than thirty years as a CHW. She played a key role in the development of the CHW Certificate Program at City College of San Francisco, where she was a frequent guest lecturer and trainer during the first two years of the program. Yvonne currently volunteers at a children's reading program and acts as an advocate for seniors in a nursing home.

The following is an excerpt from an interview with Yvonne conducted in the spring 2008 by Mickey Ellinger and E. Lee Rosenthal (www.ccsf.edu).

"I'VE BEEN DOING THIS WORK ALL MY LIFE"

YVONNE LACEY: As I think back over my history, I realize that I've been doing this work all my life. I live by this old song I heard in church as a child: "If I can help somebody as I pass along, then my living shall not be in vain."

Back when I was a dressmaker, friends would come to my shop so I could help fix a zipper or a hem, and we'd end up talking about daily problems and relationships and all that. There wasn't a week that went by that I didn't have women in there helping each other get through our daily lives.

In October 1970, I was sewing out of my home. A friend called and said, "I saw the perfect job for you!" I finally went down to the City of Berkeley's Department of Public Health and got hired as a CHW for maternal and child health. My life has never been the same.

The Maternity and Infant Care Program provided prenatal care to low-income women. It was one of the most comprehensive programs that I have ever seen up to today. There was a social worker, two CHWs, a public health nurse, a nurse practitioner, and doctors who took rotation in our clinics. That's where I learned the team concept of delivering health services. That's when I began to love this community health work. I began to really see what we could do in the community to make a difference.

Although I began the work knowing my community, I gained years of experience and training on the streets of Berkeley. I also got an education from a cherished mentor public health nurse in the department—although we fought constantly.

In the early '90s, City College of San Francisco was planning a course for CHWs and they recruited CHWs to be on the planning committee. We were planning the curriculum and trying to see the benefits of having a course, and what CHWs would get from it. In 1993, I contributed as a guest lecturer and trainer for the first groups of CHW students. I did that for two years.

After that experience I really got involved with building the CHW profession. . . . Many of us worked so hard to get more recognition for CHWs (through the American Public Health Association. When I first started attending APHA meetings in 1996, CHWs were called "the New Professionals." In 2000, we convinced APHA to change the group's name to the CHW Special Primary Interest Group (SPIG). I chaired that group for three years. It is my opinion that the chair of any CHW group has to be a CHW, not an advocate for CHWs.

From 1994 to 1998, we worked on the National Community Health Advisor Study. I was the cochair of the thirty-six-member advisory committee that included a large group of experienced CHWs. We are the only ones who really know the work that we do. With our voices we can make sure that the value of the work is known and recognized and with our voices we can lead the way to more investment in our communities.

In 2004, I was asked to cochair the CHW National Education Collaborative (CHW NEC). It was trying to bring community colleges together to have a standard competency-based training that covers the basic things that all CHWs need to know. We also helped colleges understand that CHWs have to be at the table at every stage of developing our profession. CHWs have to help plan the trainings and be involved in the teaching. Maybe having a mentorship program built into that training. I wouldn't want CHWs to lose touch with their own communities, or lose the fire and passion they have just because they earn a degree. Also, we want these colleges to understand they are training CHW leaders.

It was such rewarding work—the work I did in my thirty-seven years at the Berkeley Health Department and at the national level. You don't always see the results of the work right away. But I've gone to get gas and somebody's come up to me and said, "You're Miss Lacey, aren't you? You helped me during such and such." Or, "If it hadn't been for you I wouldn't have gone back to school." Or, "I only had that one baby, Miss Lacey, because you told me . . ." And sometime around the country I have had that same kind of confirmation from CHWs that somehow, I have touched their lives. That has made it all worthwhile. "I did touch somebody's life here." And to me that has been worth the whole thing.

2.6 TRENDS IN THE CHW FIELD

The CHW field is growing and gaining recognition. There is still an outstanding need, however, for greater respect for the skills and contributions of CHWs and increased resources to institutionalize the key roles that CHWs play in public health, health care, and related fields. As the field expands, it is important that CHWs maintain their connection and commitment to the communities they serve. Most important, CHWs must take a leading role in defining the future of their field.

RESEARCH: BUILDING THE EVIDENCE BASE ABOUT THE WORK OF CHWs

Through the 1990s, researchers conducted a number of regional and national studies of CHWs. Together, these studies demonstrated the power, value, and importance of the work that CHWs have been doing in the United States in a form that could be understood by the fields of public health and medicine.

The National Community Health Advisor Study (Rosenthal and others, 1998), which I directed in collaboration with many partners including CHWs, was carried out from 1994 to 1998 as a participatory research project: the group being studied participated in designing, analyzing, and interpreting findings. The majority of the study's advisory council were CHWs who were active participants in analyzing the data gathered. The council alone was responsible for making recommendations based on the data for the field. Many of the actions recommended by the thirty-six-member advisory council are now being taken throughout the United States. These include increased access to CHW educational programs that offer college credit and the controversial recommendation to credential CHWs.

In addition to identifying the core roles and competencies of CHWs, the study also identified the many community and clinical settings where CHWs work, including homes, schools, clinics, and hospitals. The settings in which CHWs work clearly influence the activities of CHWs. According to the California Workforce Initiative, CHWs working in clinics are more likely to perform duties focused on traditional patient care, whereas CHWs working door to door act more in the roles associated with social workers and community organizers (Keane, Nielsen, and Dower, 2004).

Early workforce studies in the San Francisco Bay Area (Love, Gardener, and Legion, 1997) inspired other regions and states to conduct similar assessments to determine the extent and roles of CHWs in local labor markets. The Annie E. Casey Foundation funded another study of the CHW workforce, looking at the potential of worker-owned CHW cooperatives (Rico, 1997). More recently, the federal government funded and coordinated the CHW National Workforce Study (HRSA, 2007). The study explored the roles and functions of CHWs in different settings and estimated that there were 120,000 CHWs throughout the United States in 2005.

In 1995, a commentary entitled "Community Health Workers: Integral Members of the Health Care Work Force" appeared in the *American Journal of Public Health* (Witmer, Seifer, Finocchio, Leslie, and O'Neil, 1995). The article's title alone stimulated attention to the field. The Institute of Medicine's landmark book, *Unequal Treatment: Confronting Racial and Ethnic Disparities in Health Care,* talked about the importance of CHWs in reducing health inequalities (Smedley, Stith, and Nelson, 2002). A study funded by the Centers for Medicare and Medicaid Services (CMS) on approaches to cancer prevention among elders of color found that CHWs were the "primary mechanism for cultural tailoring" (Brandeis University, 2003). Findings from a subsequent study may ultimately bring valuable financial resources to CHWs for the services they provide to rural and urban communities throughout the United States.

An outstanding need remains for more research to document evidence of the effectiveness of CHWs in promoting health outcomes (Giblin, 1989; Swider, 2002; Nemcek and Sabatier, 2003; HRSA, 2007). Recently, CHWs, researchers, and other stakeholders met to develop a CHW Research Agenda by and for the field (Rosenthal, DeHeer, Rush, and Holderby, 2008). At a two-day conference led by Carl Rush, conference participants identified the most important areas for additional research (complete findings may be accessed online at www.famhealth.org/researchagenda.htm):

- ✪ CHW cost-effectiveness or return on investment
- ✪ CHW impact on health status
- ✪ Building CHW capacity and sustaining CHWs on the job
- ✪ Funding options
- ✪ CHWs as capacity builders
- ✪ CHWs promoting real access to care

Research on the work of CHWs is a key building block for making the case for more resources to the field. Furthermore, a new role for CHWs is to participate in conducting research themselves, for, with, and about the communities they serve. You will learn more about conducting research with the communities you work within in Chapter Eighteen. Durrell Fox observes that CHWs have an important role to play in conducting research. He feels strongly that CHWs have already informed research and public health theories and science for decades (Rosenthal, DeHeer, Rush, and Holderby, 2008).

2.7 CAPACITY BUILDING AND EDUCATION

Capacity building refers to strengthening the knowledge, skills, and confidence of individuals—like CHWs—or communities. On-the-job training has been the cornerstone for capacity-building programs for most CHWs. More recently, college-based and some center-based programs for training CHWs have been established.

ON-THE-JOB TRAINING

On-the-job training remains the mainstay of CHW training (HRSA, 2007). Employers take responsibility for scheduling training and cover the time and costs associated with participation for their staff or volunteers. This makes a career as a CHW accessible to people from all walks of life, including those who may have had difficulty gaining employment (Jennings, 1990). Through on-the-job training, people entering or returning to the workforce can be mentored and encouraged to ensure maximum success.

At the same time, on-the-job training taxes CHW programs, as each program works with limited resources to develop staff training (Rosenthal and others, 1998). Additionally, some CHWs and administrators reported that on-the-job training was too limited and even off base (Love and others, 2004). CHWs have also reported frustration that on-the-job training was not recognized when they move from one job to another (Rosenthal and others, 1998).

FORMAL CHW CURRICULA

Many curricula and training guides have been developed for CHWs. Some programs have shared the **curriculum** (a set of classes and their content for a particular course or field of study) they developed, but no single curriculum has been adopted by the field. Among these curricula there have been numerous training materials that address specific health issues, such as diabetes, heart health, HIV disease, and prenatal health. In the early 1990s, the National Commission for Infant Mortality developed a curriculum for maternal and child CHW programs that included a guide to starting CHW programs. More recently, there appears to be a shift to curricula for developing core or foundational CHWs skills and competencies. In Minnesota, a core curriculum on CHWs was developed collaboratively by educators, employers, and CHWs (Willaert, 2005). Again, many training materials are used only by the projects that developed them, while other curriculum have been shared freely or sold for use in other CHW programs.

As of 2009, no single CHW curriculum, book, or textbook for CHWs has been adopted throughout the United States, but some resources have been widely used. *Helping Health Workers Learn*, developed by the Hesperian Foundation, has been popular, especially in international settings (Werner and Bower, 1982).

MOVING TOWARD COORDINATED CHW EDUCATIONAL APPROACHES

In the 1990s, there was a move toward center-based trainings (rather than on-the-job training), as well as college-supported educational programs for CHWs. An early example of center-based training comes from Boston's Community Health Education Center, developed by the City of Boston to respond to a citywide need for CHW capacity building. Since the 1990s, the center has provided core initial training to CHWs. It has also been a resource center for training and other materials and has served as a gathering place for CHWs, with activities like job-sharing luncheons.

Early in their history, efforts were made in some areas to assist CHWs to gain access to academic pathways and credit within college programs. Early reports of CHWs in academic settings showed that there were challenges in the college setting; some CHWs felt their competence gained through life experience and experience on the job were undervalued (Sainer, Ruiz, and Wilder, 1975).

City College of San Francisco started a CHW Certificate Program in the early 1990s. The program, designed to address some of these challenges and barriers, offered the first full-scale college credit-bearing educational opportunity for CHWs (Love and others, 2004). Building on this model and other emerging programs, Project Jump Start at the University of Arizona (1998–2002) focused on creating credit-bearing training for CHWs through four Arizona community colleges predominately serving rural communities (Proulx, 2000b). During 2004–2008, CHWs, allies, and representatives of twenty-two CHW college-based educational programs formed the CHW National Education Collaborative (CHW NEC) to advise college-based CHW programs about best practices for such programs (Proulx, Rosenthal, Fox, and Lacey, 2008). CHWs Yvonne Lacey and Durrell Fox served as the project's majority CHW Advisory Council cochairs; I was the project's codirector along with Director Don Proulx and Coordinator Nancy Collyer. In 2008, as the CHW NEC project came to an end, we generated a guidebook for the field, looking at ways colleges and other institutions can start and strengthen CHW educational and capacity-building programs.

In the City College classroom, working CHWs expand their skills and new CHWs prepare to enter the field.

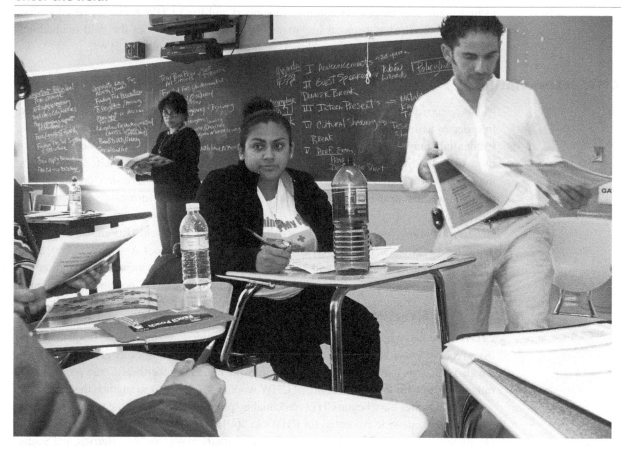

WHAT DO CHANGES IN CHW TRAINING MEAN FOR THE FIELD?

Many of the skills and personal qualities needed to excel as a CHW can be learned on the job and through life experience. The skills that lead to success in higher education do not, in themselves, translate into job effectiveness as a CHW. Veteran CHWs have often been suspicious of college-based training programs: the typical college classroom is not an avenue that is open to all community people. In addition, it is common in the health workforce that higher education credentials are set as a requirement for employment. This can limit access to employment for CHWs who are highly skilled but lack formal education. Specifically, *requirements* for college-based programs may present barriers to and adversely affect the very communities with the greatest potential to be outstanding CHWs, including low-income communities, communities of color, undocumented immigrant communities, and English language learners. At the same time, college credit and education are closely linked to employment outcomes, career advancement, and higher income. Well-designed educational programs that are accessible and that offer college credit to CHWs can provide these students with valuable opportunities for professional growth and advancement.

It is important to maintain multiple approaches to CHW education and training and to develop ways to recognize and credit the value of life and job experience. And, to the extent that college-based training becomes more widespread, it is important to ensure that these programs are accessible to CHWs financially and in their instructional approaches.

See www.chw-nec.org to learn about "Key Considerations" for starting or strengthening CHW educational programs (Proulx, Rosenthal, Fox, and Lacey, 2008). It is also important to make sure that employers continue to support and fund CHW training and education, which historically has been an important ingredient for success in the field maintaining access to many CHWs who are and become increasingly outstanding CHWs.

CHW CREDENTIALING

Many occupations use credentialing in some form, including certification and licensure, in order to assure that workers have the knowledge and skills necessary to do their jobs. Credentials may be administered by a public entity, such as a state health department, or by a free-standing organization led by members of the occupation itself. Credentialing may directly certify individuals (nurses, social workers, or CHWs) or may credential programs (agencies, clinics, training programs, institutions) that in turn assess and credential individuals.

Credentialing remains a controversial issue in the CHW field (Rosenthal and others, 1998; Keane, Nielsen, and Dower, 2004; National Human Services Assembly, 2006). Some people feel that credentialing will support the ongoing effort to increase recognition and respect for CHWs and to create stable sources of funding for CHW positions. Others question or oppose credentialing out of concern that it may keep people who otherwise have the necessary commitment, knowledge, and skills from working in the field. For example, many CHWs have had experiences, such as felony drug convictions, that would disqualify them from receiving a credential if the process is modeled after those of other professions. There are also concerns that credentialing is driven by the norms of other health care professionals rather than a genuine understanding of CHW work and a desire to strengthen the field.

Several states have begun CHW credentialing programs. Texas was the first state to create a mandatory statewide credential for CHWs in 2001; it is coordinated by the Department of Health Services with a committee that includes certified CHWs (Nichols, Berrios, and Samar, 2005). In 2003, Ohio adopted a credentialing program regulated by the state Board of Nursing. Groups in other states are considering credentialing at various levels, including credentialing individual CHWs, their trainers and/or curricula, and CHW programs.

CCSF POLICY STATEMENT ON CREDENTIALING

The City College of San Francisco Health Education Department and CHW Certificate Program strongly oppose credentialing policies that discriminate against any group of people. We oppose policies that would limit or prohibit undocumented, formerly incarcerated or non-English speakers from becoming CHWs. We also oppose efforts to require college-based certification, and support all quality CHW training programs.

2.8 CHW POLICY INITIATIVES AND SUSTAINABILITY

CHWs are usually funded by grants and in some cases by state funds or managed care contracts. Long-term, secure, or sustainable funding for CHWs is rare, but some promising changes are facilitating increased funding.

In 1989, the Health Education Training Centers (HETC) program was funded by the federal government to address Hispanic and U.S.-Mexico border health issues. It was one of the first pieces of federal legislation that identified CHWs as an integral part of the safety net system for medically underserved populations. The program ended in 2007.

In 2003, the federal Bureau of Primary Health Care's Guidance on Program Expansion, which targets mental health, substance abuse, oral health, and care management, allowed for the funding of CHW positions. This opened up options for federally funded CHCs to employ CHWs.

As noted earlier, a national demonstration project was launched in 2003 to explore the possibility of reimbursing CHW services with Medicare funding for cancer care (Capitman and others, 2003). This study could aid in leading to Medicare funding availability for CHWs.

In 2005, Congress passed the Patient Navigator and Chronic Disease Prevention Act. This legislation authorized $25 million for demonstration programs. Some consider Patient Navigators to be CHWs. Patient Navigators specialize in supporting patients with cancer or other chronic diseases in navigating the health care system to access services. The bill provided pilot funding for agencies that employ Patient Navigators, such as public or nonprofit private health centers. This federal legislation demonstrates growing support for the important roles of CHWs as guides in the health care system.

In 2007, the State of Minnesota passed legislation to reimburse CHWs under their Medicaid program. The same year, they filed for a Medicaid State Plan Amendment to authorize a broad-based reimbursement for CHW services to Medicaid recipients. Several states, including New Mexico (New Mexico Department of Health, 2003), Massachusetts (Ballester, 2005), and Virginia (James Madison University, 2006) have conducted studies on the roles and contributions of CHWs, and these and other states continue to explore options for supporting CHW integration and sustainability.

2.9 CONVENING CHWs: NETWORKS AND CONFERENCES

CHWs have organized local, state, and national networks out of the belief that they must have a strong voice in shaping the field as it evolves and to provide mutual support, mentoring, and peer learning.

DURRELL FOX, FOUNDER OF THE MASSACHUSETTS ASSOCIATION OF CHWs: In 2001 there was a crisis in public health funding in my state [Massachusetts] that deeply impacted CHWs. We had emergency budget cuts. Our state had new and long-standing outreach and prevention programs with evidence of effectiveness. Some programs that had a full year of funding were notified that funding was cut in half. Some programs were notified on a Wednesday that by Friday they would have no more funding. They had to close and lay off staff, including CHWs. We began to see a pattern where CHWs were the first to go and last to know.

Since some CHWs were already connected through training and networking we got together and said, "We've got to do something." We created the Massachusetts Association of CHWs (MACHW) to build strength, support, independence, and sustainability for CHWs. At the time, CHWs were not paid well, were disenfranchised and disconnected. We had maternal child health outreach workers, HIV outreach workers

(Continued)

funded by different agencies and not communicating with each other. You could be in a housing development stepping over other outreach workers who might be dealing with some of the same families but had no communication or coordination. This was crazy and inefficient. We didn't have enough resources to have six CHWs serving one family. So MACHW brought CHWs together to learn about what each other was doing and what communities they serve. We began to do strategic planning to help CHWs be more efficient and effective.

MACHW linked up with a couple of training programs, one in Boston (CHEC) and in Worcester (Outreach Worker Training Institute–OWTI in Worcester), and that's where we developed a way to have CHWs coming together from across the state to network, support, and learn from each other.

CHWs meet to discuss common challenges and to provide mutual support.

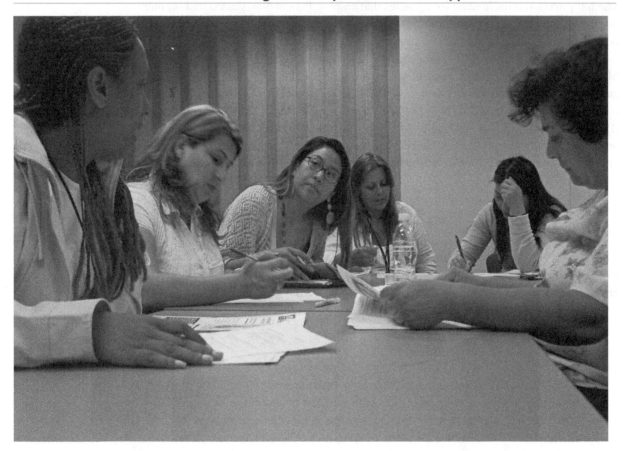

NATIONAL NETWORKS

There are five national groups in the United States that assist in regularly convening CHWs. The names of the groups and their size and capacity has varied with funding and other supports over the years, but each group works to provide leadership and opportunities for CHW networking and sharing.

1. The APHA CHW Special Primary Interest Group (CHW SPIG) In 1970, five hundred CHWs and their supporters joined together within the American Public Health Association in what was then called the New Professionals Special Primary Interest Group (SPIG). Their name was chosen in protest against the many terms used to describe them, including nonprofessional, subprofessional, aide, auxiliary, and paraprofessional (Bellin, Killen, and Mazeika, 1967; Murphy, 1972; D'Onofrio, 1970). In the year of their formation, the New Professionals wrote:

> For too long, non-degreed health workers have been left out of the mainstream of planning
> for the delivery of health services . . . and [have] gone without recognition and reward. . . .
> It is our hope that the National New Professional Health Workers will be able to change
> the status of workers across the country and thereby improve the health of the nation.
> (American Public Health Association, 1970)

In the 1980s, membership and activity in the SPIG declined. In the 1990s, the SPIG membership was small, and it was held together by longtime CHW member and SPIG leader Ruth Scarborough. I was honored in the early 1990s when she asked me to take the helm of the SPIG and assist in rebuilding it. Many CHWs and allies played a role in this effort in the 1990s, and the group grew strong once again. Through the leadership of CHWs including Yvonne Lacey and Durrell Fox, the group once again was led by CHWs and celebrating that, the name was changed from the New Professional SPIG to the CHW SPIG.

DURRELL FOX: Part of my activism on a local and national level stemmed from my observation that there were studies being funded, there were many people having long careers with big wages, good salaries, and good jobs, who were actually training us or doing a study on us, and I kept saying, "Why is it that funders give multimillions of dollars worth of training, and studies, when there are no resources to pay the CHW workforce?" For me that was another driving force behind organizing CHW leaders to focus on creating living wages and sustainable jobs for CHWs. The CHW SPIG of APHA definitely has a different flavor than many of the statewide or local networks since it is based inside of APHA with certain restrictions and parameters, but I think it was and still is today a driving force behind our national movement.

In 2001, the SPIG introduced a resolution, which was approved by the APHA Governing Council, entitled "Recognition and Support for Community Health Workers' Contributions to Meeting Our Nation's Health Care Needs." The policy outlined the roles that CHWs play in the U.S. health and human services system (Wiggins in Rosenthal and others, 1998) on behalf of communities and noted their importance to improving health and the capacity of the public health workforce (Grube-Robinson, 2001). In 2006, the SPIG added a Committee on Education and *Capacitación* to assist in guiding the field on issues of CHW education and training and possibly in the area of CHW credentialing; the SPIG has also established a committee on Policy and is active in the Governing Council of APHA (see www.apha.org).

2. The National Association of Community Health Representatives The National Association of Community Health Representatives (NACHRs) was established in the 1970s to be the voice of the more than 1,500 CHRs serving their tribal communities. Some CHRs have been supported by federal and tribal monies since the program was established in 1968. This association has twelve service area representatives, one from each of the twelve public health regions. They coordinate the activities of NACHR in collaboration with the Indian Health Service. NACHR holds a national meeting once every several years, when more than 1,000 CHRs gather to learn about other health issues and programs as well as to honor leadership and longevity in the CHR program. There are often regional CHR meetings between the national meetings (see www.nachr.net).

3. The National Association of Hispanic CHWs

The National Association of Hispanic CHWs grew out of the CHW National Network Association, based in Yuma, Arizona, at the Western Area Health Education Center. The Association was established in the West in 1992 and grew to include people from other regions, including the Midwest and New England, eventually leading it to become a national network. The annual conference is predominantly in Spanish and offers some simultaneous translation, especially for presenters in English. In 2007, the organization announced that it would officially focus on Hispanic promoters while maintaining its interest in all CHWs.

4. The Center for Sustainable Health Outreach

Since 2000, CHWs have met annually under the auspices of the national Center for Sustainable Health Outreach (CSHO), a partnership between Southern Mississippi University ("CSHO south") and Georgetown University Law School in Washington, D.C. ("CSHO north"). The CSHO Unity Conference offers an opportunity for exchange among CHWs from across the country.

5. The American Association of CHWs

CHWs and allies came together in 2006 to explore development of a national CHW leadership organization or association. This meeting led to the development the American Association of Community Health Workers (AACHWs), which is working to establish national standards and to advocate for increased recognition and resources for CHWs throughout the United States.

To learn more about these and other networks, go the Web site of the American Public Health Association at: www.apha.org/membergroups/primary/aphaspigwebsites/chw/Resources/.

STATE NETWORKS

The first statewide network of CHWs was formed in the early 1990s in New Mexico as the New Mexico Community Health Worker Association. About the same time, the Oregon Public Health Association formed a committee on CHWs that was chaired by CHWs. This committee provided leadership at the state level and nationally by working as a part of APHA.

More recently Arizona, Maryland, Mississippi, Virginia, California, Massachusetts, Florida, Minnesota, New York, Texas, and Hawaii to name a few have established statewide associations that bring CHWs together. In some states, regional and issue-specific networks have been established. In California, a group known as *Vision y Compromiso* has worked to bring together networks of *promotores* from throughout the state for conferences and to promote collaboration.

By joining together in regional, state, and national networks and associations, CHWs are claiming leadership in the development of their field, defining their roles, establishing new standards, research priorities, educational and training models, and advocating for greater recognition and increased funding.

CHAPTER REVIEW

1. Why is it so difficult to develop a common definition of CHWs and CHW roles? Why could a common definition of CHWs strengthen the field?

2. What has been the role of CHW leaders in defining and developing the CHW field?

3. Why is academic research about CHWs important to developing the CHW field? What are research priorities for the CHW field?

4. How are developments in CHW training, education, and credentialing shaping the CHW field? Why are these developments controversial?

5. How do CHW networks develop and why are they important to the future of CHWs in the United States?

6. Are there CHW networks in your city, county, or state? If not, visit the Web site of one of the national CHW networks listed in this chapter and identify its main priorities or goals.

REFERENCES

Aguirre, A., and Palacios-Waters, A. 1997. El Rio Colorado Border Vision. *Fronterieza*. Video. San Luis, AZ.

American Public Health Association. 1970. New Professionals Special Primary Interest Group. *Minutes*. Washington, DC: American Public Health Association.

Ballester, G. 2005. *Community Health Workers: Essential to Improving Health in Massachusetts, Findings from the Massachusetts Community Health Worker Survey*. Boston: Massachusetts Department of Public Health.

Bellin, L. Killen, E., M., and Mazeika, J. J. 1967. Preparing Public Health Subprofessionals Recruited from The Poverty Group Lessons from an OEO Work-Study Program. *American Journal of Public Health 57*: 242–252.

Black Panther Party Research Project. Stanford University. Accessed on April 15, 2009: www.stanford.edu

Booker, V., Grube-Robinson, J., Kay, B., Najjera, L. G., and Stewart, G. 2004. Camp Health Aide Program Overview. Working paper. Saline, MI: Migrant Health Promotion 5.

Brand, W., and Burt, C. 2006, October 8. A Legacy of Activism: Behind Fury, Black Panthers Laid Course for Social Programs. *Oakland Tribune*.

Brandeis University. 2003. Evidence Report and Evidence-Based Recommendations: Cancer Prevention and Treatment Demonstration for Ethnic and Racial Minorities. Accessed on April 15, 2009: www.cms.hhs.gov

Brownstein, J. N., Bone, L. R., and Dennison, C. R., and others. 2005. Community Health Workers as Interventionists in the Prevention and Control of Heart Disease and Stroke. *American Journal of Preventive Medicine* 29(5S1): 128–133.

Capitman, J., Bhalotra, S. M., Calderon-Rosado, V., and others. 2003. Cancer Prevention and Treatment

Demonstration for Ethnic and Racial Minorities. Prepared for U.S. Department of Health and Human Services by Schneider Institute for Health Policy. Accessed on April 27, 2008: www.cms.hhs.gov/DemoProjectsEvalRpts/downloads/CPTD_Brandeis_Report.pdf

Community Health Worker National Education Collaborative. 2007. Tucson: University of Arizona. Accessed on April 15, 2009: www.chw-nec.org/

Domke, H. R., and Coffey, G. III. 1966. The Neighborhood-Based Public Health Worker: Additional Manpower for Community Health Services. *American Journal of Public Health* 56: 603–608.

D'Onofrio, C. N. 1970. Aides–Pain or Panacea? *Pub Health Reports* 85(9): 788–801.

Eng, E., and Young, R. 1992. Lay Health Advisors as Community Change Agents. *Family and Community Health* 15: 24–40.

Giblin, P. T. 1989. Effective Utilization and Evaluation of Indigenous Health Care Workers. *Public Health Reports* 104: 361–368.

Gonzalez Arizmendi, L., and Ortiz, L. 2004. Neighborhood and Community Organizing in Colonias: A Case Study in the Development and Use of Promotoras. *Journal of Community Practice* 12(1/2): 23–35.

Gould, J., and Lomax, A. 1993. Evolution of Peer Education: Where Do We Go from Here? *Journal of American College Health* 41(6): 235–240.

Grube-Robinson, J. 2001. American Public Health Association Governing Council Resolution: Recognition and Support for Community Health Workers' Contributions to Meeting our Nation's Health Care Needs. Washington, DC: American Public Health Association.

Harlan, C., Eng, E., and Watkins, E. 1992, May 10–15. Migrant Lay Health Advisors: A Strategy for Health Promotion. Paper presented at the Third International Symposium: Issues in Health, Safety and Agriculture, Saskatchewan, Canada.

Hoff, W. 1969. Role of the Community Health Aide in Public Health Programs. *Public Health Reports* 84(11): 998–1002.

Human Resources and Services Administration (HRSA), U.S. Health and Human Services Administration, Bureau of Health Professions. 2007. Community Health Worker National Workforce Study. Accessed on April 15, 2009: http://bhpr.hrsa.gov

Indian Health Service. 2006. U.S. Department of Health and Human Services, Community Health Representative Program. Accessed one April 15, 2009: www.ihs.gov.

James Madison University. 2006. *Final Report on the Status, Impact, and Utilization of Community Health Workers.* House Document No. 9. Richmond, VA: Commonwealth of Virginia.

Jennings, W. 1990, October. Barriers to Employment for Public Health Assistance Recipients. Presented at the American Public Health Association, New York.

Julnes, G., Konefal, M., Pindur, W., and Kim, P. 1994. Community-Based Perinatal Care for Disadvantaged Adolescents: Evaluation of the Resource Mothers Program. *Journal of Community Health* 19(1): 41–53.

Keane, D., Nielsen, C., and Dower, C. 2004. *Community Health Workers and Promotores in California.* San Francisco: Center for the Health Professions.

Klitzman, R. 1997. *Being Positive: The Lives of Men and Women with HIV.* Chicago: Ivan R. D.

Larson, K. McGuire, J. Watkins, E., and Mountain, K. 1992. Maternal Care Coordination for Migrant Farmworker Women: Program Structure and Evaluation of Effects on Use of Prenatal Care and Birth Outcome. *Journal of Rural Health* 8(2): 128–133.

Love, M. B., Legion, V., Shim, J. K., Tsai, C., Quijano, V., and Davis, C. 2004. CHWs Get Credit: A Ten-Year History of the First College-Credit Certificate for Community Health Workers in the United States. *Health Promotion Practice* 5: 418–428.

Love, M. B., Gardener, K., and Legion, V. 1997. Community Health Workers: Who They Are and What They Do: A Survey of Eight Counties in the San Francisco Bay Area. San Francisco Department of Health Education, San Francisco State University. *Health Education and Behavior* 24: 510–522.

Maathai, W. 2006. *Unbowed, A Memoir.* New York: Knopf.

Mahler, H. 1978. Promotion of PHC in Member Countries of WHO. *International Health* 93: 107–113.

McFarlane, J., and Fehir, J. 1994. *De Madres a Madres*: A Community, Primary Health Care Program Based on Empowerment. *Health Education Quarterly* 21(2): 381–394.

Meister, J. S., Warrick, L. H., de Zapien, J. G., and Wood, A. H. 1992. Using Lay Health Workers: Case Study of a Community-Based Prenatal Intervention. *Journal of Community Health* 17: 37–51.

Meister, J. S. 1997. Community Outreach and Community Mobilization: Options for Health at the U.S.-Mexico Border. *Journal of Border Health* 2(4): 32–38.

Mohatt, G. and Eagle Elk, J. 2000. *The Price of a Gift: A Lakota Healer's Story.* Lincoln: University of Nebraska Press.

Murphy, M. A. 1972. Improvement of Community Health Services Through the Support of Indigenous Nonprofessional. *New York State Nurses Association* 3: 29–33.

National Human Services Assembly. Family Strengthening Policy Center. 2006. *Community Health Workers: Closing the Gap on Family's Health Resources.* Washington, DC: National Human Services Assembly.

Nemcek, M. A., and Sabatier, R. 2003. State of Evaluation: Community Health Workers. *Public Health Nursing* 20: 260–270.

New Mexico Department of Health. 2003, November 24. Senate Joint Memorial 076: Report on the Development of a Community Health Advocacy Program in New Mexico. Santa Fe: New Mexico Department of Health.

Nichols, D. C., Berrios, C., and Samar, H. 2005, November. Texas' Community Health Workforce: From State Health Promotion Policy to Community-Level Practice. *Preventing Chronic Disease* 2(special issue). Accessed on April 15, 2009: www.cdc.gov/pcd/issues/2005/nov/05_0059.htm

Norris, S. L., Chowdhury, F. M., and Van Le, K. 2006. Effectiveness of Community Health Workers in the Care of Persons with Diabetes. *Diabetic Medicine* 23(5): 544–556.

Pearl, A., and Riessmann, F. 1965. *New Careers for the Poor: Nonprofessionals in Human Service.* New York: Free Press.

Poland, M. L., Giblin, P.T., Waller, J. B., and Hankin, J. 1992. Effects of a Home Visiting Program on Prenatal Care and Birthweight: A Case Comparison Study. *Journal of Community Health* 17(4): 224–229.

Potts, D., and Miller, C. W. 1964. Community Health Aide. *Nursing Outlook* 12: 33–35.

Proulx, D. E. 2000a. Arizona's Project Jump Start: A Community College/AHEC Partnership. National AHEC Bulletin 17(Spring/Summer).

Proulx, D. E. 2000b. Project Jump Start: A Community College and AHEC Partnership Initiative for Community Health Worker Education. *Texas Journal of Rural Health* 18(3): 6–16.

Proulx, D. E., Rosenthal, E. L., Fox, D., Lacey, Y., and Community Health Worker National Education Collaborative (CHW NEC) Contributors. 2008. *Key Considerations for Opening Doors: Developing Community Health Worker Educational Programs.* Tucson: University of Arizona. Accessed on April 9, 2009: www.chw-nec.org

Pynoos, J., Hade-Kaplan, B., and Fleisher, D. 1984. Intergenerational Neighborhood Networks: A Basis for Aiding the Frail Elderly. *Gerontologist* 24: 233–237.

Ramos, R., Hernandez, A., Freirre-Pinto, J., Ortiz, M., and Somerville, G. G. 2006. Promovision: Designing a Capacity Building Program for Strengthening the Role of Promotores in HIV Aids Prevention. *Health Promotion Practice* (October): 444–449.

Rico, C. 1997. *Community Health Advisors: Emerging Opportunities in Managed Care.* Baltimore, MD: Annie E. Casey Foundation and Seedco—Partnerships for Community Development.

Rosenthal, E. L., Wiggins, N., Brownstein, J. N., Johnson, S., Borbon, I. A., Rael, R.,Guernsey de Zapien, J., Ingram, M., Meister, J., Mcleod, J., Williams, L., Lacey, Y., and Blondet, L. 1998. *The Final Report of the National Community Health Advisor Study: Weaving the Future.* Tucson: University of Arizona and Annie E. Casey Foundation. Accessed on April 15, 2009: www.rho.arizona.edu

Rosenthal, E. L., DeHeer, D., Rush, C. H., and Holderby, L. R. 2008, Fall. Focus on the Future: A Research Agenda by and for the U.S. Community Health Worker Fieldua. *Progress in Community Health Partnerships: Research, Education, and Action* 2(3): 225–235.

Sainer, E. A., Ruiz, P., and Wilder, J. F. 1975. Career Escalation Training. *American Journal of Public Health* 65: 1208–1211.

Salber, E. J. 1979. Lay Advisor as a Community Health Resource. *Journal of Health Politics, Policy and Law* 3(4): 469–478.

Satterfield, D., and Burd, C. 2002. The "In-Between People": Participation of Community Health Representatives in Diabetes Prevention and Care in American Indian and Alaska Native Communities. *Health Promotion Practice* 3(2): 166–175.

Service, C., and Salber, E. J. 1977. *Community Health Education: The Lay Health Advisor Approach.* Durham, NC: Duke University.

Smedley, B., Stith, A., and Nelson, A. 2002. *Unequal Treatment: What Healthcare Providers Need to Know About Racial and Ethnic Disparities in Healthcare.* Washington, DC: Institute of Medicine.

Swider, S. M. 2002. Outcome Effectiveness of Community Health Workers: An Integrative Literature Review. *Public Health Nursing* 19(1):11–20.

U.S. Bureau of Labor Statistics. Standard Occupational Classification. Responses to Comments on 2010 SOC, Multiple Dockets. Accessed January 2009, from www.bls.gov/soc/soc2010responses.htm.

U.S. Department of Health and Human Services, Health Resources and Services Administration. Bureau of Health Professions. 2007. Community Health Worker National Workforce Study, Rockville, MD. Accessed on April 15, 2009: ftp://ftp.hrsa.gov

Werner, D., and Bower, B. 1982. *Helping Health Workers Learn: A Book of Methods, Aids, and Ideas for Instructors at the Village Level.* Berkeley: Hesperian Foundation.

Wiggins, N. 1998. Core Roles and Competencies of Community Health Advisors. In E. L. Rosenthal and others (Eds.), *The Final Report of the National Community Health Advisor Study: Weaving the Future*, 15–49. Tucson: University of Arizona and Annie E. Casey Foundation. Accessed on April 15, 2009: www.rho.arizona.edu

Willaert, A. 2005. Minnesota Community Health Worker Workforce Analysis: Summary of Findings for Minneapolis and St. Paul. Accessed on April 15, 2009: www.heip.org

Wilkinson, D. Y. 1992. Indigenous Community Health Workers in the 1960s and Beyond. In R. L. Braithwaite and S. E. Taylor (Eds.), *Health Issues in the Black Community*, 255–266. San Francisco: Jossey-Bass.

Withorn, A. 1984. *Serving the People: Social Services and Social Change.* New York: Columbia University Press.

Witmer, A., Seifer, S. D., Finocchio, L., Leslie, J., and O'Neil, E. H. 1995. Community Health Workers: Integral Members of the Health Care Work Force. *American Journal of Public Health* 85: 1055–1058.

3

An Introduction to Public Health

Tim Berthold • Sharon Turner

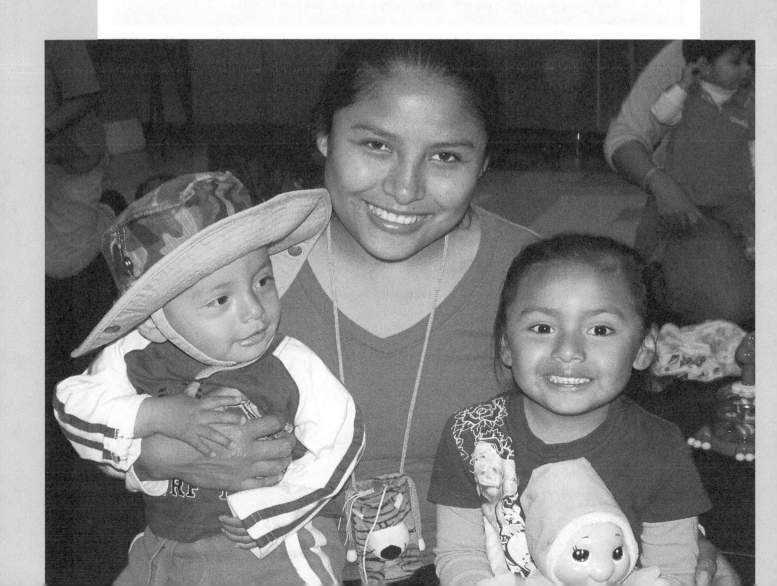

> Health care matters to all of us some of the time, public health matters to all of us all of the time.
>
> —*Former Surgeon General C. Everett Koop*

INTRODUCTION

This chapter provides a brief introduction to the complex field of public health. We focus on the concepts we believe are most essential to guiding your work as a CHW. If you are new to the study or practice of public health, you may not be familiar with some of the language used in the field. One of the goals of this textbook is to assist you in becoming more comfortable with the language of public health, so that you can actively participate in all phases of public health programs and policies: designing, implementing (putting into practice), and evaluating them, and so that you can support the communities you work with to do the same. Please note this chapter often applies the example of HIV disease to illustrate public health concepts.

WHAT YOU WILL LEARN

By studying in the information in this chapter, you will be able to:

- ✪ Define health and public health and explain how the field of public health is different from the field of medicine
- ✪ Explain how the field of public health analyzes the causes of illness and health of populations and emphasizes the social determinants of health
- ✪ Describe the ecological model of public health and apply it to specific public health issues
- ✪ Explain why public health is concerned with health inequalities
- ✪ Discuss the relationship between promoting social justice and promoting public health
- ✪ Discuss public health's emphasis on prevention
- ✪ Explain the spectrum of prevention and provide examples for each of the six levels

WORDS TO KNOW

Population	Prevalence	Infant Mortality
Epidemiology	Chronic Disease	Infectious Disease
Life Expectancy	Social Determinants of Health	Ecological Models of Health
At Risk	Interdisciplinary	

3.1 DEFINING HEALTH

Public health promotes the health and well-being of all people. There are many definitions of *health*. As you read in Chapter One, the World Health Organization (WHO) defines *health* as "the complete state of physical, mental, and social well-being, not just the absence of disease." This widely used definition encourages us to think about health broadly and in positive terms. Other definitions emphasize additional dimensions of health, such as emotional, intellectual, occupational, environmental, political, and spiritual health.

? *How do you define health?*

3.2 DEFINING THE FIELD OF PUBLIC HEALTH: KEY CONCEPTS

To define the field of public health, this chapter discusses several key concepts.

PUBLIC HEALTH IS POPULATION BASED

While the field of medicine focuses on the health of individual patients, the field of public health is concerned with the health of large groups of people or **populations**. These populations are usually defined by one or more factors, such as:

- Geographic and political boundaries (ZIP code, city, county, nation)
- Demographic characteristics such as ethnicity, gender, age, and immigration status
- Health-related data on groups with similar patterns of risk factors, illness, injury, disability, or mortality

For example, a population could be defined as women in the United States, Latina women in California, or pregnant Latina women under the age of twenty-one in the city of Oakland, California.

? *What populations do you belong to?*

? *Which populations are you most interested in working with as a CHW?*

PUBLIC HEALTH IS AN INTERDISCIPLINARY FIELD

Public health is an **interdisciplinary** field. This means that it builds on and applies a wide range of science, social science, and professional disciplines, including biology, anatomy, economics, demography (the study of populations), statistics, business, urban planning, law, anthropology, sociology, medicine, psychology, and political science.

PUBLIC HEALTH USES THE SCIENCE OF EPIDEMIOLOGY

Public health has also developed its own science of **epidemiology**, the study of the health and illness of populations.

Dr. John Snow is often called the father of modern epidemiology. He worked to stop a cholera epidemic in London in 1854. Cholera is a terrifying disease that causes extreme vomiting and diarrhea and can result in death from dehydration in a matter of hours. Today we know that disease can be spread from person to person by invisible microorganisms such as the bacteria that cause cholera and tuberculosis and viruses that cause the flu and HIV. The germ theory of disease, however, was not widely understood or believed before the turn of the twentieth century. People were not certain what caused cholera or the other common communicable diseases like smallpox, measles, and diphtheria. Many people believed that disease was spread by *miasma* or foul air identified with the conditions of poverty.

Snow had a theory that cholera was spread by contaminated water. He interviewed cholera patients and their surviving family members and studied death records. He plotted deaths from cholera on a map of London and observed that the death rate was much higher among families who got their water from the Broad Street Pump. Snow convinced local leaders to turn off the Broad Street Pump. Once the handle to the pump was removed, there was a sudden and dramatic decline in the number of local residents infected with and dying from cholera.

Chapter Seventeen, "Community Diagnosis," shows how Dr. Snow used a map to record cholera deaths in London. The chapter also demonstrates how CHWs sometimes work in partnership with local communities to create similar maps of local health risks and resources.

The methods that Snow used to investigate the cholera epidemic are still used today. They are used to study epidemics such as HIV/AIDS, tuberculosis, automobile-related accidents and deaths, and **infant mortality** (the number of children born alive who die before the age of one).

Today, public health applies a range of scientific methods, including epidemiology, in order to:

○ Identify patterns of illness, injury, disability, and death within populations
○ Analyze the causes of disease within populations
○ Compare disease rates between different populations to identify those with the highest rates of illness and death
○ Guide the development of public health programs and policies designed to promote the health of populations
○ Evaluate the effectiveness of public health programs and policies
○ Guide future investments, programs, and policies to methods that have been proven effective

Public health analyzes existing government data and gathers new information in order to analyze patterns of disease and death. In the United States, each state keeps a record of all deaths and their primary causes. These records are used to analyze the leading causes of death within a population, to compare changes in the causes of death over time, and to establish priorities for public health programs and policies. The National Center for Health Statistics, of the Centers for Disease Control and Prevention (CDC, 2005), lists the leading causes of death in the United States for 2004 as follows:

○ Heart disease: 652,486
○ Cancer: 553,888
○ Stroke (cerebrovascular diseases): 150,074
○ Chronic lower respiratory diseases: 121,987
○ Accidents (unintentional injuries): 112,012
○ Diabetes: 73,138
○ Alzheimer's disease: 65,965
○ Influenza/Pneumonia: 59,664
○ Nephritis, nephrotic syndrome, and nephrosis: 42,480 (inflammation or damage of the kidneys)
○ Septicemia: 33,373 (life-threatening infection sometimes known as blood poisoning)

An analysis of death records shows that the leading causes of death in the United States today are primarily **chronic diseases** such as heart disease, cancer, stroke, and diabetes. A century ago, in 1900, the leading causes of death were **infectious disease**s such as tuberculosis, the flu or pneumonia, and diarrheal diseases. While many people assume that the dramatic change in the leading causes of death that occurred in the twentieth century was due to new developments in the field of medicine, public health research has demonstrated the change was primarily due to passing new public policies, such as those that promoted universal schooling, improvements in sanitation and access to clean water, the minimum wage, and prohibitions against child labor.

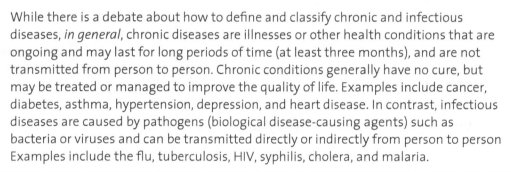

CHRONIC AND INFECTIOUS DISEASE

While there is a debate about how to define and classify chronic and infectious diseases, *in general*, chronic diseases are illnesses or other health conditions that are ongoing and may last for long periods of time (at least three months), and are not transmitted from person to person. Chronic conditions generally have no cure, but may be treated or managed to improve the quality of life. Examples include cancer, diabetes, asthma, hypertension, depression, and heart disease. In contrast, infectious diseases are caused by pathogens (biological disease-causing agents) such as bacteria or viruses and can be transmitted directly or indirectly from person to person Examples include the flu, tuberculosis, HIV, syphilis, cholera, and malaria.

Records of births and deaths are generally available for study, but it is not as easy to document the number of people living with a specific illness or disability, such as HIV disease. The field of public health uses statistical research methods to gather information from a sample (a smaller but representative number) of the population and to make reliable estimates of the number and percentage of people with a particular illness, and how rapidly the illness or other health condition is increasing within the population. Statistical methods guide researchers in determining how to gather this information, whom to gather it from, and how many people must be sampled in order to provide a reliable estimate of the number or percentage of the population who are affected.

For example, the field of public health uses scientific research methods to estimate the **prevalence** (or the percentage of a population with a health risk or condition) of HIV in populations throughout the United States and around the world. It is estimated that 1 percent or 1 out of every 100 adults in the United States is infected with HIV. In comparison, it is estimated that 20.1 percent or one out of every five adults are infected with HIV in Zimbabwe, a nation in southern Africa (all data from UNAIDS, 2007).

Epidemiologists conduct research to estimate basic health indicators that measure the health of a population. These indicators can also be used to compare the health status of different populations. The most widely used health indicators are infant mortality and life expectancy. **Infant mortality** is the estimated number of children, out of every 1,000 children born alive, who die before the age of one. **Life expectancy** is the estimated number of years that people will live. In 2007, infant mortality for the United States was estimated at 6.7 per 1,000 live births. In comparison, infant morality for Zimbabwe was estimated in 2006 at 51.12 per 1,000 live births (Henry J. Kaiser Family Foundation, 2008). In 2005, life expectancy in the United States was estimated at 75 years for males and 80 years for females. In comparison, life expectancy in Zimbabwe was estimated at 43 years for males and 42 years for females (Henry J. Kaiser Family Foundation, 2008).

? *Are you surprised by the large difference in infant mortality and life expectancy rates between the United States and Zimbabwe?*

? *What do these life expectancy and infant mortality rates tell you about the relative health of each nation?*

While CHWs are not expected to have an in-depth knowledge of epidemiology or statistics, the more you know, the better prepared you will be to participate in decisions about public health research, programs, and policies. You may wish to begin by locating and reviewing reports from your local health department on the health status of communities you belong to and are working with. This may include reports on issues such as infant mortality, diabetes, or domestic violence. Conduct an online search for the health department or department of public health in your city, county, or state and select a report to read. Identify language or information that you don't fully understand, and talk about it with a colleague.

? *What type of health statistics do you most want to learn about?*

? *How can health data guide and support your work as a CHW?*

PUBLIC HEALTH IS CONCERNED WITH HEALTH INEQUALITIES

One of the most important public health issues of our time is the growing inequality in health among different populations. Health inequalities, also referred to as *health inequities* or *disparities*, occur when one group of people experience significantly higher rates of illness and death than others (these populations are sometimes referred to as "**at risk**"). As you will read in Chapter Four, epidemiological data documents these differences in health status between nations and between different communities within the United States.

An example is the dramatic inequality in HIV prevalence between the populations of the United States and Zimbabwe presented earlier. The data underscores the critical need facing the people of Zimbabwe, where more than 20 percent of adults are living with HIV disease. Dr. Paul Farmer points out that the HIV epidemic follows patterns of class, race, and gender inequalities (Farmer, 1999). In Zimbabwe, colonialism, unequal distribution of basic economic resources, political oppression, poverty, famine, and gender oppression set the stage for HIV/AIDS.

HIV disease is also unequally distributed among populations within the United States. For example, in 2005 the AIDS case rate (or the number of people living with AIDS per 100,000) for African American women was 45.5 per 100,000, or 23 times higher than for white women. While African American women make up only 12 percent of the total population of women in the United States, they account for 66 percent of estimated AIDS cases among women (Henry J. Kaiser Family Foundation, 2007).

Health inequalities are not inevitable or due to genetic or other biological differences between populations. They are the consequence of the way a society structures access to the basic resources, rights, and opportunities that all people require in order to live long and healthy lives. To change or eliminate these inequalities will require changing social policies that determine people's access to resources such as housing, food, education, employment, health care, safety, and human rights.

Leading institutions in the United States and internationally—including the National Association of County and City Health Officials (NACCHO), Centers for Disease Control and Prevention, the Institutes of Medicine (IOM), the Office of Minority Health (OMH), and the World Health Organization—have recognized health inequalities as a public health priority.

For many of us, working to eliminate health inequalities between populations is the central challenge facing public health today. As frontline workers who often have the most contact with the communities that experience disproportionately high rates of illness and death, CHWs have a significant role to play in the movement to eliminate health inequalities.

PUBLIC HEALTH EMPHASIZES THE SOCIAL DETERMINANTS OF HEALTH

The field of public health understands the causes of illness and death differently than does the field of medicine. Traditionally, medicine focuses on the causes of disease located within the individual patient. For example, physicians want to know if a patient is infected with a specific pathogen (or disease-causing agent) such as HIV. For a patient already diagnosed with HIV disease, medicine focuses on what the patient knew, believed, or did that caused or contributed to the infection or progression of disease: Did the patient understand how HIV is transmitted? Did the patient engage in unprotected sex? Is the patient taking her medications properly?

In contrast, public health is concerned with understanding the factors that cause and contribute to patterns of illness and death among large populations of people. Public health research has demonstrated that the most significant of these factors are located at the societal level. These **social determinants of health** include economic, social, and political policies and dynamics that influence whether or not people have access to resources and opportunities essential to good health. In general, populations with less access to these resources experience higher rates of illness and death. These resources, rights, and opportunities include:

- Quality education
- Safe housing and public transportation
- Proper and sufficient nutrition
- Personal safety (from interpersonal violence and war, for example)
- Civil rights and protection from discrimination
- Employment, safe working conditions, and a living wage
- Clean water, air, and soil
- Recreational facilities and green space
- Cultural resources
- Affordable health care

? *What resources and opportunities do you consider to be essential for the health and wellness of communities or populations?*

ALVARO MORALES: Now I work for the environmental health program at a local department of public health. I investigate the health risks people are exposed to at work, at home, and in their communities. I visit families whose children have lead poisoning. These children are sick just because their families are poor, and they live in houses with lead paint. The parents are devastated. I am lucky because I have this great job, benefits in case I get sick, and when I go home at night, I know that my children will have a good meal and a safe place to sleep. It's just so unfair. People are getting sick because they live and work in bad conditions. It doesn't need to be this way. That is what is so frustrating: all of this is preventable.

PUBLIC HEALTH USES ECOLOGICAL MODELS TO UNDERSTAND AND PROMOTE HEALTH

Public health uses ecological models based on an understanding of the social determinants of health. These models guide CHWs and other public health practitioners to view individual clients in the context of their families, neighborhoods, and the broader society in which they live. While there are many different ecological models used in the field of public health, we refer throughout this book to the model presented as Figure 3.1.

Figure 3.1 shows interconnected circles representing the individual; relationships with family and friends; the neighborhood or community in which people live, work, and go to school; and the broader society.

The innermost circle represents the individual. A person's health status is influenced by his or her genetics (DNA), thoughts, feelings, beliefs, values, and behaviors. In reference to HIV disease, how people think and feel about themselves (self-esteem) and their perception of risk (youths, for example, often feel invulnerable to HIV) influence rates of infection. So do individuals' acceptance of and comfort with their own sexuality and sexual orientation, their past experiences, including their record of accomplishments, whether or not they engage in sex and drug use, and whether or not they practice safer sex (such as the regular use of condoms).

Figure 3.1 Ecological Model of Health.

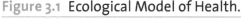

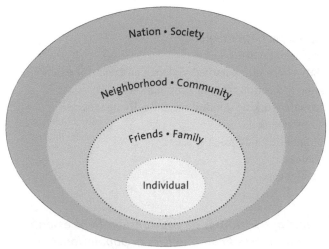

? *Can you think of other ways that individuals influence their own health?*

? *How do you influence your health?*

The next circle represents family and friends who influence health in many ways. In reference to HIV disease, for example, families have not always provided effective education or guidance in order to understand and prevent the transmission of HIV. Some families have judged, alienated, and even disowned members who are lesbian, gay, bisexual, or transgender, who engage in sex with members of their own sex, who use drugs, or who are living with HIV. Other families are supportive regardless of the identities and behaviors of their relatives. While friends sometimes encourage healthy behaviors, they sometimes promote risk taking such as the use of drugs and unprotected sex. People who are in relationships, including marriage, are sometimes pressured or threatened into doing things that they don't want to do, such as having unprotected sex. People sometimes experience physical, sexual, and emotional abuse or assault from family members, and these traumatic experiences have been shown to influence their health status and risks for HIV disease.

? *Can you think of other ways in which family and friends influence health status?*

? *How do your family and friends influence your health?*

The next circle represents the neighborhood or community we live in. Our health is strongly influenced by whether or not we have a safe home to live in, safe working conditions and a living wage, and are exposed to environmental hazards and violence. Neighborhoods and communities also influence whether or not people have access to recreational and cultural activities, public transportation to get back and forth from our homes to school, work or grocery stores and to visit with family and friends. In reference to HIV disease, some neighborhoods have community-based organizations that provide culturally appropriate outreach, education, HIV antibody testing, and counseling services, while others do not. Some communities have safe places for youths to congregate, while others do not. Some neighborhoods have lots of billboards and stores that market and sell alcohol; others do not. Some communities have good schools and job training, nearby access to jobs and social services; others do not. Living in neighborhoods that lack these basic resources results in chronic stress that causes chronic health conditions such as diabetes and heart disease and, ultimately, premature death.

? *Can you think of other ways in which a community may contribute to the risks of disease?*

? *How does the neighborhood and community you live in and belong to influence your health?*

The outermost circle in Figure 3.1 represents the nation or society we live in. It includes social, cultural, economic, and political factors that influence our health status. The decisions that our governments make about where and how to invest public funds largely determines which populations have greater access to resources such as safe housing, loans, transportation, recreational facilities, quality schools, social services, and employment opportunities. The media, including television and the Internet, may encourage risky behavior or healthy choices. Economic dynamics influence access to jobs that provide safe working conditions and a living wage.

In reference to HIV disease, most governments, including the government of the United States, have hesitated to acknowledge or take action to prevent HIV disease, often due to economic concerns (such as a negative impact on tourism) or prejudice against the populations who are most affected (such as injection drug users, communities of color, and gay men). Governments have not always provided accurate information about how to prevent HIV infections, access to HIV antibody test counseling, medical care and other services that people living with HIV need in order to live healthy and productive lives. People with HIV do not always have civil rights and protection from discrimination in housing, education, health care, and employment. Poverty rates within populations also influence health status and risks for HIV. People who live in poverty often take risks that others would not in order to survive and assist their families to survive, such as engaging in sex in exchange for food, shelter, or money. Incarceration has also been shown to facilitate HIV transmission, and the United States has the highest rate of imprisonment among industrialized nations (National Commission on Correctional Health Care, 2002). HIV disease is much more prevalent among communities characterized by poverty, histories of discrimination, violence, inadequate housing, and poor access to other basic resources.

Whether CHWs work with individuals, families, or communities, an ecological perspective is essential to guide their efforts.

? *What would you add to the ecological model presented above?*

? *Can you think of other ways that our society and our government influence our health?*

DEFINING PUBLIC HEALTH ISSUES

Public health is not only concerned with commonly understood health issues (such as cancer or tuberculosis), but with any issue that significantly contributes to patterns of illness, injury, disability, death, or wellness in a population. Public health issues are broadly defined and may include:

- Chronic diseases such as diabetes, heart disease, and cancer
- Infectious diseases such as tuberculosis, HIV/AIDS, and pneumonia
- Violence, including handgun violence, domestic violence, and war
- Mental health issues, including depression and suicide
- Disability issues and disability rights
- Racism and other forms of discrimination
- Prevention of injuries such as automobile accidents
- Occupational health issues such as exposure to toxic chemicals
- Inequalities in rates of illness or death, such as infant mortality rates
- Environmental health issues such as exposure to pesticides or other toxins and access to clean water, soil, and air
- Reproductive health issues such as access to contraceptives and prenatal care
- Access to safe and permanent housing
- Emergency preparedness

✪ Hunger and access to proper and sufficient nutrition
✪ Urban planning to promote the development of neighborhoods and cities that promote health
✪ Incarceration rates and conditions
✪ Access to drug and alcohol treatment programs
✪ Promotion and protection of civil and human rights

? *What additional public health issues would you add to this list?*

The Office of the Surgeon General of the U.S. Department of Health and Human Services (2009) has identified the following four public health priorities:

1. Disease prevention
   This includes addressing obesity, increasing physical activity, prevention of HIV/AIDS, and reducing tobacco use.
2. Eliminating health disparities
   This focuses on eliminating the higher burden of death and disease experienced by minority communities.

Refineries and other environmental hazards are more commonly located near low-income communities of color, seriously affecting their health. CHWs and other community advocates are organizing to change this.

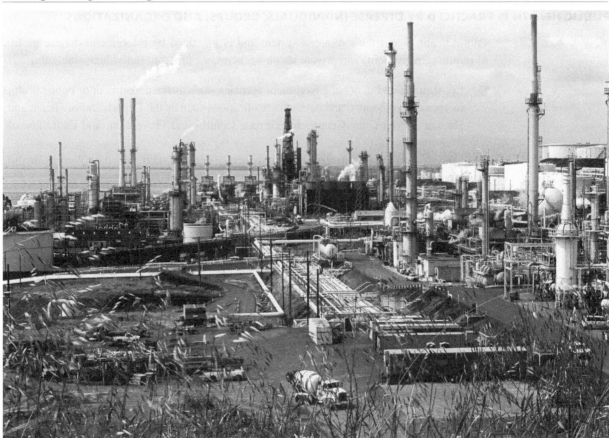

3. Public health preparedness

    This includes responding to issues such as terrorism, emerging infections (such as multi-drug-resistant strains of tuberculosis and staphylococcus), natural disasters (such as Hurricane Katrina), and mental health and resilience.

4. Improving health literacy

    Health literacy is defined as "the ability of an individual to access, understand, and use health-related information and services to make appropriate health decisions." This is identified as a priority because "more than 90 million Americans cannot adequately understand basic health information."

    The United States has also established national health goals and objectives through the year 2010. *Healthy People 2010* (www.healthypeople.gov) establishes two overarching goals and twenty-eight focus areas. The goals are (1) increase the quality and years of healthy life, and (2) eliminate health disparities.

?   *What do you think about the public health priorities and goals established by the United States?*

?   *What do you consider to be the most important public health issues facing the communities you live in and work with?*

3.3 THE PRACTICE OF PUBLIC HEALTH

PUBLIC HEALTH IS PRACTICED BY DIVERSE INDIVIDUALS, GROUPS, AND ORGANIZATIONS

Public health is not a coordinated system and is practiced by a large and diverse group of public (government) and private sector agencies, groups, and individuals, including:

- Local, state, and national government agencies, such as the department of public health in your city or county, and national organizations such as the Department of Health and Human Services, the Centers for Disease Control and Prevention, and the Office of Minority Health

- International and intergovernmental organizations such as the World Health Organization and the United Nations Children's Fund (UNICEF)

- Public and private clinics and hospitals, particularly those that provide health care services to low-income and uninsured patients. *Which clinic or hospital, if any, provides services to low-income patients in your community?*

- Colleges and universities with departments or schools of public health, health education, medicine, public policy, and social work that provide education and professional training and conduct research and advocacy related to public health. *Is there a college or university close to where you live? Does it provide education and training or conduct research or advocacy related to public health?*

- Many small and large private agencies or nongovernmental organizations including nonprofit agencies that provide health and social services to promote the health of low-income and at-risk communities (communities with increased risks for illness, disability, injury, or premature death). These may include agencies that work with youths or seniors and address issues such as domestic violence, homelessness, or drug and alcohol use. These agencies are typically funded by a range of sources, including government contracts, grants from private foundations, donations from individuals and businesses, and the fees that the agencies charge for services. *Which agencies provide services in your community?*

✪ Individuals, groups, and associations work to promote the health and welfare of low-income and otherwise vulnerable communities. Individual activists may advocate with local governments to develop policies or fund programs designed to address specific public health issues such as access to housing, nutrition, civil rights, or health care. Informal groups of people come together to advocate on behalf of particular issues, such as a group of public housing residents who advocate for the repair of hazardous living conditions. More formal associations are also active in advocating for public health and social justice. Labor unions, for example, have taken leadership in promoting occupational health and advocating for expanding access to quality health care services for the uninsured. *Can you identify individual activists, groups, or associations that are working to promote public health in your community?*

Though the practice of public health is largely invisible and not often publicized, our lives are affected by public health programs and policies every day, including programs that immunize children against infectious disease, that prevent automobile accidents and deaths, that restrict tobacco use, and that monitor the quality of our drinking water. *Can you think of other examples?*

Despite former Surgeon General C. Everett Koop's statement that "health care matters to all of us some of the time, public health matters to all of us all of the time," public health agencies in the United States have been historically underfunded, and funding continues to decline (Public Health Foundation, 1996). The vast majority of health-related funding is spent on expensive and relatively inefficient health care services (see Chapter Five). Public health professionals advocate to change the balance of these investments and to increase government spending on public health programs and policies.

Policies that affect the public's health are largely determined by the decisions that our governments make, including the level of investment in essential resources such as education, housing, transportation, food, safe working conditions, and access to health care, including mental health services. Every time your government makes a decision about where to invest public dollars, it has an impact on public health. (Everyone, regardless of citizenship status, pays taxes, including sales taxes, automobile, gasoline, and tobacco taxes.) When governments enforce civil rights, raise the minimum wage or build affordable housing, they are promoting public health. When international bodies negotiate a cease fire or treaty, they are taking action that impacts public health.

? **What decisions has your local government made in the past year that affects the health of the communities you work with?**

? **How could you and the communities you work with influence such decisions in ways that improve the community's health?**

PUBLIC HEALTH EMPHASIZES PREVENTION

One of the defining features of public health practice is the emphasis on prevention. The "upstream story" is frequently used to illustrate this point.

THE UPSTREAM STORY OF PREVENTION

Four hikers beside a river heard cries for help and saw a man struggling against the current, trying to reach the shore. They managed to save him, but just as they were pulling him to safety, along came a boy in the river, slamming against the boulders. Before they pulled the boy out, two more people swept by: the hikers barely rescued them. Exhausted, they treated the victims. Then they heard another cry for help. One of the hikers said, "That's it—I'm going upstream to investigate." The others said, "You can't! More people will need to be rescued, and we can't do it without you. If you leave, someone might drown." The hiker replied, "I want to find out why they are falling in the river, so we can find a way to stop it!"

Just like the hiker moved upstream to see what could be done to prevent people from falling into the river, public health tries to intervene "upstream" to prevent epidemics from developing in the first place. Money spent on upstream programs and policies that promote social equality and equal access to basic resources will not only save lives; they will aid in preventing the expense of caring for people who would become ill. If we apply this example to the AIDS epidemic, public health emphasizes the importance of investing "upstream" in programs and policies that will prevent new HIV infections.

Primary, Secondary, and Tertiary Prevention   Public health distinguishes among three different types of prevention. *Primary prevention* is defined as preventing the development of a disease (or other health condition) from occurring. *Secondary prevention* involves the early diagnosis and treatment of illnesses or conditions before they become symptomatic. *Tertiary prevention* involves services for those already living with symptomatic conditions to aid in delaying further progression of disease, alleviate symptoms, prevent complications, and delay death.

Applied to HIV disease, primary prevention might include both the promotion of equal access to essential resources and more targeted programs such as syringe exchange programs to provide injection drug users with clean syringes in exchange for used ones. Secondary prevention might include policies to promote access to affordable and confidential HIV antibody-testing programs for the early diagnosis of HIV disease, as well as civil rights protections from discrimination in housing and employment and affordable health care for those newly diagnosed. Tertiary prevention might include policies that promote access to free and low-cost antiretroviral medications (medications used to treat HIV disease) and social services, such as subsidized housing and meals that have proven effective in aiding to delay the progression of HIV disease.

The Spectrum of Prevention   The spectrum of prevention provides a framework for understanding different "levels" of prevention and has been widely used to guide the development of public health programs in areas such as injury prevention, violence prevention, nutrition, HIV/AIDS, and fitness (Prevention Institute, 2009).

We use the spectrum of prevention (Table 3.1) to teach CHW students about the range of public health interventions (a public health program or activity aimed at producing a change) that they may participate in.

In Table 3.2, we provide an example of how CHWs can work at each level of the spectrum of prevention. The examples provided in Table 3.2 are drawn from the HIV/AIDS field. At the end of this chapter, you will be asked to apply the spectrum of prevention to a different public health issue.

Table 3.1.   The Spectrum of Prevention.

Spectrum	Definition
1. Strengthening individual knowledge and skills	Enhancing an individual's ability to prevent injury or illness and promote safety
2. Promoting community education	Reaching groups of people with information and resources to promote health and safety
3. Educating providers	Informing health providers who will transmit skills and knowledge to others
4. Fostering coalitions and networks	Bringing individuals and groups together to work for common goals with a greater impact
5. Changing organizational practices	Adopting regulations and shaping norms within organizations to improve health and safety
6. Influencing policy and legislation	Developing strategies to change laws and policies in order to influence health outcomes

Table 3.2.   Spectrum of Prevention Examples.

Spectrum	Example
1. Strengthening individual knowledge and skills	CHWs work in a clinic and provide client-centered education and counseling to high-school-aged youths regarding how to prevent HIV and other sexually transmitted infections.
2. Promoting community education	CHWs visit local high schools and give educational presentations designed to assist youths reduce their risks for HIV infection.
3. Educating providers	CHWs facilitate trainings for the staff at a youth-serving agency on topics related to HIV prevention and how to work effectively with at-risk youths, including lesbian, gay, bisexual, and transgender.
4. Fostering coalitions and networks	CHWs facilitate the formation and planning process of a coalition of youths and youth-serving organizations interested in preventing HIV disease and providing increased access to prevention education and HIV antibody test counseling.
5. Changing organizational practices	CHWs work with local youth networks and youth leaders to advocate with local schools or school districts to provide comprehensive sexuality education; to support civil rights protections for lesbian, gay, bisexual, and transgender students; or to implement condom availability programs.
6. Influencing policy and legislation	CHWs advocate with state policymakers on behalf of new policies, such as policies to prohibit discrimination of people living with HIV or those that support syringe exchange programs, living wages, and universal health care.

? *Have you participated as a volunteer or paid staff in programs that represented one or more levels of the spectrum of prevention?*

? *Which levels have you worked at? Which levels do you hope to work at over the course of your career as a CHW?*

PUBLIC HEALTH PRACTICE IS EVIDENCE BASED

The field of public health conducts research, gathering and analyzing data to identify the populations at greatest risk for illness and premature death and to evaluate the effectiveness of public health programs and policies. This information is then used to guide future public health investments. Rather than investing money in programs or policies that we *think* will promote health outcomes among a specific population, public health encourages investments in programs and policies that have already proven to be successful with similar populations, or the adaptation and testing of similar models with different populations.

At the same time, it is important to acknowledge that political beliefs and goals sometimes undermine this process, and scientific evidence may be disregarded in the development of policies. For example, our federal government has deemphasized the use of condoms and focused on abstinence-only education despite overwhelming evidence that condoms are an effective means of preventing HIV and abstinence-only education is not (Center for AIDS Prevention Studies, 1997).

The Center for AIDS Prevention Studies (CAPS) at the University of California, San Francisco, is well respected for the research it conducts and disseminates (shares with others) on local, national, and international public health programs and policies related to HIV disease. Much of the research that CAPS conducts is in partnership with local community-based organizations and CHWs. The CAPS Web site (www.caps.ucsf) provides access to ongoing and completed research studies, reports on research findings, and resources from model programs that have been proven to be effective and may be adapted and implemented in other communities. The *Science to Community* series provides four-page summaries of research findings on a variety of issues relevant to the work of CHWs. The purpose of these reports is to make scientific findings accessible to community members and all levels of public health practitioners. A sample of reports on HIV prevention projects posted on the Web site as of March 2009 includes:

- HIV Prevention for Women Visiting Their Incarcerated Partners: The HOME Project (August 2007)
- The CHANGES Project: Coping Effectiveness Training for HIV+ gay men (June 2007)
- *Investigación Conjunta para la Prevención del VIH con Poblaciones Encarceladas y sus Familias* (December 2004)
- Prevention Strategies of HIV Positive Injection Drug Users (VENUS Study) (September 2001)
- Study of HIV Sexual Risk Among Disenfranchised African American MSM Community (March 2001)

When research demonstrates the effectiveness of an HIV-prevention program, the team at CAPS is often able to post a detailed description of the program, and the resources used, on their Prevention Tools Web page. For example, research demonstrated that The Mpowerment

Project was effective at reducing rates of unprotected anal sex among young men who have sex with men. The Mpowerment Program Model is available on the CAPS Web site, and further grant funding has allowed the team at CAPS to facilitate trainings and provide technical assistance to local communities interested in implementing the model.

CHWs benefit from keeping up-to-date with public health research about the issues you address in your work. You can learn from both successful and unsuccessful public health models to more effectively promote the health of the clients and communities you serve. The most useful research evidence will be based on program models and strategies that are very similar to your own, and with populations that are very similar to those you work with. For example, just because a diabetes management program was effective with Native American women in Arizona, a similar program may not be equally successful serving white men in New Hampshire. As we have tried to emphasize, the environment in which people live and the identities and culture of the community you serve need to be taken into consideration when you plan and provide public health programs.

Finally, as a CHW you may have opportunities to participate in public health research and will certainly have opportunities to participate in the evaluation of the programs and services you provide. We encourage you to talk with your colleagues about the program models you work with. How were they developed? Are they guided by existing research? Have they been evaluated? If so, what are the findings? If they haven't been evaluated, ask to participate in the development of evaluation methods that will assist you to learn if the programs you work for are making a positive difference to the health status of participating communities. Even if you are unfamiliar with research or evaluation methods, your experience as a CHW may be invaluable in identifying what information to gather from the community and how to gather it. (Refer to information provided in Chapter Eighteen and Chapter Nineteen for an introduction to some types of evaluation and assessment.)

PUBLIC HEALTH ADVOCATES SOCIAL JUSTICE

As public health research demonstrates, the factors that have the biggest impact on human health are social determinants, including political decisions about where and how to invest public resources. It follows, therefore, that the most powerful strategy for promoting public health is to advocate for changes to public policies that will provide equal access to the resources and opportunities that are essential to health (education, housing, nutrition, safety, civil rights, and so on). If everyone, regardless of their educational background, income, ethnicity, immigration status, or other demographic characteristics, had access to these resources and opportunities, our society wouldn't experience such high rates of infectious or chronic disease, or such pronounced inequalities in illness, death, and wellness between different populations.

We define *social justice* as the equal access to these basic human resources, rights, and opportunities.

Leading public health institutions such as the American Public Health Association, Schools of Public Health at universities such as San Francisco State and Harvard, the National Association of Local Health Directors, and the World Health Organization have all expressed their commitment to advocating for social justice as a best practice for promoting public health. For example, see *The Health and Social Justice Reader* (Hofrichter, 2003). To read about how local health departments are working to promote health justice, read *Tackling Health Inequities Through Public Health Practice: A Handbook for Action*, published by the National Association of County & City Health Officials (2007).

Anthony Iton, Medical Officer for the Alameda County Health Department in Oakland, California, says:

> In virtually every public health area . . . be it immunizations, chronic disease, HIV/AIDS . . . or even disaster preparedness, local public health departments are confronted with the consequences of structural poverty, institutional racism and other forms of systemic injustice. By designing approaches that are specifically designed to identify existing assets and build social, political and economic power among residents of afflicted neighborhoods, local public health departments can begin to sustainability reduce and move towards eliminating health inequities in low-income communities of color. Additionally, local public health agencies must simultaneously seek opportunities to strategically partner with advocates for affordable housing, labor rights, education equity, environmental justice, transportation equity, prison reform. . . . Without such a focus, local health departments will most likely only succeed in tinkering around the edges of health disparities at a cost too great to justify. (NACCHO, 2007)

One of the primary roles of all public health practitioners, including CHWs, is to advocate for social justice on behalf of and in partnership with the clients and communities you serve. Only by doing so can we change and improve the conditions that have the biggest impact on health status.

ALVARO MORALES: I've been working in public health for fourteen years now. I've learned that if we could change things so that the communities I work with—mostly low-income communities of color and immigrant communities—if they had access to things like education, housing that isn't dangerous, a job with benefits for enough money to live on, good places for my children to go to school, then we could prevent most of the health problems I see on a daily basis. People's children wouldn't get lead poisoning, and there wouldn't be so many homeless people. The communities I work with wouldn't have a life expectancy that is so much lower than others. It all comes down to working for social justice, and I'm proud to be part of that.

PUBLIC HEALTH HAS NOT ALWAYS PROMOTED JUSTICE

Unfortunately, public health is sometimes practiced from the top down: professional "experts" develop and implement programs and policies they think will promote the health of a vulnerable community. This approach has sometimes resulted in significant harm to the community. For example, the Tuskegee Syphilis Trials, an infamous public health research project, withheld treatment from African American men who were being studied to learn more about syphilis. As a result, men enrolled in the study were disabled and died. (For more information about Tuskegee, see Chapter Seven.) Unfortunately, public health history has many such examples.

? *Have your communities been harmed by public health programs or policies in the past?*

? *How do the communities you belong to view the government?*

PUBLIC HEALTH WORKS IN PARTNERSHIP WITH COMMUNITIES

At its best, public health is practiced in collaboration with the communities that have the most to gain or lose. One of the key roles of CHWs is to assist in flipping the top-down strategy just described and to partner with communities to develop public health programs and policies that represent and benefit from the wisdom, creativity, skills, and leadership of affected communities. This is important for many reasons, including:

- ✪ *It is the right thing to do.* Communities with the most to gain or lose from a public health program or policy have the right to be consulted regarding its design, management, and evaluation. The right of a community to self-determination, and a voice in the decisions that affect them, is rooted in our most fundamental beliefs in democracy.
- ✪ *Long-term effectiveness.* Public health programs and policies come and go. Programs developed with leadership from the community are much more likely to be culturally relevant and to result in significant and lasting changes.
- ✪ *Capacity building.* You may have heard the expression, "Give a person a fish and they will eat well for a day. Teach a person to fish, and they will eat well forever." A key dimension to enhancing the health of communities is to foster community leadership and skills that may be used to address other health concerns in the future.

The quality of your work as a CHW can be judged to great extent by the degree to which you establish and maintain respectful partnerships with the communities you work with and your ability to facilitate and support their leadership. (For more information about community-centered practice and the role of the CHW, please see Part Three of this textbook.)

PUBLIC HEALTH PROMOTES THE HEALTH OF THE NATURAL ENVIRONMENT

Our ancestors understood that human health was dependent upon the health of the planet. Modern societies have largely forgotten and forsaken this knowledge and often operate in ways that harm our planet, the air and atmosphere, our oceans, ground water, soil, plants, and animal species. The health of the planet and the health of human populations are integrally connected and mutually dependent, and increasingly, public health is beginning to promote both goals.

Increasingly, public health has turned its attention to global climate change. Public health practitioners are beginning to join the movement to address climate change, which will affect all populations but will have the greatest impact on low-income and otherwise vulnerable populations. Public health has an important role to play to ensure that the policies we use to reduce greenhouse gases offer health cobenefits (health benefits in addition to the benefit of addressing climate change; for example, increasing public transportation options or increasing locally grown fresh fruits and vegetables) and promote health equality. A strong public health infrastructure will also be key to handling the effects of climate change such as heat waves, floods and natural disasters, food shortages, and changes in patterns of infectious disease.

CHAPTER REVIEW

To review, answer the following questions and apply the ecological model and the spectrum of prevention to the public health issue of gun violence.

GUN VIOLENCE IN AMERICA

Between 1979 and 2001, gunfire killed ninety thousand children and young people in America (Children's

Defense Fund, 2007). The rate of death from gun violence among children under age fifteen is nearly twelve times higher in the United States than in twenty-five other industrialized countries combined (Centers for Disease Control and Prevention, 2005).

1. Apply your understanding of the ecological model to the public health issue of handgun-related homicides.

   What types of individual factors might contribute to handgun-related homicides?

   How might family and friends contribute to handgun-related homicides?

   What types of community- or neighborhood-level factors might contribute to handgun-related homicides?

   What types of societal factors contribute to handgun-related homicides?

2. How would you explain that handgun violence is considered a public health issue?

3. Imagine that you are going to work with a public health program designed to assist in preventing handgun violence in a large city. What type of public health statistics would you want to study?

4. Using the spectrum of prevention framework shown in Table 3.3, provide examples of public health strategies that CHWs can participate in to assist in preventing handgun-related violence.

Table 3.3. The Spectrum of Prevention Applied to Gun Violence in the United States.

Spectrum	Strategy
1. Influencing policy and legislation	CHW will _____
2. Changing organizational practices	CHW will _____
3. Fostering coalitions and networks	CHW will _____
4. Educating providers	CHW will _____
5. Promoting community education	CHW will _____
6. Strengthening individuals knowledge and skills	CHW will _____

5. How would promoting social justice assistance to prevent handgun violence in the United States?

REFERENCES

Center for AIDS Prevention Studies. The University of California, San Francisco. Accessed on April 11, 2009: www.caps.ucsf.eduCenter for AIDS Prevention Studies. 1997. *Should We Teach Only Abstinence in Sexuality Education?* University of California, San Francisco. Accessed on April 11, 2009: www.caps.ucsf.edu

Centers for Disease Control and Prevention. 2005. Accessed on April 11, 2009: www.cdc.gov

Children's Defense Fund. 2007. Child Watch. Protect Children, Not Guns. Accessed on April 11, 2009: www.childrensdefense.org

Farmer, P. 1999. *Infections and Inequalities: The Modern Plagues.* Berkeley, CA: University of California Press.

Hofrichter, R., Ed. 2003. *The Health and Social Justice Reader.* San Francisco: Jossey-Bass.

The Henry J. Kaiser Family Foundation. 2007. HIV/AIDS Policy Fact Sheet. Women and HIV/AIDS in the United States. Accessed on April 11, 2009: www.kff.org/hivaids/upload/6092_05.pdf

The Henry J. Kaiser Family Foundation. 2008. Global Health Facts. Accessed on April 11, 2009: www.globalhealthfacts.org/

The Institutes of Medicine. Accessed on April 11, 2009: www.ion.edu

National Association of County and City Health Officials. 2007. *Tackling Health Inequities Through Public Health Practice: A Handbook for Action.* Washington, DC: National Association of County and City Health Officials.

National Commission on Correctional Health Care. 2002. *Health Status of Soon-to-Be-Released Inmates: A Report to Congress. Vol. 1.* Washington, DC: National Commission on Correctional Health Care.

Prevention Institute. Accessed on March 30, 2009: www.preventioninstitute.org/tool_spectrum.htm

Public Health Foundation. 1996. *Measuring Expenditures for Essential Public Health Services.* Memorandum. Accessed on April 11, 2009: www.phf.org

UNAIDS. 2007. Joint United Nations Programme on HIV/AIDS. Accessed on April 11, 2009: www.unaids.org/en/

U.S. Department of Health and Human Services. *Healthy People 2010*. Accessed on April 11, 2009: www.healthypeople.gov

U.S. Department of Health and Human Services. The Office of the Surgeon General. Public Health Priorities. Accessed on March 30, 2009: www.surgeongeneral.gov

ADDITIONAL RESOURCES

American Public Health Association. Accessed on April 11, 2009: www.apha.org

International Centre for Health and Society of the University of London. Accessed on April 11, 2009: www.ucl.ac.uk/ichs

Office of Minority Health. Accessed on April 11, 2009: www.omhrc.gov

University of California, Los Angeles. School of Public Health. Department of Epidemiology. Accessed on April 11, 2009: www.ph.ucla.edu/epi

University of California, San Francisco. Center for AIDS Prevention Studies. Accessed on April 11, 2009: www.caps.ucsf.edu

University of Virginia Health System. *Bad Blood: The Tuskegee Syphilis Study*. Health Sciences Library. Accessed on April 11, 2009: www.healthsystem.virginia.edu

World Health Organization. Accessed on April 11, 2009: www.who.int

World Health Organization, Europe. *Social Determinants of Health: The Solid Facts* (2nd ed.). Accessed on April 11, 2009: www.euro.who.int

World Health Organization. WHO Commission on Social Determinants of Health. Accessed on April 11, 2009: www.who.int/social_determinants/en/

4

Promoting Health Equality

Tim Berthold

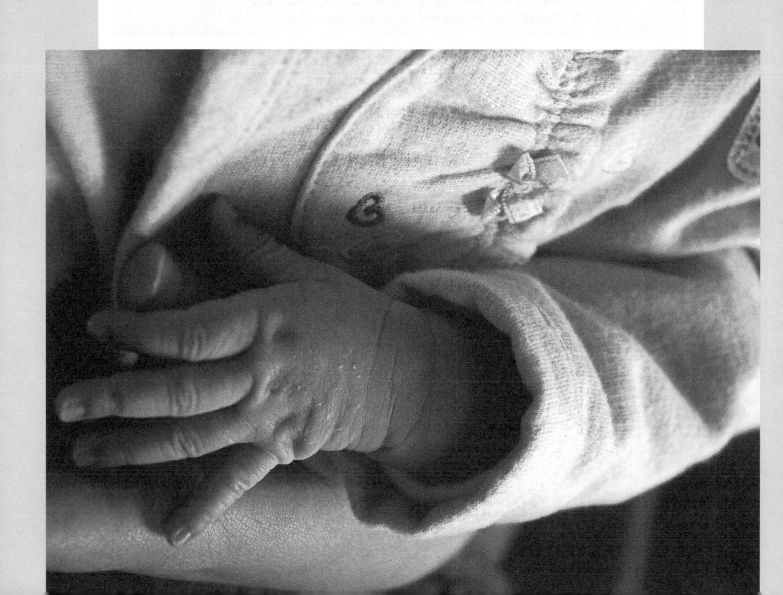

> Of all the forms of injustice, inequality in health is the most shocking and inhumane.

—Dr. Martin Luther King, Jr.*

INTRODUCTION

The United States and the world are characterized by dramatic inequalities in health. Bluntly stated, some populations get sick more often and die much earlier than others. This is not a consequence of chance or genetics, or a result of poor choices. Rather, these inequalities are socially constructed: they are the consequences of the decisions we make about the allocation of basic resources and rights that all people require in order to live healthy lives. These resources include human rights, safety, sufficient and proper nutrition, safe working conditions, a living wage, quality housing, health care, and education. It is within our power to prevent communities from experiencing excess illness and premature death.

WHAT YOU WILL LEARN

By studying the information in this chapter, you will be able to:

- ⊙ Define health inequalities
- ⊙ Discuss and analyze the data that show health inequalities among populations
- ⊙ Explain how social inequalities result in health inequalities
- ⊙ Analyze how health inequalities are harmful to our society
- ⊙ Describe and analyze how health inequalities are preventable
- ⊙ Identity and discuss the role of CHWs in preventing health inequalities and promoting health justice

WORDS TO KNOW

Child Mortality	Stress	Transphobia
Maternal Mortality	Morbidity	Food Security
Life Expectancy	Environmental Racism	
Homophobia	Environmental Justice	

4.1 DEFINING HEALTH INEQUALITY

Health inequalities, also referred to as "health disparities," are significant differences in health status between different populations. The following definition comes from Richard Hofrichter (2007) with the National Association of County and City Health Officials: "Differences in

UNNATURAL CAUSES

In March 2008, a documentary series on health inequalities premiered on public television. *Unnatural Causes* presents recent research on the causes of health inequalities and highlights local efforts to promote health justice. We strongly recommend viewing this series and reviewing the case studies, research, and educational materials posted on the *Unnatural Causes* Web site www.unnaturalcauses.org. We reference resources from the Web site throughout this chapter.

---

population health status and mortality rates that are systemic, patterned, unfair, unjust and actionable, as opposed to random or caused by those who become ill."

4.2 EVIDENCE OF HEALTH INEQUALITIES

The evidence of health inequalities between and within nations is extensive but is sometimes difficult for people to comprehend. When studying this data, we ask you to look not only at the statistics but also to think about what they imply about the lives of the people they represent.

HEALTH INEQUALITIES AMONG NATIONS

Table 4.1 documents significant differences in health status among nations. The table documents differences in **child mortality,** or the estimated number of children who die before the age of five out of every 100,000 live births; **maternal mortality,** or the estimated number of women who die as a result of pregnancy or childbirth per 100,000 live births; and **life expectancy,** or the average number of years that a population is expected to live.

The data reveal that children born in Afghanistan are 64 times more likely to die before the age of 5 than children born in Sweden or Japan (257 deaths per 100,000 compared to 4 per 100,000). Mothers in Nepal are 276 times more likely to die from complications related to pregnancy and childbirth than mothers in Sweden (830 deaths per 100,000 compared to 6 per 100,000). And people in Japan are estimated to live, on average, 46 years longer than people in Zimbabwe. These are not small or trivial differences or inequalities in health: they represent significant unnecessary death and loss to families, communities, and nations.

HEALTH STATUS IN THE UNITED STATES COMPARED TO OTHER NATIONS

As we discuss in Chapter Six, the United States spends significantly more money on health care than other industrialized nations yet ranks near the bottom in most leading health indicators. For example, in 2004, the United States spent approximately $6,096 per person on health care, compared to $19 in Afghanistan, $135 in Iraq, $2,828 in Sweden, and $2,294 in Japan (World Health Organization, 2004). While the United States spent more money on health care than any other country, it ranks only twenty-ninth among nations in terms of life expectancy and thirtieth in terms of infant mortality.

Table 4.1.　International Comparison of Health Indicators.

Nation	Child Mortality (2005)	Maternal Mortality (2005)	Life Expectancy (2006)
Japan	4	6	82
Sweden	4	3	81
United States	8	11	78
Nepal	82	830	61
Iraq	125	300	55
Afghanistan	257	1800	42
Zimbabwe	126	880	36

Source: World Health Organization, 2005, 2006.

HEALTH INEQUALITIES WITHIN THE UNITED STATES

Health inequalities exist among different populations in the United States based on ethnicity, income, education, sex, gender identity, disability, immigration status, sexual orientation, geographic location, and other factors. Inequalities based on income and ethnicity have received the most attention and have been well documented by research. There is need for more research and advocacy addressing other persistent inequalities.

INCOME, WEALTH, AND HEALTH INEQUALITY

You may not be surprised by the data that show that rich people are significantly healthier than poor people, but the extent of the relationship between income and health may hold some surprises for you. First, it is not just the very poor who die earlier than the super-rich. There is a steady and direct relationship between income and health: as annual income increases from under $10,000 to over $100,000, so too does life expectancy. Middle-class families live longer than working-class families, but not as long as the wealthy (Kawachi, Kennedy, Gupta, and Prothrow-Stith, 1999). Second, these health inequalities based on income are significant and increasing. In 1980–1982, the wealthiest residents of the United States lived 2.8 years longer than the poorest (75.8 versus 73 years). By 1998–2000, this gap had increased to 4.5 years longer (79.2 versus 74.7 years) (Singh and Siahpush, 2006).

ETHNICITY AND HEALTH INEQUALITY

Health inequalities based on ethnicity are significant and are increasing in the United States, despite our federal government's policy to eliminate health disparities. According to the federal Office of Minority Health (OMH), "Compelling evidence indicates that race and ethnicity correlate with persistent and often increasing, health disparities among U.S. populations . . . and demands national attention" (Office of Minority Health, 2009).

When we present data on health inequalities in our classes at City College of San Francisco, students often experience anger and other powerful emotions. The authors of this book share these responses, and hope they will inspire and guide us to advocate for a more just world.

The National Partnership for Action to End Health Disparities (2008), part of the U.S. Department of Health and Human Services, finds that Native Americans, Hispanics/Latinos, American Indians and Alaska Natives, Asian Americans, native Hawaiians and Pacific Islanders have higher rates of infant mortality, cardiovascular disease, diabetes, HIV infection/AIDS, cancer, and lower rates of immunizations and cancer screening than do Whites.

Table 4.2. Health Indicators for African Americans and White Americans (2004).

Population	Infant Mortality	Child Mortality	Maternal Mortality	Life Expectancy
White Americans	5.7	27	9.3	78.3
African Americans	13.2	41.8	34.7	73.1

Source: National Center for Health Statistics, 2007.

Health inequalities between Whites and African Americans have been most studied because they are the most extreme. Table 4.2 presents these inequalities.

African Americans of all ages die at higher rates than do Whites. The data presented in Table 4.2 show that African American infants are 2.3 times more likely to die before the age of 1 than are White infants born in the United States. African American mothers are 3.7 times more likely to die due to complications related to childbirth than White mothers in the United States. Finally, White Americans are expected to live 5.2 years longer than are African Americans.

Dr. David Satcher, former surgeon general of the United States, completed a study of African American death rates in 2002. The study estimated that

> 83,570 African-Americans died who would not have died if health status among African-Americans was equal to that of white Americans. This is equivalent to 229 "excess deaths" each day. That's the equivalent of one Boeing 767 being shot out of the sky and killing everyone on board every day, 365 days a year. And they are all Black. (Satcher and others, 2005)

OTHER HEALTH INEQUALITIES

Immigration Status   Health inequalities also persist in the United States based on immigration status. Immigrants are much less likely to have health insurance: in 2003, 52 percent of recent immigrants lacked health insurance, compared to 15 percent of native-born citizens (Kaiser Commission on Medicaid and the Uninsured, 2004). As a consequence, immigrants are much less likely to access basic health care services (Kaiser Commission on Medicaid and the Uninsured, 2008). Interestingly, while new immigrants tend to have better health than do native citizens of the same sex, age, income, and educational level, their health status declines the longer they live in the United States (Smedley, Jeffries, Adelman, and Cheng, 2009; Franzini, Ribble, and Keddie, 2001).

Gender   While women have a higher life expectancy than do men in most nations, they experience disproportionately higher rates of domestic violence and resulting trauma, depression, and other chronic health conditions, and they face discrimination in the diagnosis and treatment of certain health conditions (Östlin, George, and Sen, 2003; National Center for Health Statistics, 2009; Kawachi and others, 1999; United Nations Population Fund, 2009).

T G: Most of my clients have HIV, and most of them are people of color, gay men, and injection drug users—people who face discrimination on a daily basis just because of who they are. They risk losing their families, get discriminated against when they look for work, or housing, or health care and sometimes just when they are walking down the street. All of this takes a big toll on their health. It keeps them from getting basic things that they need, and after awhile, for some of them, it just sort of beats them down. They can lose confidence and faith in themselves. This is why I became a CHW—to work with other people like me who had experienced discrimination, to let them know that someone wants the best for them, and to advocate for them to be treated like they should be treated—with respect.

Sexual Orientation and Gender Identity   Health inequalities also exist based on sexual orientation and gender identity. Studies have documented increased rates of depression and attempted suicide among lesbian, gay, and bisexual youths compared to heterosexual youths (Society for Public Health Education, 2005). Transgender and gender-variant communities experience some of the highest rates of HIV infection in the United States, as well as high rates of violence, depression, and attempted suicide (National Coalition for LGBT Health, 2009; National Center for Transgender Equality, 2009). Due to persistent discrimination and related stigma against such groups, comparably little research is available regarding the health status of transgender and gender-variant communities. Fortunately, this is beginning to change.

4.3   THE CAUSES OF HEALTH INEQUALITIES

The causes of health inequalities in the United States are not well understood by the general public, the media, and some members of the medical profession. People commonly assume that these inequalities are either natural, inevitable, caused by biological or genetic differences between populations, or are the result of cultural differences or poor choices made by those with higher rates of illness and death.

Public health research has demonstrated that health inequalities are caused by social determinants, including policies that result in inequalities in income and wealth, racism and other forms of institutionalized discrimination (such as sexism and homophobia), unequal working and living conditions, and the chronic stress that accompanies lives characterized by poverty, discrimination, and low levels of personal safety and control.

Communities that experience disproportionately high rates of illness and death are suffering the consequences of continuous and systematic disadvantage and discrimination. Members of these communities work in low-wage and high-stress jobs without health insurance benefits and live in cities or counties characterized by large gaps in wealth between the rich and poor. They live in substandard housing and in neighborhoods that lack green spaces, recreational facilities, quality schools, and stores that offer affordable and high-quality fresh produce. Their neighborhoods are located near waste incinerators, power plants, oil refineries, and other sources of environmental toxins and are characterized by high rates of violence and other crimes. They often face institutionalized racism, sexism, and other forms of discrimination. All of these factors contribute to high levels of chronic stress, which takes a toll on their bodies and results in chronic illnesses such as depression, diabetes, hypertension, and heart disease. The end results of ongoing exposure to these many risk factors are increased death rates and a shortened life expectancy.

A recent study by the Department of Public Health in Alameda County, California, compared the health of a Black child born in a low-income household in the "flats" of Oakland to that of a White child born to a wealthy family in the Oakland hills. Over the course of his or her lifetime, the Black child faces the cumulative impact of poverty, racism, harmful living, educational and working conditions, and chronic stress that will reduce that child's life expectancy by nearly fifteen years compared to the White child growing up in the hills (Beyers and others, 2008).

THE ROLE OF HEALTH CARE

Communities that experience the highest rates of **morbidity** (illness) and death are more likely to lack health insurance or a regular source of health care, and individuals within such communities are more likely to face discrimination when they seek out health care services. However, lack of medical care is not nearly as influential a factor in determining health or causing health inequalities as many Americans think. Dr. David Satcher, former surgeon general of the United States says, "Although critical to eliminating disparities, access to health care only accounts for 15–20 percent of the variation of morbidity and mortality that we see in different populations in this country" (Satcher and Higginbotham, 2008).

As the gap between rich and poor in the United States has widened, health inequalities have increased.

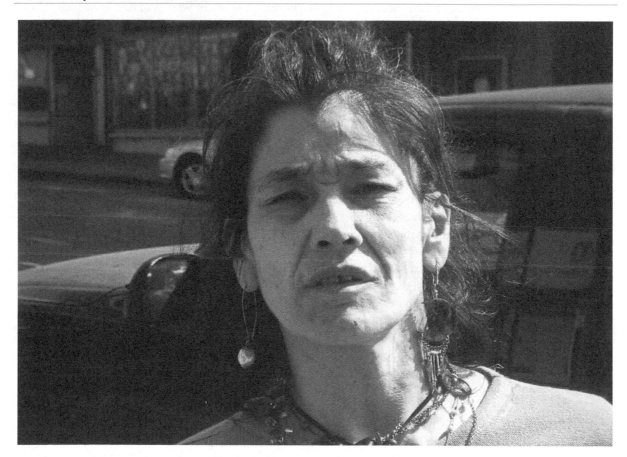

INCOME AND WEALTH

Income and wealth play a major role in determining health status. On average, individuals, families, and populations that earn less and own less have higher rates of illness and death than those who earn and own more. In addition, research has demonstrated that overall death rates increase as the gap between rich and poor increases. Cities, states, and nations with greater inequality in the distribution of wealth (a bigger gap between rich and poor) tend to have higher rates of illness and lower life expectancy overall (Kaplan and others, 1999). In other words, large inequalities in wealth are harmful to *everyone's* health. The United States has greater income and wealth inequality than any other industrialized nation in the world and significantly higher rates of mortality (including infant and maternal mortality) and lower life expectancy. In 1983, it was estimated that the wealthiest 5 percent of people owned 56 percent of all the wealth in the United States. By 1989, this had increased to 62 percent (Wolff, 1995).

RACISM AND OTHER FORMS OF DISCRIMINATION

With the exception of some Asian Pacific Islander communities, people of color in the United States generally experience higher rates of illness and death than comparable White communities. These differences are not explained by economic factors, such as higher poverty rates, nor by genetics, but by racism and discrimination.

While death rates go down for all populations as income increases, inequalities based on ethnicity persist at all income levels. The same is true for education: death rates go down as educational achievement rises, but inequalities based on ethnicity remain. For example, infant mortality rates go down as the educational achievement of mothers increases: infant mortality rates are lower for mothers who graduate from high school than for those who don't; they are lower still for mothers who graduate from college. But educational achievement cannot erase the consequences of racism: infant morality is 10.6 per 1,000 live births among African American women who have completed college, but just 6.8 per 1,000 births among white mothers with an eighth grade education (National Center for Health Statistics, 2002).

Many people, including representatives from the media and medical community, think that the comparatively poor health status of communities of color must be due to innate genetic differences. Yet public health research has clearly shown that social factors play the most significant role in determining health and causing inequalities.

The O'odham people, Native Americans who live in southern Arizona, experience extremely high rates of diabetes, a leading cause of death in the community. Many people assumed that such high rates were caused by biological or genetic factors, but research has shown that diabetes was rare among the O'odham people hundreds of years ago. The current high rates of diabetes are associated with a history of genocide and displacement and policies that have eroded territory and autonomy. These policies resulted in the loss of access to water sources for irrigation, resulting in the loss of agricultural practices and traditional diets. The community became dependent upon the federal government for hand-outs of packaged and processed foods. In other words, the epidemic of diabetes among the O'odham is the result of public policies, not genetics (California Newsreel, 2009).

Even medical providers have assumed that African Americans experience higher rates of hypertension or high blood pressure based on genetic differences. But research has shown that people in West Africa, the region of Africa that was the center of the slave trade, have very low rates of hypertension (Cooper and others, 2005).

Similarly, African American infants have lower birth weights than White infants (low birth weight places these children at risk for a wide range of health conditions). However, while the infants of new African immigrants to the United States weigh as much as White infants, the children born to the next generation of African immigrants weigh less than White infants. With time and exposure to social conditions in the United States, birth weight among people of African descent decreases (David and Collins, 1997; Collins, Wu, David, 2002).

David Williams, profession at the University of Michigan explains:

> It is important to note that the pathways of race are linked to the structure of society and to social experience – not to biology or genetics. We have known for some time that racial categories do not represent much biologic distinctiveness, and they are unlikely to be a major explanation for health disparities. (Center for the Advancement of Health, 2003)

Research has also documented a strong connection between exposure to racial discrimination and poor health: African Americans and Asian Americans who reported a higher rate of exposure to racism were found to have higher rates of various health conditions, including hypertension and cancer (Smedley, Jeffries, Adelman, and Cheng, 2009; Taylor and others, 2007; Troxel, Matthews, Bromberger, and Sutton-Tyrrell, 2003; Gee, Spencer, Chen, and Takeuchi, 2007; Mays, Cochran, Barnes, 2007; McCracken and others, 2007).

Racism also influences the level and quality of health care services that patients of color receive. Among older patients who qualify for Medicare, patients of color receive fewer visits, cancer screening, flu shots, and necessary heart bypass surgery and are more likely to experience preventative amputations and radical cancer surgery than White patients (Gornick, 2003). While this may not be due to conscious racism and discrimination, the effect is the same: patients of color receive poorer-quality health care than White patients. The National Partnership for Action to End Health Disparities (2008) recognizes that patients of color receive substandard health care due to many causes, "including patient-provider miscommunication, provider discrimination, stereotyping or prejudice."

Racism also results in limited access to other basic resources for people of color, including bank loans, housing, education, and employment:

> Educational, housing and wealth-accumulating opportunities have been shaped by a long history of racism that confers economic advantage to some groups while disadvantaging others. For example, studies of hiring have consistently found that employers prefer white candidates over African American ones, even when their qualifications are identical. In fact, one study even found that fictitious white applicants with a felony record were preferred over Black applicants with no criminal history. And low socio-economic status translates into poorer health. (Smedley, Jeffries, Adelman, and Cheng, 2009)

SEGREGATION

Many Americans still live in highly segregated neighborhoods (neighborhoods without much ethnic diversity). Some studies have found that segregation in American cities is similar to that under apartheid in South Africa, with a sharp divide between the neighborhoods where Whites and communities of color live. Segregation has been found to negatively influence economic opportunities, education, access to quality housing, affordable and nutritious food and green spaces, exposure to environmental hazards, crime, and rates of incarceration (Smedley, Jeffries, Adelman, and Cheng, 2009).

ENVIRONMENTAL RACISM

Communities of color are much more likely than White communities to be exposed to environmental toxins and other pollutants that are harmful to human health. This is known as **environmental racism**. Waste incinerators, landfills, and oil refineries are more likely to be located in or nearest to neighborhoods with a majority population of color. These same communities are more likely to be exposed to lead-based paint in their homes and hazardous chemicals and conditions at work.

The **environmental justice** movement grew in the 1980s and is defined as:

> The right to a decent, safe quality of life for people of all races, incomes and cultures in the environments where we live, work, play, learn and pray. Environmental justice emphasizes accountability, democratic practices, equitable treatment and self-determination. Environmental justice principles prioritize public good over profit, cooperation over competition, community and collective action over individualism, and precautionary approaches over unacceptable risks. Environmental justice provides a framework for

communities of color to articulate the political, economic and social assumptions underlying why environmental racism and degradation happens and how it continues to be institutionally reinforced. (Asian Pacific Environmental Network, 2002)

The environmental justice movement has been led by the communities most at risk and has resulted in changes in national and state policies. In 1994, President Bill Clinton signed the Executive Order on Environmental Justice that requires federal agencies to take action to reduce environmental racism. The struggle continues to enforce national and state policies.

SEXISM, HOMOPHOBIA, AND TRANSPHOBIA

Research has found that women's health status is also linked to their overall social status. When women are able to participate more actively in politics, are employed at a fair wage, and live in areas that support reproductive rights (access to birth control and family planning services), they experience lower mortality and disability rates (Kawachi and others, 1999).

Less research has been done about the health impacts of **homophobia** (fear of and prejudice against homosexuals or people who have romantic or sexual feelings or relationships with people of the same sex) and **transphobia** (fear of and prejudice against transgender people or people who may have sex, gender, or gender expression that is different from that assigned to them at birth and may identify with one or more, or none, of a long and growing list of terms used to describe gender identity). However it is clear that both homophobia and transphobia results in discrimination and violence perpetrated against lesbian, gay, bisexual, transgender, and gender-variant people and increased health risks (National Coalition for LGBT Health, 2009).

WORKING CONDITIONS, STATUS, AND CONTROL

For many communities, living and working conditions contribute to higher rates of illness and death. People who work longer hours for low wages, lack benefits, are exposed to hazardous conditions or chemicals, face threats of job loss or reduced pay, or work in environments characterized by conflict with management experience higher rates of chronic stress and higher rates of chronic illness (Taylor and others, 2007).

Research has shown that it is not just income and working conditions that influence health but also people's level of status and control. Though people often think of management jobs as particularly stressful, professional status affords greater autonomy and job security, resulting in less chronic stress and disease. Workers who are lower down the management hierarchy, who have less decision-making power and less control over their own work hours, process, and pay suffer higher rates of illness and death (Marmot and others, 2005; Job Stress Network, 2009).

LIVING CONDITIONS

People who live in wealthier communities generally experience better health than do those who live in low-income areas:

Residents of middle- and upper-income communities typically have access to high-quality housing, an abundance of shops, parks, health-care services and transportation. In poor neighborhoods, these resources are less likely to be available. Consequently, the lower one is on the SES [socioeconomic status] continuum, the greater amount of hassle and time needed to address basic tasks of living. Further contributing to the chronic stress of lower SES communities are characteristic such as police-documented higher crime rates. (Taylor, Repetti, and Seeman, 1999)

A recent study documents higher rates of diabetes in low-income communities that have a higher ratio or percentage of fast-food restaurants and convenience stores. Communities with a higher ratio of grocery stores and produce (vegetable and fruit) vendors had lower rates of diabetes (California Center for Public Health Advocacy, 2007).

EXPOSURE TO CHRONIC STRESS

All people experience demanding or challenging situations or events that result in **stress**. When faced with these circumstances situations, our bodies release hormones such as cortisol and epinephrine that prepare us to respond quickly (sometimes called the "fight or flight response"). But when people experience stress responses on a chronic or ongoing basis, it takes a destructive toll on their health: "If there is no physical outlet for the 'fight or flight' stimulus, emergency-response chemicals remain in the body, causing depression, increased susceptibility to infection, diabetes, cholesterol and fat buildup and high blood pressure" (Center for the Advancement of Health, 2003).

Studies have clearly shown that people who live in poverty, who work physically demanding but low-wage jobs, who live in poor housing in crowded neighborhoods with few parks and recreational resources, who experience institutionalized racism and other forms of discrimination, or who are constantly exposed to violence or threats of violence are likely to experience chronic stress. Over time, chronic stress harms our bodies and results in chronic health conditions like depression, diabetes, respiratory infections, hypertension, and heart disease that in turn cause premature death (MacArthur Foundation, 2008).

RAMONA BENSON: I worked with a young lady who was on CalWORKs [a public benefit program]. She found a job but was fired after three months. I actually thought she shouldn't have been working: she was so stressed out trying to raise two children while having major relationship problems. CalWORKs said, "You have to come in here and you have to work." But that just added new stress, and nothing was done to help her cope with it.

At her job, when it was time to do effective communication, it was really hard for her. Her anxiety kicked in. She ran into a problem with a coworker and didn't have conflict resolution skills. There was a big blow up, and she got fired.

So now she'll get cut off from CalWORKs. So she's not gonna have her rent, and she's eventually gonna get evicted. Then she'll be running around from house to house looking for a place for her and her kids to lay their heads. Her stress is gonna heighten to where maybe she's gonna start using drugs to try to manage this stress. Then CPS [Child Protective Services] is eventually gonna come in there and her family is gonna be threatened. I mean, I hope all this doesn't happen, but I've seen it too many times before.

4.4 HEALTH INEQUALITIES ARE HARMFUL TO OUR SOCIETY

Social inequalities and resulting health inequalities harm our society in the following ways:

- ✪ Some communities suffer increased rates of preventable illness and death.
- ✪ The society as a whole experiences worse health and lower life expectancy.
- ✪ Losses to our economy and our democracy occur when poor health and premature death prevent people from fully participating. It is estimated that U.S. businesses lose more than $1 trillion a year due to chronic illness of employees and reduced productivity (California Newsreel, 2009).
- ✪ Health insurance premiums are more expensive.
- ✪ Fewer resources are available to be invested in social programs such as education or housing.
- ✪ Social conflict and instability increase.
- ✪ Chronic stress, which is toxic to human health, increases.
- ✪ Social and health inequalities are inconsistent with deeply held values of fairness, justice, and peace.

? *Can you think of other reasons why health inequality is harmful to our society?*

? *What evidence would you provide to support your opinion?*

4.5 PROMOTING HEALTH EQUALITY

While the U.S. Department of Health and Human Services has identified eliminating health disparities as a key goal for the nation, "these goals remain largely symbolic and unprioritized" (Hofrichter, 2003). In fact, many health inequalities are increasing.

Promoting health equality requires swimming far upstream against the tide of social policies that are producing larger inequalities in income, wealth, and health status. It will require addressing the true root causes of inequalities: challenging racism and other institutionalized forms of discrimination and improving access to safe and healthy neighborhoods, housing, education, and other basic resources.

We can look to other nations for examples of how to reduce health inequalities. Sweden has promoted health and health equality through public policies that establish higher taxes and invest this money to provide universal access to basic resources. Education through college is free to all citizens. So are health care, child care, family leave, and other resources that promote public health.

We can also look to our own history for inspiration. During the first part of the twentieth century, average life expectancy in the United States increased by approximately thirty years. This was not achieved primarily by new advances in medicine but by advocating for new social policies that improved working conditions and wages and increased access to education and civil rights.

Successful advocacy for policies that promote social justice requires supporting the participation and leadership of representatives from communities that currently suffer the consequences of health inequalities, including low-income communities of color. It also requires building broad-based coalitions of diverse stakeholders who can work together. This includes maintaining partnerships between those working in public health and those working in areas such as affordable housing, urban planning, **food security** (or access to affordable and nutritious food), worker's rights, and civil and human rights, including women's rights.

Increasingly, public health professionals are pushing for social justice policies as a way to eliminate health inequalities and enhance the health of all communities. David Williams of the University of Michigan argues for "increasing opportunities, providing education and training for better jobs, investing in our schools, improving housing, integrating neighborhoods, giving people more control over their work—these are as much health strategies as diet, smoking and exercise" (Center for the Advancement of Health, 2003).

POLICIES DESIGNED TO PROMOTE HEALTH EQUALITY

Public health professionals have identified a wide range of public policies designed to promote health equality. For the purposes of this chapter, we summarize and provide key examples from California Newsreel's *Policy Guide* and the *Unnatural Causes* documentaries produced for public television. (A list of policy recommendations can be found at www.unnaturalcauses.org.)

Policies designed to promote health equality include those that:

1. *Promote understanding of the social determinants of health:* such as educating decision makers and the general public about how patterns of inequality in the larger environment–where we live, work, and play–influence inequalities in health.

2. *Improve income and reduce wealth inequalities:* such as raising the minimum wage to a livable level; increasing income supports, including unemployment insurance; ensuring secure retirement and pension plans and expanding access for nonstandard workers; supporting the right to organize; and repealing tax cuts and loopholes for the rich.

3. *Improve the physical and built environment:* such as creating more low-cost housing; creating more safe and inviting parks and green spaces; providing appropriate clean-up and removal of toxic material; and providing reliable and low-cost public transit.

4. *Promote racial justice:* such as strengthening and rigorously enforcing existing antidiscrimination, voting rights, and equal opportunity laws; desegregating schools and neighborhoods; providing resources for jobs and educational access and retention; monitoring and eliminating environmental health threats; addressing arrest and sentencing discrimination and promoting rehabilitation in corrections facilities; increasing access, quality, and cultural competence of medical care and social services; and protecting the civil rights of undocumented workers. And we would advocate broadening this proposal to include promoting justice and civil rights for all communities, including women, lesbian, gay, bisexual, transgender, and intersex communities.

5. *Promote better working conditions:* such as strengthening and reinforcing occupation health and safety laws; legislating paid sick leave (including parental and family leave) and vacations; and removing unfair barriers to unionization and strengthening collective bargaining.

6. *Improve conditions for children:* such as guaranteeing universal quality preschool and day care; providing quality public schooling and safe places to play; and ensuring good nutrition and preventive (health) care.

7. *Improve social inclusion:* such as strengthening democratic decision making, community organizations, and opportunities for civic engagement; strengthening laws against discrimination and segregation; and investing in jobs and public infrastructure in resource-poor communities.

8. *Improve education:* such as reforming school financing to equalize school spending and access to quality K–12 education, and improving teacher compensation, training, and support.

9. *Improve food security and quality:* such as providing affordable and nutritious food for all, especially the most vulnerable; limiting fast food and alcohol outlets; and supporting sustainable agriculture and local food production, especially organics.

10. *Improve public and sustainable transportation:* such as giving precedence to cycling and walking; discouraging out-of-town malls and residential sprawl; and improving public transit.

11. *Use health impact assessments (HIAs):* such as requiring the use of HIAs to evaluate the consequences of proposed development and policy initiatives on population health.

12. *Provide universal health care:* such as supporting guaranteed and culturally competent, quality health care, access and treatment for all.

? *Can you think of other policies that would promote health equality?*

PROJECTS THAT WORK TO PROMOTE HEALTH EQUALITY

ADVOCATING LIVING WAGE POLICIES

How much people earn has a strong impact on their health and the health of their families. In July 2009, the minimum wage in the United States increased to $7.25 per hour. Someone who works full time (40 hours a week for 52 weeks per year) at $7.25 an hour would earn $15,080 in a year—seldom enough to cover the costs of rent, food, transportation, clothing, health care, and other basic expenses for an individual, much less a family.

Since the mid-1990s, coalitions in more than 140 cities have successfully advocated for living wage ordinances. Living wage policies require local companies that receive public funds to pay their workers enough to keep them and their families above the poverty level. Some policies also require companies to hire people from the local community and to provide workers with vacation and sick leave (Reynolds, 2006).

Increasingly, public health professionals and local health departments have actively participated in living wage campaigns, joining broad-based coalitions made up of diverse community members and other stakeholders, including labor unions, churches, and other faith-based organizations. By improving pay, increasing workers' ability to pay for basic needs, and reducing stress, living wage policies promote the health of workers and their families and reduce health inequalities.

The City of San Francisco passed a living wage ordinance requiring companies to pay workers $11 an hour. The San Francisco Department of Public Health supported the ordinance (Reynolds, 2006) and estimated that it would result in:

✪ Lower mortality for both men and women
✪ A measurable decrease in depression

- ✪ A measurable reduction in sick days
- ✪ An increased chance of completing high school for the children of covered workers
- ✪ A reduction in the risk of childbirth outside of marriage for daughters of covered workers

? *What are minimum wages for the state and/or city where you live?*

? *Are they high enough to keep a family above the poverty level?*

? *Are groups in your city or region organizing to advocate for a living wage ordinance?*

REDUCING MATERNAL AND CHILD HEALTH INEQUALITIES: THE BERKELEY BLACK INFANT HEALTH PROJECT

Babies who weigh less than 5.5 pounds at birth are considered low birth weight and face significantly increased risks of developing a range of health problems including asthma, cerebral palsy, hypertension, cardiovascular disease, and learning disabilities. In 1995, the rate of low-weight births in Berkeley, California, was 42 per 100,000 live births for White children and 166 per 100,000 live births for Black children. Black infants were four times more likely than White infants to be born with low birth weight. At the time, this was the largest inequality in any U.S. city of comparable size (City of Berkeley, 2002).

The City of Berkeley evaluated the causes of this inequality and recognized that "being at risk for having a low birth weight baby is not a genetic predisposition but is due to many factors, including stress, that may be related to discrimination and racism" (City of Berkeley, 2002).

In response, the public health department developed the Berkeley Black Infant Health Program, based on a community empowerment model. Residents were supported to create community action teams that engaged in ongoing planning, organizing, and advocacy campaigns to promote changes in local policies and the creation of new programs. CHWs were hired to conduct health outreach to invite pregnant and parenting women to participate in an ongoing support group. The group combined health education and stress reduction with empowerment.

Rᴀᴍᴏɴᴀ Bᴇɴsᴏɴ: In our group we talk about relationships, including relationships with mothers, with the baby's father, and a circle of friends. We talk about how to create support in our lives and to provide it to others. We talk about finances, education, racism, stress reduction, personal and community empowerment—and how to have a healthy baby. If our moms aren't stressed, if they have support in their life and are empowered to advocate for themselves, to navigate systems and ask for what they need, that will help their pregnancy and help them to raise a healthy baby.

Berkeley's Black Infant Health Program successfully reduced unequal infant mortality rates.

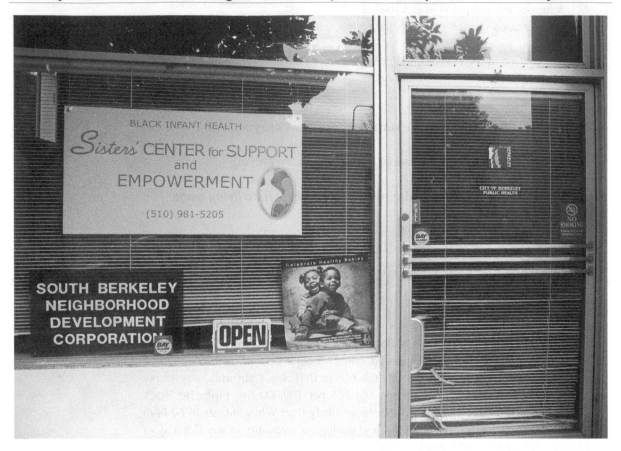

By 2007, ten years after the Black Infant Health Program was started, the inequality in rates of low birth weight between Black and White babies had been reduced from 4-to-1 to 2-to-1. Although Black babies in Berkeley were still twice as likely as White babies to be born with low birth weight, significant progress had been made. The program continues to work to eliminate these inequalities.

?   *What are public health professionals and activists doing in your local communities to promote health equality?*

?   *What policies and programs exist that are designed to reduce higher rates of illness and death among vulnerable communities?*

4.6 THE ROLE OF CHWs

CHWs play an important role in promoting social justice and health equality, whether they are assisting individuals or families to access essential services, facilitating support groups, or engaged in community organizing campaigns. Part Three of this textbook provides greater detail about the work that CHWs do at the community level, and

Chapter Twenty-Two presents the competencies that CHWs require in order to facilitate grassroots community organizing and advocacy efforts.

Many CHWs work with others to advocate for social policies that will promote greater social and health equality. CHWs encourage communities that face the highest rates of illness and premature death to fully participate in these efforts, assisting to ensure that new policies and programs are based in the reality and vision of those communities.

When we confront health inequalities and other forms of injustice, we may feel overwhelmed, depressed, or hopeless. Historian Howard Zinn (2004) reminds us of the key role that hope and faith play in keeping us moving forward to create a better and more just world:

> To be hopeful in bad times is not just foolishly romantic. It is based on the fact that human history is a history not only of cruelty but also of compassion, sacrifice, courage, kindness. What we choose to emphasize in this complex history will determine our lives. If we see only the worst, it destroys our capacity to do something. If we remember those times and places— and there are so many—where people have behaved magnificently, this gives us the energy to act, and at least the possibility of sending this spinning top of a world in a different direction. And if we do act, in however small a way, we don't have to wait for some grand utopian future. The future is an infinite succession of presents, and to live now as we think human beings should live, in defiance of all that is bad around us, is itself a marvelous victory.

Nancy Krieger and Annie-Emanuelle Birn (1998), public health researchers and advocates, write:

> To declare that social justice is the foundation of public health is to call upon and nurture that invincible human spirit that led so many of us to enter the field of public health in the first place: a spirit that has a compelling desire to make the world a better place, free of misery, inequity, and preventable suffering, a world in which we all can live, love, work, play, and die with our dignity intact and our humanity cherished. (p. 1603)

? *Who inspires you to work for social justice and health equalities?*

? *What brings you hope?*

CHAPTER REVIEW

1. You are talking with a friend, family member, or client about your work as a CHW. How would you explain the following concepts, *in your own words:*
   - What are health inequalities?
   - What causes health inequalities?
   - Why are health inequalities harmful to our society?
   - What can we do to eliminate health inequalities?
2. Conduct research to answer the following questions about health inequalities in the area where you live:

   - Where can you find statistics on health inequalities that impact your city, county, state, or nation?
   - Which communities in your city or county face health inequalities?
   - What organizations are working to eliminate these disparities and to advocate for social justice?
   - What policy changes are these organizations advocating for?
   - What else needs to happen in your local area in order to promote health equality?
   - What role can you play in these efforts?

REFERENCES

Asian Pacific Environmental Network. 2002. Accessed on April 12, 2009: www.apen4ej.org/issues_what.htm

Beyers, M., and others. 2008. Life and Death from Unnatural Causes: Health and Social Inequity in Alameda County. Alameda County Public Health Department. Accessed on April 12, 2009: www.acphd.org

California Center for Public Health Advocacy. 2007. Designed for Disease: The Link Between Local Food Environments and Obesity and Diabetes. Accessed on April 12, 2009: www.publichealthadvocacy.org/designedfordisease.html

California Newsreel. Unnatural Causes . . . Is Inequality Making Us Sick? Accessed on April 12, 2009: www.unnaturalcauses.org/

Center for the Advancement of Health. 2003, May. The Forgotten Population: Health Disparities and Minority Men. *Facts of Life: Issue Briefings for Health Reporters* 8(5). Accessed on April 12, 2009: www.cfah.org/factsoflife/vol8no5.cfm

City of Berkeley. 2002. *Health Status Report* 8(5). Accessed on April 12, 2009: www.ci.berkeley.ca.us

Collins, J. W., Wu, S-Y., and David, R. J. 2002. Differing Intergenerational Birth Weights Among the Descendents of U.S.-Born and Foreign-Born Whites and African-Americans in Illinois. *American Journal of Epidemiology 155*: 210–216.

Cooper, R. S., and others. 2005. An International Comparative Study of Blood Pressure in Populations of European vs. African Descent. *BMC Medicine* 3: 2.

David, R. J., and Collins, J. W. 1997. Differing Birth Weights Among Infants of U.S.-Born Blacks, African-Born Blacks, and U.S.-Born Whites. *New England Journal of Medicine* 337: 1209–1214.

Franzini, L., Ribble, J. C., and Keddie, A. M. 2001. Understanding the Hispanic Paradox. *Ethnicity and Disease* 11: 496–518.

Gee, G. C., Spencer, M. S., Chen, J., and Takeuchi, D. 2007. A Nationwide Study of Discrimination and Chronic Health Conditions Among Asian Americans. *American Journal of Public Health* 97: 1275–1282.

Gornick, 2003, May. Vulnerable Populations and Medicare Services: Why Do Disparities Exist. *American Journal of Public Health* 93(5): 753–759.

Hofrichter, R. 2003. The Politics of Health Inequities: Contested Terrain. In *Health and Social Justice Reader.* San Francisco: Jossey-Bass.

Hofrichter, R. 2007. *A Brief Lexicon for Health Equity and Social Justice.* Washington, DC: National Association of

County and City Health Officials. Accessed on April 12, 2009: www.naccho.org

Job Stress Network. Accessed on April 12, 2009: www.workhealth.org

Kaiser Commission on Medicaid and the Uninsured. 2008, September. Key Facts. The Uninsured and the Difference Health Insurance Makes. Accessed on April 12, 2009: www.kff.org

Kaiser Commission on Medicaid and the Uninsured. The Henry J. Kaiser Family Foundation. 2004, November. Health coverage for immigrants. Accessed on April 12, 2009: www.kff.org/uninsured/upload/Health-Coverage-for-Immigrants-Fact-Sheet.pdf

Kaiser Commission on Medicaid and the Uninsured. The Henry J. Kaiser Family Foundation. 2008, March. Five Basic Facts on Immigrants and Their Health Care. Accessed on April 12, 2009: www.kff.org/medicaid/upload/7761.pdf

Kaplan, G. A., Pamuk, E. R., Lynch, J. W., Cohen, R. D., Balfour, J. L. 1999. Inequality in Income and Mortality in the United States. In I. Kawachi, B. P. Kennedy, and R. G. Wilkinson (Eds.), *The Society and Population Health Reader: Income Inequality and Health,* 50–59. New York: New Press.

Kawachi, I., Kennedy, B. P., Gupta, V., and Prothrow-Stith, D. 1999. Women's Status and the Health of Women and Men. In I. Kawachi, B. P. Kennedy, and R. G. Wilkinson (Eds.), *The Society and Population Health Reader: Income Inequality and Health,* 474–491. New York: New Press.

Krieger, N., and Birn, A.-E. 1998. A Vision of Social Justice as the Foundation of Public Health: Commemorating 150 Years of the Spirit of 1848. *American Journal of Public Health 88*: 1603–1606.

MacArthur Foundation. 2008. *Reaching for a Healthier Life: Facts on Socioeconomic Status and Health in the U.S.* Research Network on Socioeconomic Status and Health. Accessed on April 12, 2009: www.macses.ucsf.edu.

Marmot, M., and others. 2005. Health and the Psychosocial Environment at Work. In M. Marmot and R. G. Wilkinson (Eds.), *Social Determinants of Health,* 97–130. Oxford: Oxford University Press.

Mays, V. M., Cochran, S. D., and Barnes, N. W. 2007. Race, Race-Based Discrimination, and Health Outcomes Among African-Americans. *Annual Review of Psychology* 58: 201–225.

McCracken, M., and others. 2007. Cancer Incidence, Mortality, and Associated Risk Factors Among Asian

Americans of Chinese, Filipino, Vietnamese, Korean, and Japanese Ethnicities. *California Cancer Journal for Clinicians* 57: 190–205. Accessed on April 12, 2009: http://caonline.amcancersoc.org/

National Center for Health Statistics. Centers for Disease Control and Prevention. 2009. Accessed on April 12, 2009: www.cdc.gov/nchs/data/

National Center for Health Statistics. Centers for Disease Control and Prevention. 2007. *Summary List of Trend Tables by Topic.* Accessed on April 12, 2009: www.cdc.gov/nchs/data/hus/hus07.pdf#summary

National Center for Health Statistics. Centers for Disease Control and Prevention. 2002. Accessed on April 12, 2009: www.cdc.gov/nchs/data/

National Center for Transgender Equality. Accessed on April 12, 2009: www.nctequality.org/Issues/health.html

National Coalition for LGBT Health. Accessed on March 2009: www.lgbthealth.net/resources2.shtml

National Partnership for Action to End Health Disparities. 2008. U.S. Department of Health and Human Services. A Strategic Framework for Improving Racial/Ethnic Minority Health and Eliminating Racial/Ethnic Disparities. Accessed on April 12, 2009: www.omhrc.gov/npa

Office of Minority Health& Health Disparities. Centers for Disease Control. About Minority Health. Accessed on April 12, 2009: www.cdc.gov/omhd/

Östlin, P., George, A., and Sen, G. 2003. Gender, Health, and Equity: The Intersections. In Richard Hofrichter (Ed.), *Health and Social Justice: Politics, Ideology, and Inequity in the Distribution of Disease. A Public Health Reader,* 132–156. San Francisco: Jossey-Bass.

Reynolds, D. 2006. Using Living Wage Campaigns to Benefit Public Health. In D. Reynolds (Ed.), *Tackling Health Inequities Through Public Health Practice: A Handbook for Action,* 155–166. Washington, DC: National Association of County and City Health Officials.

Satcher, D., Fryer, G. E. Jr., McCann, J., Troutman, A., Woolf, S. H., and Rust, G. 2005. What If We Were Equal? A Comparison of the Black-White Mortality Gap in 1960 and 2000. *Health Affairs* 24: 459–464. Accessed on April 12, 2009: http://content.healthaffairs.org/cgi/content/full/24/2/459.

Satcher, D., and Higginbotham, E. J. 2008. The Public Health Approach to Eliminating Disparities in Health. *American Journal of Public Health* 98: 400–403.

Singh, G. K., and Siahpush, M. 2006. Widening Socioeconomic Inequalities in U.S. Life Expectancy 1980–2000. *International Journal of Epidemiology* 35: 969–979. Accessed on April 12, 2009: www

.ingentaconnect.com/content/oup/ije/2006/00000035/00000004/art00969

Smedley, B., Jeffries, M., Adelman, L., and Cheng, J. *Race, Racial Inequality and Health Inequities: Separating Myth from Fact.* Briefing Paper. Accessed on April 12, 2009: www.unnaturalcauses.org

Society for Public Health Education. 2005. Resolution on Eliminating Health Disparities Based on Sexual Orientation. Accessed on April 12, 2009: www.sophe.org/content.sexres.asp

Taylor, S. E., Repetti, R. L., and Seeman, T. 1999. What Is an Unhealthy Environment and How Does It Get Under the Skin? In I. Kawachi, B. P. Kennedy, and R. G. Wilkinson (Eds.), *The Society and Population Health Reader: Income Inequality and Health,* 351–378. New York: New Press.

Taylor, T. R., and others. 2007, July. Racial Discrimination and Breast Cancer Incidence in Black Women: The Black Women's Health Study. *American Journal of Epidemiology* 166: 46–54.

Troxel, W. M., Matthews, K. A., Bromberger, J. T., and Sutton-Tyrrell, K. 2003. Chronic Stress Burden, Discrimination, and Subclinical Carotid Artery Disease in African American and Caucasian Women. *Health Psychology* 22: 300–309.

United Nations Population Fund. Accessed on April 12, 2009: www.unfpa.org/gender

U.S. Department of Health and Human Services. 2008, March. *Healthy People 2010.* Accessed on April 12, 2009: www.healthypeople.gov

Wolff, E. 1995. *Top Heavy: A Study of the Increasing Inequality of Wealth in America. A Twentieth Century Fund Report.* New York: Twentieth Century Fund Press.

World Health Organization. World Health Report 2004. Annex Table 5 Selected national health accounts indicators: measured levels of expenditure on health 1997–2001. http://www.who.int/whr/2004/annex/topic/en/annex_5_en.pdf

World Health Organization. World Health Report 2005. Annex Table 1 Basic indicators for all Member States. http://www.who.int/whr/2005/annex/annexe1_en.pdf

World Health Organization. World Health Report 2006. Annex Table 1 Basic indicators for all Member States. www.who.int/whr/2006/annex/06_annex1_en.pdf

Zinn, H. 2004, September 20. The Optimism of Uncertainty. *The Nation.* Accessed on April 12, 2009: www.thenation.com/doc/20040920/zinn

ADDITIONAL RESOURCES

Bay Area Regional Health Inequalities Initiative. Accessed on April 12, 2009: www.barhii.org/.

Environmental Justice/Environmental Racism. Accessed on April 12, 2009: www.ejnet.org/ej/

Hofrichter, R., Ed. 2006. *Tackling Health Inequities Through Public Health Practice: A Handbook for Action.* Washington, DC: National Association of County and City Health Officials. Accessed on April 12, 2009: www.naccho.org.

Institute of Medicine. 2002. *Unequal Treatment: Confronting Racial and Ethnic Disparities in Health Care.* Washington, DC: National Academies Press.

Kaplan, G. A., Pamuk, E. R., Lynch, J. W., Cohen, R. D., and Balfour J. L. 1999. *Inequality in Income and Mortality in the United States.* In I. Kawachi, B. P. Kennedy, and R. G. Wilkinson (Eds.), *The Society and Population Health Reader: Income Inequality and Health,* 50–59. New York: New Press.

LaVeist, T. A., Ed. 2002. *Race, Ethnicity and Health: A Public Health Reader.* San Francisco: Jossey-Bass.

Mayberry, R. M., Mili, F., and Ofili, E. 2002. Racial and Ethnic Differences in Access to Medical Care. In Thomas A. LaVeist (Ed.), *Race, Ethnicity and Health: A Public Health Reader.* San Francisco: Jossey-Bass.

National Association of City and County Health Officers. 2002. *Resolution to Promote Health Equity.* Accessed on April 12, 2009: http://archive.naccho.org.

5

An Introduction to Globalization and Health

Tim Berthold • Sharon Turner •
Alma Avila-Esparza • Mickey Ellinger

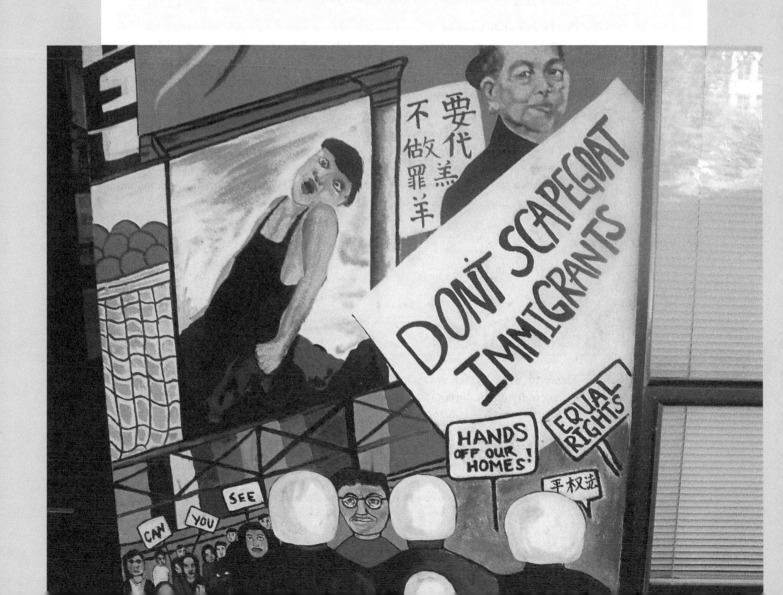

Development has to be concerned with advancing human well-being and human freedom.

—*Amartya Sen*

INTRODUCTION

Globalization refers to the increasing connections—including economic, legal, technological, scientific, and cultural connections—between people and countries throughout the world. There is a great debate taking place among diverse stakeholders about the goals and policies that guide these connections. The dominant model of globalization has promoted rapid economic growth and expansion throughout the world. Critics advocate for a new form of globalization based on the promotion of human rights, social justice, an end to world hunger, and preservation of the natural environment.

Globalization is a large and complex topic. We have included this introduction because globalization has a significant impact on the health and welfare of the poorest and most vulnerable communities throughout the world—the very communities whom CHWs work with and advocate for.

WHAT YOU WILL LEARN

By studying the information in this chapter, you will be able to:

- ✪ Define globalization
- ✪ Describe the key players, goals, and policies that have guided the dominant form of globalization
- ✪ Analyze the consequences of globalization for poor communities and nations
- ✪ Identify and discuss alternative models of globalization
- ✪ Describe how the global justice movement is working to oppose the dominate model of globalization and to advocate for social justice
- ✪ Describe how CHWs can participate in creating a world that promotes the health and well-being of all communities
- ✪ Discuss the connections between the work that CHWs do in their local communities and the work of the global justice movement

WORDS TO KNOW

Gross Domestic Product

5.1 DEFINING GLOBALIZATION

The term *globalization* was introduced in the 1990s to describe increasing connections among individuals, corporations, and nations around the world. The Levin Institute defines *globalization* as

> a process of interaction and integration among the people, companies, and governments of different nations, a process driven by international trade and investment and aided by information technology. This process has effects on the environment, on culture, on political systems, on economic development and prosperity, and on human physical well-being in societies around the world. (Globalization101.org)

GLOBALIZATION AFFECTS OUR LIVES EVERY DAY

We are increasingly connected to others throughout the world in many ways. We talk on the phone to relatives in other countries. We use the Internet to shop, watch YouTube videos, and conduct research. We watch television shows that are broadcast to hundreds of countries throughout the world. Many of the products we buy at a large supermarket have traveled thousands of miles and across national borders. We receive news of environmental devastation from all parts of the globe. Our concerns about access to sufficient food, shelter, human rights, education, and health care are shared by other public health professionals and activists in every nation.

Globalization is often talked about as a relatively modern development, dating from the 1940s, the end of World War II, and the establishment of the United Nations. But global connections have existed and increased throughout history. Travel, trade, and migration have spread science and technology, warfare, occupation, colonialism, knowledge, new products, and culture throughout the world.

> Around 1000 A.D., the global reach of science, technology, and mathematics was changing the nature of the old world. . . . The high technology in the world of 1000 A.D. included paper, the printing press, the crossbow, gunpowder, the iron-chain suspension bridge, the kite, the magnetic compass, the wheelbarrow and the rotary fan. A millennium ago, these items were used extensively in China—and were practically unknown elsewhere. Globalization spread them across the world, including Europe. A similar movement occurred in the Eastern influence on Western mathematics. The decimal system emerged and became well developed in India between the second and sixth centuries; it was used by Arab mathematicians soon thereafter. These mathematical innovations reached Europe mainly in the last quarter of the tenth century. . . . Playing an important part in the scientific revolution that helped to transform Europe. (Sen, 2002)

Globalization is also represented by the rise of colonialism, as European nations competed to occupy and rule nations throughout the world, controlling large areas of Africa, Asia, the Pacific Islands, and North, Central, and Latin America.

Globalization can take many forms. However, the primary debate about globalization is taking place between those who support and those who oppose the dominant model promoted by international financial institutions (IFIs). These two very different perspectives are sometimes referred to as "globalization from above," determined by wealthy corporations and governments, and "globalization from below," led by diverse coalitions of grassroots activists and organizations such as labor unions, student and environmental groups, public health, human rights and women's organizations.

5.2 WHY IS GLOBALIZATION IMPORTANT FOR CHWS TO UNDERSTAND?

We encourage CHWs to learn more about globalization because it affects the lives and health status of the clients and communities you work with and challenges the values that guide your profession. As we describe later, globalization policies have resulted in increased social and health inequalities and devastating harm to our natural environment.

The struggle to define the type of globalization that connects people throughout the world will determine whether the gap between rich and poor people continues to widen, whether the communities you represent continue to experience higher rates of illness and death, and the very survival of our natural environment. The struggle over globalization really comes down to the question: "What kind of world do we want to create?"

It can be challenging to develop a global vision, to start thinking about the world as a whole. We recommend a two-minute video—entitled *Miniature Earth* (www.minatureearth .com)—as a great introduction to thinking globally. It asks us to imagine that the world is represented by a village of a hundred people. Out of this global village of one hundred people:

- ✪ Forty-three lack access to basic sanitation.
- ✪ Eighteen lack access to improved water.
- ✪ Thirteen are hungry or malnourished.
- ✪ Fourteen can't read.
- ✪ Twelve have a computer.
- ✪ Eighteen people struggle to live on $1 or less a day.
- ✪ Fifty-three people struggle to live on $2 or less each day.
- ✪ Six people own 59 percent of the wealth.
- ✪ If you have a refrigerator, a bed, and a roof over your head, you are richer than 75 percent of the population.
- ✪ If you have a bank account, you are one of the thirty wealthiest people.

The video ends with the following words: "Do your best for a better world."

While you may not always be aware of it, the work you do in your own community is also being carried out in cities, towns, and rural areas throughout the world. CHWs and other activists are working to prevent homelessness, malnutrition, domestic violence, infectious and chronic illness, and to provide compassionate and culturally competent care to those who are already sick or dying. They are organizing and advocating for access to housing, nutrition, safe working conditions, fair wages, health care, education, and other forms of social justice.

? *What kind of a world do you want to create?*

5.3 THE DOMINANT MODEL OF GLOBALIZATION

When people talk about globalization today, they are usually referring to what emerged as the dominant model of globalization in the twentieth century. This model was developed at the end of World War II and is represented by the policies of international financial institutions such as the World Bank and the International Monetary Fund (IMF). These institutions aided in financing the reconstruction of Europe after the war and continued to provide loans to poorer or less-developed nations to spur economic development. In 1995, the World Trade Organization (WTO) was formed; it plays a leading role in determining the policies that govern world trade, economic development, and globalization.

The dominant model of globalization (or globalization from above) has emphasized economic development at the expense of other goals. Success has primarily been measured by increases to a nation's **gross domestic product** (GDP), or the total value of all goods and services produced within a country in a year or other given period of time. Rapid economic growth has been promoted by policies designed to remove barriers that limit economic production and free trade. These policies have often included limiting the role of government by privatizing state-owned industries and services including utilities, banks, and schools; reducing government spending on social services; and reducing government regulation of private corporations, including laws that govern labor practices and protect the environment.

Proponents of the dominant model have argued that rapid economic growth should be first priority for all nations. The dominant model has assumed that economic growth will eventually pay off (or trickle down) to benefit societies as a whole, providing increased employment, access to new consumer goods, reduced poverty and hunger, and improved health status.

THE KEY PLAYERS

Globalization from above has been led by the world's largest and wealthiest corporations, investors, governments, and international financial institutions. These players cooperate to advance the same agenda: the expansion of global markets and economic production designed to increase the GDP of nations and profits for private corporations.

The World Bank and the International Monetary Fund The World Bank and the International Monetary Fund are IFIs that make large loans to countries on the condition that they agree to follow certain economic policies (described later). In 2006, the World Bank alone managed over $200 billion (in U.S. dollars) in outstanding loans and made new loans totaling $28.9 billion to more than eighty nations. The World Bank and the IMF are governed by their member nations, but voting power is based on the size of each nation's economy and financial contributions; so policies are dominated by the wealthiest countries, such as the United States.

The World Trade Organization The World Trade Organization was established in 1995. It sets and enforces the rules of international trade and strives to eliminate "barriers to trade." These barriers to trade are often laws and regulations that protect worker's rights, salaries, and working conditions, the environment, and access to food, water, health care, and other public services. WTO rules, which can take precedence over national law, are backed up by the threat of trade sanctions. If a conflict arises between national policies and trade interests, the dispute may be settled by a WTO tribunal.

Transnational Corporations Large multinational or transnational corporations (TNCs) are perhaps the chief beneficiaries of the policies promoted by the dominant model of globalization. The latter half of the twentieth century saw a rapid increase in the number of corporations that no longer operated within the territories of a nation but produced, bought, and sold products internationally, operating in several or many nations at once. TNCs are guided by basic economic principles that seek to produce goods at the lowest possible cost and sell them for the greatest profit. They are engaged in what has been called the "race to the bottom" as they move around the world seeking the cheapest labor, the least restrictive labor laws, the most favorable tax policies and tariffs. The wealth and power of TNCs has been dramatically increased by the policies of the World Bank, the IMF, and the WTO.

KEY POLICIES OF GLOBALIZATION

Globalization from above has been promoted by policies and activities designed to increase economic growth. In order to qualify for further loans or debt relief from the

World Bank and the IMF, nations must agree to a set of conditions that have often included privatization, deregulation, and trade liberalization.

Privatization   Until the later part of the twentieth century, most national governments owned basic services, including transportation and utilities such as water, electricity, telephone, and public transportation. This began to change, however, as the IMF and other IFIs advocated for these services to be provided by private companies. They argued that private corporations would be able to provide better quality services at lower cost. As a result, basic services have been taken out of the hands of the public and the government and given to private corporations. Supporters of privatization are committed to increasing the number of good and services that will be taken over by the private sector, including garbage collection, education, and health care.

NOT A DROP TO DRINK: PRIVATIZING WATER IN BOLIVIA

Access to safe drinking water is one of the most essential resources for human life and the public health. But as water has become a scarce resource, the private water industry, dominated by a handful of TNCs, has developed to profit from water scarcity. In Bolivia, South America's poorest country, nearly two-thirds of the population lives below the poverty line, annual per capita income is about $950, and safe drinking water is limited. In 2000, the World Bank pushed the Bolivian government to privatize their water system as a condition for borrowing additional money. A private company based in London started selling water in Bolivia, and prices quickly tripled. For the poor majority in Bolivia, buying water cost nearly half their income. Without access to affordable and clean water, poor communities were at increased risk for infectious disease and death. Unable to survive under the burden of the new water prices, the public staged protests and forced the government to cancel the private water contract (Public Citizen, 2000).

Deregulation   Governments regulate privately owned companies to prevent discrimination, control how much the public can be charged (such as phone rates), what companies can and cannot own (for example, can banks also own insurance companies?), and what companies must tell their investors. In the twentieth century, under pressure from consumers and trade unions, government regulations also enforced safe working conditions and the right to form unions. Government regulation has traditionally regulated privately owned utilities and basic services such as airlines and other forms of public transportation, telephone, gas, and electricity companies. In the 1990s, many public utilities were deregulated in the United States and throughout the world. Deregulation eases restrictions and increases the power of corporations that provide essential services to the public. These policies have often harmed consumers, resulting in higher prices and undermining health and safety regulations.

Many critics blame deregulation policies for the economic recession that began in the United States in 2008 and quickly spread worldwide. The recession has resulted in new calls to end or limit policies that promote deregulation of financial institutions such as the banks that made the subprime mortgage loans that precipitated the current economic crisis.

Trade Liberalization   Trade liberalization allows goods and services to move from one country to another without paying tariffs or extra fees. For example, in 1994, the North American Free Trade Agreement (NAFTA) went into effect among the United States, Mexico, and Canada and eliminated trade barriers between these three countries. Supporters argue that NAFTA has increased the market for U.S. products and provided Canada and Mexico with options to buy cheaper products. Critics argue that the flood of cheap imports from the United States has harmed Mexican industries and will lead to higher prices in the long term. Many U.S. companies have moved outside the country to take advantage of lower wages in Mexico, resulting in the loss of an estimated three million jobs for U.S. workers. Some argue that this has benefited Mexico by providing new jobs, while others point out that these are low-paying jobs and workers have no chance of advancement and are sometimes subject to exploitation. In addition, the profits return to the United States rather than remaining in Mexico to assist the country to develop further (American Jewish World Service, 2005).

Other conditions imposed upon nations accepting loans or debt relief from IFIs have included:

- Increased production for export to other countries, including the use of cheap labor to produce goods and the export of natural resources and agricultural products (even in nations with persistent hunger and undernutrition)
- Reduced production of basic goods that people, especially the poor, need to survive, such as grains and other foods
- Promotion of "labor flexibility," permitting layoffs and suspension of the minimum wage and other labor laws
- The creation of special "enterprise zones" that are not subject to the labor rules and regulations of the host country, where workers, often women, work long hours assembling clothes, shoes, toys, and other consumer goods for export to the rich countries
- The removal of subsidies that make basic goods, including rice, beans, and other common food items, affordable
- Elimination of price controls that keep certain goods affordable for poor and working families
- Reduced access to credit or loans to smaller producers, including small farmers
- Balanced budgets through reducing basic social services, such as transportation, education, and health care, and increasing fees for these services
- A decline in the value of a country's own national currency as compared to the U.S. dollar

For many years, the IMF, the World Bank, and other IFIs imposed conditions on countries accepting loans through structural adjustment policies (SAP). Structural adjustment policies came under such criticism that they were abandoned in the mid-1990s and replaced by a new requirement for countries to develop a Poverty Reduction Strategy Paper (PRSP). PRSPs were supposed to lead to economic growth that benefited the poor and to limit conditions from IFIs. However, critics argue that PRSPs are simply structural adjustment by another name, and that the IMF and other IFIs still impose similar conditions upon nations receiving loans (Molina, 2008; Bretton Woods Project, 2008; Nag and Salimullah, 2006; Mutume, 2003; Zulu, 2003; CIDSE-Caritas International, 2004; Abugre, 2000). A recent report "finds that IMF loans carry an average of 14 structural conditions each . . . including privatization . . . as well as other conditions prescribing regressive taxation" (Molina, 2008).

5.4   THE CONSEQUENCES OF GLOBALIZATION

It is important to acknowledge that the dominant model of globalization has generally been successful at increasing economic growth and has led to positive outcomes, including increased literacy rates, average income, life expectancy, and access to sanitation and safe drinking water, for many countries and populations (World Bank, 2009; United Nations Development Programme, 2008).

However, these benefits have not been equally shared. Indeed, inequalities in income, wealth, access to basic resources, and health status between nations and among their populations have only increased. Globalization policies and increased economic production have also come at great cost to our natural environment.

Leading concerns about the consequences of globalization from above include:

- Increasing concentrations of wealth and gaps between rich and poor
- Increasing national debt
- Declining access to basic resources, including education, housing, food, water, and health care, for the poorest populations
- Failure to address food security issues and to prevent widespread hunger and malnutrition
- Rising inequalities in health status, including infant mortality and life expectancy
- Declining wages, working conditions, and rights for many workers and the failure to prevent child labor
- Forced migration and internal displacement of populations
- Erosion of human rights and the status of specific populations, including women, low-income workers, and indigenous communities
- Environmental devastation
- Increasing wealth and power of private corporations and diminished power for national governments
- Erosion of democratic participation and governance. Globalization increases the power and influence of international financial institutions like the IMF and WTO over that of national governments. Individuals, communities, and organizations have less ability to participate in or influence these international institutions than they do local or national governments (see Stiglitz, 2007)
- Increasing global instability and concerns with safety, conflict, and war

? How has globalization affected your nation, community, and family?

? What have some of the benefits been?

? Do you have other concerns about the consequences of globalization?

INCREASED INEQUALITIES IN INCOME AND WEALTH

The United Nations acknowledges that the gap between rich and poor is increasing, including the gap between rich and poor nations and between rich and poor people within nations. It is estimated that the richest 2 percent of the world's population owns more than 50 percent of the global wealth, while the poorest 50 percent own less than

1 percent (Davies and others, 2006). The United Nations Development Programme (2008) reports that

> the gains from global growth are being highly unequally distributed. In 2007, over a billion people had almost no income (the equivalent of a dollar a day or less for each). They typically spent more than half of what they did earn on food for their families, leaving even less for shelter, water, education and health care. . . . In the latter decades of the 20th century, there was a widely held view that a rising tide of global economic integration would lift all boats. Some developing countries have indeed been lifted up and are now sailing ahead so fast that they are starting to catch up with developed countries. But many other poor nations have been left behind by the tide, and are not yet able to navigate global seas. A similar thing is happening within most countries: the benefits of growth are not reaching large parts of the population.

Despite the most accelerated period of economic growth in human history, hundreds of millions of people across the globe still live in extreme poverty and struggle to survive. In sub-Saharan Africa, it is estimated that the number of people living on less than $1 per day doubled between 1981 and 2001 (from 164 million to 313 million), and the number living on $2 per day or less nearly doubled (from 288 million to 516 million) (Labonte and Schrecker, 2007). In the period from 2001 to 2003, it is estimated (Worldwatch Institute, 2008) that

- More than 12 percent of the global population experienced chronic hunger.
- Twenty percent of the world's population lacked access to clean drinking water.
- Forty percent lacked access to basic sanitation.

Globalization policies have also resulted in a rapid increase in the number, wealth, and power of transnational corporations. In 2000, it was estimated that there were more than 40,000 corporations in the world whose activities crossed national boundaries and who were active in international markets through 250,000 foreign affiliates (Anderson and Cavanagh, 2000). Two hundred corporations now control well over a quarter of the world's economic activity. Of the 100 largest economic entities in the world, 51 are corporations; only 49 are countries.

While globalization policies have resulted in reduced pay for many low-income workers, the pay for corporate executives has increased significantly. Average income for chief executive officers (CEOs) of large U.S. companies was $10.8 million in 2007, more than 364 times as much as an average American worker (Anderson and others, 2007). The highest-paid managers of equity and hedge funds (investment bankers) earned an average of $657.5 million each in 2007. While the minimum wage in the United States was increased to $5.85 in 2007, this is 7 percent less than it was in 1997, when inflation (or increases in the price of basic goods and services) is taken into account. Over the same period of time, the pay of executives increased by nearly 50 percent (United for a Fair Economy, 2007).

INCREASING NATIONAL DEBT

Loans from the World Bank, the IMF, and other financial institutions to support economic development have resulted in extreme debt for many nations. Debt for the world's poorest nations increased from $25 billion in 1970 to $523 billion in 2002. Debt among poor nations was estimated at more than $1.5 trillion in 2007 (Stiglitz, 2007). Over the same period of time, the debt for African nations has increased from $11 billion to $295 billion (Shah, 2005). Debt payments for Uganda equal 44 percent of all earnings from exported goods; they equal 50 percent of all export earnings for the Republic of the Congo (Global Exchange, 2007).

NATIONAL DEBT IS LIKE FAMILY DEBT

Many families have large debts at high interest rates. In order to pay off these debts and prevent the loss of their homes and other assets, families have to reduce other expenses. They may cut back on their budgets for food, clothes, transportation, health care, education, or recreational activities for their children. These choices are similar to those that poor nations face when they have a large debt. To make payments on their debt, nations are forced to cut expenses elsewhere, including basic services for the poor, such as education, health care, food subsidies, and transportation.

The business models and products of transnational corporations are often unresponsive to basic human needs.

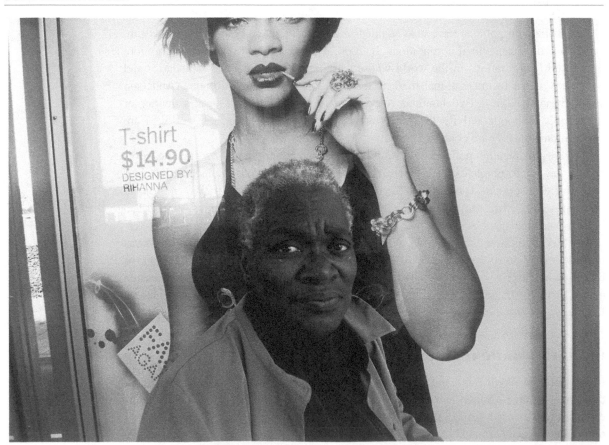

AN INCREASE IN CHILD LABOR

Globalization policies that seek to promote economic growth often do so without sufficient concern for labor practices. In some parts of the world, these policies have resulted in increased use of child labor.

GROWING FOOD INSECURITY, HUNGER, AND MALNUTRITION

The world faces a growing food crisis. In 2008, the United Nations estimated that 854 million people are "food insecure" around the world, meaning that they do not regularly have enough to eat and consequently face hunger and malnutrition (World Food Programme, 2008). Food prices increased nearly 40 percent worldwide in 2007, with the price of grains increasing 42 percent and the price of dairy products by 80 percent (UN Food and Agricultural Organization, 2008). Prices have risen so dramatically that millions of people around the world are starving and protests have broken out in many countries. In Haiti, for example, the official minimum wage is $1.80 per day, but 55 percent of the population lives on just 44 cents each day and cannot afford to purchase sufficient amounts of rice and other basic staples (Lendman, 2008). As the number of people throughout the world dependent upon food aid increases, the United Nations estimates cost of feeding them is $30 billion a year (UN Food and Agricultural Organization, 2008).

The global food crisis has only intensified with the global recession that began in the fall of 2008. As economic activity declines, along with employment opportunities and wages, more low-income individuals and families are at risk of hunger and starvation.

Malnutrition increases vulnerability to illness and is the leading cause of child death around the world. Every day, approximately 16,000 children die from hunger-related causes (Bread for the World, 2008). Hunger and malnutrition are also common within the United States: the number of Americans facing food insecurity increased from 31 million in 1999 to 36.3 million in 2003. These figures include 13 million children and 16.7 percent of families with children (Children's Defense Fund, 2005).

INDIA: CHILD LABOR ON THE RISE IN COTTON FIELDS

More than 416,000 children under the age of eighteen, of whom almost 225,000 are younger than fourteen, are involved in child labor in India's cottonseed production. . . . According to the report, more than thirteen Indian companies and two multinationals, Monsanto and Bayer, are involved in this "modern form of child slavery." The biggest among the Indian seed companies, Nuziveedu, Raasi, Ankur and Mahyco (a joint venture partner of Monsanto), make use of around 200,000 children who are employed by the farmers to whom they have sub-contracted the cultivation of Bt cotton seeds. (Reddy, 2007)

While the world food crisis is the result of multiple factors, globalization has contributed in several key ways. Critics argue that globalization policies, including the use of subsidies, have shifted agricultural production away from small farmers who grow food for local use and toward corporate agribusinesses that use large farms to grow crops for export, for use as biofuels, and to raise cattle for beef production (Bello, 2008; Nichols, 2008; Dossani, 2008; Bretton Woods Project, 2008; Mittai, 2007; Stokes, 2008). A concern for short-term economic profits has undermined investments in sustainable models for regional production and consumption. Peter Timmer, an economist and expert on food security, commented that "the mindless liberalization mentality at the World Bank, the

U.S. Agency for International Development, and among my fellow economists misses the fact that food is a biological necessity as well as a commodity" (Stokes, 2008).

POPULATION DISPLACEMENT AND MIGRATION

Globalization policies have resulted in increased migration away from rural areas and poor countries. People are forced to leave their homes out of economic necessity to look for employment in wealthier countries. It is estimated that 36 million people immigrated to other countries between 1990 and 2005, with more than 90 percent migrating to industrialized nations (Globalization 101, 2008).

ALVARO MORALES: I came to the United States from Guatemala for many reasons. I wanted to be with my family, and I wanted better economic opportunities. When I left Guatemala, so many people, including students like myself, were being kidnapped and disappeared and killed—that is what was going on around me. This was the time when millions of people fled Central America because of the wars in Guatemala and El Salvador and Nicaragua. We were just trying to find a safe place to live.

Today I work in San Francisco with day laborers. They are mostly immigrants like me who came to this country for the same reasons I did. Because they are undocumented, they stand on the streets looking for work. One of the places they do this in San Francisco is on César Chávez Avenue. But the neighbors who live there are complaining that the day laborers are a nuisance, that they crowd the street, they say they are worried about what they will do to their children. It makes me so angry, because the day laborers are the same human beings that these neighbors pay to build their houses, to clean their houses, to cook their meals and take care of their children. But these neighbors want to kick them off the streets. And I think about where the day laborers come from, about the conditions that they are escaping from. They just want the same things as everyone else—they want to be safe to work and earn a living so that they can support their families. They want their children to grow up in safety and to have a chance for a better life. It is ironic and upsetting that this is all happening on a street named after César Chávez, a man who fought all his life to support the rights of immigrants who work in our farms, who grow and pick the food that we eat every day.

ENVIRONMENTAL DESTRUCTION

Global economic output increased 18 times over the course of the twentieth century, reaching $66 trillion in 2006 (Worldwatch Institute, 2008). Economic production has devastated the natural environment and resulted in the highest level of carbon dioxide in the atmosphere in 650,000 years; global warming; threats of species extinction; over-fishing and the death of 20 percent of the ocean's coral reefs; depletion of forests, ground-water, atmospheric space, petroleum, and other natural resources; water and air pollution (Worldwatch Institute, 2008).

Increasingly, policymakers are beginning to realize that globalization has been based on outdated economic models that fail to take environmental factors into consideration. For example, calculations of GDP fail to calculate the considerable economic costs to a country from overuse or exhaustion of natural resources, such as timber, and of environmental devastation resulting from economic activities such as the use of large areas of land for raising cattle, for mining, and for corporate agriculture that relies on petrochemicals to increase production. As the Worldwatch Institute (2008) states, "National economies and the global economy of which they are a part . . . are becoming their own worst enemies."

HEALTH CONSEQUENCES

While health status generally continued to improve throughout the world in the twentieth century, this has not been true for all nations or populations. For example, while life expectancy has increased in most nations, it has declined in others: between 1990 and 2006, life expectancy declined from 64 to 56 years in Iraq; from 62 to 43 years in Zimbabwe; and from 59 to 42 years in Lesotho (World Health Organization, 2008a).

Globalization policies have also resulted in increased and startling inequalities in income and wealth. As we discussed in Chapters Three and Four, inequalities in income and wealth are harmful to human health: they result not only in greater inequalities in health status but are also associated with higher average rates of illness and premature death overall (Kawachi, 1999).

Inequalities in health status have also increased. For example, Table 5.1 shows that women in the United States are 2.75 times more likely to die as a consequence of pregnancy or childbirth than are women in Australia. Women in Angola are 350 times more likely to die from the same causes as women in Australia.

IMPACT IN THE UNITED STATES

While globalization policies have benefited some regions, populations, and corporations within the United States, critics argue that it has also led to the following consequences:

- Restructuring of employment opportunities away from industrial production and factory jobs to the services sector
- Less job security and more temporary jobs without benefits

Table 5.1.   Inequalities in Health Status Across Nations.

Nation	Infant Mortality Rate (No. of infants who died before the age of 1 per 1,000 live births in 2006)	Child Mortality Rate (No. of children who died before the age of 5 per 1,000 live births in 2006)	MaternalMortality Rate (Maternal deaths per 100,000 live births in 2005)	Life Expectancy (2006)
Australia	5	6	4	82
United States	7	8	11	78
Guatemala	31	41	290	68
Cambodia	65	82	540	62
Haiti	60	80	670	61
Angola	154	260	1,400	41

Source: World Health Organization, 2008a.

- ✪ Loss of jobs as transnational corporations move production oversees in search of cheaper labor
- ✪ The real value of most wages remain the same or decline when inflation is taken into consideration. It is estimated that real income will decline significantly for American workers during the next ten to twenty years (Bivens, 2007)
- ✪ Increasing poverty (Berkowitz, 2007) and rapidly increasing costs of living, including costs of food, housing, and health care
- ✪ Increasing subsidies and tax breaks for large corporations
- ✪ Cuts to government services including welfare, health care, and aid to the disabled
- ✪ Erosion of worker benefits, including health insurance and pensions, as more companies decide not to provide health insurance or to increase the share of costs for workers
- ✪ Increasing inequalities in income and wealth
- ✪ Increasing inequalities in health status

? *How has globalization affected the communities where you live and work?*

? *Have there been changes to the local economy and to job opportunities?*

THE 2008–2009 GLOBAL RECESSION

In the fall of 2008, an economic crisis began in the United States, linked to subprime mortgage lending. This crisis quickly developed into a global recession (a significant decline in economic activity over an extended period of time). According to the United Nations Conference on Trade and Development (2009), "the world economy is mired in the severest financial crisis since the Great Depression." Economic growth is expected to slow dramatically worldwide in 2009 (United Nations Conference on Trade and Development, 2009; The World Bank, 2009).

While the causes of the global recession are complex, many critics point to the failure of globalization policies, including the deregulation of financial markets. The United Nations Conference on Trade and Development (2009) argues that factors that led to the current global economic crisis include "financial deregulation driven by an ideological belief in the virtues of the market has allowed 'innovation' of financial instruments that are completely detached from productive activities in the real sector of the economy." Levinson (2009) attributes the recession to "the combustive concoction of free market fundamentalism, corporate-dominated globalization, stagnant wages, growing inequality, greed, excessive leverage and financial innovations such as securitization."

The global recession will negatively affect the economies of many nations and result in the closure or downsizing of many businesses and the loss of many jobs. However, the consequences of the current economic crisis will be especially harmful for poorer nations and the poorest communities within all nations. Advocates call for a resurgent global justice movement working to restructure the vision, goals, ethics, and strategies of globalization to focus on promoting more equitable access to basic resources including water, food, health care, and human rights.

? *How has the global recession affected you, your family, and your community?*

5.5 ALTERNATIVE MODELS OF GLOBALIZATION

> I am not anti-globalization. I am very pro-globalization! I believe that globalization is such a good thing that it would be awfully bad if only some people benefited from it and not others. We need to improve the distribution of benefits between and within countries, between classes, and between urban and rural areas.

> *—Amartya Sen, 2002*

Globalization is inevitable, and its pace has increased dramatically in the past twenty years through the use of new technologies. But the values, goals, and policies that guide globalization are open to debate. So too are the indicators or types of data that are used to measure and evaluate the progress or success of globalization and national development.

ALTERNATIVE VISIONS AND GOALS FOR GLOBALIZATION

People throughout the world are organizing to oppose the dominant model of globalization and may participate in what are known as the anti-globalization, counter-globalization, alternative globalization, or global justice movements. These movements present a diverse range of alternative visions and goals for globalization including:

✪ An end to hunger and chronic malnutrition

✪ The promotion of social justice, including equal access to resources essential to human life such as food, shelter, water, education, employment at a living wage, and safety from violence

✪ Sustainable development that promotes the rights and autonomy of local communities and protects natural resources including the earth's rivers, oceans, groundwater, soil, forests, animal and plant species, and atmosphere and prevents further global warming

✪ Human rights, including protections for women, children, indigenous communities, and other oppressed groups; social and economic rights to education, employment, safe working conditions; and a living wage, housing, and health care

✪ Peace and safety, including the absence of war, institutional, and interpersonal violence

✪ Improved health for all and the elimination of persistent health inequalities between nations and populations within nations

✪ Increased democracy, including the meaningful participation of low-income residents and communities in making substantial decisions about their future

? *What should the goals of globalization be?*

HOW THE CONSEQUENCES OF GLOBALIZATION ARE EVALUATED

Critics question not only the goals, values, and policies of globalization, but also the indicators that are used to measure its success and consequences. The dominant model of globalization is most commonly measured by growth or changes to gross domestic product and GDP per capita (or per person) (Stiglitz, 2007). Critics argue that GDP is an inaccurate, incomplete, and misleading indicator of national development and globalization for several key reasons:

1. The GDP of many nations continues to rise despite national catastrophes such as famine and war. For example, the GDP per capita in Sudan has increased by approximately 23 percent since 2000, yet 600,000 residents faced famine, 400,000 were killed as a result of the conflict in Darfur, and 2.5 million were displaced from their homes (Worldwatch Institute, 2008).

2. GDP per capita does not reflect how income is divided or shared within a nation. To calculate GDP per capita, the total value of economic production is simply divided by the total population. GDP per capita in the United States was estimated at $41,890 in 2005, but this hides that fact the United States has the greatest inequality in income of all industrialized nations: the richest 300,000 Americans earned as much as the poorest 150 million. In 2005, the entire value of the increase in GDP went to the richest 10 percent of the country, while the poorest 90 percent earned less income than the year before (Worldwatch Institute, 2008).

3. The field of economics has developed considerably in the past sixty years. Today, economists take many more factors into consideration when estimating the value of economic activities. Economists argue that GDP is an inaccurate depiction of a national economy because it fails to include a range of activities that contribute to the economy (such as household work, investments in higher education, and maintaining roads and other transportation infrastructure) and completely fails to factor into the calculations substantial costs to an economy, including the costs of pollution, depletion of nonrenewable resources, of crime and underemployment.

Over the past several decades, a wide variety of other indicators have been identified and promoted as alternatives for evaluating the success and consequences of globalization. For example, the Genuine Progress Indicator (GPI) estimates both economic contributions and deductions or costs. In 2004, the GDP for the United States was estimated at $10.7 trillion, but the GPI was estimated at $4.4 trillion, or less than half the value of the GDP. This was largely due to the inclusion of big costs to the environment and the economy, such as the depletion of nonrenewable resources ($1.76 trillion) and carbon emissions damage ($1.18 trillion) (Talberth, 2007).

The United Nations Development Programme uses eight goals—called the "millennium development goals"—to assess national, regional, and global development:

1. Eradicate extreme poverty and hunger
2. Achieve universal primary education
3. Promote gender equality and empower women
4. Reduce child mortality
5. Improve maternal health
6. Combat HIV/AIDS, malaria, and other diseases
7. Ensure environmental sustainability
8. Develop a global partnership for development

Increasingly, organizations are creating alternative indicators that take multiple factors into consideration rather than relying on just one type of data. For example, the *Human Development Index* (HDI) includes estimates of life expectancy, adult literacy (reading and writing) rates, school enrollment (in primary or elementary school, high school, and college), and GDP per capita. The *Gender-Related Development Index* expands upon the HDI by comparing data for all factors for both female and males. The *Human Poverty Index* (HPI) estimates the extent of poverty in a nation; the probability of living to ages forty and sixty; the percentage of the population who cannot read and write; and the percentage of the population who lack access to safe drinking water and children who are underweight for their age. The *GINI coefficient* is widely used to measure the distribution of income within a population. Nations with a higher GINI coefficient have greater income inequality or a larger gap between rich and poor than nations with a lower GINI coefficient. The *Environmental Sustainability Index* (ESI) is a combination of twenty-one distinct environmental factors that support sustainable development, including existing environmental resources, efforts at conservation, and past and present levels of pollution (Socioeconomic Data and Applications Center, 2008). Since 1972, the country of Bhutan has been using *Gross National Happiness* (GNHI) as an indicator for the success of national development. The index is based on Buddhist principles and evaluates progress made in terms of equity, conservation of the natural environment, preservation of cultural values, and good governance (Gross International Happiness, 2008).

? *How should national development and globalization be measured and evaluated?*

GLOBALIZATION GUIDED BY HUMAN RIGHTS

Many people have called for globalization to be based on and guided by a commitment to preserving and protecting human rights. The Universal Declaration of Human Rights (1948) was established by the United Nations. The Universal Declaration includes thirty Articles that reflect a broad and comprehensive vision of human rights. The articles not only address rights to freedom of association and expression but also economic and social rights to employment, fair wages, union representation, housing, food, and medical care.

For example, Article 23 states, "Everyone who works has the right to just and favorable remuneration [pay] ensuring for himself and his family an existence worthy of human dignity, and supplemented, if necessary, by other means of social protection," and "Everyone has the right to form and to join trade unions for the protection of his interests."

Article 25 is often referenced as a guide for globalization. It reads:

> Everyone has the right to a standard of living adequate for the health and well-being of himself and of his family, including food, clothing, housing and medical care and necessary social services, and the right to security in the event of unemployment, sickness, disability, widowhood, old age or other lack of livelihood in circumstances beyond his control.

Article 26 addresses rights to education.

Globalization based on human rights would better protect the rights of world's poorest nations and communities and promote their access to basic resources such as education, employment characterized by safe working conditions and a living wage, food, housing, health care, and safety.

A farmer's market.

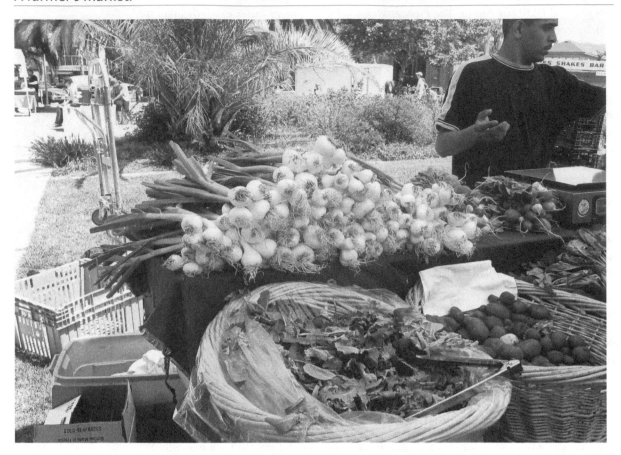

GLOBALIZATION AS SUSTAINABLE DEVELOPMENT

Sustainable development is an alternative approach to economic development. Sustainable development is characterized by a concern for the environment, for increased participation and control by local communities, and diminished dependency on outside experts, funding sources, and corporations. The World Commission on Environment and Development defines *sustainable development* as "meeting the needs of the present without compromising the ability of future generations to meet their own needs" (United Nations, 2008).

PROMOTING GLOBALIZATION THROUGH FAIR TRADE

You may have heard of "fair trade" products, such as certain brands of coffee or sugar. While *free trade* seeks to produce goods for the cheapest price, maximizing the profits of private corporations, *fair trade* policies produce goods and services by paying workers a reasonable wage and providing fair and safe working conditions. Fair trade seeks to build the capacity of local producers, to preserve local environments, and to promote gender equality (World Fair Trade Organization, 2009).

5.6 ORGANIZING FOR ALTERNATIVE MODELS OF GLOBALIZATION

Individuals, communities, organizations, and nations all over the world are organizing to oppose the dominant model of globalization and to promote social justice.

These "global justice movements" take many different forms. We share just a few examples here.

THE PEOPLE'S HEALTH MOVEMENT

The People's Health Movement (PHM) is a coalition of grassroots public health and social justice activists around the world, including many CHWs. The PHM calls on all nations to return to the goals and principles of the Alma-Ata Declaration made by the United Nations in 1978. Alma-Ata established the goal of Health for All by the year 2000 and influenced public health policies and programs throughout the world (World Health Organization, 2008b). PHM views health as a human right and is guided by commitment to social justice, peace, and ecologically sustainable development. Key objectives include promoting the participation of local communities and organizations in the development, implementation, and evaluation of health policies and programs. The PHM is organized through eight different assemblies throughout the world and publishes a newsletter about its activities (www.phmovement.org).

THE CHIPKO MOVEMENT

Chipko is an example of an early environmental movement—named for the Hindi word variously translated as to "hug," "cling," or "stick"—that advocated for a different path to economic development. In the 1970s, the Indian Government's Forest Department provided private companies with logging contracts throughout the country. Women from rural villages in the Himalayan mountain ranges of northern India came together to resist the logging of their ancestral forests. The forests were integral to the economy and culture of local communities, and logging often resulted in the destruction of the vulnerable ecology of the Himalayan slopes. The forests literally held the mountains together, preventing erosion and flooding. When contractors came to cut down trees in the state of Uttar Pradesh (now Uttarakhan), bordering Nepal and Tibet, local women ran to the forests, hugged the trees, and refused to move. The women declared their willingness to die in order to preserve the forests. The Chipko movement was born. The movement spread, and the women developed songs to promote their message: "What do the forests bear? Soil, water and pure air" (Joshi, 1982). Chipko activists argued that economic development should not come at the expense of the environment or the livelihood of local communities. The movement was successful in turning back loggers from several forest areas in India and raising public awareness about environmental issues and sustainable development. Chipko is representative in many ways of the global justice movement today that prioritizes environmental preservation and is often lead by women. One of the participants in the Chipko movement, Vandana Shiva, has emerged as a leader of the global environmental and justice movements.

OTHER MOVEMENTS

The World Social Forum is not an organization but "an open meeting place where social movements, networks, NGOs and other civil society organizations opposed to neoliberalism and a world dominated by capital or by any form of imperialism come together to pursue their thinking, to debate ideas democratically, for formulate proposals, share their experiences freely and network for effective action."

Poor communities in rural areas are organizing for access to their own land for subsistence agriculture. In Brazil, the *Landless Workers Movement* (LWM) has successfully obtained title to land for hundreds of thousands of families. (Landless Workers Movement, 2009).

Direct action to protest the policies of the World Bank, the IMF, and the WTO has included the protests in Madrid of the fiftieth anniversary of the IMF and the World Bank in 1994, the protests in Seattle during the 1999 meeting of the WTO, and many more.

Grassroots activists throughout the world have led the struggle to make antiretroviral medications accessible to millions of poor people living with AIDS. The struggle challenged patent rights that protected the profits of large pharmaceutical corporations that manufacture AIDS medications and effectively denied treatment to the majority of people around the world infected with HIV. This grassroots campaign was ultimately successful in changing national and international policies and trade agreements, dramatically reducing the price of medications, and making HIV treatment more accessible for poor patients and nations. The struggle continues, however, to make HIV prevention, testing, and treatment accessible to all communities throughout the world (Global Treatment Access, 2008).

5.7 THE ROLE OF CHWS IN GLOBALIZATION

Your work as a CHW with local communities is connected in many ways to the work of other CHWS throughout the world and to the efforts described earlier of people working to promote an alternative model of globalization. You are likely to share common goals: promoting public health, human rights, social justice, and respect for the environment. You are also likely to use similar strategies in your work, including community organizing and advocacy.

Some CHWs in the United States are actively engaged in working with health workers all over the world. One exchange project or *intercambio* connects the Tobacco Free Project (TFP) of the San Francisco Department of Public Health to nongovernmental organizations around the world in order to "reduce the global impact of the multinational tobacco companies by holding them to the same standards both nationally and internationally" (San Francisco Department of Public Health, 2007). Through this *intercambio*, TFP partnered with community-based organizations and CHWs from Togo, Senegal, Ecuador, El Salvador, Colombia, India, Thailand, Uganda, Nigeria, Sierra Leone, Hong Kong, and other countries to survey youth in their communities, develop educational videos, and advocate for adoption of new tobacco policies. The partnerships provided grassroots support for the adoption of a global tobacco control treaty, the Framework Convention for Tobacco Control (World Health Organization, 2008c), which limits marketing of tobacco products and sponsorship of events and organizations by tobacco companies.

This book is designed to provide you with knowledge and skills for working at both the client and community levels. By supporting low-income and otherwise vulnerable clients and communities to take actions that improve their health and welfare, by raising your voice to advocate for increased access to basic resources and rights, you are working to create a new world based on social justice and human rights.globalization guided by human rights.

?
How might globalization influence your work as a CHW?
What connections do you see between the work that CHWs do in your community and country and the global justice movement?

CHAPTER REVIEW

1. Conduct research (online, in the library, or by conducting interviews) to learn more about the impacts of globalization where you live.

   - How has globalization impacted the local economy? Have certain types of jobs been reduced or eliminated, such as manufacturing or factory jobs? Have new employment opportunities been created? Have the wages of most workers stayed the same, increased, or declined in comparison to the cost of living? Have employment benefits changed? What about health insurance?

   - Where is the food that you purchase and eat grown? Can you buy locally grown food in your town?

   - Has globalization increased migration to or from your local area? Which immigrant communities live in your city or county? What nations are they from? What challenges do new immigrant communities face?

   - How has globalization affected the cultures, languages, food, and arts in your community? How has it influenced your own understanding of the world?

2. Imagine that you are having dinner with a family member or close friend. They ask you what you are studying. In your own words, how would you explain the following concepts:

   - What is globalization?
   - Who sets the rules and policies for globalization?
   - What are the primary goals of the dominant form of globalization?
   - Why are so many people organizing to oppose and change globalization policies? What are their primary concerns?
   - What alternatives do the critics of globalization propose?

3. What is your vision for globalization? What do you think the goals of globalization should be?

4. The indicator most commonly used to measure the outcomes and consequences of globalization (and national development) is GDP or GDP per capita. Many people have criticized the use of this economic indicator. A wide range of alternative indicators have been developed. Some of these alternatives have been reviewed in this chapter. Please develop your own indicator to measure the consequences or outcomes of globalization in your community or nation. What will you call this new indicator? What types of data will you include in this indicator and why?

REFERENCES

Abugre, C. 2000. Still SAPping the Poor: A Critique of IMF Poverty Reduction Strategies. London: World Development Movement. Accessed on April 12, 2009: www.wdm.org.uk/news/archive/19992001/PRSP_critique.htm

American Jewish World Service. 2005. Addressing Global Poverty: International Aid, Debt Relief, and Trade Justice. Accessed on April 12, 2009: www.ajws.org

Anderson, S., and Cavanagh, J. 2000. Top 200: The Rise of Corporate Global Power. New York: Global Policy Forum. Accessed on April 12, 2009: http://globalpolicy.igc.org/socecon/tncs/top200.htm

Anderson, S., and others. 2007. Executive Excess. Washington, DC: Institute for Policy Studies. Accessed on April 12, 2009: www.ips-dc.org

Bello, W. 2008, May 16. How to Manufacture a Global Food Crisis: Lessons from the World Bank, IMF, and WTO. Amsterdam: Transnational Institute. Accessed on April 12, 2009: www.tni.org/detail_page.phtml?act_id=18285

Berkowitz, B. 2007. Ten Years After Welfare Reform Recipients Decline While Poverty Rate Increases. Accessed on April 12, 2009: www.mediatransparency.org/story.php?storyID=184

Bivens, L. J. 2007, October 10. Globalization and American Wages: Today and Tomorrow. Washington, DC: Economic Policy Institute. Accessed on April 12, 2009: www.epi.org

Bread for the World. 2008. Hunger Facts International. Accessed on April 12, 2009: www.bread.org

Bretton Woods Project. 2008, June 17. Agribusiness vs. Food Security: The Food Crisis and the IFIs. Accessed on April 12, 2009: www.brettonwoodsproject.org/print.shtml?cmd[884]=x-884–561820

Children's Defense Fund. 2005, June 2. Over 13 Million Children Face Food Insecurity. Accessed on April 12, 2009: www.childrensdefense.org/site/DocServer/foodinsecurity2005.pdf?docID=482

Davies, J. B., and others. 2006. The World Distribution of Household Wealth. Helsinki, Finland: United Nations University. Accessed on April 12, 2009: www.wider.unu.edu/publications/working-papers/research-papers/2007/en_GB/rp2007-77/

Dossani, S. 2008, June 26. *Africa's Unnatural Disaster*. Washington, DC: Foreign Policy in Focus.

Global Exchange. 2007. Accessed on April 12, 2009: www.globalexchange.org/campaigns/wbimf/facts.html

Global Treatment Access. 2008. Accessed on April 12, 2009: www.globaltreatmentaccess.org

Globalization 101, A Project of the Levin Institute. Accessed on April 12, 2009: www.globalization101.org/uploads/File/Migration/migrall.pdf

Gross International Happiness. Accessed on April 12, 2009: www.grossinternationalhappiness.org

International Federation for Alternative Trade. 2007. Accessed on April 12, 2009: www.ifat.org/

Joshi, G. 1982. The Chipko Movement and Women. Delhi, India: People's Union for Civil Liberties. Accessed on April 12, 2009: www.pucl.org/from-archives/Gender/chipko.htm

Kawachi, I. 1999. *The Society and Population Health Reader: Income Inequality and Health*. New York: New Press.

Landless Workers Movement. Accessed April 12, 2009; www.mstbrazil.org

Labonte, R., and Schrecker, T. 2007. Globalization and Health. Accessed on April 12, 2009: www.globalizationandhealth.com.

Lendman, S. 2008, April 21. Global Food Crisis: Hunger Plagues Haiti and the World. Montreal: Global Research. Accessed on April 12, 2009: www.globalresearch.ca/PrintArticle.php?articleId=8754

Levinson, M. 2009, Winter. The Economic Collapse. *Dissent* 56(1): 61–66.

Miniature Earth. 2008. Accessed on April 12, 2009: www.miniature-earth.com.

Mittai, A. 2007, February 22. Free Trade Doesn't Help Agriculture. Washington, DC: Foreign Policy in Focus. www.fpif.org/fpiftxt/4021.

Molina, N. 2008, April. Europe Questions IFIs on Conditionality: Whose Outcome? London: Bretton Woods Project. Accessed on April 12, 2009: www.brettonwoodsproject.org/print.shtml?cmd[884]=x-884-561068

Mutume, G. 2003, February. A new anti-poverty remedy for Africa? Adjustment policies weaken PRSP goals, critics charge. *Africa Recovery* 16(4). Accessed on April 12, 2009: www.un.org/ecosocdev/geninfo/afrec/vol16no4/164povty.htm

Nag, N. C., and Salimullah, A.H.A. 2006, April–June. Structural Adjustment or Poverty Reduction? An Overview of Bangladesh's I-PRSP. *Asian Affairs* 28(2): 5–23.

Nichols, J. 2008, April 24. The World Food Crisis. *The Nation*. Accessed on April 12, 2009: www.thenation.com/doc/20080512/nichols

The People's Health Movement. Accessed on April 12, 2009: www.phmovement.org

Public Citizen. 2000. Water Privatization Case Study: Cochabamba, Bolivia. Accessed on April 12, 2009: www.citizen.org/documents/Bolivia_(PDF).PDF

Reddy, C. P. 2007, October 1. Business Standard. Accessed on April 12, 2009: www.corpwatch.org/article.php?id=14726

San Francisco Department of Public Health, Tobacco Free Project. Accessed on April 12, 2009: http://sftfc.globalink.org/

The Tobacco Free Project, San Francisco Department of Public Health. 2004. Health Before Tobacco Profits: An *Intercambio* to Stop the Globalization of Tobacco. Case Study. Accessed on April 12, 2009: http://pcsd.neda.gov.ph/susdev.htm

Sen, A. 2002. How to Judge Globalism: Global Links Have Spread Knowledge and Raised Average Living Standards. But the Present Version of Globalism Needlessly Harms the World's Poorest. *American Prospect* 13(49): A2.

Shah, A. 2005. The Scale of the Debt Crisis. Global Issues. Accessed on April 12, 2009: www.globalissues.org/TradeRelated/Debt/Scale.asp

Stokes, B. 2008, June 7. Food Is Different. *National Journal*. Accessed on April 12, 2009: www.nationaljournal.com/njmagazine/print_friendly.php?ID=cs_20080607_0606

Socioeconomic Data and Applications Center. 2008. Accessed on April 12, 2009: http://sedac.ciesin.columbia.edu/es/esi/

Stiglitz, J. E. 2007. *Making Globalization Work*. New York: Norton.

Talberth, J., Cobb, C. and Slattery, N. The Genuine Progress Indicator, 2006: A Tool for Sustainable Development. Redefining Progress. 2007. http://www.rprogress.org/publications/2007/GPI%202006.pdf

Universal Declaration of Human Rights. 1948. Accessed on April 12, 2009: www.udhr.org/UDHR/default.htm

United for a Fair Economy. 2007. Executive Excess 2007: The Staggering Social Cost of U.S. Business Leadership. Accessed on April 12, 2009: www.faireconomy.org

United Nations Conference of Trade and Development. World and Economic Situation and Prospects, 2009. http://www.unctad.org/Templates/webflyer.asp?docid=10852&intltemID=2874&land=1

United Nations Development Programme. 2008. Accessed on April 12, 2009: www.undp.org

United Nations, Food and Agriculture Organization. 2008, September. Briefing Paper: Hunger on the Rise. World Food Situation. Accessed on April 12, 2009: www.fao.org/newsroom/common/ecg/1000923/en/hungerfigs.pdf

United Nations. 2009. The Global Economic Crisis: Systemic Failures and Multilateral Remedies. Accessed on April 12, 2009: www.unctad.org/en/docs/gds20091overview_en.pdf World Bank. 2008. Accessed on April 12, 2009: www.worldbank.org

United Nations. Report of the World Commission on Environment and Development. December 11, 1987. www.un.org/documents/ga/res/42/ares42-187.htm

World Bank. 2009, March. Swimming Against the Tide: How Developing Countries Are Coping with the Global Crisis. Accessed on April 12, 2009: http://siteresources.worldbank.org/NEWS/Resources/swimmingagainstthetide-march2009.pdf

World Commission on Environment and Development. 2008. New York: United Nations. Accessed on April 12, 2009: www.un-documents.net.

World Food Programme. 2008. Hunger Facts. Accessed on April 12, 2009: www.wfp.org

World Fair Trade Organization. Accessed June 2009. www.wfto.org.

World Health Organization. 2008a. Accessed on April 12, 2009: www.who.int/whosis/whostat/2008/en/index.html

World Health Organization. 2008b. Alma Ata Declaration. Accessed on April 12, 2009: www.who.int/hpr/NPH/docs/declaration_almaata.pdf

World Health Organization. 2008c. WHO Framework on Tobacco Control. Accessed on April 12, 2009: www.who.int/fctc/en/

Worldwatch Institute. 2008. Accessed on April 12, 2009: www.worldwatch.org

Zulu, J. J. 2003. PRSP—A Critique and Commentary of the PRSP as a Panacea to Poverty Alleviation and the Development Crisis in Zambia. Paper presented at the ZCTU/FES Workshop on General Orientation to the PRSPs and the Zambian PRSP Process. Accessed on April 12, 2009: www.jctr.org

ADDITIONAL RESOURCES

Association for Women's Rights in Development. Accessed on April 12, 2009: www.awid.org

Brazil's Landless Workers Movement. Accessed on April 12, 2009: www.mstbrazil.org

Bretton Woods Project. 2004. Bank and Fund Evaluation Vindicates PRSP Critics. Accessed on April 12, 2009: www.brettonwoodsproject.org

Delaney, J. 2008, May 7. Globalization: Future Job Loss a Problem. *Epoch Times*. Accessed on April 12, 2009: http://epoch-archive.com/a1/en/us/lax/2008/05-May/08/full.pdf

Fair Trade. Accessed on April 12, 2009: www.fairtrade.org

Farmer, P. 2005. *Pathologies of Power: Health, Human Rights, and the New War on the Poor*. Berkeley: University of California Press.

Global Education. Accessed on April 12, 2009: www.globaleducation.edna.edu

Global Footprint Network. Accessed on April 12, 2009: www.footprintnetwork.org

Global Justice Movement. Accessed on April 12, 2009: www.globaljusticemovement.org

Global Policy Forum. 2000. Accessed on April 12, 2009: www.globalpolicy.org

Greider, W. 1997. *One World, Ready or Not: The Manic Logic of Global Capitalism*. New York: Touchstone.

Hertz, N. 2003. *Global Capitalism and the Death of Democracy: The Silent Takeover*. New York: Harper Business.

International Monetary Fund. Accessed on April 12, 2009: www.imf.org

International Rivers Project. Accessed on April 12, 2009: www.inernationalrivers.org

Meadows, D. H., and others. 1972. *The Limits to Growth*. New York: Universe Books.

Sustainability Institute. Accessed on April 12, 2009: www.sustainer.org

National Center for Health Statistics, CDC. Accessed on April 12, 2009: www.cdc.gov

National Network for Immigrant and Refugee Rights. Uprooted: Refugees of the Global Economy. Accessed on April 12, 2009: www.nnirr.org

People's Health Movement. Accessed on April 12, 2009: www.phmovement.org

Redefining Progress. Accessed on April 12, 2009: www .rprogress.org

Sustainable Scale Project. Accessed on April 12, 2009: www.sustainablescale.org

Tabb, W. K. 2002. *Unequal Partners: A Primer on Globalization*. New York: New Press.

Weissman, R. 2005. Victories! Justice! The People's Triumphs over Corporate Power. *Multinational Monitor*. Accessed on April 12, 2009: http://multinationalmonitor.org

World Social Forum. Accessed on April 12, 2009: www .forumsocialmundial.org

World Trade Organization. Accessed on April 12, 2009: www.wto.org

6

An Introduction to Health Care and Health Policy in the United States

Len Finocchio • Ellen Wu

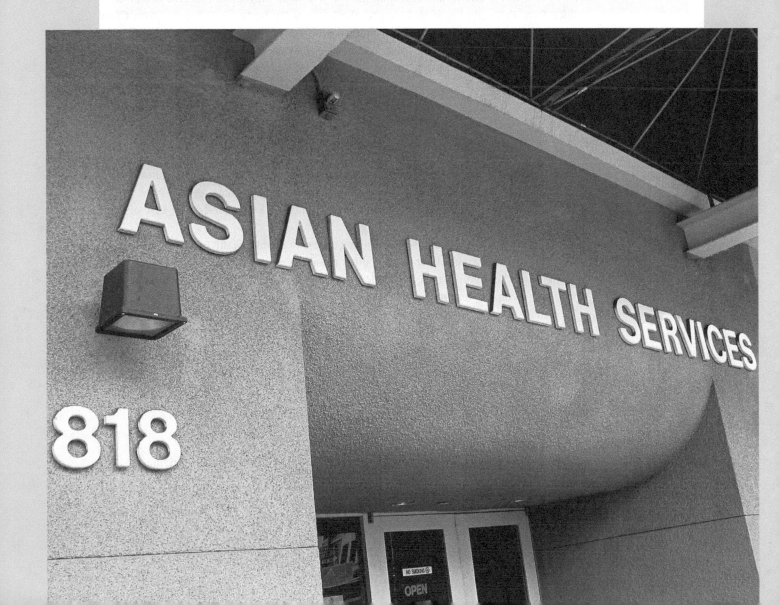

Health care is a human right. Reform of the health care system must provide universal access and ensure a single standard of health care, regardless of ethnicity, residency, citizenship, or employment status, including care for persons without an established residence.

—*California Pan Ethnic Health Network*

INTRODUCTION

Our health care system is very complicated. As you will learn in this chapter, people in the United States have no legal right to health care services, as do individuals in most other wealthy nations. Receiving care in the United States generally requires having health insurance (through your job, a government program, or by purchasing it) or money to pay for care directly. Even with insurance, some groups, such as immigrants or people with disabilities, experience challenges getting care.

The United States spends more money on health care per person than any other country. Yet even though we spend more than $2 trillion each year on health care, we are generally less healthy and live shorter lives than people in other industrialized countries.

Most of the clients and communities you will work with do not receive health insurance from their employers and cannot afford to pay for health care directly. As a CHW, you will guide clients through our complicated system to assist them in getting the right health care from the right providers. You can also play an important part by advocating for changes to our health care system that will make care more accessible to everyone.

WHAT YOU WILL LEARN

By studying the information in this chapter, you will be able to:

- Explain how health care services are financed or paid for in the United States
- Describe who provides health care services in the United States
- Analyze why health status in the United States ranks so far behind that of other nations
- Explain the role of CHWs in expanding access to quality health care services
- Identify health care programs and other resources that serve low-income clients
- Discuss how public policy is made, including policies about access to health care for low-income communities
- Analyze some of the factors that have prevented the establishment of universal access to health care in the United States
- Discuss and provide examples of how CHWs can participate in the public policy process

WORDS TO KNOW

Universal Health Care	Stakeholders	Scope of Practice
Premiums	Deductible	Grassroots Organizing
Copayments	Safety Net	

6.1 WHAT HEALTH CARE "SYSTEM" DO WE HAVE?

WHAT A HEALTH CARE SYSTEM SHOULD DO

The goal of any health care system is to organize and pay hospitals, health professionals, drug manufacturers, and others so that people can get preventive care to stay healthy and quality medical care when they are sick or injured. The definition of a *system* is a "group of objects or an organization forming a network especially for distributing something or serving a common purpose" (Merriam-Webster, 2009).

In most countries with large economies, the national or federal government ensures that the health system serves all people equally. They do this by passing laws to (1) make access to health care a legal right for all persons; (2) collect taxes to pay for services; and (3) regulate providers and other parts of the system so that people receive quality health care services.

While the structure of these **universal health care** systems (systems that provide health care for everyone) vary, people living in a country with a universal health system, such as Canada, Sweden, Japan, or France, are guaranteed access to necessary medical care. Using tax dollars, the government budgets what it will spend on health care and negotiates prices for services. Care is coordinated among clinics, hospitals, doctors, and other providers through centralized systems. The government also sets priorities about which services are most important to ensure the overall health and well-being of the population, with an emphasis on promoting the health of *all* people.

THE NONSYSTEM WE HAVE

The United States is the only country with a large, industrialized economy that does not have a universal health care system. Health care in the United States is not organized into a coherent "system" in which all the different components work together to achieve a common goal. Instead, health care in the United States is a complicated and uncoordinated mix of parts with few common goals and no central leadership. As a result, people in the United States are not served equally, and many, especially low-income working families, do not get health care when they need it.

In 1946, the World Health Organization (WHO) declared that "The enjoyment of the highest attainable standard of health is one of the fundamental human rights of every human being without distinction for race, religion, political belief, economic or social condition." Yet there is no legal right to health care for all persons in the United States. Rather, access to health services depends upon having health insurance from your job, qualifying to receive it from a government program, or buying insurance or services directly with your own money. About two out of three Americans get health insurance from their employers, and one in five from a government insurance program like Medicare or Medicaid (see Figure 6.1). *This leaves one in every six people, or about 47 million Americans, without any health insurance at all.*

Since there is no central coordination of health care in the United States, influence and control comes from many places, mostly governments, employers, and insurance companies. The federal government is solely responsible for health insurance for the elderly (Medicare). State governments, along with federal aid, are responsible for programs serving some low-income patients; these programs vary from state to state. Local governments, like cities and counties, can be responsible for health care for some people in need.

Each employer decides if and how much they will pay for health insurance for their employees, and there are very few rules guiding what they offer. Most large employers offer very good benefits, including health insurance, retirement plans, and so on. Small businesses are less likely to offer health insurance, because these benefits are very expensive

Figure 6.1 Health Insurance in the United States (2006).

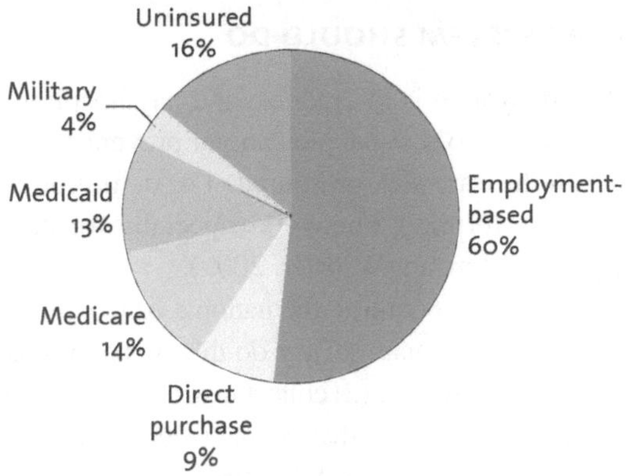

Note: The percentages total more than 100 percent, as some people can be covered by more than one type of insurance during the year.

Source: DeNavas-Walt and others, 2007.

and increasing in cost every year. The number of employers in the United States who offer health insurance to their employees has been steadily declining over the past decade due to increasing costs. At the same time, the cost to employees has been increasing through escalating **premiums** and rising **copayments**. These are the out-of-pocket expenses that we pay to cover part of the costs for insurance (premiums are usually paid monthly) or a share of costs for receiving services at a clinic or hospital or for medications (copayments).

Health insurance companies offer insurance products to governments, employers, and individuals. Nationwide, there are dozens of insurance companies offering hundreds of different insurance plans, so choosing among them can be difficult.

Other organizational influence and control of the health care system comes from the providers of health care, like physicians, hospitals, and manufacturers of drugs, technology, and medical devices. Physicians in particular exert a lot of control because they make most of the decisions about what health care services people get. Hospitals control some of the system in the way they organize services and employ the health care workforce. Big drug companies produce new drugs and influence consumption and spending on those drugs through their marketing to doctors and consumers.

While federal and state governments do create laws governing many aspects of health care delivery, the U.S. system relies heavily on market forces to determine how health services are delivered and paid for, and who gets them. In fact, there is frequent tension between the role of the government and market forces in shaping the system, how it works, and whom it serves.

Market forces in health care do not work like they do in other sectors of the economy. For example, when you shop for a new cell phone, you can easily compare prices and quality to make an informed decision about which one to buy. In health care, it is difficult to compare prices and quality. In addition, you may not have a choice of where you go for health care services, so "shopping around" doesn't really apply.

? *Can you think of other differences between health care and other products or services that are bought and sold in the United States?*

? *Should health care be a right or a product that people have to buy?*

HOW MUCH DO WE SPEND AND WHAT DO WE GET?

One of every six dollars in the U.S. economy (or about 16 percent) is spent on health care (California Healthcare Foundation, 2007). This totals more than $2 trillion (yes, trillion!), or about $7,000 per person living in the United States (see Figure 6.2).

WHY IS HEALTH CARE SO EXPENSIVE IN THE UNITED STATES?

There are many factors that contribute to an expensive system. Our population is growing, so more people are using services. We are also living longer and using more expensive services later in life. Our system encourages the creation and use of expensive medical technology. In addition, many **stakeholders** (individuals or groups with a stake of interest in a particular issue or policy), such as health plans, pharmaceutical companies, and some hospitals, are making a profit from our health care system. More money is also spent on administration and on marketing or promotion of health care in the United States than in countries with universal health care systems.

As the government spends more of its total resources on health care services, less funding is available to be invested in other areas such as education, housing, or social services that promote the public's health. The costs to businesses that provide employees with health insurance benefits have also increased, often putting them at a disadvantage in the global economy. As a result of increasing costs and other factors, the number of uninsured people in the United States keeps growing.

WHAT DO WE GET FOR ALL THE MONEY WE SPEND?

The United States spends more on health care than any other industrialized countries, yet we rate poorly for many national health indicators established by the World Health Organization. For example, in 2006, the infant mortality rate for the United States (the number of babies, out of one thousand born, who will not live to their first birthday) was 6.86 deaths per live births, and for this key health indicator our nation ranked twenty-ninth in the world.

Figure 6.2 Health Care as a Share of Gross Domestic Product.

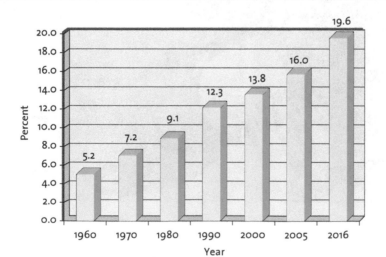

Note: Gross domestic product is the total value of all goods and services produced by a nation in a year.

Source: California HealthCare Foundation, 2007.

There are many elements of the U.S. health care system that are among the best in the world. The overall health of the country has improved over the past century and continues to do so each year, due in large part due to public health programs, medical services, and health education. Our most basic measure for improved health is that we live much longer than we did fifty years ago.

This progress, however, has come with several important consequences. Our longer lives mean we have more people with chronic diseases and disabilities living a long time. Our system is not well coordinated to take care of people with complicated long-term needs.

The successes of the public health and medical systems have not benefited all people in the country equally. In general, people of color and poor people are more likely than Whites and middle-income people to experience barriers to getting services, and when they do get them, the services are often of poorer quality. Low-income people and people of color are more likely to have chronic diseases, disabilities, and live shorter lives. For example, African Americans are more likely than Whites to die from stroke, heart disease, and cancer (National Center for Health Statistics, 2006). (For more information, review Chapter Four.)

Despite the achievements of high-end medical care in the United States, millions of people still go without access to basic health care services.

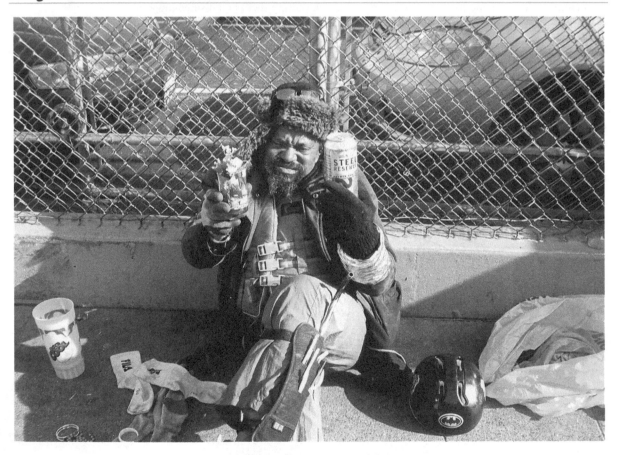

These inequalities are the result of many factors, including health insurance coverage. Since most people in the United States receive their health insurance through their employers, and since people of color in the United States experience inequalities in education, employment, and advancement, non-Whites are more likely to be uninsured

Figure 6.3 Health Care Spending in Selected Countries.

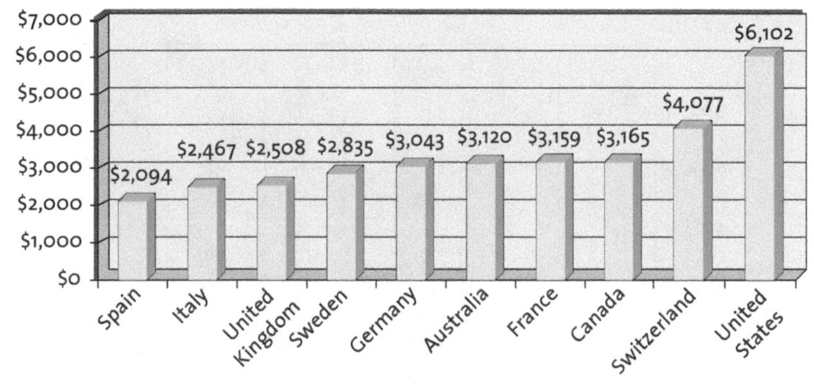

Bar chart: Spain $2,094; Italy $2,467; United Kingdom $2,508; Sweden $2,835; Germany $3,043; Australia $3,120; France $3,159; Canada $3,165; Switzerland $4,077; United States $6,102. Y-axis from $0 to $7,000.

Source: OECD, 2006.

or underinsured. Nearly one in three Latinos in the United States is uninsured. When compared to Whites, all other racial and ethnic groups are more likely to be uninsured (DeNavas-Walt and others, 2007).

While the quality of health care in the United States can be excellent, the care delivered every day to the average person is mediocre at best. Research has shown that adults get only recommended preventive, acute, and chronic care about half the time they visit their providers (McGlynn, Asch, Adams, Keesey, Hicks, DeCristofaro, and Kerr, 2003). In addition, there are many medical errors made each year, with as many as 98,000 people dying each year by accident (Institute of Medicine, 2000). We are making progress at improving health care services, but we still have a very long way to go.

Though we spend more than any other developed country in the world (see Figure 6.3), other countries generally have healthier people who live longer than Americans. In addition, they report that they are much happier about their health care systems and the care that they receive.

6.2 HOW DO WE PAY FOR HEALTH CARE?

? *If you have health insurance, how much does it cost each year, including the costs of copayments, deductibles, and premiums?*

? *Has the cost increased in the past several years?*

FINANCING

Where does all of the money come from to pay for insurance, hospital visits, lab tests, and physician care? Nearly half of all health care dollars come from the local, state, and federal taxes that support public programs such as Medicare, Medicaid, the State Children's Health Insurance Program (SCHIP), and local programs for the uninsured. The other half comes from the private sector, mostly from employers (California Healthcare Foundation, 2007). During the past 40 years, the proportion (percentage) of public dollars paying for health services has increased, while the proportion of private dollars has decreased (see Figure 6.4).

Figure 6.4 Proportion of Public and Private Health Care Expenditures (1960–2006).

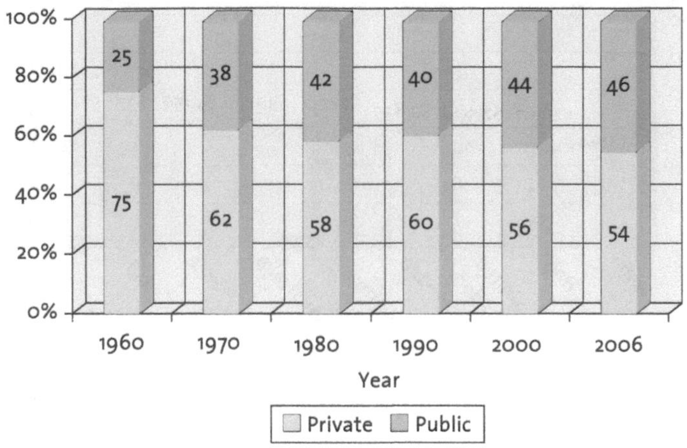

Source: Center for Medicare and Medicaid Services, 2007.

HEALTH INSURANCE

Most health care dollars are not paid directly to medical providers, but through health insurance companies. The primary goal of insurance is to spread the financial risk for an unexpected, random event, such as an accident or serious illness, across a large group of people. A good example is car insurance. The consumer is one of many people who pay a set amount, usually monthly, to an insurance company for "coverage." This regular payment is called a *premium.* If that insured driver has an accident, that person will be required to pay an initial fixed amount (**deductible**), and the insurance company will pay the rest of the cost of repair. The likelihood of an unexpected event is small, but one may cost a great deal when it occurs. The larger the group of contributors, the more effectively the insurance system works. In universal systems of care, everyone contributes, and everyone is insured.

In the United States, health insurance is very important in determining our access to health care services and the quality of those services. Most people can't afford to pay for their health care out of pocket because the costs are so high. Numerous studies have shown that people with health insurance are more likely to have a doctor (primary care provider) whom they visit regularly and are more likely to get preventive care services. The insured are also more likely to be treated earlier for health conditions and, as a result, have lower mortality.

EMPLOYER-BASED HEALTH INSURANCE

More than 60 percent of people with health insurance in the United States get it through their employers. And yet, the majority of people who are uninsured are employed but do not receive health insurance benefits from their employer, or they cannot afford to participate in their employer-sponsored health benefit.

GOVERNMENT PROGRAMS

Although the U.S. government has not committed to financing health insurance for *everyone,* it has identified specific populations that are particularly vulnerable and need assistance in accessing health care. As a result, there are certain groups of people who are able to receive health care through government programs, paid for by taxes. The two major public programs are Medicare and Medicaid, which were established in 1965. A third program, the

State Children's Health Insurance Program (SCHIP), was created in 1997 to provide health coverage for low-income children. These programs are probably the most common form of insurance and access to health care for the clients typically served by CHWs.

Medicare   Medicare is a federally funded and administered program that provides universal medical care for the elderly. Generally, someone is eligible for Medicare if they are sixty-five years or older and are a citizen or permanent resident of the United States. In 1972, the government also included coverage for people who are disabled or have end-state renal (kidney) disease. Medicare has four different parts:

1. *Medicare Part A* covers hospital care, skilled nursing facilities, hospice care, and home health care related to hospital services. Part A is automatic, which means that people are enrolled once they turn 65 without filling out any paperwork or paying any money.
2. *Medicare Part B* covers the costs of physicians' services, outpatient care, and other medical services that Part A doesn't cover, in addition to preventive care. Medicare Part B works like insurance, with premiums, copayments, and deductibles. Copayments are the amount that we pay for each health care visit or medical prescription.
3. *Medicare Part C* is known as Medicare+Choice or Medicare Advantage. It is a program that started as a pilot in the late 1990s that authorized new Medicare health plans to increase beneficiaries' choices of where they receive health care services while controlling costs.
4. *Medicare Part D* is the newest part of the Medicare program; it was established through the Medicare Modernization Act of 2003 and was implemented in 2006. Up until that time, a major health care cost for seniors—prescription drugs—was not covered. Seniors had to qualify for Medicaid (discussed next), or purchase Medigap or supplemental insurance in order to be able to afford their prescriptions. The cost of drugs can be very expensive and continues to increase annually, and they are difficult for low-income patients, especially people living on fixed incomes, to afford. A fixed income is one that will not continue to increase over time. Seniors who receive Social Security or pensions will continue to receive the same dollar amount over time, even as the costs of medicines and other products continue to increase.

Medicare does not cover long-term care, dental, or vision services, although some health plans offer these benefits as well as Medigap plans. (Medigap plans provide coverage for services not provided by Medicare.) More information about Medicare can be found at the Center for Medicare and Medicaid Services Web site (www.medicare.gov/MedicareEligibility).

Medicaid   Medicaid was designed to aid some but not all low-income individuals and families to get health care. Medicaid is funded by both the federal and state governments and administered by the state. The federal government provides general guidelines for the program, and each state develops specific ones, which results in different eligibility requirements and benefits from state to state. But generally, the following individuals and families are eligible for Medicaid (Foundation for Health Coverage Education, 2008):

- Those who meet the requirements for Aid to Families with Dependent Children (AFDC) program
- Children five years old and younger whose family income is at or below 133 percent of the federal poverty level (FPL). The 2009 FPL for a family of three is $18,310 (more information about the FPL is presented later in this chapter).
- Pregnant women whose family income is below 133 percent of the FPL
- Recipients of Supplemental Security Income (SSI)

✪   Recipients of adoption or foster care assistance

✪   Only people who are U.S. citizens or permanent residents

The basic medical services provided by Medicaid are hospital, nursing home care, preventive care, family planning, labs, and x-rays. The money to pay for Medicaid comes from the general revenue funds of both the federal and state governments. The majority goes to pay for services for the elderly who are poor.

You can find general information about Medicaid at the Medicaid Web site (www. cms.hhs.gov/MedicaidGenInfo) and information about Medicaid for each state (www.statehealthfacts.org).

? *Who is eligible for Medicaid in your state?*

? *What are the income eligibility requirements?*

? *How often do people have to reapply for Medicaid?*

State Children's Health Insurance Program   SCHIP is funded by both the federal and state government and administered by the states. There are three different ways that a state could implement SCHIP: (1) expand their Medicaid program to children who previously did not qualify; (2) create a separate program; or (3) combine the two options. Like Medicaid, the federal government provides general guidelines for the program, and each state develops specific ones. Generally, children whose family income is below 200 percent FPL qualify, although some states have expanded SCHIP to above 200 percent, and others are also covering parents of the children in SCHIP.

Basic services that must be provided by all states include well-baby and well-child care, immunizations, and emergency services. Most states provide a comprehensive benefit package, and some even include vision and dental services.

The funding for SCHIP is from the federal and state general revenue. When the program began in 1997, the federal government authorized $40 billion over a ten-year period. Because of its success, more funding has been necessary to sustain the program. Unlike Medicare and Medicaid—programs that do not have budget or time constraints—when SCHIP reached the end of its ten-year approval period, it needed to be reauthorized, and funding for SCHIP had to be included and approved in the federal budget. In 2007, Congress passed legislation to reauthorize SCHIP twice, but both times President George W. Bush vetoed it.

On January 14, 2009, President Barack Obama signed the SCHIP reauthorization, extending the program until September 2013, when it will need to be reauthorized again. Many gains were achieved in this version, including expanding coverage to an additional four million children, which will be paid for by an increase in the federal tobacco tax, removing the five-year waiting period for legal immigrant children and pregnant women, and improving the benefit package for dental and mental health services.

For more information about the State Children's Health Insurance Program, go to www.cms.hhs.gov/MedicaidGenInfo and www.statehealthfacts.org.

? *Who is eligible for SCHIP programs in your state?*

? *How much of the insurance premium do families have to pay?*

? *What do you think the income eligibility requirement should be—*
200 percent of FPL or higher, and why?

Other Government Programs   Other public programs, such as the Veterans Administration program and Indian Health Services, provide health care. In addition to these federal programs, states, counties, and cities are developing initiatives to provide coverage. Massachusetts is the first state to approve new laws and programs with the goal of universal coverage, and the City and County of San Francisco are the first to try to ensure that all residents have a "medical home" to get basic medical care. As a working CHW, you should become familiar with the government health care programs in your area and those that serve the populations you work with.

THE FEDERAL POVERTY LEVEL

Because so many policies use the federal poverty level (FPL) to determine eligibility, it is important to understand how this guideline affects the lives of individuals and families. It is especially relevant to the clients and communities with whom CHWs work. Many people consider the FPL to be an outdated measure that fails to take into account the reality of today's families. For example, the poverty line does not take into account the cost of child care in determining what makes up a family's basic needs. It also does not take into consideration the high cost of living in some regions and states. The federal poverty line is updated each year. The guidelines for 2009 are presented in Table 6.1.

In 2009, the poverty line for a single adult was $10,830. It was $14570 for a household with two adults, and $22,050 for a family of four (the FPL is higher in the states of Alaska and Hawaii). A report found that a single adult in California requires an annual income of $28,336—more than double the amount of the federal poverty line (California Budget Project, 2007)—to cover basic expenses. This is equivalent to an hourly wage of $13.62, which is almost twice as much as the minimum wage in California. The findings also show that a single parent with two children needs an annual income of $59,732 and that a family with two working parents with two children needs an annual income of $72,343 to support a modest standard of living. A modest living for a family of four in California costs more than three times the official poverty level.

As of July 2009, the federal minimum wage was $7.25 per hour (some states have set higher minimum wages). Someone who works full time, 40 hours a week, 52 weeks a year, will earn $15,080 in a year.

Table 6.1 **2008 HHS Poverty Guidelines**

Persons in Family or Household	48 Contiguous States and D.C.	Alaska	Hawaii
1	$10,400	$13,000	$11,960
2	14,000	17,500	16,100
3	17,600	22,000	20,240
4	21,200	26,500	24,380
5	24,800	31,000	28,520
6	28,400	35,500	32,660
7	32,000	40,000	36,800
8	35,600	44,500	40,940
For each additional person, add	3,600	4,500	4,140

Source: Federal Register, Vol. 73, No. 15, January 23, 2008, pp. 3971–3972.

?   *In your city or county, can a family of four making $22,050 a year afford basic needs, including rent, food, clothes, transportation, and health care?*

?   *What is the minimum wage in your city or state? What do you think about the level at which the federal government draws the poverty line?*

?   *Where would you draw the line, and why?*

6.3   WHO PROVIDES HEALTH CARE SERVICES?

As you have read in the previous sections of this chapter, money to pay for health services comes from the government, employers, or individuals. Insurance companies take these dollars and pay the providers of health services when we use them. Hospitals and physicians develop contracts with insurance companies to provide health care services for a negotiated price. We spend the majority of our health care dollars on hospitals and physicians. Figure 6.5 shows the distribution of all health care spending.

HOSPITALS

Hospitals provide a wide range of health care, from basic primary care to very high-tech and expensive specialty care. Most hospitals have both outpatient facilities, or clinics, and inpatient services. In clinics, people receive services for health care needs that are not serious. Most clinics accept all types of insurance, including government-sponsored ones. In a clinic, your visit may last a few minutes or up to a few hours. Inpatient care, where you stay overnight, is for more complicated needs that require specialists and high-tech interventions like surgery. Inpatient care is typically very expensive. A hospital stay usually costs around $3,000 per day, *plus* the cost of services provided by physicians.

Figure 6.5   Where We Spend Money in the Health Care System.

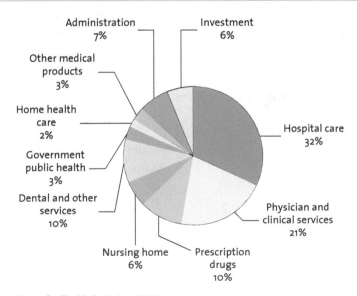

Source: National Center for Health Statistics, 2006.

General hospitals provide a wide range of services. Specialty hospitals focus on specific services, such as cardiology or children. Many communities have at least one hospital, and it is commonly an important source of employment. However, there are many communities, including Native American nations, without hospitals. Hospitals link with many other services and providers, such as physician groups, laboratories, imaging services, and long-term care facilities such as nursing homes. Hospitals may also serve as teaching sites for nurses, CHWs, allied health providers, and physicians.

Some hospitals have emergency departments to treat life-threatening conditions. In large urban areas, emergency departments are commonly used by the uninsured and some insured persons as their primary source of health care. Emergency departments make up one part of what is the health care **safety net** through which those without insurance seek care. *Safety net* is the term used to refer to those parts of the system that provide care to people without insurance or the ability to afford health care, or difficulty finding an accessible practitioner.

Approximately one in three hospitals is a public, or government-owned, facility (see Figure 6.6). Paid for largely through taxes, public hospitals have an obligation to serve the poor, and they play an important safety net role for people who are uninsured. Public hospitals take care of more than half of the nation's uninsured and low-income patients (National Association of Public Hospitals, 2007). In addition to public hospitals, the safety net includes community health centers (discussed next) and nonprofit hospitals that have a legal obligation to provide a community benefit such as care to the uninsured. In return for providing free care to some patients, nonprofit hospitals typically receive additional tax benefits.

Of those hospitals that are privately owned, half are not-for-profits. For-profit hospitals are more likely to be specialty hospitals and serve a more narrow population, nearly all of which is insured.

? *Where do uninsured patients in your city or region go to receive health care?*

? *Does your city or region have a public hospital, a community health center, a free clinic?*

Figure 6.6 Types of Hospitals.

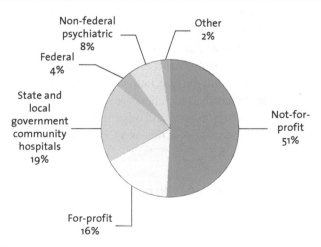

Source: American Hospital Association, 2007.

PHYSICIANS AND THEIR PRACTICES

Most people using the health care system visit their doctors about three times per year (National Center for Health Statistics, 2006). People with insurance see a primary care doctor for most of their needs and will go to specialists for more complicated treatments. Of all 813,000 physicians in the United States, about 40 percent are primary care doctors and 60 percent are specialists (Health Resources and Services Administration, 2008). We spend more than $400 billion, or one in every five health care dollars, on doctors' services (National Center for Health Statistics, 2006).

Until the 1980s, physicians in the United States primarily worked in individual private practices. Patients would make an appointment and come to the office, using their insurance or paying cash for the visit. It is now more common for physicians to work in large private group practices that provide business management services. Most group practices focus on a single specialty, such as family medicine or dermatology, but there are also group practices that have many different specialties under the same roof.

Physicians do not typically work directly for hospitals but are given "privileges" to admit their patients into hospitals. Because of this relationship, hospitals compete for patients by offering the latest technology, best nurses, and nicest facilities. Payers, such as Medicare and private insurance companies, pay physicians separately for their services, typically in a fee-for-service manner in which doctors get paid for each service they provide.

Physicians have the broadest **scope of practice** of all health professionals and generally direct the medical care that each patient receives. *Scope of practice* refers to the skills and services that professionals are qualified and competent to provide. Other health professionals typically take direction from physicians who are often team leaders. You will learn about the scope of practice for CHWs in Chapter Eight.

COMMUNITY HEALTH CENTERS

The more than six thousand community health centers across the country form an important part of the health care delivery system (NACHC, 2006). *Community health centers often serve as the only affordable and accessible source of care in a community.* These not-for-profit outpatient clinics have a mission to serve the neediest in every community: 40 percent of their patients are uninsured, and 35 percent have Medicaid or SCHIP.

These centers receive most of their funding from Medicaid, a combination of state and federal dollars, and federal grants that support their services to the uninsured. Most of the clinics provide primary care services, some specialty services, and some dental and mental health services. They are especially committed to and capable of providing culturally and linguistically competent health care services.

Like public hospitals, community health centers play a critical role in the health care safety net; they primarily serve low-income individuals, persons of color, the uninsured, immigrants, and those on Medicaid. These clinics are often the only source of health care for these populations, particularly in rural and other medically underserved areas. If you work within the health care system in your role as a CHW, you will often work in connection with these clinics.

? *Where are the closest community health centers in your city or county?*

? *What types of services do they provide?*

? *What communities do they serve?*

? *Do they have special programs for clients who speak languages other than English?*

Some of Lee Jackson's clients need treatment for substance abuse, or need mental health care, or other intensive services. He finds that the safety net doesn't catch everyone—there aren't enough clinics and treatment centers to meet the need.

> LEE JACKSON: There just aren't enough services. Ask anyone in the health field; you have too many homeless people and you have too many people with substance abuse problems and you have too many people that are mentally ill that don't get services. I see this every day I walk through the poor neighborhoods where my clients live. . . . Some people want things right away, but it just doesn't work that way. I tell them, "You have to be patient and make all of your appointments. I will be there with you to take you to your appointment, but the key factor is you have to show up." Some people are just at a point in their life where they're incapable of getting to their appointment because they're multiply diagnosed: they might have HIV disease, and substance abuse and mental health issues to deal with. They just have too many things going on.

HOW HEALTH CARE PROVIDERS WORK TOGETHER

Some providers, such as large physician group practices, hospital chains, and managed care plans, tend to work closely together. Some community health centers work closely with public hospitals, since both contribute to the health care safety net in a community.

But overall, the pieces of the U.S. health care system do not fit together very well, and health care is not well coordinated. Coordination is very important for people with chronic diseases, because the management of such conditions requires the services of many different providers. A person with diabetes, for example, may need to consult with their primary care provider, the endocrinologist, the ophthalmologist, the podiatrist, the neurologist, the cardiologist, the urologist, the dentist, and the nutritionist.

In some systems, the patient medical record is kept on paper and is largely inaccessible to the patient. Providers at the same office or hospital can add to the record, but when a patient goes to another clinic or laboratory for a service, the information might not be entered right away. When information is not kept all together in one place in a timely way, providers are not fully up to date on a patient's care. This can lead to poor quality of care and sometimes dangerous mistakes. It can be highly frustrating to patients who are doing their best to navigate the system to get the health care services that they need.

MANAGED CARE

Despite the overall poor coordination within the health care system, there have been some improvements over the past twenty-five years. In particular, managed care insurance plans have been established that aim to organize medical services and payment to offer better care at a lower cost. Managed care developed in response to many pressures, including spiraling health care costs, poor coordination of patient's health care, and the need to focus on health promotion and disease prevention. All managed care plans use similar mechanisms to coordinate care and manage costs, the most common being primary care providers as "gatekeepers" to services. In other words, you have to see your primary care provider before you can access other health services.

THE ROLE OF CHWs IN HEALTH CARE

CHWs are increasingly being recognized as a vital part of the health care system and are hired to work in clinics and hospitals as part of a health care team. Whether they work for a hospital, clinic, local health department, or community-based organizations, CHWs often work to ensure that clients understand their health and receive the best health care possible. For example, CHWs:

- Provide outreach to assist community members to understand and access health care services available in their communities
- Link people to health care services and follow up to ensure that clients understand their health issues and treatment
- Provide health education to assist individuals, families, and communities in learning about health and factors that affect their health and well-being
- Assist clients in enrolling in health insurance programs such as SCHIP for the children of low-income families
- Act as navigators, assisting clients to figure out how to access the proper providers and services within a clinic, hospital, or health plan
- Advocate for clients within the health care organizations and systems to aid in ensuring that they are provided with culturally competent services, including, for example, interpretation services
- Provide client-centered health education and counseling services to assist clients to understand their health conditions and treatment regiments, how to follow treatment guidelines, and how to make changes that promote their health

? *Can you think of other ways that CHWs work within the health care "system" to promote health?*

The United States has a long history as a nation of immigrants. However, the health care system does not have enough bilingual and bicultural providers or trained interpreters. Phuong An Doan-Billings describes how Asian Health Services is handling the language issues that arise when serving a multiethnic and multilingual population.

PHUONG AN DOAN BILLINGS: The patient navigator program at Asian Health Services is an attempt to respond to community feedback. Our agency is located right in the middle of Chinatown, so there's a lot of Chinese patients that come in, and because there's a lot of Chinese, we had to hire a lot of Chinese-speaking workers. We set up patient navigators to help patients from other communities who also have language needs, such as Korean, Vietnamese, and Cambodian patients. The navigators can assist with check in, check out, receiving phone calls, referrals, everything. Before, everything went to the patient service representative (the receptionist), and then to the interpreter. If the interpreter was in the exam room with a doctor, and a phone call came in, the receptionist was usually a Chinese-speaking person, and if the patient was not Chinese-speaking, they both would have difficulty. So the patient navigator actually assists the patient to navigate through our system. They also work closely with the community liaison unit, doing outreach to immigrant populations to help them understand about our services.

6.4 WHAT DO WE WANT FROM THE SYSTEM AND HOW DO WE GET IT?

THE CHALLENGES TO FIXING OUR HEALTH CARE SYSTEM

There have been attempts by at least seven presidents over the past hundred years to achieve some form of universal health care in the United States. The arguments for universal care include increasing access to health care for all people, decreasing health inequalities and health care costs, promoting economic productivity through a healthy workforce, and protecting against catastrophic financial losses from unpredicted health expenses.

Why, then, have attempts to establish a universal health care system in the United States failed? How did we end up with a health care nonsystem in which so many go without insurance and health care? There are many cultural, economic, and political values and forces that shape all our major institutions, including government, education, and health care systems.

We deeply value individualism in the United States, and people are expected to succeed for themselves in all aspects of life—education, career, business, family, and even health. While our nation has prospered in many ways, including the development of a large economy, a vigorous legal system, science, and the arts, the emphasis on *individual* success often means that our social values, or how we take care of each other, are less of a priority. This contributes to economic, social, and health inequalities between the "haves" and the "have-nots." The United States is one of the most unequal industrialized nations in the world in terms of the distribution of wealth, access to basic resources, and health status.

Government plays an important role in the health care for the U.S. population, but it is one that is limited to a few groups determined most in need. This limited role reflects a deep mistrust of government and a preference for marketplace solutions for most economic and social challenges. As a result, health care is primarily regarded as a commodity or product like any other that is bought and sold, rather than a basic right.

Another reason that we have not developed a universal health care system is that most providers of health care services, like doctors, hospitals, insurance, and pharmaceutical companies, resist major changes to the current system, as they stand to lose money and control.

Our entrepreneurial spirit and inventiveness itself is another factor. It leads the United States to highly value technology and science. As a result, our health care system focuses on using advanced and expensive technology to treat illnesses once people have them, rather than to prevent illness from developing in the first place.

In addition, we are a diverse society. While this diversity is the very strength of our nation, it makes bringing people together to agree on common goals difficult. Because we have different views about health, individualism, and the role of government, finding agreement on one health care system for all people has been highly challenging.

Finally, the way our government is structured, with checks and balances, makes the process of passing public policies slow, with many opportunities for a policy to be rejected. The process of how public policies are decided is outlined in the next section of the chapter.

Despite these obstacles to implementing a universal system nationwide, efforts continue at the state, local, and federal levels.

WHAT CAN WE DO TO FIX OUR HEALTH CARE SYSTEM?

To change the health care system to provide better care for more people, we must get involved with how health policy is made. *Policies* are rules that guide how something works. Families often set household policies, including curfews and bedtimes for children. Many people and organizations develop and advocate for policies that impact our health care system. For example, the Center on Medicare and Medicaid Services writes regulations that govern how these two major public programs (Medicare and Medicaid) are run. States have ballot initiatives through which people can vote on policy. The local school board can pass a health and fitness plan for schools. In order to achieve a better health care system, we need to understand the process of how policies are made and seek opportunities to influence these policies.

HOW A BILL BECOMES A LAW

The most public form of public policy is legislation, or a bill. At the federal level, the three policymaking bodies are Congress, made up of the House of Representatives and the Senate, and the administration (Office of the President). The idea for a bill can originate from a legislator in the House or Senate or from the president. Sometimes an organization or individual has an idea and works with a legislator to introduce it. The bill is introduced in either the Congress or the Senate, is given a number, and is assigned to different committees. Most national health bills will be assigned to go to the Health, Education, Labor, and Pensions Committees. Any bill that requires funding must go through the Appropriations Committee (to "appropriate" or allocate the funding) or the Finance Committee. A bill can be assigned to more than one committee. In order for the bill to "pass," it must pass each of the committees and then pass a vote by the full house. One of the reasons it is so difficult to pass policy is that opponents have multiple opportunities to defeat it.

Once the bill passes the first house (the house it originated from), it goes through the same process in the second house. Only if it passes both the Congress and the Senate does it go to the president for his or her signature (see Figure 6.7). At the state level, legislation gets passed using a similar process and is signed by the governor.

At more local levels, the process is not as complicated. If the policy is related to your county, the policymaking body might be a board of supervisors or the county commissioners. If the policy is related to your city, the decision makers may be the city council members or aldermen. Usually these groups hear public testimony about a specific issue and then take a vote on it at their meeting. These meetings are generally open to the public.

This is a system of "checks and balances," and no single governing body has complete control. While this system is important to prevent an authoritarian government, it also makes it difficult for policy to get passed, because it requires much negotiation and many compromises.

? *Have you ever participated in the public policy process by supporting or opposing specific legislation or policies?*

? *Can you identify current proposals for legislation (local, state, or national) that would affect the health of communities you belong to or work with?*

? *Who is speaking out to support the interests of these communities?*

Figure 6.7 How a Bill Becomes a Law.

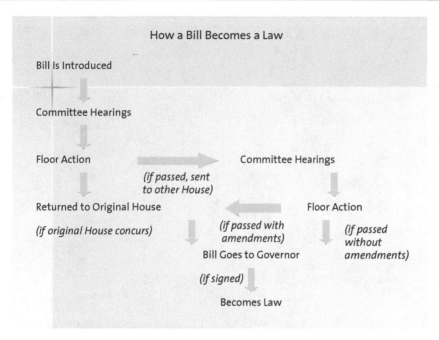

Source: The Legislative Counsel, State of California, 2009.

WHAT REGULATIONS ARE AND WHO MAKES THEM

Changing public policy through the administrative regulatory process is less familiar to most people, but perhaps more important than legislation. This is because most of the details about how laws will be implemented (put into practice) are decided through the administrative process. Administrative policies do not require legislative action, and they can be influenced by advocacy efforts of consumers, communities, CHWs, and organizations that represent their interests.

Many administrative agencies are required by law to get public comments on their initial draft regulation. The key is to be on their mailing or e-mail list to get their notifications. At the federal level, the largest agency responsible for health and health care related services is the U.S. Department of Health and Human Services (DHHS). Other key agencies include the Center for Medicare and Medicaid Services (responsible for Medicaid, Medicare, and SCHIP), the Food and Drug Administration (FDA), and the Health Resources and Services Administration. There are similar agencies at the state level. And at the local level, the board of supervisors and city council develop administrative regulations through ordinances.

THE POLITICS OF CHANGING HEALTH POLICY

There are many stakeholders with different interests and perspectives trying to influence the health care system, and this makes negotiations and compromise extremely challenging. A *stakeholder* is anyone who has an interest in the outcome of a decision (usually a policy change). Some stakeholders are well organized and have a lot of money to invest in their advocacy efforts; others do not. Stakeholders in our health care system include:

- Individuals, families, and communities
- Physicians

Improving access to quality health care for everyone requires changing health care policies.

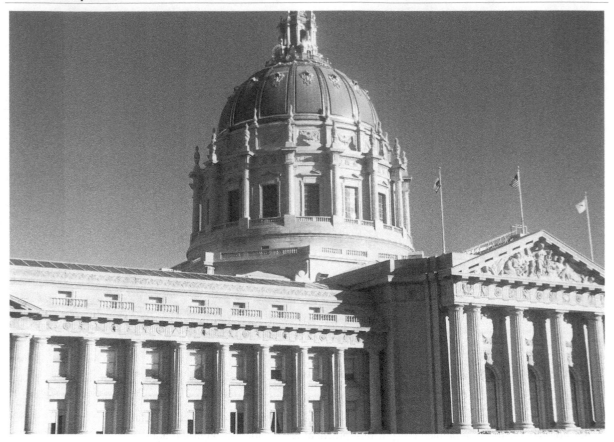

- ✪ Hospitals
- ✪ Health plans
- ✪ Pharmaceutical companies
- ✪ Businesses
- ✪ Unions
- ✪ Advocacy organizations representing patients and communities

Each of these stakeholders has a unique view of the health care system and how it should be "fixed," and they lobby to influence changes to policy. Some, like insurance and pharmaceutical companies, have substantial resources to spend on advocating for their position, and others, like consumers, low-income communities, and the advocacy organizations that represent them, do not.

? *How might the interests of consumers (or patients) be different from the interests of pharmaceutical companies or health plans?*

? *What is the primary concern of patients?*

? *What are the primary concerns of insurance companies and other stakeholders?*

THE ROLE OF CHWs IN GRASSROOTS ORGANIZING AND ADVOCACY EFFORTS

Part Three of this textbook focuses on the role that CHWs play in facilitating community-level intervention and organizing efforts. Just as CHWs may serve as links between communities and health care systems, they may also link communities to the public policy process, assisting to mobilize grassroots participation and leadership. **Grassroots organizing** efforts are characterized by the participation of the communities that will be most affected by the proposed policies.

CHWs often play a vital role in supporting communities to organize and advocate for policy changes on the local, state, and national levels. While CHWs may themselves become visible leaders in these efforts, speaking to the media or testifying before policymakers, their primary role is to support community members to raise their own voices in support of social change. We will address these roles in greater detail in Chapter Twenty-Two.

CHWs may contribute to changing public policies in the following ways:

- ✪ Conduct research on health inequalities and outstanding needs in the community
- ✪ Facilitate a community diagnosis in which community members identify their own resources and needs (see Chapter Eighteen)
- ✪ Conduct outreach, education, and mobilization to inform community members and voters about important health issues
- ✪ Participate in media advocacy efforts by talking to reporters and writing opinion pieces or letters to the editor
- ✪ Testify to policymakers who are considering legislation on specific health issues important to your community
- ✪ Participate in public meetings and rallies on health issues
- ✪ Write letters to legislators, regulators, and providers about issues of concern in your community
- ✪ Collect stories about important health issues or encourage your clients to share their stories and speak out
- ✪ Partner with other advocacy organizations and collaborations working on issues of importance
- ✪ Train and support community members to engage in direct advocacy efforts, including protests, media advocacy, and testifying before policymakers

? *Can you think of other ways that CHWs can participate in efforts to advocate for new public policies?*

? *Have you ever participated in such advocacy efforts?*

? *What was your role?*

? *What policies is your local community currently advocating to change?*

PROPOSALS FOR FIXING OUR HEALTH CARE SYSTEM

Nearly two-thirds of Americans believe that the federal government should take on reforming our health care system (Kaiser Family Foundation, 2008). While most Americans increasingly agree that everyone should have a right to affordable, quality health care, we do not agree on how to reach this goal. There are several models that have been proposed for improving the health care system.

Single Payer   Single payer proposals insure *everyone*, in one common insurance risk pool, usually with the government paying providers directly for services. Single payeris the only model that provides universal coverage; it is used in Canada and throughout Europe. This model would save money overall, through the government's ability to negotiate lower rates and decrease administrative costs.

Employer Mandate   Employer mandate proposals require all employers to provide insurance to their employees. Often the requirements for employers are based on the size of their company, the amount of their payroll, and they may differentiate between full-time and part-time employees. This model builds on our current employer-based system and has received increased attention as more employers are dropping health insurance benefits or asking employees to pay a larger share of the costs. However, employer mandate is difficult to pass because most employers are against such a requirement, and a federal law, the Employee Retirement Income Security Act (ERISA), prohibits states to regulate employers health insurance and has been used to overturn state initiatives to enact employer mandates. Hawaii and Massachusetts and the City of San Francisco are currently the only states or local counties that have an employer mandate.

Expansion of Government Programs   Many people argue for expanding existing public programs to cover more people by changing the eligibility. For example, proposals have included expanding Medicaid to adults without children who make less than a certain percentage of the federal poverty level, changing the age of Medicare eligibility from sixty-five to sixty, or raising the income eligibility threshold, such as from 200 percent to 250 percent. Generally, people are in favor of expanding public programs but are concerned about the financing of the programs.

Market-Driven Solutions   Though only 9 percent of people who are insured purchase health coverage themselves, some proposals for health care reform focus on individual purchasing as their solution. For example, medical savings accounts (MSA) provide incentives for people to save money in a tax-deductible account in order to pay for their own medical bills. However, these accounts discourage the use of preventive care services and are generally affordable only to people with higher incomes. If someone gets seriously ill, the cost of medical care could still exceed what they can save in an MSA. Inability to pay medical bills has long been the number one reason for personal bankruptcy in the United States.

Individual Mandate   Another policy option gaining in popularity, recently implemented in Massachusetts, is an *individual mandate*, which requires everyone to have health insurance. One of the concerns with an individual mandate is that most people cannot afford to purchase a comprehensive health insurance plan on their own. Some policymakers understand this dilemma and couple an individual mandate with subsidies to aid the low income, tax credits for the middle income, and exemptions when there is no affordable health insurance available or when an individual or family experiences hardship.

CONSIDERATIONS FOR ALL HEALTH REFORM PROPOSALS

Questions to ask when analyzing proposals for health care reform and the impact on your clients include:

- ✪ Who will be covered and who will be left out (for example, what about immigrants)?
- ✪ Who is participating, funding, and leading efforts to advocate for these proposals? Are low-income communities and the uninsured represented in these efforts?

- Who will benefit financially from the initiative?
- What is the defined benefits package? What health care services will people be able to receive, and what services will not be covered?

The United States will continue to debate proposals for health care reform. Low-income communities, the organizations that serve them, and CHWs can play a vital role in determining the direction of health care reform and advocating for reforms that provide full access to quality and affordable care for all communities.

? *What is your proposal for how to improve the U.S. health care system?*

? *Do you support any of the proposals presented here, or do you favor other solutions?*

CHAPTER REVIEW

1. You have been asked to make a presentation to a local community group about the health care system. How will you answer the following questions from the community:
   - How many people lack health insurance in the United States?
   - What is universal health care?
   - How does the U.S. health care system compare with those of other countries? Do we have the healthiest society?
   - Why is health care in the United States more expensive than in other countries?
   - What types of health insurance programs are available to low-income people?
   - What can we do to change the system and to get better health care for our community?
   - If you could make any changes you wanted to the U.S. health care system, what changes would you make and why?
2. Identify the following resources for low-income and uninsured clients in your community, city, or county:

   - Which hospitals provide care to uninsured patients? Do these hospitals publicize their policies and make it easy for uninsured patients to access free care?
   - Are there free clinics in the city or county?
   - Where and how can people with limited English proficiency access health care? Are there clinics or hospitals that provide services in languages other than English or that provide trained health care interpreters?
   - Where can clients go to enroll in Medicaid, Medicare, or SCHIP programs? What are the eligibility requirements for these programs in your state?
   - What local organizations are advocating for expanded access to quality health care for low-income and other vulnerable communities?
   - What policies are currently being debated in your city or county that will have an impact on access to health care services?

REFERENCES

American Hospital Association. 2007. *Health and Hospital Trends*. Accessed on April 10, 2009: www.aha.org/aha/resource-center/Statistics-and-Studies/fast-facts.html

California Budget Project. 2007. *Making Ends Meet: How Much Does It Cost to Raise a Family in California.*

Accessed on April 10, 2009: www.cbp.org/pdfs/2007/0710_mem_003.pdf

California Healthcare Foundation. 2007. *Snapshot: Health Care Costs 101, 2007 Edition.* Accessed on April 10, 2009: www.chcf.org/topics/healthinsurance/index.cfm?itemID=132421

DeNavas-Walt, C., Proctor, B., Smith, J., and U.S. Census Bureau. 2007. Income, Poverty, and Health Insurance Coverage in the United States: 2006. *Current Population Reports,* 60–233. Washington, DC: U.S. Government Printing Office.

Foundation for Health Coverage Education. 2008. *The 2008 U.S. Federal Poverty Level.* Accessed on April 10, 2009: www.coverageforall.org/pdf/FHCE_FedPovertyLevel.pdf

Institute of Medicine. 2000. *To Err Is Human: Building a Safer Health System.* Washington, DC: National Academy of Sciences.

Kaiser Family Foundation. 2008, October. *Kaiser Health Tracking Poll: Election 2008.* Accessed on April 10, 2009: www.kff.org/kaiserpolls//h08_posr102108pkg.cfm

McGlynn, E., Asch, S., Adams, J., Keesey, J., Hicks, J., DeCristofaro, A., and Kerr, E. 2003. The Quality of Health Care Delivered to Adults in the United States. *New England Journal of Medicine* 348: 2635–2645.

Merriam-Webster's On-Line Dictionary. Accessed on September 30, 2007: www.m-w.com/dictionary/system

National Association of Public Hospitals. 2007. *Characteristics of NAPH Members.* Accessed on April 10, 2009: www.naph.org/Content/NavigationMenu/ About_Our_Members/Characteristics_of_NAPH_ Members/Characteristics_of_NAPH_Members.htm

National Center for Health Statistics. 2006. *Health, United States, 2006 with Chartbook on Trends in the Health of American*s. Hyattsville, MD: National Center for Health Statistics.

The legislative Counsel, State of California. A guide for Accessing California Legislative Information on the Internet. January 2009. http://www. leginfo.ca.gov/ guide.html

U.S. Department of Health and Human Services, Center for Medicare and Medicaid Services. 2007. *National Health Expenditure Data.* Accessed on April 10, 2009: www.cms.hhs.gov

U.S. Department of Health and Human Services, Health Resources and Services Administration. 2008. *Physician Supply and Demand: Projections to 2020.* Accessed on April 10, 2009: http://bhpr.hrsa.gov/ healthworkforce/reports/physiciansupplydemand/ currentphysicianworkforce.htm

The World Health Organization. 1946. Preamble to the World Health Organization's Constitution. Accessed on April 10, 2009: www.who.org

ADDITIONAL RESOURCES

California Pan Ethnic Health Network. Accessed on April 10, 2009: www.cpehn.org

Henry J. Kaiser Family Foundation. Accessed on April 10, 2009: www.statehealthfacts.org

National Association of Community Health Centers. Accessed on April 10, 2009: www.nachc.com/ about-our-health-centers.cfm

World Health Organization. Accessed on April 10, 2009: www.who.org.

7

Practicing Cultural Humility

Abby Rincon

I have a dream that one day my child will be judged not by the color of his skin, but by the content of his character.

—*Dr. Martin Luther King Jr.**

INTRODUCTION

All CHWs work with clients and communities with cultural backgrounds and identities that are different from their own. Even if you work in the same community you live in and belong to, some of the clients you work with will come from a different generational, economic, professional, ethnic, religious, or linguistic background or will have a different gender, gender identity, or sexual orientation than you do.

This rich diversity that surrounds us also poses challenges. As CHWs, how can we learn to work effectively with all clients? What if we don't know much about people who are lesbian, gay, transgender, Muslim, Christian, or disabled? Some of us were raised in households where stereotypes and prejudice existed, and maybe we struggle with some of those "old tapes" playing in our heads.

Unfortunately, along with celebrating our rich diversity, we must recognize that many of us have faced discrimination because of who we are. Whether because of conscious, unconscious, or structural bias, some of us have enjoyed greater access to resources and rights than others. In the communities where CHWs most commonly work, many people haven't had equal access to opportunities, including education, safety from violence, affordable housing, civil rights, sufficient food, job training programs, recreational and cultural programs, and culturally competent health care. As a result, these communities often face higher rates of illness and death.

As CHWs, we are committed to becoming compassionate providers to people of all backgrounds. One chapter will not make you an expert in doing this, but by studying the concepts, questions, knowledge, and skills included in this chapter, you can enhance your understanding and ability to respond to the complexities of cultural diversity. This chapter invites you to make a commitment to become a lifelong learner and practitioner of cultural humility.

This chapter starts by presenting some of the demographic changes and other key issues that shape the context for community health work. The second half of the chapter presents definitions, useful models for client interactions, and ends with an invitation to develop your own plan that will assist you to continue learning.

WHAT YOU WILL LEARN

By studying the material in this chapter, you will be able to:

- Explain the changing demographics in the United States and how this affects the work of CHWs
- Discuss how historical and institutional discrimination affects the health of targeted communities and influences their work with public health providers
- Define the concept of cultural humility
- Analyze the importance of becoming lifelong learners and practitioners of cultural humility
- Discuss and analyze concepts of traditional health beliefs and practices and how they may influence the delivery of services to clients

Reprinted by arrangement with The Heirs to the Estate of Martin Luther King Jr., c/o Writers House as agent for the proprietor New York, NY. *Copyright 1963 Dr. Martin Luther King Jr; copyright renewed 1991 Coretta Scott King*

✪ Identify, analyze, and apply models for practicing cultural humility and conducting client-centered interviews regarding health issues, including the Tool to Elicit Health Beliefs and the LEARN Model

✪ Create a personal learning plan in order to become a culturally effective CHW

WORDS TO KNOW

Cross-Cultural	Demography	Demographic
Sexual Orientation	Structural Racism	Structural Discrimination
Gender Identity		

7.1 WHY PRACTICING CULTURAL HUMILITY IS SO IMPORTANT

Many clients and communities face bias and discrimination when they attempt to access health and social services and, as a result, receive fewer services and services of poorer quality. As we addressed in Chapter Four, this is a significant reason for persistent health inequalities. In order to be successful in your ultimate goal of promoting health equality and social justice, you must develop your capacity to reach and provide quality services to diverse communities (do **cross-cultural** work). Indeed, this is one of the primary reasons why CHWs are trained and hired.

As CHWs, it's important to acknowledge what we don't know about cultural diversity. This is the first step toward improving our ability to work with people effectively, regardless of their identity and life experience. Intellectually, we have the ability to absorb new information about cultures, subcultures, power, privilege, and oppression. This forms one aspect of cultural diversity training. However, to fully understand cultural diversity, we must undertake a personal journey. Learning how to work effectively across cultures is not just an intellectual endeavor: we must open our hearts as well as our minds in order to develop cultural humility.

This process requires a willingness to acknowledge our pain and past hurts and those of others as well as acknowledging our own biases and judgments about others. This may be uncomfortable and may provoke strong emotion. In these moments, it can be helpful to stay humble and remember that we have all made mistakes and are capable of personal growth and change. Learning about cultural diversity can be a challenging, lifelong, and transformative journey.

Practicing cultural humility isn't easy and can be deeply challenging. It requires:

✪ Studying histories of oppression and discrimination
✪ Closely examining our own assumptions and prejudices about people who come from different communities than our own
✪ Learning to put our own assumptions aside when working with others
✪ Engaging respectfully with all clients and recognizing that they are our guides in determining their own cultural identity, values, knowledge, behaviors, and decisions

7.2 THE CULTURALLY DIVERSE CONTEXT FOR COMMUNITY HEALTH WORK

Ismael Reed has said that, as a society, the United States is unique in the world because "the world is here." In America, "the cultures of the world crisscross" on a daily basis (Takaki, 1993, p. 16).

? *Think about where you fit in this multicultural mix.*

? *Were you born in the United States?*

? *What about your parents and grandparents?*

? *What about your neighbors, the people you encounter at the grocery store, the bank, in your children's schools?*

? *What are the languages, cultures, and other identities of the students in your classes and the people in your community?*

? *What about the people who are your local politicians or in charge of large businesses and government institutions?*

The 2000 U.S. Census and the studies that followed provided data that assists us to better understand demographic changes we are experiencing. **Demography** is the study of human populations, their composition, structure, and change. **Demographic** information about people may include age, sex, gender identity, ethnicity, primary languages, immigration status, **sexual orientation** (whether people are romantically and sexually attracted to people of the same or opposite sex or both), disability status, income, religious or political affiliations, and so on. The most dramatic of these demographic changes occurred in states where the percentage of people of color (people who do not identify as White or Caucasian) rose above 50 percent of the total population: Hawaii (75 percent), New Mexico (57 percent), California (57 percent), and Texas (52 percent).

According to demographers, the changes we are experiencing result from increased immigration from all over the world, different age patterns for the largest ethnic/racial groups, and different fertility (or birth) rates among these same groups. We have experienced increases in groups with the youngest median ages that are more likely to be starting families (for example, Latinos, Asians, immigrants of all ethnic/racial origins), and decreases among groups whose median ages are higher and therefore are not likely to be starting families. In both rural and urban areas, White communities have a higher percentage of people who have reached retirement or will reach retirement in the next five to ten years. For this reason, the percentage of White Americans in the total population will continue to decline as the percentage of people of color and new immigrants increases.

In 2006, the Census Bureau reported that the nation's minority population totaled 98 million, or 33 percent of the total population of 296.4 million. In the current decade, Latinos, who number 42.7 million, became the second largest ethnic/racial group in the country, ahead of African Americans (39.7 million), Asians (14.4 million), American Indians and Alaska Natives (4.5 million), and native Hawaiians and other Pacific Islanders (990,000).

By 2006, 300, or 10 percent of the 3,000 counties in the United States also had majorities of color. With 7 million (71 percent of the total population), Los Angeles County had the largest population of color in the country.

Over the next twenty to thirty years, these dynamics will result in even more dramatic changes in the cultural mix of the country and every state. For example, demographers now project that by the year 2040, Latinos will be on the verge of becoming the majority population in California, the largest state in the nation. Around the same time, the United States will become a no-majority country, as no one single ethnic or racial group will be larger than 50 percent of the total population.

These statistics should allow you to understand why it is so critically important to take steps to increase your understanding of cultural diversity and to build your skills as a culturally humble CHW. And this is only taking into consideration race or ethnicity, and in the broadest terms: each of the categories of the Census Bureau includes a wide array of ancestral countries of origin, cultural backgrounds, tribal affiliations, customs, religions, or life experiences. Along with these demographic changes comes a rich linguistic diversity as well. It is estimated that there are between six and seven thousand languages spoken in the world. Multilingualism is an important consideration in working within the diversity around us.

Add to this rich diversity of cultures the differences emerging from life experiences and opportunities, such as poverty, political experience, and educational opportunity, and individual differences, such as gender identity, disability, family history, or sexual orientation.

HISTORIES OF DISCRIMINATION

Your ability to work effectively with diverse communities will also depend on your willingness to examine how larger societal practices influences health status. As CHWs, we must be ready to understand the impact of discrimination based on ethnicity, nationality, immigration status, sex, gender identity, sexual orientation, and other identities on the lives and health status of the clients and communities you work with.

Racial discrimination is an integral part of U.S. history. African Americans/Blacks, Latinos, American Indians, Pacific Islanders, and some Asian groups are disproportionately represented in the lower socioeconomic ranks of our multicultural society. Racial discrimination across generations has also meant that a greater majority of children of color attend lower-quality schools; more adults of color work in lower-paying jobs; and disproportionate percentages of Black and Latino males end up in our prison systems. Ultimately, racial discrimination results in higher rates of illness and lower life expectancy (see Chapter Six). The government and institutional policies that created these inequalities in the past and that sustain them in the present are referred to as structural racism. **Structural racism** means that inequities are built into the key systems of a society, such as the educational, legal, employment, housing, and health car systems.

Other groups in the United States have also experienced individual and **structural discrimination**. For example, women still experience unacceptable levels of domestic violence. In the workforce, they receive less pay and fewer opportunities for promotion and experience higher rates of sexual harassment. Structural discrimination still prohibits people from marrying their same-sex partners and discharges individuals from the military based on their sexual orientation. As a CHW, you will work with many clients who have experienced discrimination in their lives.

? *Can you think of other examples of structural racism or structural discrimination?*

? *How might structural discrimination have affected a client you are working with?*

? *Have you experienced structural discrimination?*

The field of public health itself harbors notorious instances of racism and other forms of discrimination, instances that have led some people to have a deep mistrust of the public health system. One of the most painful episodes of this kind involves a clinical study of the effects of untreated syphilis conducted on African Americans. In 1932, the Public Health Service, a branch of the U.S. government, carried out an infamous study known as the "Tuskegee Study of Untreated Syphilis in the Negro Male." This study focused on the effects of untreated syphilis among African American men in Macon County, Georgia. For more than forty years, African American men who had the disease were given a placebo (a treatment that the patient does not know is ineffective) for what they were told by the U.S. government was "bad blood." They were each given $50 to participate in the study, offered a decent burial when they died, and were under the impression that the treatment for "bad blood" was helpful. Even though in 1942 it was well known that penicillin could cure syphilis, it was never offered to the men in the study. As a result, many of the men died, and others were disabled.

The Tuskegee study was officially ended in 1972 after it was exposed and publicized by the media. However, the memory of this unethical study, a blatant form of racism, remains strong in many African American communities. On May 16, 1997, President Bill Clinton issued a formal apology on behalf of the nation to the family members of the men who took part in this study.

Another example is the role of the U.S. government in the sterilization of women in Puerto Rico. When the United States assumed governance of Puerto Rico in 1898, the U.S. government worried that overpopulation of the island would lead to disastrous social and economic conditions. In 1937, a law was passed to implement a "population control program."

Rather than providing Puerto Rican women with information and access to alternative forms of safe, legal, and reversible contraception, the U.S. government actively promoted the use of permanent sterilization through tubal ligation (tying off the fallopian tubes). Women were pushed toward having *la operacion* through door-to-door visits from health workers, with financial subsidies, and by favoritism toward sterilized women from industrial employers. Sterilization was not only provided by government clinics but also by factories where women provided cheap labor for overseas corporations. Rather than pay women maternity leave and benefits, factories did the calculations and found that by providing "operations" they would save millions of dollars.

Without informed consent, many women didn't understand that sterilization through tubal ligation was permanent. The phrase "tying the tubes" made women think the procedure was easily reversible. In 1936, 6.5 percent of Puerto Rican women had been sterilized. By 1953, 20 percent of women had had the operation, and by 1980, 30 percent had been sterilized. When word of this practice got out to the public, Puerto Rican community leaders and others were outraged.

Our government and health care institutions have a history of discriminating against many communities. Another example is the systematic discrimination that lesbian, gay, bisexual, transgender, and intersex (LGBTI) communities have experienced in health care, education, employment, and housing. Transgender communities lack civil rights protections at the federal level and in most states. When transgender and gender-variant people seek assistance from health professionals, their very identity may be pathologized and labeled as "gender identity disorder." Rather than providing transgender clients with the health care they seek, health professionals may diagnose their identity as an illness and, in some cases, have committed transgender clients against their will to mental wards or hospitals.

Actions such as these destroy public trust and create barriers between the communities who have experienced discrimination and our public health system. While you as a CHW don't have the power to undo history, you can work to ensure that gaps in your own knowledge, attitudes, and professional competencies do not cause further harm to your diverse clients.

? *What are your thoughts and feelings when you read about the government-sanctioned Tuskegee study or the sterilization of Puerto Rican women?*

? *How do you think these actions have affected Black and Puerto Rican communities?*

? *Are you aware of current structural or institutional injustices that harm people of color or other communities?*

? *How might these injustices influence your work as a CHW?*

? *How can you work to build trusting relationships with communities that have experienced such injustices?*

7.3 DEFINING AND UNDERSTANDING CULTURE

In essence, culture includes the beliefs, behaviors, attitudes, and practices that are learned, shared, and passed on by members of a particular group. Medical anthropologist C. G. Helman defines *culture* as:

> a set of guidelines, (both explicit and implicit) that individuals inherit as members of a particular society, and that tell them how to view the world, how to experience it emotionally, and how to behave in it in relation to other people, to supernatural forces and gods, and the natural environment. (Helman, 1994)

According to Judith Carmen Nine Curt (1984):

- Culture cannot be shed.
- Every cultural detail is incredibly old.
- Culture functions in "out-of-awareness."
- In order to understand others, we must first understand our own culture.
- Culture is better understood by observing and studying the cultures of others.
- Cultures are neither better nor worse, simply different.
- Every human being is bound by his or her culture.
- In order to be free from the hidden constraints of culture, we must study it.
- This study is new in our society and our educational world.
- Behind the differences among people, there are basic similarities, such as love, family, loyalty, friendship, joy, and the belief in transcendence.

Culture is not static—it doesn't stand still. It is dynamic, constantly changing and evolving with us. Culture is also multifaceted. It incorporates and includes ethnic identity, immigration status and experience, sexual orientation, gender identity, religion or spirituality, social class, family background, language, physical ability, traditions, and much more.

Keep in mind that it is not unusual for people to have more than one ethnic identity. For example, someone who has an African American father and an Asian mother may identify with both African American and Asian ethnic groups. But is this person's cultural identity based solely ethnic roots and traditions? Probably not. This same individual may have other cultural affiliations that she has stronger ties to than her ethnic identity (for example, gender identity, class status, immigration status). For example, an elderly, gay, Latino male potentially shares experiences with four different cultural groups. For this reason, it's important as CHWs to allow our clients to define their cultural identities for themselves.

Gender identity is an important cultural consideration. Simply stated, **gender identity** is someone's own sense of being female or male, both or neither, and what that means to him or her. Gender identity is an internal perception and may not be visibly apparent to others.

Culture and identity have many dimensions.

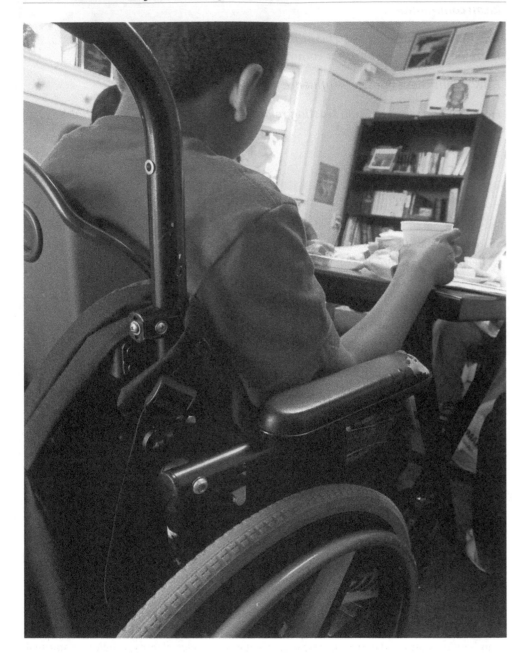

Social definitions of what it means to be a man and what it means to be a woman vary across cultures. Like racial stereotypes, gender stereotypes and assumptions can be deeply harmful.

? *Have you ever had someone ask you, "Where are you from?" or "What are you?"*

? *Have you ever had someone mistakenly assume one of your cultural identities?*

? *How did this make you feel?*

? *How did you react?*

?
> *How do you define your cultural identities?*

?
> *Does this change depending upon the circumstances?*

It may be tempting to review the anthropology and social science literature to gather descriptions of different cultures so that we can categorize our clients into one group or another. But there is no simple definition or set of categories we can refer to in order to easily understand our diverse clients and communities. Instead we must add culture (and cultural diversity) to the core professional competencies we work constantly to improve—like keeping up with technology. And we must always respect and support the right of the clients and communities with whom we work to define their own cultural identities.

7.4 BUILDING CULTURAL SELF-AWARENESS

Take a few minutes to answer the following questions.

1. What types of clients/communities do you think might have the greatest difficulties in accessing health or social services? Why?
2. What types of clients and communities do you lack experience with and knowledge about?
3. What types of clients or communities may you be less comfortable working with? Why?
4. How can you keep your personal attitudes and feelings from influencing the way you work with diverse clients?
5. What can you do to acknowledge your own stereotypes and prejudices? Why is this an important step to becoming an effective CHW?
6. Is it okay to be uncomfortable at times with clients of a particular cultural identity, or does this make you an unskilled CHW?
7. Is it okay to talk with your colleagues when you find that you are challenged in working with a client?
8. How can you learn to accept critical feedback about your work with diverse clients?

Now take a moment to reflect on your answers. Becoming aware of your own perceptions of others, your attitudes and behaviors, will aid you to work and live in a more culturally appropriate and sensitive manner. All of us have ideas and beliefs about people based on our upbringing and the prejudices that were passed on to us by our families.

Self-reflection is a powerful process through which to understand our own backgrounds and our own "hot-button issues"—the strong feelings, attitudes, and values that may arise during our work with others and that can have a negative influence on our ability to counsel a client effectively. Can you identify opportunities and areas for further learning? Are there communities that you are less comfortable working with and need to learn more about?

Taking the additional step of acknowledging when your group is the beneficiary of unearned privilege (for example, White people, males, heterosexuals, physically able) may be more challenging, because we are socialized to assume that our experiences are shared by others around us—that everyone has access to the same level of benefits enjoyed by all. It is hard to know what we don't know. Congratulate yourself on your willingness to see where you still have room to grow. Cultivating a high degree of self-awareness is the first major step in becoming a culturally effective CHW.

7.5 BUILDING CAPACITY AS CULTURALLY EFFECTIVE CHWs

Cultural and linguistic competence is defined as: a set of congruent behaviors, attitudes, and policies that come together in a system, agency, or among professionals that enables effective work in cross-cultural situations" (National Prevention Information Network, 2009).

By participating in ongoing education and training, you can learn about diverse cultures and skills for working effectively across cultures. Principles of cultural competence include the abilities to:

- Define culture broadly
- Value clients' cultural beliefs
- Recognize the importance and complexity of language interpretation
- Facilitate learning between providers and communities
- Involve the community in defining and addressing service needs
- Collaborate with other agencies
- Professionalize staff hiring and training
- Institutionalize cultural competency training and standards

A WORD OF CAUTION

Some cultural diversity and competency materials and trainings may do more harm than good. They teach seemingly definitive information about specific cultural groups. The assumption is that once people have learned about Mexican American (or other cultural group) culture and traditions related to health issues such as diet, death and dying, or sexuality, they will then *know* how to provide more sensitive or culturally competent services to members of that community. From our perspective, there are several key problems with this approach:

- It promotes the idea that human populations and cultures can be deeply and accurately understood by reading a few books or participating in a few trainings or another course of study.
- It essentializes culture by assuming that there is such a thing as *the* Mexican American culture or *the* Mexican American diet. In reality, there is tremendous diversity within Mexican American or Chicano cultures or Vietnamese or Italian American cultures, or within any other culture.
- It fails to recognize, honor, and appreciate the tremendous richness and complexity of what we call culture.
- It may foster the very stereotypes that have proven so harmful in the past.
- It focuses on knowing specific information about the cultures, beliefs, and customs of others rather than the process and interaction between providers such as CHWs and the clients and communities they serve.
- It ignores power differences between people of different identities or cultural backgrounds (such as a CHW and a client).
- It fails to focus our attention on our own cultural traditions, values, and beliefs, and how these may cause us, unintentionally, to make assumptions about the beliefs, values, feelings, and behaviors of others.

Though learning about different cultures can certainly strengthen your understanding of the communities you work with, *assuming that we understand or know something definitive about other cultures* can result in harm to our clients and communities. When we assume that we understand where others are coming from, we may fail to ask for or to listen to the information that they provide.

To illustrate, let's consider the following scenario. Your agency sends you to a training that focuses on the "Cultural Health Beliefs and Practices of the Hmong Community." The training is two days in length and exposes you to knowledgeable speakers, including doctors, CHWs, and anthropologists. They provide detailed information about Hmong history, culture, and customs and address the challenges Hmong immigrants face in the United States. You leave with a sense of having a solid understanding of the Hmong population and the most pressing health issues the community faces. There is a danger that the next time you encounter a Hmong client, you will assume to know a lot about her. You may not ask appropriate questions and fail to learn important information about the client and her health. As a result, the client may not receive an accurate assessment, relevant health education, case management services, or referrals from you.

While there is considerable value in knowing as much as possible about the cultures of the communities that you will work with, we should learn and apply this new information with the understanding that all clients are unique individuals with unique sets of circumstances. The cultural competency trainings that are available for health care professionals can be a useful part of the ongoing educational process, but they are just part of the lifelong journey of becoming a culturally humble CHW.

7.6 DEFINING CULTURAL HUMILITY

What is the difference between cultural competence and cultural humility?

According to Melanie Tervalon and Jane Murray-Garcia (1998), the primary difference between cultural competence and cultural humility is that

> cultural humility incorporates a lifelong commitment to self-evaluation and critique, to redressing the power imbalances in the physician-patient dynamic, and to developing mutually beneficial and non-paternalistic partnerships with communities on behalf of individuals and defined populations. (p. 123)

We prefer the concept of *cultural humility* as a guide for CHWs because of the emphasis it places on power relationships and understanding our own cultural identities first.

Cultural humility is about being flexible and humble enough to:

- Engage in self-reflection and self-critique, including reflection about our own assumptions and biases
- Understand that our own culture is no better than any other— all cultures deserve our respect
- Admit when we don't know about the culture and social context of our clients
- Seek out resources that may broaden our understanding of the various cultures of the communities and clients we serve
- Recognize that only the client is the expert about her own culture, values, and beliefs
- Place our assumptions aside when working with others, and ask clients and communities to share their own experiences, knowledge, resources, needs, and priorities with us so that we may best support their health and well-being

By practicing cultural humility with our clients, we build a welcoming and respectful working partnership. In this partnership, we recognize that we need to learn about the client's experience, culture, values, beliefs, and behaviors, and we remember that the way to do that is to ask and to listen deeply to what they tell us.

TRANSFERENCE OF POWER

An important component of cultural humility is a heightened awareness of the *transference of power* when clients work with caregivers. While this concept has mostly been applied to the physician/clinician and patient scenario, it has important implications for CHWs as well. Traditionally, during a health care appointment, the health care provider asks most of the questions and leads the appointment with what they think is most important to talk about and or ask about.

Reflect on your last appointment with your health care service provider:

- Who asked most of the questions?
- Were the questions the ones you wanted to answer in order to get to the problem and/ or issue at hand?
- Were you able to fully express yourself, or did you find the appointment limiting?

Changing our approach can make it possible for the visit to be client-centered and to support the client to take the lead in identifying the concerns that are most important to them. This is what is known as a *transference of power.* While some questions need to be asked to begin the client intake or interviewing session, we want to create an atmosphere that invites and supports the client to tell her story and assert her needs. This transference of power allows the client to be the expert and the CHW or other caregiver to be the student. This produces a powerful change in the caregiver-client dynamic.

How can the CHW facilitate this transference of power? Client-centered interviewing and counseling are the best approaches for changing the power dynamic. This is a skill based on the concept of cultural humility. Chapters Eight through Twelve provide detailed information about the client-centered approach, but let's start here by reviewing a particularly helpful model for interacting with clients.

Please note that several of the models introduced later in this chapter (the explanatory model, tools to elicit health beliefs, and the LEARN model) were developed to be used by physicians or other clinicians in health care settings. However, these tools and many of the questions may be adapted and used by CHWs to guide their work with clients.

THE EXPLANATORY MODEL

The explanatory model, developed by anthropologist Arthur Kleinman, is a client-focused health assessment that is respectful of the clients' views, perceptions, and definitions of *their* current concerns (Kleinman, 1980). Rather than imposing our own understanding of health conditions and related behavior, Kleinman recommends asking clients basic questions (what, why, how, and who) about their illness, to learn about their own experience and understanding.

Questions that may be used in the explanatory model include:

1. *What* do you call the problem?
2. *What* are the signs and symptoms of the illness that you are experiencing?
3. *What* are your concerns or fears?
4. *Why* do you think this illness or problem has occurred?
5. *How* does the illness affect you and your family?
6. *How* do you think the sickness should be treated?
7. *How* do want us to assist you?
8. *Who* do you turn to for assistance?
9. *Who* should be involved in decision making?

Interactive client interviewing techniques will enable clients to tell you about the primary issue at hand and assist you to understand how their cultural identities come into play.

Think about the following scenario with Luisa M.

CLIENT SCENARIO: LUISA M.

Luisa M. comes to your agency and you are the first one to see her. Luisa is a recently arrived immigrant from Honduras and currently works as a domestic helper during the day and at night she washes dishes at a restaurant. She has three children, all living with her mother in Honduras. She has limited English language proficiency, wants to take ESL classes, and thinks she might be pregnant.

In the client interview, you learn of the many facets of Luisa's life. Because Luisa tells you about what is most pressing for her at this time, you learn that she has an undocumented immigrant status and she is very fearful of being deported; she is also very worried about being unable to support her family back home. As result she has trouble sleeping at night and suffers from severe stomach aches. Finally, you learn that one of the reasons she left Honduras was to escape from a domestic violence situation and now has severe anxiety, which she refers to as *nervios* (nervousness).

You started the interview most concerned with her pregnancy and wanting to assist her with prenatal care; however the new information that you learned means that you will need to learn more about her *nervios,* whether she may be experiencing post-traumatic stress (PTS), and how her severe stomachaches may affect her prenatal nutritional plan.

If you practice cultural humility and view learning about a client's reality as part of your core competencies, a client will tell you what her multiple cultural identities are. Only she is qualified to tell you what is most important to her. Listening in a nonjudgmental and compassionate manner, as well as validating her, will be critical to establishing trust, learning what is really going on for her, and creating a positive encounter so that she will return for a follow-up visit.

WHAT IF YOU MAKE A MISTAKE?

Cultural humility is an approach that acknowledges the limits of our understanding and our tendency to make mistakes when working with clients. Consider this scenario:

A CHW is working with a client in a health education session. The client has diabetes and her health has been getting worse. The client is from a cultural group that is different from that of the CHW. Throughout the session the CHW is compassionate; however the client reacts negatively to the manner in which the CHW explains certain health information, particularly the information about healthy nutrition and eating. While the client doesn't say anything, the information the CHW presents is directly in conflict with the client's dietary traditions and family practices. The client feels that the CHW is trying to change her diet and doesn't understand or respect her traditions. Visibly offended and upset, the client leaves the session early.

(Continued)

Afterward, the CHW spends time thinking about what happened with the client, and talks with his supervisor. Through an examination of the session, the CHW and the supervisor determine that it is likely that the client was offended. The CHW realizes that he did not take time to ask the client about her own dietary beliefs and practices before presenting her with guidelines for a healthy diet, and is committed to doing so when working with future clients.

The CHW demonstrated cultural humility by acknowledging and desiring to learn about the problem, by acknowledging his mistake, and seeking to improve his skills. In this case, the CHW is "flexible and humble enough to then re-assess a new the cultural dimensions of the experiences of each client" (Tervalon and Murray-Garcia, 1998).

? *Have you ever been offended by assumptions that a health care or social services provider made about you or a family member?*

? *What else could you do to demonstrate cultural humility in working with the clients described above?*

7.7 UNDERSTANDING CULTURAL HEALTH BELIEFS

Every cultural group has its own beliefs, values, and practices related to health issues, such as pregnancy and birth, death and dying, gender roles, familial responsibility, disease causation, religion and spirituality, traditional healing, and alternative healing practices. Your cultural group is no exception to this rule.

? *What are the health beliefs in your family or culture?*

? *Where did your family go to receive health care?*

? *What were the home remedies for illnesses?*

? *How were they used?*

? *What do you still practice today?*

? *Were there health topics or issues that were considered "taboo" or were forbidden to discuss?*

Earlier we discussed why CHWs must exercise caution and not generalize or stereotype about people from any cultural groups. Yet CHWs must still acknowledge and appreciate that individuals are indeed members of one or more cultural groups and may hold values rooted in those cultures. As CHWs, our goal should be to bring an open mind and to listen deeply to "where the client is coming from."

TOOL TO ELICIT HEALTH BELIEFS IN CLINICAL ENCOUNTERS

Arthur Kleinman's Tool to Elicit Health Beliefs in Clinical Encounters is an excellent resource for working with a client to define a health belief (Kleinman, 1980). Though it was developed to inform the work of nurses, physicians, and other clinicians, Kleinman's tool is also applicable to the work of CHWs.

1. What do you call your problem? What name does it have?
2. What do you think caused your problem?
3. Why do you think it started when it did?
4. What does your sickness do to you? How does it work?
5. How severe is it? Will it have a short or long course?
6. What do you fear most about your sickness?
7. What are the chief problems that your sickness has caused for you?
8. What kind of treatment do you think you should receive?
9. What are the most important results you hope to receive from the treatment?

CHWs are not expected or required to be experts about the cultural health beliefs of their diverse clients. Rather, as a regular part of their practice, CHWs learn about these beliefs from their clients. Clients will answer these or any other questions based on their own belief systems, attitudes, and values.

THE LEARN MODEL

Another useful model when working with diverse clients is the LEARN model of Cross Cultural Encounter Guidelines for Health Practitioners (Berlin and Fowkes, 1983):

LEARN:
L: listen with sympathy and understanding to the client's perception of the problem
E: explain your perceptions of the problem
A: acknowledge and discuss the differences and similarities between the perceptions of the client and the CHW
R: recommend resources
N: negotiate agreement

The LEARN model acknowledges cultural health beliefs held by the client and allows for CHWs to share what they know about a specific health condition. Neither perception is negated or devalued, and both are acknowledged and incorporated into the session. Both are taken into consideration as clients choose a course of action to promote their health.

As CHWs engage with their clients in this fashion, they are aiding their clients to preserve their own cultural health belief systems. Remember, however, that what may be true about some or most individuals from a particular cultural group, region, or country may not be true of all people who come from the same background. According to the *Provider's Guide to Quality and Culture* (Management Sciences for Health, 2009), as you work with diverse clients, keep the following in mind:

- ✪ People from rural areas may have been living a more traditional lifestyle than people who have been living in urban areas.
- ✪ Economic status and education vary greatly among people within a cultural group or people who come from the same country.
- ✪ People from the same country may have migrated to the United States for very different reasons, including seeking economic opportunity, escaping religious or ethnic persecution, fleeing civil strife, or joining relatives in America.
- ✪ Generational differences may exist among people of different ages within the same cultural group and may include different belief systems.

TRADITIONAL HEALTH PRACTICES

Given that 40 percent of the U.S. population are new immigrants or the children of immigrants, many people have recent experiences with traditional healing methods. Traditional health practices are different from the biomedical or Western medicine approaches used by nurses, physicians, and other health care providers in clinics and hospitals in the United States. Biomedical approaches are commonly said to focus more on treating disease than promoting health. Interestingly, many of today's biomedical treatments for disease are derived from traditional healing practices throughout the world, though this is not widely understood or acknowledged. Traditional health practices are often discounted or viewed as dangerous by Western medical providers. However, the recognition of traditional health practices is growing in the United States in two ways:

1. *Alternative medicine.* Traditional health practices are used instead of Western medicine (in the United States, the medical profession classifies any health practice that is different from its own biomedical model as "alternative"). Examples of alternative medicine are the use of acupuncture to treat asthma and the use of a special diet and herbs to treat cancer instead of being treated with radiation or chemotherapy.

2. *Complementary medicine.* In this approach, Western or biomedical practices are integrated and provided along with one or more other health traditions (such as Ayurvedic, chiropractic, acupuncture, or Chinese medicine). Some medical schools and hospitals in the United States are beginning to recognize and support complimentary medicine.

? *What traditional health practices are you familiar with?*

? *Do you know of clinics or hospitals in your area that practice complimentary medicine?*

? *What has your experience been with biomedical and alternative medical traditions?*

The following scenarios illustrate how traditional healing practices or cultural health beliefs may affect the care provided by health institutions.

*   A young Cambodian mother brings her eight-year-old daughter to a health center with a fever and bad cough. Upon the physical examination, the clinician discovers multiple red marks across the child's chest and back. The clinician could mistake this as a sign of parental child abuse. However, it is not. The mother practices "coining," a traditional, common practice in Southeast Asia. Coining entails rubbing heated oil on the skin and vigorously rubbing a coin over the area in a linear fashion until a red mark is seen. This is used to allow a path by which a "bad wind" can be released from the body. People use this method to treat a variety of minor ailments, including fever, chills, headache, colds, and cough.

*   At a hospital, the nursing staff alerts a doctor about a patient who is agitated. The nurses want the doctor to order medication to calm the patient down, since he does not want to stay in bed. He is an elderly Japanese man who became upset and "uncooperative" because his bed was situated in the direction used to lay out the deceased in traditional Japan.

* A patient is seen at a health clinic for persistent, abdominal pain. The clinician suspects a stomach ulcer, prescribes medication, and sends the patient to speak with the CHW about following a new dietary regimen, eating several small meals throughout the day to minimize stomach acid buildup and pain. As the CHW explains the diet prescribed by the doctor, the patient remains quiet and appears uninterested. Finally, at the end of the session, the CHW asks if he has any questions. The man doesn't have any questions, but states that he is Muslim, this is Ramadan, and he cannot follow the prescribed diet. Ramadan is the ninth month of the Islamic lunar calendar, and every day during this month, Muslims around the world spend the daylight hours in a complete fast. Muslims abstain from food, drink, and other physical needs during the daylight hours as a time to purify the soul, refocus attention on God, and practice self-sacrifice.

Having the awareness and sensitivity to work effectively with diverse people is a critical skill for the twenty-first century. CHWs often play a vital role in aiding clients to access alternative or complimentary medicine and to advocate for these choices with Western or biomedical providers. As cultural brokers who build "bridges" between poor and underserved communities and health care providers, CHWs can play a role in assisting to foster a mutually respectful and cooperative partnership between biomedical providers and providers of other traditions.

7.8 ROLES AND RESPONSIBILITIES OF CULTURALLY EFFECTIVE CHWS

In Chapter One, you read about the core roles of CHWs. Here, we look at those roles again and provide an example or idea for how to apply cultural humility. As you read, think of examples of your own.

1. Cultural mediation between communities and health and social services systems:
   - Share cultural information about your clients with their clinical providers. Inform them about any cultural needs, practices, attitudes, or beliefs that affect the client's health or treatment, as well as any economic issues and political factors. This will allow these providers to understand and treat their clients and patients more effectively.
   - *What else might you do, in your role as cultural mediator?*

2. Providing direct services and referrals:
   - As you provide services, ask yourself if the questions or suggestions you provide are culturally biased. For example, when you ask questions about diet, are you referring to the diet of a particular culture or culture? Are your questions inclusive?
   - Be familiar with resources in the community that are culturally or linguistically appropriate. Assist your clients in navigating the system in the best way possible for them. Know which languages are spoken at various agencies for your clients who have limited English proficiency.
   - *What else might you do, in your role providing services and referrals?*

3. Providing culturally appropriate health education and information:
   - Participate in local cultural events and opportunities to increase your knowledge and cultural humility skills.
   - Support clients to understand their health and medical care by providing easy-to-understand health advising and health education materials in the appropriate language and literacy level. Don't assume everyone can read.
   - Create a checklist to guide you in providing health education. For example, did you remember to ask the client how she understands her illness? Did you acknowledge his cultural traditions respectfully? Did you avoid professional jargon and technical words that the client may not understand?
   - *What else might you do while providing health education and information?*

4. Advocating for individual and community needs:
   - Are providers in your agency communicating in a culturally and linguistically appropriate fashion? If not, advocate for a continuing education training so that staff can learn more effective ways of communicating with the clients and assist them to better understand the cultural beliefs, attitudes, and norms of the people they serve.
   - Advocate for your agency to expand its capacity to provide services in multiple languages and to use qualified health care interpreters.
   - Advocate for agency forms to be changed to be inclusive of lesbian, gay, bisexual, transgender, and intersex identities.
   - *What else might you do to advocate for your clients' and communities' cultural needs?*

5. Assuring that people get the services they need:
   - By welcoming all clients, putting your cultural assumptions aside, and inviting them to share their experiences, knowledge, concerns, and questions, you will form a positive alliance intended to promote their health and link them with necessary services. Be patient. Learn to take the client's lead.
   - Learn to work with qualified interpreters.
   - *What else might you do to address culture issues that come between people and the care they really need?*

6. Building individual and community capacity:
   - Invite community members to provide input into the design of the services you provide. Facilitate a focus group to determine, for example, if community is comfortable with the idea of support groups, or would social events be a better way to build mutual support? Adapt your ideas to what will work for *this* community.
   - Work with community members to learn new skills—such as how to conduct a community diagnosis—that will enhance their capacity to take action to promote their own health.
   - *What else might come up as you work to build individual and community capacity? How might you address those cultural differences effectively?*

CULTURAL DIVERSITY: IT'S PERSONAL, IT'S PROFESSIONAL, AND IT'S RIGHT

Cultural diversity is not something to tolerate but to embrace and celebrate. Diversity brings richness to our society and keeps our work as CHWs fascinating, dynamic, and rewarding.

As you continue with your training and your career, remember to keep an open mind and an open heart. Respect and honor the differences of the clients and communities you have the opportunity to work with. Demonstrate compassion and nonjudgmentalism along the way.

CHWs continue to participate in trainings to advance their skills in working across cultures.

How does race politics impact public health & the work of CHWs?

Tonight's Agenda

6:10 • Attendance
6:15 • Worksheet #2
6:30 • 'Angela Story'
6:40 • Review CHW skills
7:00 • BREAK
7:10 • Cultural Humility
7:20 • Video "AIDS in the Barrio"

Go ahead and take risks, expand your understanding of what cultural diversity means, ask the hard questions of yourself, challenge yourself to look at and question your own bias and assumptions! Acknowledge your own limitations and mistakes. At times you may not be comfortable in this journey. But the very moments when you are most uncomfortable may be your greatest opportunities for personal and professional growth.

CHAPTER REVIEW

As in any other area of professional development (the process of learning new or enhancing existing professional knowledge and skills), building our capacity to practice cultural humility requires planning. The following questions and strategies for learning are based on a suggested approach from California Tomorrow's *Change Starts with the Self* (Chang, Femenella, Louie, Murdock, and Pell, 2000). Spend some time answering the preliminary questions. Then identify steps you will take to strengthen your knowledge and skills over the next three to six months.

1. What three strengths do I bring to this work on cultural humility? In what ways could I build on these strengths?

2. What three gaps (or challenges) do I want to work on?

3. Did any data, discussions, definitions, principles, or questions in this chapter provoke a strong emotional reaction for me? What are those feelings? What can I do to respond to my feelings in a way that honors my own experiences and perspectives and at the same time assists me to understand and honor the experiences or perspectives that are provoking those feelings?

4. Over the next six months to a year, what activities could I undertake to strengthen my capacity to work across differences of race, class, culture, and language?

● Read the following books or articles: _____
_____

● View the following films or videos (in fictional movies, look especially for movies made *by* members of a culture, *about* their own culture): _____
_____

● Meet with and discuss these issues with:
_____

- Attend a lecture or presentation on: _____
  _____

- Participate in the following training or work-shops: _____
  _____

- Participate in the following cross-cultural community events: _____
  _____

- Join or organize a small discussion or study group focused on: _____
  _____

- Volunteer with the following organization that promotes or organizes cross-cultural work in my community: _____
  _____

- Join or support the work of the following organization that advocates or organizes for the cultural diversity or equity concerns of a group that is marginalized or discriminated against in my community:_____
  _____

- Other activities:_____
  _____

5. What resources would I draw on to assist me in these activities? Who can I go to in my orga-nization or agency to seek support and guidance in carrying out my learning plan? Which friends, family members, and colleagues do I feel most comfortable talking with about these issues, and why?

I will sit down again on the following date to evalu-ate my progress and development and to update my learning plan.

REFERENCES

Berlin, E. A., and Fowkes, W. C. Jr. 1983. A Teaching Frame-work for Cross-Cultural Health Care—Application in Family Practice, in Cross-Cultural Medicine. *Western Journal of Medicine* 139: 934–938. Accessed on April 12, 2009: http://www.pubmedcentral.nih.gov/picrender.fcgi?artid= 1011028&blobtype=pdf

Chang, H. N.-L., Femella, T. S., Louie, N., Murdock, B., and Pell, E. 2000. *Walking the Walk: Principles for Building Community Capacity for Equity and Diversity: Accompanying Tool Change Starts with the Self.* Oakland, CA: California Tomorrow.

Helman, C. G. 1994. *Culture, Health and Illness.* Oxford: Butterworth-Heinemann.

Kleinman, A. 1980. *Patients and Healers in the Context of Culture: An Exploration of the Borderland Between Anthropology, Medicine, and Psychiatry.* Berkeley, CA: University of California Press.

Management Sciences for Health. Provider's Guide to Quality and Culture. Accessed on April 12, 2009: http://erc.msh.org.

National Prevention Information Network. Cultural Competence. Accessed on April 12, 2009: www .cdcnpin.org.

Nine Curt, C. J. 1984. *Non-Verbal Communication in Puerto Rico* (2nd ed.). Cambridge, MA: Assessment and Dissemination Center.

Takaki, R. 1993. *A Different Mirror.* New York: Little, Brown.

Tervalon, M., and Murray-Garcia, J. 1998, May. Cultural Humility Versus Cultural Competence: A Critical Distinction in Defining Physician Training Outcomes in Multicultural Education. *Journal of Health Care for the Poor and Underserved* 9(2):117–125.

ADDITIONAL RESOURCES

Henry, W. A. III. 1990, April 9. Beyond the Melting Pot. *Time.*

CHW Skills and Core Competencies: Working with Clients

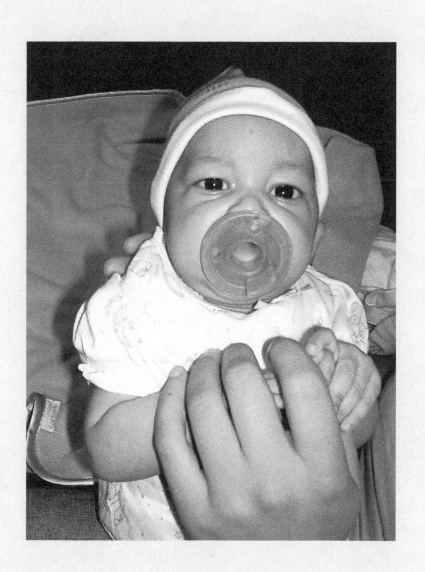

8

Guiding Principles for Working with Individual Clients

Tim Berthold • Edith Guillén- Nuñez

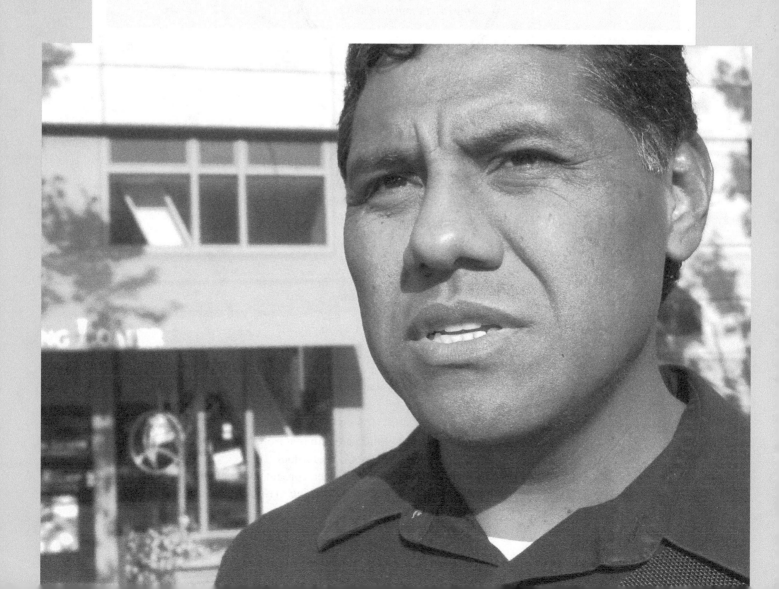

As a CHW, you will have many questions about your role, the services you should or should not provide to clients, and how best to facilitate their health without doing harm to them or others. Typical questions may include:

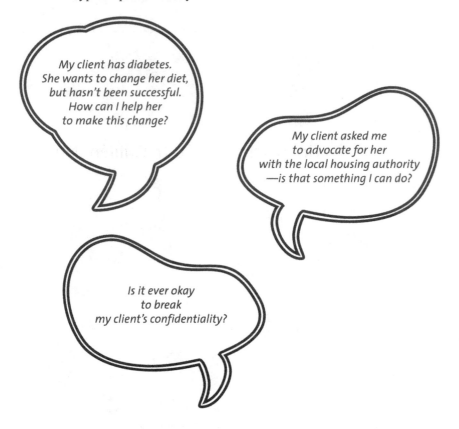

INTRODUCTION

Part Two of this textbook addresses the competencies that CHWs use when working with individual clients. Chapter Eight presents five guiding principles that shape all the work you may do with individual clients, including:

- Ethical guidelines
- Self-awareness
- Scope of practice
- Understanding behavior change
- Client-centered practice

WHAT YOU WILL LEARN

By studying the information in this chapter, you will be able to do the following:

Ethics

- Define *ethics* and explain how ethics are different from laws
- Discuss key articles in the AACHW Code of Ethics
- Apply ethical guidelines relating to informed consent and confidentiality
- Use the Framework for Ethical Decision Making to resolve ethical questions

Self-Awareness

- ✪ Define *self-awareness*
- ✪ Explain the importance of self-awareness to the work of CHWs
- ✪ Identify three or more activities that you can use to increase self-awareness

Scope of Practice

- ✪ Define *scope of practice*
- ✪ Identify competencies that may lie within and outside the scope of practice of CHWs
- ✪ Discuss competencies that may sometimes lie within and sometimes outside the CHW scope of practice
- ✪ Explain the potential consequences of working outside of the CHW scope of practice
- ✪ Respond appropriately and effectively when confronted with a challenge regarding your scope of practice as a CHW

Understanding Behavior Change

- ✪ Identify behaviors that clients may wish to change
- ✪ Apply the ecological model to analyzing individual, family, community, and societal factors that influence behavior and behavior change
- ✪ Discuss and analyze four common mistakes that CHWs make when supporting clients to change behaviors

Client-Centered Practice

- ✪ Discuss the central concepts of client-centered practice
- ✪ Explain the value of working from client strengths
- ✪ Discuss implicit theory and how you will develop your own implicit theories of behavior change

WORDS TO KNOW

Ethics	Professional Boundaries	Boundary Crossing
Dual or Multiple Relationships	Treatment Adherence or Compliance	Relapse
	Media Advocacy	
External Resources	Internal Resources	
Informed Consent	Confidentiality	

8.1 ETHICAL GUIDELINES FOR CHWs

INTRODUCTION

This section presents ethical guidelines for CHWs, drawing on a range of sources, including the Code of Ethics newly developed by the American Association of Community Health Workers (AACHW). We will highlight several key ethical issues and present a framework for ethical decision making. As you read the ethical guidelines presented here, keep in mind that they are meant to be a resource and a guide to standards of conduct and practice in the profession. However, they do not provide an answer for every dilemma you will encounter. Consult your supervisor for additional information, including relevant laws, that will govern your conduct in the program, agency, and state where you are working.

DEFINING ETHICS

Ethical standards provide guidance for professionals regarding "right conduct," and what to do when faced with a challenge or dilemma. Most professions establish a code of ethics in an attempt to standardize behavior and professional accountability.

COMMON ETHICAL CHALLENGES

CHWs are motivated by a deep and abiding commitment to promoting the health and welfare of the clients and communities with whom they work. No CHW wants to cause harm to their clients. Sometimes, however, CHWs face professional situations in which it isn't clear how to achieve these goals and what course of action to take. Examples of these ethical challenges include:

- Your supervisor assigns you to provide a service that you haven't been adequately trained to provide. What should you do?
- A homeless client with two children is late for an important medical appointment. They have no money to get to their appointment. Can you give them money for a bus ticket? Or take them to the appointment in your car? What should you do?
- A client with HIV disease informs you that she hasn't disclosed her HIV status to her partners, and she is continuing to have unprotected sex. One of these partners is also a client. What should you do?
- A former client asks you out on a date. You are single, available, and interested. What should you do?
- You observe a coworker using drugs on the job. What should you do?
- A client offers to loan you $3 so you can take the bus home. You forgot your wallet, and could definitely use a loan. What should you do?
- A client reports that her boyfriend has been beating her and threatening to hurt her children. She doesn't want anyone else to know. What should you do?

ETHICS AND VALUES

How you decide to handle an ethical dilemma will be influenced by your values. Values are beliefs and attitudes about what matters in life. Values vary from individual to individual and are influenced by culture, community, family upbringing, personal experiences, and society. Values guide the decisions we make every day, including how we treat others.

Examples of values that are at the core of the work that CHWs perform include honesty, respect, integrity, open-mindedness, self-determination, acceptance, trust, and tolerance.

At times, however, the personal values of CHWs may be in direct conflict with the values of clients and the ethical guidelines of the profession. Knowing your own values is a tremendous resource for identifying and resolving these potential conflicts.

ETHICS AND THE LAW

Ethics and the law are integrally related, yet distinct.

Ethics is about doing what is morally right. Codes of ethics attempt to standardize professional behavior and accountability. They are designed to inform clients and the public about the types of services they can expect to receive from professionals, and to ensure that clients are protected from inappropriate conduct or abuse from professionals. Typically, codes of ethics address issues such as informed consent, confidentiality, professional training, protections against discrimination, and maintaining clear professional boundaries with clients.

Laws are established by governments to prevent and punish behavior that is destructive to a society's well-being. Laws define the minimal standards that a society will tolerate that are enforced by government (Corey, Corey, and Callanan, 2007). Laws include statutes, regulations, agency policies and procedures, and court decisions and may be local (city laws), state, federal (national), or international. The consequences of breaking a law tend to be more severe than a violation of a professional code of ethics. For example, the penalty for breaking the law can include imprisonment, whereas the penalty for violation of a professional code of ethics may include being fired from your job or barred from future employment in your field. Keep in mind that violations of the law and of the professional code of ethics can impact your reputation and relationship with your colleagues, community, clients, and ultimately yourself. Additionally, violations of ethical guidelines are sometimes also legal violations. For example, if you break the confidentiality of a client by disclosing her HIV positive status to another without written consent, you are violating both your ethical guidelines and laws that protect the privacy of people with HIV disease.

Chapters One and Two of this book explained that the CHW profession in the United States is still in the process of seeking formal recognition, status, and financing mechanisms. The first truly national organization for CHWs has only recently been established. This organization, the American Association of Community Health Worker (AACHW), has developed the field's first formal code of ethics. The AACHW acknowledges that these ethical guidelines are new and may undergo further refinement over time.

THE AMERICAN ASSOCIATION OF COMMUNITY HEALTH WORKERS CODE OF ETHICS

CODE OF ETHICS FOR CHWs

A Community Health Worker (CHW) is a frontline public health worker who is a trusted member of and/or has an unusually close understanding of the community she or he serves. This trusting relationship enables the CHW to serve as a liaison/link/intermediary between health/social services and the community to facilitate access to services and improve the quality and cultural competence of service delivery. A CHW also builds individual and community capacity by increasing health knowledge and self-sufficiency through a range of activities such as outreach, community education, informal counseling, social support, and advocacy.

Purpose of This Code

The CHW Code of Ethics is based on and supported by the core values adopted by the American Association of CHWs. The Code of Ethics outlined in this document provides a framework for CHWs, supervisors, and employers of CHWs to discuss ethical issues facing the profession. Employers are encouraged to consider this Code when creating CHW programs. The responsibility of all CHWs is to strive for excellence by providing quality service and the most accurate information available to individuals, families, and communities.

(Continued)

The Code of Ethics is based upon commonly understood principals that apply to all professionals within the health and social service fields (e.g., promotion of social justice, positive health, and dignity). The Code, however, does not address all ethical issues facing CHWs and the absence of a rule does not imply that there is no ethical obligation present. As professionals, CHWs are encouraged to reflect on the ethical obligations that they have to the communities that they serve, and to share these reflections with others.

Article 1. Responsibilities in the Delivery of Care

CHWs build trust and community capacity by improving the health and social welfare of the clients they serve. When a conflict arises among individuals, groups, agencies, or institutions, CHWs should consider all issues and give priority to those that promote the wellness and quality of living for the individual/client. The following provisions promote the professional integrity of CHWs.

1.1 Honesty

CHWs are professionals that strive to ensure the best health outcomes for the communities they serve. They communicate the potential benefits and consequences of available services, including the programs they are employed under.

1.2 Confidentiality

CHWs respect the confidentiality, privacy, and trust of individuals, families, and communities that they serve. They understand and abide by employer policies, as well as state and federal confidentiality laws that are relevant to their work.

1.3 Scope of Ability and Training

CHWs are truthful about qualifications, competencies, and limitations on the services they may provide, and should not misrepresent qualifications or competencies to individuals, families, communities, or employers.

1.4 Quality of Care

CHWs strive to provide high quality service to individuals, families, and communities. They do this through continued education, training, and an obligation to ensure the information they provide is up-to-date and accurate.

1.5 Referral to Appropriate Services

CHWs acknowledge when client issues are outside of their scope of practice and refer clients to the appropriate health, wellness, or social support services when necessary.

1.6 Legal Obligations

CHWs have an obligation to report actual or potential harm to individuals within the communities they serve to the appropriate authorities. Additionally, CHWs have a responsibility to follow requirements set by states, the federal government, and/or their employing organizations. Responsibility to the larger society or specific legal obligations may supersede the loyalty owed to individual community members.

Article 2. Promotion of Equitable Relationships

CHWs focus their efforts on the well-being of the whole community. They value and respect the expertise and knowledge that each community member possesses. In turn, CHWs strive to create equitable partnerships with communities to address all issues of health and well-being.

2.1 Cultural Humility

CHWs possess expertise in the communities in which they serve. They maintain a high degree of humility and respect for the cultural diversity within each community. As advocates for their communities, CHWs have an obligation to inform employers and others when policies and procedures will offend or harm communities, or are ineffective within the communities where they work.

2.2 Maintaining the Trust of the Community

CHWs are often members of their communities and their effectiveness in providing services derives from the trust placed in them by members of these communities. CHWs do not act in ways that could jeopardize the trust placed in them by the communities they serve.

2.3 Respect for Human Rights

CHWs respect the human rights of those they serve, advance principles of self-determination, and promote equitable relationships with all communities.

2.4 Anti-Discrimination

CHWs do not discriminate against any person or group on the basis of race, ethnicity, gender, sexual orientation, age, religion, social status, disability, or immigration status.

2.5 Client Relationships

CHWs maintain professional relationships with clients. They establish, respect, and actively maintain personal boundaries between them and their clients.

Article 3. Interactions With Other Service Providers

CHWs maintain professional partnerships with other service providers in order to serve the community effectively.

3.1 Cooperation

CHWs place the well-being of those they serve above personal disagreements and work cooperatively with any other person or organization dedicated to aiding provide care to those in need.

(Continued)

3.2 Conduct

CHWs promote integrity in the delivery of health and social services. They respect the rights, dignity, and worth of all people and have an ethical obligation to report any inappropriate behavior (e.g., sexual harassment, racial discrimination, etc.) to the proper authority.

3.3 Self-Presentation

CHWs are truthful and forthright in presenting their background and training to other service providers.

Article 4. Professional Rights and Responsibilities

The CHWs profession is dedicated to excellence in the practice of promoting well-being in communities. Guided by common values, CHWs have the responsibility to uphold the principles and integrity of the profession as they assist families to make decisions impacting their well-being. CHWs embrace individual, family, and community strengths and build upon them to increase community capacity.

4.1 Continuing Education

CHWs should remain up-to-date on any developments that substantially affect their ability to competently render services. CHWs strive to expand their professional knowledge base and competencies through education and participation in professional organizations.

4.2 Advocacy for Change in Law and Policy

CHWs are advocates for change and work on impacting policies that promote social justice and hold systems accountable for being responsive to communities.

DISCUSSION OF KEY ETHICAL CONCEPTS

There are certain ethical issues and concepts that CHWs frequently encounter in the course of their work. These include informed consent, confidentiality, and maintaining healthy professional boundaries.

Informed Consent   Informed consent is related to Article 1.1 Honesty and Article 3.3 Self-Presentation in the AACHW Code of Ethics. **Informed consent** is the obligation to provide clients with all the information they need in order to make a sound decision about whether or not to participate in a program, service, or research study. This should include information about anything that could be potentially difficult for or harmful to the client including issues of cost, insurance, expectations, program requirements for participation, limitations of program services, and confidentiality.

One of the reasons we highlight informed consent as an ethical issue is because there is a long history of failing to fully inform clients about the services they are receiving, and of coercing clients into services they may not be interested in. Notorious examples include the Tuskegee Syphilis Trials and programs that sterilized Puerto Rican women, discussed in Chapter Seven.

Policies that advance public health and well-being enable CHWs to provide better care for the communities they serve.

4.3 Enhancing Community Capacity

CHWs assist individuals and communities move toward self-sufficiency in order to promote the creation of opportunities and resources that support their autonomy.

4.4 Wellness and Safety

CHWs are sensitive to their own personal well-being (physical, mental, and spiritual health) and strive to maintain a safe environment for themselves and the communities they serve.

4.5 Loyalty to the Profession

CHWs are loyal to the profession and aim to advance the efforts of other CHWs worldwide.

4.6 Advocacy for the Profession

CHWs are advocates for the profession. They are members, leaders, and active participants in local, state, and national professional organizations.

4.7 Recognition of Others

CHWs give recognition to others for their professional contributions and achievements.

Informed consent is an ongoing responsibility of CHWs. We recommend that you review the informed consent policies used by the programs you work for. Is all relevant information shared with clients in order to assist them in deciding whether or not to participate in services? Is the information presented in a way that your clients can understand? Is the same information provided to clients who speak languages other than English? If not, the ethical principle of informed consent has been devalued.

Confidentiality   Article 1.2 of the AACHW Code of Ethics addresses confidentiality. **Confidentiality** protects a client's communication with a CHW and forms an essential component in building a trusting and productive professional relationship. Unless clients are confident that the CHW will not disclose their information to others, they will be reluctant to share personal information.

SERGIO MATOS: Our access to communities is based on trust. We can't betray that trust. That trust defines us and it defines our role in these communities. And we're not at liberty to betray that trust for program goals or any other reason.

CHWs should address issues of confidentiality and its limits with new clients before services begin or before clients have an opportunity to disclose personal and intimate information. This should include an explicit discussion of the exceptions that would cause the CHW to "break" a client's confidentiality and report private information to others, including a supervisor and legal authorities such as the police or local child protection services. It is essential for CHWs to explain confidentiality and its limits using clear and accessible language, and to make sure that clients understand the concept and policy before addressing other topics in detail.

RAMONA BENSON: I had this big problem when I was starting out as a CHW, because some of my clients would say things to other providers, things that they thought were private, and then the provider would say: "I'm a mandated reporter. I have to report that to the authorities." That is the wrong way to handle things, especially with the ladies I work with. They have experienced so much racism and discrimination that it is already hard for them to trust people—and I know why! So when I start working with a client at the Black Infant Health Program, I always tell them up front what the rules are and what kind of information I will have to report to others. They have a right to know, and it's a matter of respect.

In general, CHWs do not share private information about their clients with others, including the client's identity (such as the client's name or Social Security number), unless the client provides written consent. However, there are several important exceptions to this rule that limit a CHW's ability to keep a client's information private. If clients disclose information about harm or the threat of harm to themselves or others, CHWs may have an ethical or legal obligation to report this to a third party, such as their supervisor, the local department of human services (such as a child protective services or elder abuse division), or the police. The types of harms that could require a breach of confidentiality include, for example, physical and sexual abuse and suicide. In such circumstances, CHWs have an ethical obligation not only to the client, but to anyone who may be harmed. This ethical obligation requires them to report the harm or threat of harm in order to protect the safety and health of the victim or potential victim.

When CHWs face a situation in which they must break the confidentiality of a client, we recommend that you consider if and how you may be able to involve the client in the reporting process. This can aid in preserving a positive working relationship between the client and the CHW. The decision about whether or not to participate, of course, must be left to the client. In cases of mandated reporting, it is important that the CHW fully and accurately understand the consequences of such reporting and be prepared to discuss these with the client. When necessary (or possible) the CHW may seek supervisory support in these situations.

Consider the case of a CHW working at a health clinic serving youths (see the featured example).

This is a highly challenging situation. In the example provided, the CHW clearly explained the rules of confidentiality and its limits and took time to listen to the client's questions, concerns, and feelings. The CHW also provided the client with several choices and supported her decisions. Ultimately, the CHW and the client acted together to report the sexual abuse to the authorities and to contact additional resources (the rape crisis center).

ETHICS AND THE LIMITS OF CONFIDENTIALITY

At the clinic, multiple signs are clearly posted explaining the limits of confidentiality. The CHW begins all client sessions by reviewing the limits of confidentiality and describing the types of information that cannot legally be kept private, including physical and sexual abuse and intended suicide.

After discussing the limits of confidentiality, a fifteen-year-old female client discloses that she is being sexually abused by her stepfather. Legally and ethically, the CHW has a clear duty to report this information to local law enforcement authorities. Despite having discussed the limits of confidentiality previously, the client begs the CHW not to make a report: the client is scared about what her stepfather and mother might do.

The CHW listens to the client's experience and concerns, and offers validation and support. The CHW then explains the duty to report the sexual abuse to the police. The CHW emphasizes concern for the client's safety and welfare. The CHW also explains why it would be wrong not to make a report: they have an obligation to do everything they can to protect clients from harm. Failing to report the abuse could send a message to the client that she shouldn't talk about what is happening to her or that the sexual abuse is acceptable or somehow doesn't matter.

The CHW calmly explains the need to call the police immediately, and asks the client if she would like to make the call or to wait with the CHW and speak with authorities at the clinic. The client is also free to leave, although she and her parents will be contacted later by the police. The client decides to listen in on the call to the police. The CHW also asks the client if she would like to call the local rape crisis center and explains the type of services they offer. The client calls the local rape crisis center with the CHW, explains what is happening, and asks for a rape crisis counselor to come to the clinic to be her advocate when she speaks with the police. Throughout this process it is important to assess the client's safety and make an appropriate plan to prevent further harm to her or others.

While the situation was stressful for the client, providing her with choices also aided in giving back to her a measure of control. This is an important feature of working with victims of trauma. It is also a central feature of client-centered practice, discussed below.

? *What do you think of the way in which the CHW handled this situation?*

? *Is there anything else you would want to do?*

? *Anything you would want to do differently?*

Establishing and Maintaining Professional Boundaries Establishing and maintaining appropriate professional boundaries allows CHWs to better protect the welfare of clients, themselves, employers, and the community. Examples of professional boundary issues are: a CHW's self-disclosure of personal information to a client (see Chapter Twenty), physical contact with a client, romantic or sexual involvement with a client, and managing dual or multiple relationships with clients. A dual or multiple relationship exists when you have another type of relationship or connection with someone who is also a client. For example, a client may be a former coworker, a neighbor, a friend of a family member, or a member of your church, synagogue, or mosque.

CHWs confront potential boundary dilemmas frequently, including offers of gifts from clients, requests from clients to borrow money, or invitations to develop a romantic relationship. Whether it is lending a client $1.50 for bus fare, giving your client a ride in your car to an appointment, being invited to become the godmother to the client's daughter, or seeing a client at your neighborhood grocery store or school, it is sometimes difficult to know what to do.

?   *Can you think of other situations that fall within a boundary dilemma?*

Professional boundaries   are defined as limitations or ethical guidelines that a professional establishes within working relationships. Boundaries may be fluid and flexible depending on the situation. Establishing professional boundaries can assist both the CHW and the client to clearly define their working relationship. Identifying what you can or cannot do for the client is an important part of building trust in your relationship. Your clients should know what to expect from your behavior at the outset of the relationship. The moment when a CHW deviates from a strictly professional role is known as a **boundary crossing.**

CHWs frequently develop warm, close relationships with their clients.

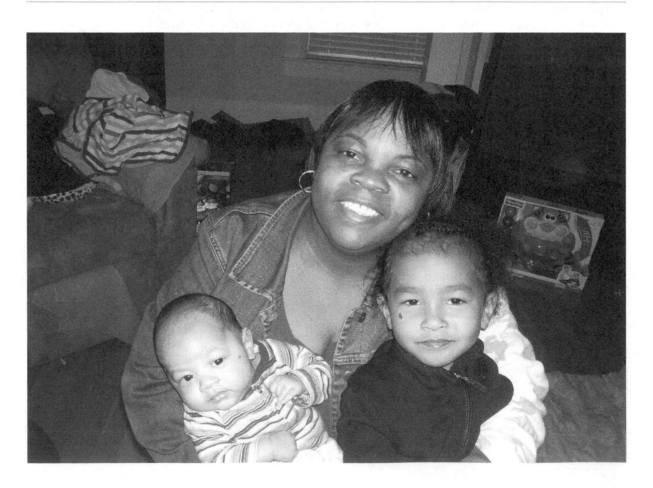

Not every boundary crossing is unethical. Because CHWs often work in the same community where they live, it is difficult to avoid dual relationships with clients. In fact, those relationships may be part of what makes the CHW a "trusted member of the community." CHWs must stay aware of their influential position with respect to clients, however, and avoid exploiting the trust of clients. Understand that some dual relationships can impair professional judgment or increase the risk of harm to clients. The guiding principle here should be: What is in the best interest of the client? If it could be harmful for a client to work with a CHW with whom the client has a dual relationship (member of the same social circle or religious community), then the CHW should refer that client to a colleague.

Looking at the principles outlined in the Code of Ethics can provide some clarity or guidance about the boundary issue you are facing. There are also questions that you can ask yourself as you reflect on the boundary dilemma: Who benefits from the boundary crossing? Is the boundary crossing necessary? Did the client receive informed consent about the potential risks involved in the boundary crossing? How will the boundary crossing affect the relationship? Am I being objective? Is there a cultural context to consider in this situation? As always, if you have questions about when and where to draw healthy professional boundaries with clients, consult with your colleagues and, most importantly, your supervisor.

AN EXAMPLE OF A BOUNDARY CROSSING

I made the mistake of giving a homeless client $10 to get some food. It was raining hard, and she and her son hadn't eaten that day. I just felt powerless to offer anything meaningful. They got a meal at Carl's Jr.® and were able to sit there away from the rain. But from then on, every time I saw the client, she kept asking me for money. I had to explain that I couldn't give her money again, and why. She never understood this, however, because I gave her money before. We were never able to get past this situation, and eventually I had to stop working with her and refer her to a colleague. She was really angry with me, and I can understand why. I messed up.

—Anonymous

In the situation described above, the CHW gave money to a client motivated by concern for her and her child, and possibly out of guilt ("I felt powerless to offer anything meaningful"). While on the surface, offering money to a family in need may seem like a kind thing to do, it is an example of boundary crossing, and in the long run, it may be harmful to the client, the CHW, the community, and the agency that the CHW works for. When the CHW gave money to the client, their relationship changed. From then on, the client saw the CHW as a potential source of money. The CHW, of course, was not able or willing to continue to give money to the client. The CHW also wasn't able to change the relationship back to the way it was before, or to continue providing effective client-centered services. If the agency found out that the CHW was giving money to clients, it would likely take disciplinary action that could include termination (firing the CHW). Once word gets out that a CHW is giving away cash, this is what other clients will come to expect and demand. It also undermines the reputation of the program and the agency that the CHW works for.

? *What do you think about this ethical challenge? What could the CHW have done differently?*

? *What are the guidelines regarding the exchange of money at the agency you volunteer or work for?*

HOW ETHICAL CHALLENGES AFFECT CHWs

The types of situations that raise ethical issues are often deeply stressful for CHWs and other helping professionals. It is difficult to witness clients in distress and at risk of harm, particularly when it isn't easy to figure out what the best course of action is. Ethical challenges may also place you in conflict with a client. For example, you may learn that your client is abusing her or his children, and have an ethical obligation to report this abuse to the authorities.

Don't forget to pay attention to your own feelings and concerns when you are in the midst of an ethical challenge. Try to develop an awareness of how these situations affect you, and develop skills to manage your stress (Chapter Fourteen).

PHUONG AN DOAN BILLINGS: Some Asians don't set the boundaries like we do in the United States. One of our doctors was approached and asked to lend some money to a Vietnamese patient. He doesn't speak much Vietnamese, so he came and told me. I said, "Leave it for me. Let me handle it." I came to talk to the patient. I talked to her with real care, like a sister, so that I didn't upset her—if I talked like a professional, it would upset her. And I said, "I understand you have real difficulty, so we have a few agencies that can provide urgent relief. You let me know what you need, and I will look around for you. But don't approach a doctor like that. Here in America, we don't do it that way."

A FRAMEWORK FOR ETHICAL DECISION MAKING

It isn't always easy to know how to respond to an ethical challenge or problem. We want to share a framework for thinking through such challenges and deciding how to respond. This is just one of many ways to frame the process of making ethical decisions.

This model is based on work by Gerald Corey (Corey, Corey, and Callanan, 2007) and asks that you consider issues that are important when evaluating conflict in relationships. The model has seven steps with questions designed to assist you to reflect deeply about the ethical problems you confront. You are asked to consider yourself, your client, your supervisor, your colleagues, and the community when examining each of the steps in the model. As you review each step, consider its importance in the work that you do with clients and in your community. The questions that you choose to answer can vary depending on the ethical challenge you are facing, your experience with similar ethical challenges, time, and other limitations. Once you have sufficient practice and familiarity using the framework's seven steps, you will be able to develop your own process in thinking through such dilemmas.

Step 1: Describe the Problem or Dilemma   Write down as much as you know about the problem or dilemma. The following questions may assist you to gather relevant information:

- ✪ What has happened so far?
- ✪ What are your sources of information about the problem—the client? Your own observations (what you have seen or heard—not your judgment or opinions)? Reports of facts from others?
- ✪ When did you first become aware of the problem? Is this a new situation or an ongoing problem?

✪ Who is involved? Who else knows about the problem?

✪ What have you learned from the client about the client's experience, opinions, and concerns? What does the client want to see happen?

✪ Do cultural differences play a role in this problem? Are you making assumptions—based on your own cultural perspective—about others who are involved in this situation?

✪ What have you done so far in relation to the problem?

Try to consider the experiences and values of your client, your agency and supervisor, your community, and yourself. Pay attention to your intuition, which could be the reason that you are thinking through this ethical problem.

Step 2: Review Relevant Ethical Guidelines or Codes   Review the CHW Code of Ethics for guidance about the problem. Are there any Principles in the CHW Code of Ethics that address the problem? For example, does the situation raise concerns about confidentiality, scope of practice, or discrimination?

Step 3: Review Applicable Laws and Regulations   Are there any laws or regulations that speak to the issues in the problem? Are there any issues in the problem where you may be breaking the law if you don't address it, or vice versa? Does the situation involve any allegations of harm or violence? Don't forget to review your agency's policies and procedures.

Step 4: Seek Consultation   Consult supervisors, colleagues, and other professionals who may assist you in processing ethical problems. It is important to receive consultation because a third person, preferably someone removed from the problem and more experienced in the field, can offer feedback, support, and most important, assist you in thinking through the situation. When you seek consultation, remember to maintain client confidentiality. Explain the situation, but leave out the client's name and identifying details.

Step 5: Consider Possible and Probable Courses of Action   What possible courses of action can you take in response to the ethical challenge you face? Do you need to do anything at all? If it is appropriate and feasible, include your client as part of this discussion. If the challenge is one that you consider serious, however, and may result in harm to a client or other party, consult your agency's policies and your supervisor.

Step 6: Outline Possible Consequences of Decisions   Reflect on and write down the possible consequences of the various choices that you identified during Step 5. How might these courses of action and decisions impact the client, the agency, the community, and yourself? Might these decisions lead to further harm to any party? Again, consider inviting your client into this conversation about the consequences that may have an impact on the client's life and, as always, consult other CHWs and your supervisor if you are uncertain about your various options.

Step 7: Decide on What Appears to Be the Best Course of Action   When you think you've identified the best course of action, spend a little time reviewing and evaluating it first. Questions to consider may include: How does this choice fit with the ethical code? Will anyone be harmed by this course of action? How would I feel if my actions became public knowledge? Did I practice cultural humility? How were my client's cultural values and experiences taken into consideration? How were my own values affirmed or challenged? What did I learn from the struggle to resolve this ethical dilemma?

The goal of this seven-step framework is to assist in guiding you through the ethical decision-making process when you are faced with challenging dilemmas. It is important to engage in self-reflection throughout the steps so that you think about balancing all of the various needs involved in the problem. Implementing the framework takes practice.

8.2 SELF-AWARENESS

In Chapter One we introduced self-awareness as an essential quality and skill for CHWs, as well as an ethical responsibility. A lack of self-knowledge can significantly undermine your ability to provide client-centered and culturally competent services. When CHWs and other helping professionals are unaware of their own experiences, values, and beliefs, they are at risk of letting these personal issues guide their work. When our own issues begin to influence the way we view and work with others, we may end up causing harm to people whom we intend to assist.

THE IMPORTANCE OF SELF-AWARENESS

When our own issues are present, powerful and unresolved, we may not be fully aware that they are influencing our ability to listen to, work with, and support others. We may unconsciously guide, direct, or pressure clients to talk about or avoid certain topics, to consider certain options, to make choices that are more about our own needs than those of the client.

For example, a CHW who is uncomfortable with aspects of human sexuality may communicate this discomfort to clients. A CHW with strong values and beliefs about reproduction, including pregnancy, abortion, and adoption, may impose these beliefs on a client who is pregnant. CHWs with a history of substance use may have difficulty separating their own experiences and beliefs from those of clients who are currently using drugs. CHWs who have been exposed to trauma, such as child abuse or sexual assault, may become restimulated and overwhelmed by their own memories and responses when working with clients who have also survived trauma. CHWs who are unaware of what triggers their anger and defensiveness are less prepared to handle these emotions when they are triggered during interactions with clients.

? *Can you think of other examples of how a CHW's own issues may interfere with the ability to work effectively with clients and communities?*

? *Have you ever worked with a helping professional who seemed uncomfortable or judgmental about your identity or behaviors?*

? *Can you identify past experiences or personal issues that could be triggered through your work as a CHW?*

Developing self-awareness is a lifelong task. It involves an ongoing process of identifying and working to better understand yourself, including:

- *Life experiences:* divorce, incarceration, immigration, chronic illness, the deaths of family and friends, discrimination, and other challenging experiences
- *Values and beliefs:* values and beliefs about reproduction, religion, substance use, sexuality, and death and dying

✪ *Prejudices:* Each of us has grown up in a community or a society that values certain groups of people more than others based on factors such as ethnicity, nationality, religion, age, immigration status, sex, gender identity, sexual orientation, and disability status. While many of us don't want to acknowledge it, growing up surrounded by prejudice influences our own thoughts, feelings, and behavior, often in subtle ways. We may be more comfortable working with certain groups of people than others, and we may provide more attention and better services to some types of clients than others. Examining our assumptions and prejudices is an essential first step in developing the ability to provide equal treatment and quality services to all clients and communities without discrimination.

SELF-EVALUATION

No matter how much you already know about yourself and others, you can always learn more. Please reflect on the following questions:

✪ What types of situations may trigger strong emotion or judgment in you? What triggers your anger or defensiveness? When do you find it most difficult to listen to others? When are you most tempted to tell others what to do?

✪ What health and health-related topics are you least prepared to address with clients? For example: How prepared are you to deal with experiences of trauma such as exposure to war, domestic violence, child abuse, and sexual assault?

✪ What health behaviors are you less familiar or comfortable with? For example: Which aspects of human sexuality are you least prepared to address effectively with clients?

✪ What populations are you less familiar with and least prepared to work with? Are you equally capable of working effectively with men and women? With people of all sexual orientations? With people of all gender identities? People of all ages including children, teenagers, and seniors? People who do not speak the same language as you? Are you comfortable working with interpreters?

ENHANCING SELF-AWARENESS

We encourage you to take an active approach to increasing your self-awareness. There are many ways to do this:

✪ Self-reflection:
Make time to think about your own life experiences, beliefs, and values.

✪ Learn to identify issues that come up in the course of your work:
With time and practice you will begin to notice when your own issues arise in the course of your work with colleagues or clients. Successful CHWs learn how to note this and put the issue or issues aside in the moment. They continue to focus on the client or group they are working with, and after their work is done, they take time to reflect on what happened and how they can best move forward to learn more about these issues.

✪ Journaling:
All CHWs document their work with clients and communities. Many CHWs also keep a separate journal to write about their own work experiences, including their accomplishments, challenges, insights that assist them to better understand themselves, and questions that emerge through practice.

✪   Counseling, supervision:
      All CHWs should receive regular supervision. This is an opportunity to talk further
      about your own issues in order to better understand them and to enhance your ability
      to ensure that they don't interfere with your work. You may also seek to participate in
      counseling or therapy outside of the work environment to enhance self-awareness and
      to address particularly challenging issues.

✪   Classmates, colleagues, family, and friends:
      Talk with someone you trust and who can support your effort to better understand the
      issues that may get in the way of client- and community-centered practice.

✪   Training and other professional development opportunities:
      Seek out opportunities to learn more about the communities you work with, the topics
      and issues that arise in your work, and how to enhance cultural humility and client-
      centered skills.

✪   Continuing your formal education:
      You may take courses at a local college or university on issues that will assist you to
      better understand yourself, your own community and history, and how to work effec-
      tively with communities that are different from your own. This may include vocational
      or academic courses in psychology, ethnic studies, art, or history.

8.3 SCOPE OF PRACTICE

Scope of practice is a concept commonly used in most practices, including the health
and mental health fields, to determine which skills workers are competent to perform
on the job and which lie outside their expertise. For example, doctors are trained to
diagnose illness and to prescribe treatment, including medications. These functions
lie within their scope of practice. But doctors are not trained to provide legal advice
(within the scope of practice of attorneys-at-law) or to install an electrical circuit in
your home (within the scope of practice of electricians); these competencies lie outside
their scope of practice.

Scope of practice is also an ethical issue, and relates to several of the ethical principles introduced above, including Article 1.3: Scope of Ability and Training.

More established professions, such as medicine and social work, have well-developed
scope-of-practice guidelines. Because the CHW field is still in development, however, it
lacks well-defined guidelines. For CHWs, this lack of formal guidelines significantly complicates the challenge of determining which skills or competencies you can and cannot
practice. Unfortunately, the topic of scope of practice may not be raised with a CHW until
someone—usually a supervisor or colleague from another profession, such as nursing or
social work—tells the CHW that they shouldn't have done something on the job. We hope
this chapter will assist you to understand and to clarify your scope of practice and to prevent conflict with colleagues and supervisors.

As we discussed in Chapters One and Two, the CHW field is not always recognized or
adequately respected by other professions. Other occupations often try to limit the scope of
work of CHWs, questioning the ability of CHWs to provide certain types of services. As
their numbers grow, however, CHWs are negotiating a clearer and more expanded scope
of practice.

The role and the work of CHWs can appear to be so large and all-encompassing that it
feels overwhelming. Understanding where your role begins and ends, and when to make a
referral to another professional, can provide clarity and comfort to CHWs and assist you to
prevent mistakes that may harm your clients, your agency, and your own career. The scope

of practice for CHWs varies considerably from one place to another, and may depend on a variety of factors, such as:

- State and local laws (including employment, mandatory reporting, and Medicaid reimbursement statutes)
- The agency, program, and supervisor you work for. (Some agencies, for example, may train CHWs to facilitate training or to provide treatment adherence counseling while others do not.)
- The type of health issue you focus on. (For example, CHWs who work in the HIV/STI field may be trained to provide HIV antibody test counseling or to draw blood.)
- Your background, training, and skills
- Your own level of comfort and competency
- Overlapping scopes of practice of other colleagues such as nurses, medical assistants or medical evaluation assistants, senior health educators, and social workers
- Politics and competition among occupations for control, recognition, and pay
- The context of the work, including issues raised by clients

One way to think about scope of practice is to brainstorm a list of competencies that CHWs are commonly trained to provide and therefore competent to perform, and competencies that are generally considered to lie outside the scope of practice of CHWs. These are not definitive lists and may vary in your state, agency, or health program.

The following competencies generally lie *within* the CHW scope of practice:

- Providing culturally and linguistically appropriate health education and information
- Providing informal counseling and peer support
- Recruitment of clients or study participants, including the provision of informed consent
- Conducting initial interviews with new clients
- Supporting clients to access services
- Supporting clients in better understanding their own questions, resources, knowledge, and options for action and services
- Supporting clients in communicating their questions or concerns
- Supporting clients in developing and implementing a plan to reduce risks and to enhance their health
- Supporting clients in changing behaviors
- Providing case management services (although some have challenged the use of this term and would reserve case management for nurses, social workers, and other licensed professionals) and referrals
- Community organizing and advocacy. (Some CHWs work for agencies that encourage and support community organizing and advocacy for policy changes, although some do not. Even if this is not a formal part of your job, many CHWs are engaged in community organizing outside of their paid job with local, national, or international organizations.)

?

What other competencies do you think generally lie within the CHW scope of practice?

The following competencies are considered to lie *outside* the CHW scope of practice:

- Diagnosing illness
- Prescribing treatment or medication
- Counseling severely mentally ill clients (although CHWs will often provide outreach, peer support, health education, and case management services to clients living with severe mental illness)

✪ Providing therapy (rather than peer counseling)
✪ Providing advice on legal or medical issues

? *What other competencies do you think generally lie outside the CHW scope of practice?*

It is generally easiest to determine competencies that lie within or outside of the CHW's scope of practice. However, there are a number of competencies that are sometimes considered to lie within and sometimes outside of the scope of practice, depending on the factors identified above (state law, policies of the employer, professional politics, and training). In order to avoid confusion, conflict with colleagues, and harm to your clients, seek clear guidance from your supervisors regarding what you are and are not permitted to do on the job.

The following competencies may require specialized training and *sometimes lie within* and *sometimes outside* the scope of practice of CHWs.

Counseling   While some professionals argue that CHWs shouldn't perform "counseling" and object to the use of this term, there is a strong tradition of CHWs and others providing peer counseling, including reproductive health and HIV/STI counselors and the example of domestic violence and rape crisis centers. In many agencies, CHWs are trained to use motivational interviewing and other client-centered counseling skills with clients.

Interpretation and Translation Services   Bilingual CHWs are frequently asked to interpret oral conversations between clients and providers, or to translate written documents from one language to another. Some CHWs and their employers have advocated for CHWs to provide these services. Others have advocated for interpretation and translation services to be provided only by those with specialized training or certification because the potential consequences of mistakes made during interpretation or translation can be harmful for clients.

Treatment Adherence or Compliance Counseling   Increasingly, CHWs work in partnership with clinicians to support clients in understanding and following treatment guidelines—sometimes referred to as **treatment adherence or compliance**. For example, CHWs at San Francisco General Hospital work with families to aid them to better understand their children's asthma medications and know how to use them properly to prevent symptoms. The CHWs work under the close supervision of a nurse practitioner.

Accompanying Clients   CHWs may accompany clients during sessions with physicians or other professionals to lend support or provide advocacy.

Media Advocacy   Some organizations train and support CHWs to take a lead role in media advocacy—working with print, radio, TV, or other media to promote programs, policies, or health information—while others do not.

Facilitating Training or Community Education Sessions   CHWs may facilitate a presentation at a local juvenile hall on the topic of domestic violence or a training for medical providers on working with patients living with HIV disease.

Facilitating Social or Support Groups   There are different points of view regarding the level of education or training required to facilitate groups. Some groups may be facilitated by licensed professionals, others by CHWs.

Crisis Intervention   CHWs may provide crisis intervention or work with a client in crisis, such as a client recently exposed to sexual assault or domestic violence or someone who is thinking of suicide.

On the one hand, some professionals argue that CHWs do not have sufficient training to provide these services, and the risk of inadvertently causing harm to clients is too great. These advocates believe that clients in crisis should be referred as soon as possible to licensed professionals.

On the other hand, some CHWs and professionals argue that CHWs can be trained to provide crisis intervention services. They argue that it is not possible for many clients in crisis to be seen by a licensed clinical provider. These advocates also point to the rape crisis and domestic violence movements as models for the provision of culturally competent crisis intervention services by unlicensed staff.

Research Projects   CHWs may provide assistance with research projects as interviewers or focus group facilitators.

Determining Eligibility Status   CHWs may assist in determining the client's eligibility for state and federal Medicaid, Family Health Plus, Child Health Plus, Healthy Families, Medi-Cal, and other programs.

? *What other competencies do you think may sometimes lie within or outside of the CHW scope of practice?*

T G: There have been lots of times when other professionals have tried to tell me that I'm not qualified to provide some kind of service just because I don't have a graduate degree. A social worker at the hospital told me that I shouldn't call myself a case manager. I told her that was my title—prevention case manager. And I told her that my work was funded by the State AIDS Office, and that they could look on the CDC (Centers for Disease Control and Prevention) Web site to learn more about how CHWs do case management. It made me angry, but I also had to stay professional, because I know that I will continue to refer clients to that social worker.

WHY CHWs MAY WORK OUTSIDE THEIR SCOPE OF PRACTICE

CHWs may be motivated to work outside of their scope of practice by the desire to assist their clients. CHWs may do this when they perceive that their clients are at risk and lack access to important resources and services, such as health care or legal assistance. CHWs sometimes get caught up in the dangerous notion that it is their responsibility to rescue their clients or solve their clients' problems.

? *Can you think of situations where you might be tempted to exceed your scope of practice?*

Consequences of Working Outside of Your Scope of Practice   Imagine that a CHW:

- Advises a client about cancer treatment
- Provides a client in a domestic violence situation with legal advise about whether or not to file a report or to seek an order of protection
- Provides ongoing counseling to a highly suicidal client

? *What might happen to the client? To the CHW? To the agency? To the community?*

When CHWs step outside of their scope of practice, they risk doing harm to their clients and to themselves. CHWs do not have the required training or licensure to diagnose or treat medical conditions, to provide legal guidance, or to provide therapy to a suicidal or severely mentally ill client. For example, giving advice (rather than information) about cancer treatments could result in a client seeking inappropriate, ineffective, or harmful treatments. Under such circumstances, CHWs should refer the client to a medical provider.

Stepping outside of your scope of practice may negatively affect your professional reputation and could result in disciplinary action and the loss of your job. When you step outside of your scope of practice, you are likely to be usurping (taking over) the role of other professionals, such as nurses or social workers, and this may damage your relationship with these colleagues.

Providing services that you are not competent or licensed to provide may also seriously damage the reputation of your program or agency. News that a CHW has done something unethical or has harmed a client will travel quickly in the community and could result in diminished support for an important agency or program.

Exceeding your scope of practice also breaks trust with the communities that CHWs pledge to support. Most of the communities that CHWs serve have already experienced a long history of harmful treatment by health, medical, education, law enforcement, or other government agencies or representatives. Each betrayal takes a toll on the community and makes it harder for them to establish trusting relationships with service providers.

What to Do When You Are Uncertain About Your Scope of Practice

- Review your job description and your agency's policies regarding your scope of practice.
- If you are not certain that a certain duty lies within your scope of practice, *don't do it*, and seek guidance from your colleagues and supervisor.
- Examine the potential for causing harm to clients or communities.
- Be aware of your own risk factors for exceeding your scope of practice. For each of us, there may be particular types of situations or clients that may motivate our desire to go above and beyond the call of duty and may tempt us to step outside of our professional boundaries. *What are your risk factors?*
- Clearly explain to your client what services you can and cannot provide.
- Don't let the client be your guide regarding scope of practice. Some clients, out of an understandable desire to meet their needs, may try to pressure you to step outside of your scope of practice. Hold firm to your scope of practice and your ethical guidelines.
- When questions arise, ask for support and guidance from colleagues and your supervisor, as appropriate.

What to Do When You Disagree with How Your Scope of Practice Is Defined

As we noted above, professionals sometimes disagree about which competencies are within or outside of a CHW's scope of practice. As a result there may be times when you disagree with how your scope of practice is defined by your agency, your supervisor, or your colleagues.

Sometimes, a supervisor or colleague might ask you to perform tasks that you have not been trained to do. At other times, you may find that your agency has defined a scope of practice that is too restrictive and that keeps you from providing services that you are truly competent to provide.

Handle these challenges in a way that preserves the safety of your clients as well as your own professional reputation and that of the program and agency you work for. Take this as an opportunity to advocate *within* your agency and with your supervisor for changes to your scope of practice. This might involve educating your colleagues and your supervisor about CHWs and their role and about your training, experience, and skills. It might involve finding out from your supervisor what additional training he or she would like you to have in order to provide certain services. It is likely to involve advocating for increased opportunities for professional development.

As CHWs organize on a local, state, and national level, they will be better able to advocate for recognition of their competencies and contributions, an expanded scope of practice, and increased pay.

8.4 UNDERSTANDING BEHAVIOR CHANGE

Perhaps the most common role for CHWs is supporting the behavior change efforts of individual clients. While supporting people in changing behavior and reducing health risks may sound relatively straightforward, the process of changing behavior, and the art of supporting others in doing so, is a complex and challenging task. For these reasons, we introduce here some basic information and guiding principles about human behavior and the behavior change process. Chapter Ten will build on this information and present skills for conducting behavior change counseling.

WHICH BEHAVIORS DO PEOPLE TYPICALLY ATTEMPT TO CHANGE?

These behaviors may include:

- Patterns of eating (including disordered eating) and nutrition
- Patterns of exercise
- Parenting practices (such as effective discipline)
- Screening for cancer (including regular self-exams for breast and testicular cancer)
- Stress management
- Adherence or compliance to treatment guidelines (such as remembering to take medications at the proper times and in the proper doses)
- Sexual behaviors (such as regular and effective contraceptive use and safer sex practices)
- Smoking, alcohol, and drug use (reducing or eliminating use)
- Anger management
- Driving (such as driving within the speed limit and not under the influence of alcohol or other substances)

? *Can you think of other behaviors to add to this list?*

YOUR EXPERIENCE WITH BEHAVIOR CHANGE

Before you begin to think about how to support others in changing their behaviors, we would like you to reflect on your own experiences. If possible, take time to discuss your responses with a friend or colleague.

- Which behaviors have you tried to change?
- What motivated you to change your behavior?
- Was it easy to make changes?
- Did change happen all at once?
- What factors supported you in making change?
- What got in the way of successful behavior change?
- Were you able to maintain change over time?
- Did you ever **relapse** or return to the old behavior you had hoped to change? If so, what influenced this? How did you feel when you relapsed?
- After a relapse, were you able to try again to change your behavior? How? What helped?

Most of us have struggled over the course of our lives to change certain behaviors: to stop smoking, to exercise regularly, to eat healthier, to turn in homework assignments on time, or to change the way we talk with loved ones when we are angry. We know from our own experience how challenging and frustrating it can be to make and sustain behavior change. If it were easy to change behavior, our society wouldn't experience such high rates of violence, cancer, heart disease, diabetes, HIV disease, or automobile accidents.

FACTORS THAT INFLUENCE BEHAVIOR: DEVELOPING AN ECOLOGICAL APPROACH

Imagine that you are working with a client who has expressed the desire to:

- Change his diet in order to manage diabetes and prevent heart disease
- Use condoms regularly to reduce the risks of sexually transmitted infections
- Leave a relationship characterized by abuse

Despite good intentions, clients may fail to meet their own expectations and may relapse for various periods of time to the very behaviors or situations they were attempting to change. *Why is changing behavior so difficult? What gets in the way?*

Table 8.1 identifies some of the factors that may get in the way of successful behavior change. These factors correspond to the ecological model presented in Chapter Three and include individual, family and friends, neighborhood and community, and societal factors.

The table illustrates how a wide range of factors may influence the health and behavior of your client and complicate their efforts to change. We have categorized these factors at the level of the individual, family and friends, neighborhood or community, and the broader society or state. These factors will always depend on your client's identity (including life experiences, gender, age, ethnicity, nationality, immigration status, primary

Table 8.1 Factors That Get in the Way of Behavior Change: An Ecological Model.

Client Example	Individual Factors	Factors Related to Family and Friends	Neighborhood and Community Factors	Societal Factors: Media, Economics, and Politics
The client wants to leave a relationship characterized by violence and threats of violence.	A long history of abuse—beginning as a child Lack of self-esteem Loneliness and fear of being on one's own Lack of formal education and job skills Age Love for the partner who hurts the individual Perceived need to preserve the family Shame about having stayed in the relationship so long; worried about what others will think *Other possibilities?*	Pressure from family and friends not to be single Judgment from friends about being with an abusive partner Cultural norms and attitudes A history of incarceration related to drug use *Other possibilities?*	Isolation from the spiritual community that used to be a source of faith and comfort Domestic violence is accepted as normal by many members of the local community Lack of job training and employment opportunities that could assist with independence Lack of social services, including services for victims of domestic violence *Other possibilities?*	Discrimination based on ethnicity, nationality, immigration status, gender, sexual orientation, or other identity Poverty Lack of government support for educational and social service programs for low-income communities Lack of funding for victims of domestic violence, including counseling, legal assistance, and affordable transitional housing *Other possibilities?*

language, sexual orientation, disability status, and so on) and social context. Social context refers to the reality in which people live, and includes their families, friends, workplaces, homes, and economic, cultural, and political dynamics affecting their neighborhood, city, state, or nation.

The list of factors provided in Table 8.1 is not meant to be exhaustive: it doesn't include every possibility. When students at the City College of San Francisco brainstorm a list of factors that influence behavior, the list typically fills up six to eight large pieces of flip chart paper and includes over a hundred distinct items. Additional factors that influence the ability of our clients to successfully change behaviors may include the following:

Individual Factors

- Emotions, such as embarrassment, shame, guilt, fear, love, or loneliness
- Desire for love, intimacy, and a sense of belonging
- Dependency—economic or emotional—on others
- Pleasure (the desire for pleasure, including pleasure from sex or drug use)
- Lack of confidence in the ability to succeed
- Thoughts, including self-defeating thoughts (such as "I always mess up," "I won't be able to," "I don't care what happens . . . ")
- Self-esteem (how we think and feel about ourselves)
- Spiritual, religious, or metaphysical "faith," meaning, or purpose
- Knowledge relevant to behavior change (such as information about nutrition)
- History—what has happened before—including history of successful behavior change and history of trauma such as domestic violence and sexual assault
- Long-established patterns of behavior, including risk behaviors such as drinking or using drugs when under stress
- Choices, including choices regarding education, relationships, drug use, sexual behavior, nutrition, and so on
- Lack of formal education and employment skills

Family and Friends

- Level of family support and conflict
- Isolation
- Peer pressure—from friends and sexual partners
- Sense of belonging
- Healthy romantic and sexual relationships
- Exposure to violence in relationships with family or others

Neighborhood and Community Factors

- Social identity and sense of belonging to a defined community
- Availability of community-based resources such as health and social services agencies, good schools, faith-based institutions including churches and mosques, recreational and cultural programs including parks and after-school programs for youths, affordable and healthy food, public transportation, affordable housing

⊙ Working conditions, including exposure to hazardous chemicals, low pay and lack of benefits, conflict with management, and other sources of stress

⊙ Relative presence of potentially harmful dynamics and resources, such as a large number of bars and liquor stores; drug sales; or crime, including property theft, assault, gang-related activity, and violence

⊙ Support from helping professionals, such as CHWs (or harmful interactions with helping professionals)

⊙ Cultural or religious support or rejection

⊙ Social norms and expectations

⊙ Stigma and prejudice against one's identity or behaviors

Societal Factors

⊙ Prejudice and discrimination based on ethnicity, nationality, immigration status, language, gender, gender-identity, sexual orientation, level of education, disability, age, history of incarceration, and so forth

⊙ Government policies, including those determining access to necessary services such as safe housing, healthy nutrition, effective schools, after-school programs, health insurance, employment, drug treatment programs, residency or citizenship, health education programs, and civil rights

⊙ Criminal justice approach to drug use, rather than a harm-reduction approach (people locked up for using drugs rather than provided with treatment and services to reduce harm)

⊙ Economic policies and forces influencing wages, working conditions, employment benefits, and access to resources

⊙ Corporate promotion of products such as fast food, low-mileage cars, or handguns

⊙ Media promotion of harmful attitudes and behaviors

⊙ Political events, including global economic practices and war

⊙ Natural influences (often influenced by human actions) including natural disasters such as Hurricane Katrina

? *What do you think of these lists? Is there anything you would like to add? Is there anything listed here that you question or would like to see changed or omitted?*

As discussed in Chapter Three, research in the field of public health has demonstrated that social context and ecological factors influence human health far more significantly than the genetics, knowledge, or behavior of individuals. In order to become effective agents of change, CHWs must learn to view individual clients within the broad social context in which they live. An ecological approach to understanding and facilitating behavior change examines both the factors that an individual may be able to control, and the broader social, economic, cultural, and political factors that influence her choices, behavior, and health.

COMMON MISTAKES IN ATTEMPTING TO FACILITATE BEHAVIOR CHANGE

Before introducing resources designed to facilitate effective behavior change, we want to address several common mistakes that CHWs and other helping professionals often make when working with clients. We encourage you to understand what these mistakes are, and why we suggest that they may undermine your effective work with clients. The four common mistakes are:

1. Relying on information alone
2. Giving advice
3. Blaming the client
4. Failing to address issues of accountability

As we address each of these common mistakes in turn, we will apply them to the case of working with a client named L.

THE CLIENT "L."

L. was recently diagnosed with gonorrhea and is worried about getting infected with HIV. L. is shy around people she or he is attracted to, and feels embarrassed in sexual situations when not drinking or using drugs. L. doesn't regularly use condoms and isn't comfortable negotiating safer sex. L. wants to change these behaviors, but doesn't feel confident that she or he can.

Common Mistake #1: Relying on Health Information Alone   Often, CHWs and other helping professionals, including nurses and physicians, work from the assumption that if they provide a client with clear and accurate information about a health condition, and what they can do to prevent the condition or improve their health, the client will apply that information to change the behavior.

For example, a CHW working with L. may focus on providing information about STIs and how to prevent them:

C HW: Gonorrhea is one of the most common sexually transmitted infections or STIs. You can contract it from unprotected vaginal, anal, or oral sex. Fortunately, gonorrhea is a bacterial STI and can be effectively treated with antibiotics. If you don't get treated with antibiotics, and complete that treatment, a gonorrheal infection can result in a range of complications including sterility: the inability to have children. To prevent infection with gonorrhea or other STIs in the future, practice safer sex. This may include no penetrative oral, vaginal, or anal sex; monogamy with a committed and trusted partner who has been tested and proven to be free of STIs; and the use of latex condoms every time you have sex. . . . (And the CHW goes on—and on!—providing information about safer sex, testing, and treatment of STIs.)

While the information provided is accurate, in most cases it is unlikely to motivate the client to make immediate, significant, and lasting behavior change. It is common for people who fully understand the health risks of certain behavior, such as unprotected sex or smoking, to continue these behaviors. It is likely, for example, that L. already knows a lot about STIs and how to use condoms. L. doesn't necessarily lack information: other factors are influencing L.'s behavior and getting in the way of successful behavior change.

? *Have you ever encountered a health care or other helping professional who focused exclusively on providing you with health information?*

? *How does this type of approach work for you?*

? *Do you think that this type of approach will be effective with most clients?*

? *Why or why not?*

We don't recommend this approach because:

- ✪ It is unlikely to result in effective and lasting behavior changes.
- ✪ The CHW dominates the session in providing information and does not make space for the client to share knowledge, questions, concerns, and ideas.
- ✪ This approach assumes that the client doesn't have complete or accurate knowledge about the health issue.
- ✪ It minimizes the difficulty of making changes in behaviors and doesn't provide meaningful support to assist in that process.
- ✪ The client may feel condescended or "talked-down" to, particularly if the CHW doesn't take time to acknowledge what the client already knows and to talk about the challenges of behavior change in a more realistic way.
- ✪ The client may feel frustrated by the encounter and less likely to return to this or other similar providers in the future.

Please note: We want to underscore that the critique we offer here is not about the value of providing health information. Indeed, a vital role of CHWs is to educate clients about health conditions, under the guidance of other health professionals and within their scope of practice. CHWs provide health information to clients and assist them to better understand health conditions, their risks, and the options for reducing these risks. The problem arises when CHWs don't first assess what the client already knows, and when they assume that accurate health information alone is sufficient to support their clients in making healthy and lasting behavior changes.

Mistake #2: Giving Advice   Many helping professionals provide advice to clients about what they should and shouldn't do, and sometimes what they should think and feel. For example, a CHW working with L. may make the following types of statements:

- ✪ "If you haven't been treated yet, you should go to a clinic immediately to get a prescription for the right antibiotic. Let's call up City Clinic right now to make an appointment."
- ✪ "You shouldn't feel embarrassed about sex, it's just a natural part of life."
- ✪ "You need to start using condoms every time you have sex, regardless of the circumstances." All you need to say is, "I don't have unprotected sex. My health is too important to me to take a risk."
- ✪ "I think you should go to a drug and alcohol recovery group. I facilitate a support group on Thursday nights for women/men like you. It starts at 4 PM."

In this example, the CHW not only wants to tell the client what to do ("Go to City Clinic" or "Attend a recovery support group"), they even want to tell L. what to feel ("You shouldn't feel embarrassed") and what to say ("All you need to say is . . .").

? *Have you ever encountered a health care or other helping professional who liked to give you advice?*

? *How does this type of approach work for you?*

? *Do you think that this type of approach will be effective with most clients?*

? *Why or why not?*

We don't recommend this approach because:

- ⊘ It is unlikely to result in effective and lasting behavior changes.
- ⊘ It assumes that clients cannot determine for themselves what to do to promote their health. It assumes that clients require an "expert" to guide their behavior.
- ⊘ It may undermine the client's autonomy and sense of competency. It fosters dependence on others.
- ⊘ Many clients do not like to be told what to do. Such an approach may cause them to lose trust in and respect for health care and other helping professionals and could result in avoiding services in the future.

Sometimes, we fall into a pattern of giving advice without even noticing it, generally out of a desire to be supportive. While providing advice may be an appropriate thing to do in your family or with your friends, it isn't something that we recommend you do with clients. Be aware of the words you use and cautious about the times when you find yourself using phrases such as:

- ⊘ You should . . .
- ⊘ You need to . . .

Please note: There are many occasions when we encourage CHWs to share suggestions with clients about choices that they may make. Rather than telling a client what to do, however, we encourage you to present the choices as options for the client to consider. Instead of saying "You should," try:

- ⊘ Have you thought about?
- ⊘ Have you considered?
- ⊘ What do you think about . . . ?
- ⊘ I'd like to share a suggestion with you, something to consider as you decide what you want to do . . .

Mistake #3: Blaming the Client   Sometimes CHWs or other helping professionals focus primarily on the choices that clients make which contribute to their health risks. Unfortunately, this focus on what clients have done or are doing that increases their health risks may be accompanied by a tendency to blame clients for the resulting health risks or conditions. This approach is deeply influenced by political and media messages that tend to blame people for unfortunate circumstances, including poverty and poor health outcomes. For example, when people engage in risky behaviors, others blame them. When people try but don't succeed in changing behaviors, they may be blamed again. Sometimes, when people are diagnosed with cancer, diabetes, HIV disease, or other health conditions, they are blamed yet again. This perspective may unduly influence the approach and tone that CHWs take when working with individual clients. This strong cultural tendency toward blaming has been well documented (Ryan, 1976).

Blaming the client is manifested both in the tone with which a CHW communicates \with a client and the content of what is said (and what is not addressed). For example, a CHW influenced by a "blaming the client" approach, may ask or make the following types of questions and statements when working with L.:

- Why are you having sex with so many partners?
- Why aren't you more concerned about a sexually transmitted infection?
- Don't you know what gonorrhea can do to your body?
- If you don't stop having anal sex, you are going to end up with a disease that is a lot worse than gonorrhea.
- If you can't talk with your partners about using condoms, you shouldn't be having sex: No Glove, No Love!
- Why are you so embarrassed about sex? It is just a natural part of life.

? *Have you ever encountered a health care or other helping professional whoseemed to be blaming you in some way?*

? *How does this type of approach work for you?*

? *Do you think that this type of approach will be effective with most clients?*

? *Why or why not?*

We don't recommend this approach because:

- It is unlikely to result in effective and lasting behavior changes.
- It assumes that the client's health and behavior are determined 100 percent by the client.
- It fails to recognize social, political, economic, and cultural relationships and dynamics that influence our knowledge, attitudes, choices, and behaviors.
- It fails to recognize how difficult it is to change certain behaviors such as alcohol and drug use, diet, and sexual behaviors.
- It isn't the proper role of CHWs to pass judgment on clients.
- It is likely to provoke feelings of embarrassment, shame, or anger in the client, especially if they have often been judged by others in the past.
- It is likely to prevent the formation of a trusting, supportive, and lasting relationship with the CHW.
- It may discourage a client from returning to the same agency for services or from accessing services elsewhere.

○ It may be harmful to your client. Blaming people for poor health or for the inability to change behaviors is generally counterproductive; it contributes to a lack of confidence and may diminish their hope in the possibility of change. One of the key roles of CHWs is to carry hope for positive change for the clients and communities you work with, especially during difficult times when they are discouraged.

RAMONA BENSON: I don't put the blame on the client when she doesn't do something. She's probably blaming herself already. I look at the whole picture. I look at the system, too. Did the health care system treat her right? Give her an appointment on time? Cancel that appointment? Get her a prescription that she needed for her baby? Charge her too much? Mix up her health insurance?

Mistake #4: Failing to Address Issues of Accountability   Like everyone, your clients will sometimes make decisions and engage in behaviors that may be harmful to their health or the health of others. When this occurs, you will be faced with the question of how to respond. Unfortunately, many CHWs and other helping professionals fail to take advantage of this opportunity and do not ask clients to talk about what they are doing that may be harmful to their health. This common mistake may be thought of as the flip side of "blaming the client." In order not to make judgments about clients, the CHW may simply be silent, may focus the discussion on what clients are doing well to promote their health, or may otherwise avoid the conversation.

Some of reasons for making this common mistake may include:

○ A mistaken notion that the role of the CHW is always to accept and support everything their client *does* (rather than always accepting and supporting *the client*, but not necessarily the behavior or choices)
○ Being uncomfortable with confrontation or conflict
○ Fear of insulting, angering, shaming, or otherwise harming the relationship with the client

? *Have you ever encountered a health care or other helping professional who failed to talk with you about things that you were doing that could be harmful to your health or to others?*

? *How does this type of approach work for you?*

? *Do you think that this type of approach will be effective with most clients?*

? *Why or why not?*

We don't recommend this approach because:

○ It is unlikely to result in effective and lasting behavior changes.
○ It deprives the client of an opportunity to reflect in a deep way about behaviors that may be harmful to themselves or others.

- It does not respect your client's ability to address challenging issues.
- It sends and reinforces a message that the client should not discuss these issues.
- It may result in increased shame and guilt regarding the behaviors.
- It increases the likelihood that clients will continue to engage in the behavior and will indeed cause harm to themselves or others (imagine, for example, that your client has untreated gonorrhea and is continuing to have unprotected sex with others).
- It violates your code of ethics to do no harm to the client or others.
- It may discourage a client from returning to the same agency for services or even from accessing services elsewhere.

An alternative:

Rather than avoiding the situation, we encourage you to address these concerns directly and respectfully with the client. For example, when working with L., a CHW may say something along the lines of:

CHW: "L., you told me that you want to prevent getting another STI in the future, and that you are having sex without a condom. How do you feel about this? (Stop and listen.) What influences you to have unprotected sex in these moments? (Stop and listen.) What do you think you can do to change this dynamic?

More guidance will be provided regarding how to gently confront clients in Chapter Ten.

8.5 CLIENT-CENTERED PRACTICE

In the section above, we have focused on common mistakes we hope you will avoid when working with clients. In this section, we will introduce concepts that we do recommend to guide your work in supporting clients in changing health behaviors.

There are a wide range of resources that CHWs and others use to guide their work with individual clients to facilitate behavior change. Because there are so many resources, including theories of and strategies for behavior change, it is not possible to address all of them in detail here. Indeed, a number of textbooks are devoted entirely to the topic of behavior change, such as *Health Behavior and Health Education: Theory, Research and Practice, Third Edition* (Glanz, Rimer, and Lewis, 2002). As our textbook is based on the CHW Certificate Program at City College of San Francisco, it will provide detailed descriptions of resources that are used in our program. In Chapter Ten, we will cover models and techniques commonly used by CHWs to conduct behavior change counseling, including the states of change, harm-reduction and risk-reduction counseling, and motivational interviewing. Each of these, however, is an example of a client-centered approach to facilitating behavior change. This is an overarching principle that we hope will guide all of the work that you do with individual clients.

The client-centered approach views CHWs as facilitators who support clients to make changes that promote their health. This approach recognizes that in order for these changes to be most valuable, effective, and long-lasting, they must come from the client and the community, not from providers or outside "experts." In other words, it is not the role of the CHW to tell clients or communities what to believe or what do in order to promote their health. Rather, your role is to support clients and communities in carefully analyzing the factors that both harm and promote their health, in identifying possible choices or courses of action and their consequences, and in developing and implementing a plan for individual or community-level change.

HIV prevention groups in Zimbabwe (I-TECH, 2005) use the diagram in Figure 8.1 to depict client-centered practice.

Figure 8.1 **Big Ears, Big Eyes.**

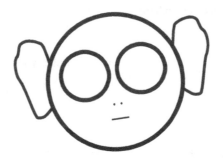

This diagram depicts a CHW who is working with a client. The big ears show a CHW who is listening carefully and deeply to the client. The big eyes indicate that the CHW is carefully observing the client and the surrounding world (social context). The small mouth indicates that the CHW is careful not to talk too much during the session. Rather than dominating the discussion, the CHW uses techniques such as open-ended questions designed to provide clients with an opportunity to reflect on their life and their health, to explore their experiences and feelings, and to identity actions that will reduce harm and promote their health and well-being.

Client-centered practice is also strength-based. While traditional approaches have often focused primarily or exclusively on the client's risk behaviors and lack of resources, a client-centered approach seeks greater balance. It emphasizes the internal and external resources that a client already has. **External resources** are often easier to identify. They are the resources that lie outside of the client and may include family and friends, stable housing, a trusted primary health care provider, spiritual faith or religious tradition, or a secure job at a living wage. **Internal resources** reside within the client, and may include knowledge, skills, talents, experiences, wisdom, courage, compassion, personality, sense of humor, interests, abilities, and past successes. The client-centered practitioner always looks for and acknowledges a client's internal and external resources and supports clients in using and building on these resources to promote their health.

Client-centered practice does not mean that CHWs should always agree with or support everything that a client says or does. While CHWs should provide unconditional regard for clients, CHWs do not provide unconditional approval of their behaviors. Some of your clients will continue to do things that may be harmful to themselves or others. These are the times for CHWs to intervene, to ask questions, to challenge clients, and to pose alternatives for consideration. As we learned earlier, occasionally CHWs will have an ethical and legal obligation to report these behaviors (if they include suicide or child abuse, for example). You also have a responsibility to gently confront clients about behaviors or decisions that concern you, such as skipping medical treatments, engaging in unprotected sex, smoking, or sharing needles to inject drugs. Knowledge and skills for how to address these issues in a client-centered way will be addressed in the chapters that follow.

Am I Doing Client-Centered Work?   To assess whether or not you are doing client-centered work, reflect on the following questions:

- Am I providing clients with the space and the opportunity to voice their true feelings and opinions?
- Are clients making health decisions that truly reflect their own ideas, values, and reality?
- Am I dominating the discussions with clients? Am I talking more than my clients are?
- Am I bringing my own agenda into the clients' sessions?
- What is getting in the way of my ability to truly listen to clients?

ALVARO MORALES: I started out doing a lot of HIV antibody test counseling that really trained me in the client-centered approach. My job was to work with a client to assess their own risks for HIV infection—and what they could realistically do to reduce those risks. I would ask pretty straightforward questions that just gave them a chance to talk, to identify their own resources, and anything else that they might want to learn or to get access to . . . like drug treatment or syringe exchange or parenting classes, anything. I still use this approach anytime I am working with clients and even when I am working with communities, because the same skills that you use to listen to clients and to support them to figure out what they can do to improve their health, it's the same thing you do to support communities to figure out what they want to do to improve things on a bigger level.

An Application of Client-Centered Counseling   Above, we discussed four classic mistakes that CHWs might make when working with a client named L. Here, we wish to show how a client-centered approach could be used to work with the same client.

Using a client-centered approach, a CHW may ask a range of questions over the course of one or more sessions. These questions should not be asked all at once, but as appropriate and in response to what the client says. They may include:

Assessing Knowledge

- Can you tell me what you know about STIs and how to prevent them?

Questions About Specific Behaviors

- Are there particular times or situations when you notice that you are more likely not to use condoms? What is it about these situations that makes it more difficult for you to use condoms?
- Can you tell me about a time when you did negotiate condom use or another type of safer sex? What made this possible? What was this like for you?
- It seems that when you are sexually attracted to someone, it is harder for you to talk with them about using condoms—is that right? Why do you think this is so?

Deep listening is the essence of client-centered counseling.

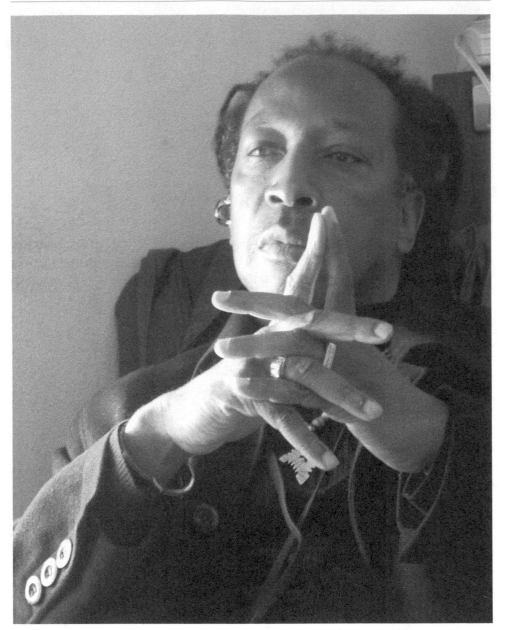

Assessing Resources

⭐ What kind of support do you have to make these changes in your life? Is there a par-ticular family member or friend you feel comfortable confiding in?

⭐ Do you have a good source of health care? Where do you usually go? Do you know about the free health clinic? What has your experience been with these medical providers?

⭐ Can you tell me about a time when you were successful at making a change in your life?

Assessing Readiness

✪ What is it like for you to talk about these issues with me?

✪ How important is it to you to start using condoms more frequently when you have sex?

✪ It sounds like you are ready to try talking about condom use with your sexual partners—is that right?

✪ Would you like to meet and talk with me again?

Identifying Actions to Promote Health

✪ What can you start to do now to reduce your risk for STIs?

✪ What will you try to do differently in your next relationship?

✪ What will assist you to reduce risks for sexual transmission of HIV?

The CHW may make the following types of statements, as appropriate:

✪ I'm glad that you talked with me tonight, and that you went to a clinic to get tested for STIs. It can take a lot of courage to get tested.

✪ I just want to let you know that you decide what we talk about together. I will ask you some pretty personal questions, including questions about your sex life, but it is completely up to you whether or not you want to answer or talk about these issues. I will respect whatever you decide about this.

✪ I talk with a lot of people who find it difficult to negotiate safer sex and condom use. Most people don't grow up being taught how to talk about sex. I think most people find it embarrassing at first.

✪ I'd really like to talk with you again. You can always find me here on Saturday nights. You can also call me at (gives business card and number).

This CHW asks open-ended questions designed to assist clients to reflect on their knowledge, behaviors, and feelings; their risks for HIV infection; and what they are ready to do to reduce these risks. The CHW doesn't judge clients' behavior or tell clients what to do, say, or feel. The CHW assesses and affirms the positive steps that clients have taken and aids in identifying their resources. While the CHW does affirm the efforts that clients are making to understand and change their behavior, the clients do most of the talking.

IMPLICIT THEORY

When most people think of theory, they think of theories like those mentioned above (stages of change, motivational interviewing) that have been written down and published in books or articles. Implicit theory refers to the concepts that each of us develop—in this instance related to behavior change—based on our own life and work experience. Over time, CHWs develop implicit theories about behavior change through the course of their work with hundreds of clients through the course of thier work with hundreds of diverse clients. Typically, we don't have the opportunity to conduct research on these theories or to publish them, and they are not formally recognized by others working in the public health field.

The Implicit Theories Project investigated beliefs about behavior change among CHWs doing HIV prevention work in the San Francisco Bay Area. Researchers from the University of California, San Francisco (UCSF) reported that CHWs develop their own theories about risk behaviors and the factors that influence behavior change based on their work with clients and communities (Freedman and others, 2006). The theories developed by CHWs often shared common ideas, including an emphasis on the influence of social context (or environmental factors) and the importance for clients of having a sense of community. Researchers also highlighted the importance of implicit theories to the development of effective community-based programs and services.

We strongly encourage you to continue to develop your own implicit theories as you build your career in the community health field. We encourage you to reflect deeply about the question of why people behave the way they do, and what supports people to change behaviors that are harming their health or the health of others. Consider the following resources for developing your own implicit theories:

- Examine your own biases and reflect on how your own identity, experience, and culture may influence your ideas about behavior and behavior change (you may wish to refer to Chapter Seven).
- Research and read about theories of behavior change.
- Attend local workshops and classes that address issues related to behavior change.
- Ask your colleagues what they have found works in supporting the behavior change of clients.
- Share your implicit theories with colleagues, engaging in dialogue and refining your beliefs over time.
- Most important, don't forget to ask, and to listen carefully to, what your clients believe motivates their behavior and supports their ability to create lasting changes.

You will learn more about client-centered practice and how to apply it in your work with clients in Chapters Nine, Ten, Eleven, and Twelve.

CHAPTER REVIEW

ETHICAL GUIDELINES

To review, revisit some of the questions posed at the beginning of this section on ethics. For example:

- A client asks to borrow $10 to get something to eat. What should you do? How will you explain your decision to the client?
- A client with HIV disease informs you that she hasn't disclosed her HIV status to her partners, and she is continuing to have unprotected sex. One of these partners is also a client. What should you do?

1. Which articles in the AACHW Code of Ethics apply to these situations?
2. Apply the Framework for Ethical Decision Making to one or more of these situations:

    Step 1. Identify and describe the problem or dilemma.

Step 2. Review the relevant ethical guidelines or codes.

Step 3. Know the applicable laws and regulations.

Step 4. Obtain consultation.

Step 5. Consider possible and probable courses of action.

Step 6. Outline possible consequences of decisions.

Step 7. Decide on what appears to be the best course of action.

SELF-AWARENESS

Review the questions posed earlier in the chapter for self-evaluation, such as: What populations are you less familiar with and least prepared to work with?

SCOPE OF PRACTICE

- What is scope of practice (SOP), and why is it important for CHWs to understand?

✪ Identify specific examples not used in the text-book of the following:

- One CHW task that is clearly within their SOP
- One CHW task that is clearly outside of their SOP
- One task that may or may not be within their SOP
- What factors may determine whether or not this task is within the CHW's SOP? What could the CHW do to determine whether the task was within their SOP?

✪ What may happen when CHWs exceed their scope of practice?

PROMOTING BEHAVIOR CHANGE

Apply the ecological model to the issue of binge drinking. A client gets drunk on the weekend, blacks out, and can't remember what happened or what he or she did. Identify factors that influence behavior and may get in the way of successful behavior change at the following levels:

- Individual factors
- Family and friends
- Neighborhood and community factors
- Societal factors

✪ How might the "blaming the client" approach be used when working with the client who is binge drinking?

✪ Why would you discourage a new CHW from using the "blaming the client" approach?

CLIENT-CENTERED PRACTICE

✪ How would you briefly explain the central concept of client-centered practice to a new CHW?

✪ What does it mean to apply a strength-based approach to your work with clients, and how is this different from traditional approaches?

REFERENCES

Corey, G., Corey, M. S., and Callanan, P. 2007. *Issues and Ethics in the Helping Professions* (7th ed.). Belmont, CA: Thomson Brooks/Cole.

Freedman, B., Binson, D., Ekstrand, M., Galvez, S., Woods, W. J., and Grinstead, O. 2006. Uncovering Implicit Theories of HIV Prevention Providers: It Takes a Community. *AIDS Education and Prevention*

18(3): 216–226. Accessed on March 27, 2009: http://www.caps.ucsf.edu/CAPS/about/pdf/ITarticleAEP.pdf

Glanz, K., Rimer, B. K., and Lewis, F. M., eds. 2002. *Health Behavior and Health Education: Theory, Research and Practice, Third Edition.* San Francisco: Jossey-Bass.

Ryan, W. 1976. *Blaming the Victim.* New York: Vintage Books.

ADDITIONAL RESOURCES

International Training and Education Center on HIV (I-TECH) and the Ministry of Health and Child Welfare, Zimbabwe. 2005. Integrated Counselling for

HIV and AIDS Prevention and Care: Training for HIV Primary Care Counsellors. Unpublished training manual.

9

Conducting Initial Client Interviews

Tim Berthold • Mickey Ellinger

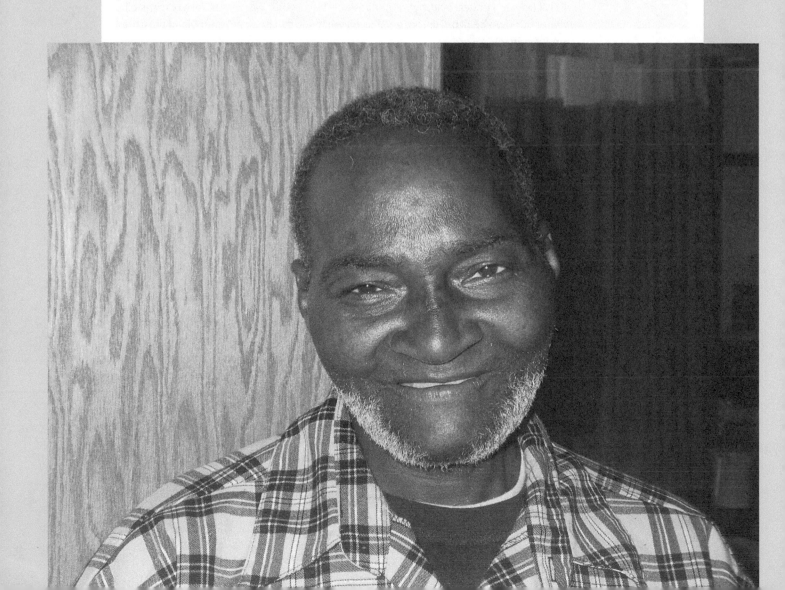

CASE STUDY: ARNOLD

Arnold Winters is fifty-two years old and was recently released from prison after completing an eight-year sentence related to drug use. During his stay in prison, Arnold developed hypertension (high blood pressure) and it still isn't under control. He doesn't feel that he received good health care in prison, and the food and lack of exercise only worsened his health. Arnold really wants to make changes in his life: he wants to stay in recovery and reunite with his family, particularly his children and grandchildren. He also wants to find a job. A friend referred him to The Good Health Center. It is close to where he is staying in his cousin's garage.

Arnold fills out a form at The Good Health Center, providing a reason for the visit, and his latest blood pressure readings. The receptionist tells Arnold to take a seat and wait for his name to be called. He is fifteen minutes early for his appointment. An hour later, Arnold's name is called, and he is escorted to an interview room by a CHW.

CHW (says): "Hi, I'll be doing your intake today to see if you qualify for our services. I see here that your blood pressure has been really high. How did you let it get so out of control?"

Arnold (says): "Well, the biggest factor was being in prison for the past eight years. It was hard to take care of myself there, and the health care wasn't so good either."

CHW (says): "I understand, but our philosophy here is that we need to take responsibility for our own health. Our focus will be on what you can do to get your blood pressure under control."

Arnold (*thinks*): "The only way you can *understand* is if you've been in prison. Have you been in prison?"

Arnold (says): "Well, I guess that's why I came, to get some help figuring it all out. I've started exercising, and I'm trying to eat good, but it's hard when you don't have any money. I mostly eat at the soup kitchen at Temple Church."

CHW (says): "Maybe I could put you in Keith's group. He's another one of our clients and he's also an ex-convict."

Arnold (*thinks*): "Here we go again with the 'ex-convict' label. That isn't who I am!"

Arnold (says): "Okay."

INTRODUCTION

Think about a time when you have been a new client or patient at a clinic, hospital, or social services agency. What was your initial interview like? How did you feel during the interview, and how did you feel about the clinic or agency afterward? What did the person who was interviewing you say or do to make the interview more (or less) comfortable and productive for you?

This chapter addresses how to conduct an initial interview with a new client who may be interested in participating in a particular program, service, or research study. These interviews are often the first contact that a client has with an agency, and the CHW's first opportunity to develop a positive connection or rapport with that individual or family. These initial client interviews may also be referred to as client intakes or client assessments. For the purposes of this chapter, we will focus on conducting initial interviews to determine eligibility and participation in a particular health-focused program or service.

Guidelines for conducting research interviews tend to be much more extensive and strict, and the format, questions, and policies for research interviews vary widely. If you are hired to conduct research interviews, you will be trained to follow detailed procedures.

Our approach to client interviewing is informed by the guiding principles covered in Chapter Eight. Our goal is to prepare you to conduct an ethical, client-centered interview that stays within the scope of practice for CHWs.

WHAT YOU WILL LEARN

By studying the information in this chapter, you will be able to:

- Describe the types of initial client interviews that CHWs are likely to conduct
- Explain confidentiality policies to a client
- Obtain informed consent for an interview
- Build rapport with a new client
- Conduct a client-centered interview, including the use of open- and closed-ended questions
- Conduct a strength-based assessment, and explain why this is so important
- Explain the importance of documentation and specific strategies for taking notes during an interview
- Close an initial interview effectively

WORDS TO KNOW

Body Language   Closed-Ended Question   Open-Ended Question
Resilience

9.1 AN OVERVIEW OF CLIENT INTERVIEWING

In general, CHWs conduct initial interviews with new clients in order to:

- Assess and determine whether the client is eligible for and interested in participating in the services provided by a particular agency or program
- Complete an initial assessment of the client's resources, risks, and needs
- Obtain informed consent for participation in a research study, and in some cases, to initiate the research interview

The questions that you will ask, the length of the interview, and the forms used to document information about the client will vary depending on the purpose of the interview and the type of program or service that the client is interested in. Initial interviews may be fairly simple or very complex, and may consist of ten to fifty or more questions. Some interviews are conducted in one session lasting fifteen to forty-five minutes or longer, and others take place during more than one session. The longest interview forms and most complicated procedures are used by research studies that may be conducted over multiple sessions.

During an initial interview, you will gather a range of information from the client. You will probably ask for basic demographic data such as date of birth, gender, gender identity, ethnicity, primary languages, address, income, and family status. This demographic information is sometimes sensitive in nature, and we will offer suggestions about how and when to gather it. You may also ask questions about the client's health status, including questions about their knowledge, attitudes, and behaviors in relation to a specific health condition or concern such as diabetes, hepatitis C, or a type of cancer. Interviews may also include questions about the client's support system; prior experience with similar programs and agencies; the client's current condition and concerns; and the client's expectations regarding the program or service your organization offers.

The type of questions you ask during initial interviews will vary depending on the program you are working for and the specific health issues you are addressing. As you may imagine, the questions asked by CHWs working with a domestic violence agency will be different from those working for a perinatal health, drug counseling, diabetes management, or mental health program. Some questions may be highly personal in nature. For example, interviews regarding clients' risks for HIV disease typically include questions regarding their history of drug use and sexual behaviors.

You will use a form or forms, provided by your employer, to document the information that you learn from the client. Suggestions for how to document the interview are provided toward the end of this chapter.

Initial interviews or assessments may be stressful for a client. Clients may be worried that they or their family members won't qualify for services. They may have been mistreated or disrespected by health or social services providers in the past, and be worried about being judged by the interviewer. Clients may have engaged in activities that are illegal, such as drug use or prostitution, and be worried about whether telling you about such activities will be held against them. Undocumented immigrants may be worried about their security and the possibility that they will be reported to immigration authorities.

?   *Can you think of other concerns or sources of anxiety for new clients?*

?   *For example, what might contribute to Arnold's stress as he prepares for his interview at The Good Health Center?*

?   *What might he be hoping for?*

?   *What might he be worried about?*

?   *What experiences might he have had before, at other agencies or clinics, including in prison?*

As a CHW, your primary goals for an initial client interview are to:

- Welcome the client to the agency, and make the person as comfortable as possible during the interview process
- Build a positive initial connection
- Clearly describe and explain the interview process and related services that the client may be eligible for
- Clearly explain confidentiality and its limits
- Obtain informed consent from the client in order to conduct the interview, and in order to decide whether to participate in a particular program
- Assess not only the client's risk factors, but also the internal and external resources that promote their health
- Listen and respond to the client's questions and concerns
- Provide guidance and support to the client in making decisions about their next steps including whether to enroll in specific programs or research studies

? *What other goals might you have when you conduct an initial*
client interview?

A REMINDER ABOUT SCOPE OF PRACTICE

Your scope of practice may limit the type of questions you are qualified to ask and the type of information you gather during an interview. For example, when CHWs conduct a client interview at a hospital or health center, medical providers will assess medical conditions, such as hypertension or diabetes. In this context, the role of the CHW is to work in partnership with medical providers who will be responsible for diagnosing medical conditions and prescribing treatment. When working as part of a team, be sure to clarify your role and scope of practice with your supervisor and your teammates.

THE STRUCTURE OF A CLIENT INTERVIEW

A client interview, like a good story, has a distinct beginning, middle, and end.
   The *beginning* of the client interview consists of:

- Welcoming the client and assisting the person to feel as comfortable as possible
- Introducing yourself, your agency and program, and the purpose of the interview
- Explaining the interview process and the types of information that you hope to learn
- Explaining confidentiality and its limits
- Obtaining informed consent to conduct the interview and initiate services
- Building rapport

   The *middle phase* of the interview usually consists of:

- Gathering detailed information from the client required in order to determine eligibility for the health program, service, or research study
- Answering the client's questions and concerns
- Assessing the client's risk factors, as well as the internal and external resources they bring to the task of improving their health
- Building rapport

   The *ending phase* of the interview usually consists of:

- Determining enrollment or participation in the program or service in question
- Providing other referrals, as appropriate
- Identifying the next steps for the client (such as scheduling a follow-up appointment)
- Asking if the client still has any outstanding questions or concerns
- Closing the interview in a way that affirms and respects the client

JUGGLING ALL THE ELEMENTS OF THE CLIENT INTERVIEW

It can be challenging to juggle all of the essential elements of an initial client interview. You have a lot to accomplish in a relatively short period of time. From a client-centered perspective, the most important thing about the interview is to listen and respond to the client's priority concerns. While you may feel pressure from your supervisor to complete the interview and all of the required paperwork, if you in turn pressure the client to answer your questions and respond to your priorities, you may undermine the working relationship. Remember to be patient with the client and yourself. If necessary, you can always schedule another time to complete your intake questions and forms.

9.2 THE BEGINNING OF THE INTERVIEW

In most, but not all cases, the interview will serve as your first interaction with a prospective client, and it may be that person's first interaction with anyone from the agency you work for. Making a positive first impression on the client is important to conducting a productive interview. It is the first step toward establishing an ongoing working relationship, and it increases the chances that the client will return to the agency to participate in the services you provide.

? *What makes you feel comfortable and welcomed when you go to a new agency for services?*

? *Do you think Arnold felt comfortable with the CHW who interviewed him?*

? *Do you think he would trust the CHW to support him to reach his health goals?*

? *Is he likely to participate in programs, or to recommend the agency to others?*

BUILDING A POSITIVE CONNECTION WITH CLIENTS

Your success as a CHW will be influenced by your ability to create and maintain a positive, trusting relationship with the clients you serve. While trust will largely be based on the quality of services that you and your organization provide, it will also depend on how clients feel they are treated by you and by others who deliver those services. The personal style that you bring to your encounters contributes to building a trusting professional relationship. This personal style may include, for example, your tone of voice, your smile and sense of humor, and how you listen to clients and acknowledge their accomplishments and their challenges. Never fake your approach or style of working with clients: be true to your own experience, values, and personality.

Some of the clients you work with will have personal histories that include abuse, violence, discrimination, homelessness, addiction, and incarceration. Many clients have also had bad experiences with helping professionals, and these may influence their interactions with you. Some clients may observe you closely to see if you are going to be yet another person who in some way disrespects or puts them down. While you can't do anything to change the past, you can treat your clients with the respect and dignity they deserve and work to build a professional alliance that supports their health. We cannot emphasize enough the vital importance of building a warm and respectful relationship with your clients: it is the foundation for all the work that you and the clients will do together.

THE INTERVIEW SPACE

A great interview can start before you say your first word, by simply setting the stage for privacy and respect. In the real world, not all client interviews take place in a quiet, comfortable, and private room. Often, the interviews will take place in the middle of waiting rooms, in homes, in shelters—or even outside, on the street or in a park. No matter where the interview takes place, you can find ways to make the best of a less than private situation to assist the client feel safer and more comfortable.

If you are working in a setting that is not ideal for conducting an interview, acknowledge this and ask the client to aid you in determining the best location for your conversation:

"How about sitting down together on that bench over there in the corner: it seems a little less noisy and more private. Would that work for you? Do you have another suggestion for where we can talk?"

If you do have access to an individual office for conducting interviews, think about what you can do with the materials and budget at hand to make it as inviting as possible. Does the office have a comfortable chair for clients? Can you decorate the space? Is there a place for a client's children to sit and play while you conduct an interview? Can you purchase or seek donations of children's books or toys? Can you offer clients a glass of water, a cup of tea, or a snack? This kind of attention to detail will show your clients that you care about them and your work.

Seating arrangements can affect the relationship between you and the people you're interviewing. Asking a client to sit on the other side of your imposing desk may create a feeling of formality and distance that could get in the way of building rapport or connection. Sitting next to a client during an interview may create a more relaxed atmosphere and allow the information you write down to be shared. Think about the options available to you, and talk with colleagues about how they set up their interview space.

? *What sort of an office makes you feel most comfortable?*

? *How would you decorate an office—with very little money— where you conduct client interviews?*

? *How would you handle the interview space when doing street outreach?*

INTRODUCING YOURSELF TO A CLIENT

You may have noticed that Arnold was never properly introduced to the CHW he met with. Introduce yourself to your clients: tell them your name, job title (if this is the first meeting), what you will cover during your meeting, and how you would like to be addressed. For example:

"Hi, it's a pleasure to meet you. My name is Lucy Chang, and I'm a community health worker here at the clinic. I'll be talking with you today about our asthma management program. Please call me Lucy."

Sometimes people try to use a "professional" tone of voice that may seem impersonal, cold, or robotic to a client. We encourage you to be yourself, and to welcome a new client like you would a visitor to your home. Smile. Reach out to shake hands if appropriate. Use a warm and friendly tone of voice.

Greet the client, and if you know it, call them by name—it may be written down in an appointment book. In clinic or agency settings, it generally conveys respect to address clients by their last names—Mr. Dorman, Ms. Lee, Mrs. Ramaya—until or unless they ask you to address them differently. If they are using a name different from the one you have written on the appointment form, clarify which name they would like to use in the documents you prepare and what name they would like to be called by. If you are ever unclear as to how to address new clients, ask them how they would like to be addressed.

"Good morning, Mrs. Sanchez, how are you today? Should I call you Mrs. Sanchez, or do you prefer to be called by a different name?"

By asking the clients what name they would like to be called, you are demonstrating respect and flexibility, and your willingness to take their guidance. This sets a positive tone for a client-centered interview.

DETERMINE THE LANGUAGE OF SERVICE

You may be conducting an interview in English, Spanish, American Sign Language, Farsi, Cantonese, or another language. Be sure to ask clients what their primary language is. You may need to provide them with an interpreter, if available, or find someone who speaks their language to conduct the interview. Don't proceed with the interview if you are not truly fluent in the language of service. This is essential so that no mistakes are made that could be harmful to the client's health or welfare.

ASK CLIENTS WHAT THEY WANT TO ACHIEVE

A good way to begin an interview is to ask some version of: "What brings you here today?" This gives clients an opportunity to share what they hope to get out of the meeting. They can ask about the type of services they are most interested in, and mention anything else that is on their mind. This, too, conveys your concern for the client.

EXPLAIN THE INTERVIEW

Let the client know what to expect, by clearly explaining:

- The purpose of the interview
- How long it may take
- The type of information you will ask them for
- How this information will be used

The rest of the interview session will soon shift, with you asking questions and then listening, and the client speaking most of the time. You will speak more at the beginning of the interview, however, and must take time to explain the interview process. You will also explain confidentiality and obtain informed consent. For example, you might say:

"I understand that your daughter Christa has asthma. I'm here to talk with you about her asthma and to see how we might work together to improve her health. This first meeting will take about half an hour. Do you have that much time today?"

(Assuming the client is prepared to spend half an hour with the CHW, continue . . .)

"I have a number of questions to ask about Christa and your family. The questions are about her symptoms, any medication she may be using, problems that she and you may be facing that influence her health—things like that. If I ask you a question that you would prefer not to talk about, please let me know, and I promise to respect your wishes. Will you feel comfortable letting me know if you don't want to talk about something?"

(Client responds.)

"You will see me writing down the information that you tell me on this client intake form. (Show the client the form, even if they are unable to read.) At the end of the interview, we can decide together whether our Pediatric Asthma Program would be a good fit for Christa and your family.

If you do decide to participate in the program, the information I document will be placed in a file to be shared with your service provider. Do you have any questions about the interview before we begin?"

EXPLAIN THE CONFIDENTIALITY POLICY

Confidentiality was introduced in Chapter Eight, as one of the most important ethical obligations for CHWs. Part of this obligation is learning how to clearly explain confidentiality and its limits to your clients. You must do this at the beginning of your first session or interview with new clients, before they have an opportunity to tell you something that you may have to report to others.

Telling a family that an interview is confidential is not sufficient. Clearly explain what confidentiality means. Tell the client who will have access to the information you document. Check with your supervisor to be sure that you understand the confidentiality policy and protocols at your agency.

While in general you are able to promise that the client's information will be kept private, there are important exceptions to this rule. For example, if you learn that any of your clients have harmed or are intending to do harm to themselves or others, or have been harmed by others, you have a duty to report this information. The harms that we refer to include suicide, child abuse, sexual abuse, physical assault, or threats.

Earlier, we suggested that when you welcome a new client, you ask: "What brings you to the clinic today?" However, if clients starts to talk about a subject that you may need to report to legal authorities, we suggest that you interrupt them and take time to clearly explain the limits of confidentiality. If you don't explain this up front, and a client discloses a situation that you have a legal and ethical obligation to report, it is likely that they client may feel set up or betrayed. This is likely to destroy all hope of establishing trust.

The CHW might say something such as:

"I want to hear more about your daughter's asthma. But before we start to talk about that in greater detail, I need to explain our policy on confidentiality."

"Everything that you tell me will be kept private. It will go into your client file here at the clinic. Only your service providers here, including the nurse practitioner, respiratory therapist, and community health worker will have access to the information in your file. They will not share this information with other service providers unless they talk with you first, and you sign a form giving them permission to share this information with others."

Take your time. Don't rush this. Maintain eye contact and a friendly tone of voice. Pay attention to your client's body language and signs that the person may not understand you.

"However, there are a couple of exceptions to this policy that I need to discuss with every new client. If a client ever tells me that they are harming themselves or others or are being hurt by someone else, then by law I have to tell my supervisor, and they may have to tell law enforcement authorities. By hurting themselves or others we mean things like sexual or physical abuse or suicide. As a health worker, if I learn that someone is in danger, I can't keep silent. Do you understand? Do you have any questions about the privacy of what we talk about today?"

If you doubt that clients fully understand you, ask them to tell you what they understand about the privacy or confidentiality policy. This is the best way to be certain that you have been clear. For more information about confidentiality and ethics, please refer to Chapter Eight and, most important, remember to share any questions or concerns you may have with your supervisor.

? *How would you explain the concept of confidentiality to a client?*

OBTAIN INFORMED CONSENT

Before you conduct an interview or provide services to a client, you need the client's informed consent. Informed consent means that the client fully understands what the interview or service will consist of, and gives permission to participate in the interview or program in question. Generally, the client is asked to give informed consent in writing.

The biggest mistake a CHW can make is to rush this process. Sometimes clients are told to: "Sign your name here so that we can do the interview [or *before you start the program*]." This is *not* informed consent! In order to be certain that clients understand what the interview will consist of, explain it to them in simple language, then ask them to tell you what they have learned. "Mrs. Sanchez, I want to be sure that you understand what this interview is all about before I start. Can you tell me what we will talk about and how the information will be used?"

If the client does not fully understand what the interview will consist of (the types of questions you will ask, how the information will be used, and the limits of confidentiality), review the information again. Check to see if they have any questions or concerns: "I don't want to rush you. Before we begin the interview, do you have any questions for me?"

Note: Review your agency's policies about informed consent. Depending on the program you work for, there may be an age of consent for minors and guidelines for working with people who are developmentally disabled or mentally ill. In some instances, a parent or legal guardian must be consulted. People who are noticeably drunk or high on drugs cannot provide consent for services.

BE AWARE OF BODY LANGUAGE AND TONE OF VOICE

You and the client will communicate not only with words, but also through **body language** and tone of voice. Our facial expressions, how close we sit to others, how we hold our body and our arms, and the degree of eye contact we maintain often convey important messages about what we are thinking or feeling. The tone of our voice also tends to change with emotion and may invite connection or create distance. Try to build an awareness of the tone of voice and body language that you and your clients use.

Be cautious, however, about assuming that you understand what is meant by a particular physical expression such as avoiding eye contact, crossing arms over the chest, frowning, or rolling the eyes. Body language is influenced by cultural as well as individual differences. With experience, you will become more skilled in noticing the body language of others, and as appropriate, talking with your clients about them. For example: "I notice that whenever you talk about your father-in law, your expression seems to change. I wonder what you are feeling when we talk about him. Is there anything else you would like to say about this?" Remember that many people are unaware of their body language. Don't push clients to talk further about this or anything else if they don't want to.

? *How might your tone of voice and body language work to build a connection with clients?*

? *How might it get in the way of building a connection?*

Body language can show that we are truly paying attention to clients.

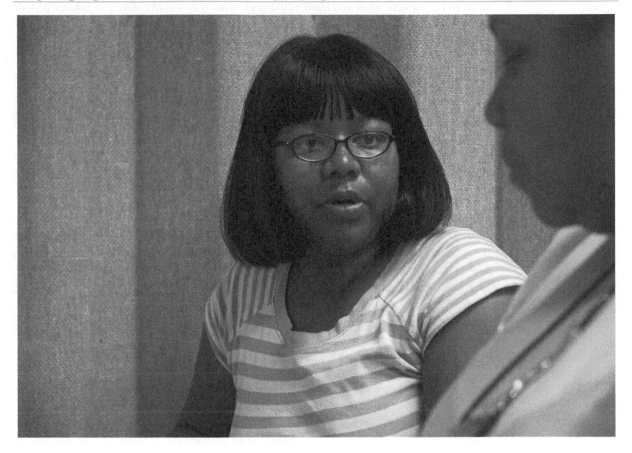

9.3 THE MIDDLE OF THE INTERVIEW

The middle of the interview is when you gather and provide information that will assist you and your clients in determining whether they should participate in a particular health program or service. Various techniques can assist you to gather and provide this information in effective, client-centered ways.

PHUONG AN DOAN BILLINGS: I try to understand people who come to us with a lot of problems. Sometimes they don't say all that's going on for them. When the doctors ask them, "How you feel today? How are you?" they'll say, "I'm good," but there's a lot inside that they cannot say. But because we CHWs are one of them, we are community people, and we use our client-centered skills. They can confide in us. They can tell us how they really feel.

LISTEN TO AND FOCUS ON THE CLIENT

Gathering the right information is an important part of providing quality services to clients. However, you don't have to be rigid in the way you gather information. Your focus should be on the client or family in front of you rather than on the form waiting to be filled out. If you are interviewing people from a different community or culture from your own, take time to be sure that you are paying attention to cultural differences. Ask the questions on the form and document what you learn as the conversation flows. Maintain eye contact periodically even while taking notes, and be sure to explain why you are taking notes. For example, "I want to make sure I can tell the nurse exactly what you're telling me in your own words."

T G: The forms are not the most important part of the interview. I want to make sure my families are doing okay. I check in with them first, and we talk. Most of the time, I get all the information I need by just talking with them. No one wants to be grilled with question after question.

Before you begin to interview clients, check the forms your organization uses for assumptions that could make someone uncomfortable, such as assumptions about gender, gender identity, or who makes a family. If the forms you have been asked to use are biased, talk with your supervisor. When you are working with your clients, practice cultural humility. Frame your questions in ways that respect all kinds of individuals, and all kinds of families. Asking a client to tell you about their family, for example, is preferrable to asking: "Are you married or single?"

USE LANGUAGE THAT IS ACCESSIBLE TO THE CLIENT

If you use words or phrases that your client doesn't understand, you will undermine your ability to conduct an effective interview. Similarly, if you present detailed information that a client already understands, you may also undermine rapport. A good way to start is to ask clients what they already know about a topic. For example: "Can you tell me what you already know about mammograms?" or "Can you tell me what you remember about the HIV antibody test?" If you use medical terms, such as mammogram, sputum, or antibody test, be sure to explain them using everyday language. Try to avoid using acronyms (initials or words made out of initials, like SSI or WIC), at least until you have first spelled them out and explained them (Social Security Income; Women, Infants, and Children). As you talk with clients, periodically check in to see whether they understand, by asking them to explain the information to you.

SHOW THAT YOU CARE

Create an atmosphere of mutual respect and trust by showing genuine interest, concern, and empathy. Allow time for people to talk, tell their stories, and explain their problems. If the client sounds upset, check in with the person:

"It sounds like you are upset. Do you want to take a break before we move on?" or

"It sounds like you had a really bad experience at the emergency room. It can be difficult to see your child so sick and not be able to do anything about it. Let's try to figure out what happened, and what can be done to prevent this from happening in the future."

GATHERING DEMOGRAPHIC INFORMATION

The demographic information that you will gather (information such as date of birth, nationality, ethnicity, sex, gender identity, family status, address, income, health insurance, and so on) can be highly sensitive. It can be awkward to ask for this type of information: it isn't something that you would ordinarily ask someone. For these reasons, we suggest that you don't start an interview by asking for demographic information. Even though these questions tend to be placed at the very beginning of the forms you use, you may want to leave them until later in the interview, after you have established a connection with the client. You could also ask clients to fill out the information themselves and then review it together (although keep in mind that not all of your clients will be able to read or write). As always, be respectful of the client's right not to answer any of the questions that you ask.

TIME MANAGEMENT

Part of your job is to juggle providing client-centered services with the need to complete the interview questions, all within the time frame that you and the client have allotted for your meeting. With practice, you will learn to listen to your client and to be aware of the time that remains in your session. If you scheduled forty minutes, are you on track to finish the interview on time? Would it be possible to finish on time without unduly interrupting the client's agenda or damaging your rapport? If so, call this to the client's attention and make this decision together: "Arnold, I don't mean to interrupt, but we have about fifteen minutes left, and I think we can complete the intake form in that time. Should we move on to the next set of questions?"

Sometimes, however, priority issues may emerge for the client during the course of the interview, and these are the most important issues for you to address in the moment. If and when this occurs, acknowledge this to the client. "Arnold, we have about fifteen minutes left, and I'd like to keep talking with you about your family. Is it okay with you to finish the intake interview next time?"

RESPECT YOUR CLIENT'S RIGHT TO PRIVACY

While it is your job to ask questions, clients have a right to decide what information they will and won't share with you. This is especially true with questions about immigration, welfare, substance use, sexuality, traumatic experiences, and any issue that may have legal consequences that may range from loss of housing to deportation. Even if you maintain confidentiality about such issues, the fears of your clients need to be respected. If you ask a sensitive question and you sense that the client is uncomfortable, move on—don't try to push or force an answer.

"These questions can be difficult to talk about. I don't want to push you to talk about anything that you may not want to discuss with me. Do you want to skip this question"

ASSESSING CLIENT RESOURCES: A STRENGTH-BASED APPROACH

Generally, you will be asked to assess clients' health risks and current needs including, for example, their needs for housing, legal assistance, mental health counseling, and health education. The forms will guide you in asking these questions.

However, helping professionals often focus primarily or exclusively on clients' problems, including what they have or haven't done that may increase their risks for disease or disability. In contrast, client-centered practice also focuses on the positive accomplishments and attributes, and the **resilience** (or ability to face and handle challenges) of clients and communities. Every client has done something positive to promote their own health and survival or that of their family.

When working with clients, assess them for both external and internal resources that promote their health and wellness. External resources are sometimes easier for CHWs and clients to talk about. These are resources that lie outside of the individual and may include, for example, family and friends, spiritual or religious community, cultural traditions, a "good" job, a safe home, health insurance coverage, or a skilled medical provider. Internal resources are those that lie within the client and may include, for example, previous life accomplishments, a sense of humor, spiritual or religious faith, intelligence, creativity, integrity, the ability to be a good friend, commitment to family, vocational skills, or the ability to survive difficult life challenges. For more information about external and internal resources, please refer to Chapter Fourteen.

Every client you will work with has both external and internal resources, though, at times, it may be difficult for the client or the CHW to see these resources.

During a class at City College of San Francisco, a CHW student raised her hand to say: "All this stuff about resources sounds good in theory, but I'm working with homeless heroin addicts. I'm working with one man who has been out on the streets for almost ten years. I don't think he has any of these resources!" In response, the other students in class validated her experience ("sometimes it is really hard to see the positive things"), and offered suggestions for how to move forward with the client. For example, classmates asked:

* "He must have been doing something right just to be able to survive the streets for so long. What has kept your client alive on the streets for almost ten years?"
* "What do you like about this client?"
* "If he isn't in touch with any of his family, does he have any friends out on the streets?"
* "What else—other than heroin—is important to this client? What else does he really care about?"

As a consequence of this classroom discussion, the student began to view her client in a different way and to understand that he did, indeed, have both internal and external resources. For example, the client, no matter how bad he was doing, always asked how she (the student) was doing: he had tremendous capacity to be kind to others. He also had a buddy, and they watched out for each other on the street, sharing places to sleep, drugs, and food.

At appropriate points in the interview, ask questions and create opportunities to focus on the client's strengths. There are many ways to do this. Ask clients who or what they care about, or what gives them pleasure. They may not be able to answer these questions readily, or may simply say: "Nothing gives me pleasure anymore," or "Heroin is the only thing." You might ask: "What has kept you going all these years?" or "What did you do to survive . . . (the war in your country, being homeless, losing your family)?" Ask about and document a client's external and internal resources, even if this is not part of your agency's interview form.

Reflect back the resources and strengths that you observe in your client. For example, you might say something like: "I respect how you have managed to survive all you have gone through. It takes a lot of strength and creativity to keep going in the face of such great loss." A few kind words can mean a lot to a client who is struggling, and acknowledging a client's strengths often makes it more possible for that person to do so as well. These words have to be authentic, though, and true to the strengths you observe in a client.

One of the key roles for CHWs is to hold onto hope for your clients, even in times when they can't hold it for themselves. Recognizing your clients' strengths and assisting them to draw upon those strengths as you work together should underlie all of your interactions with your clients.

? *Think about Arnold, the client introduced at the beginning of the chapter. Based on the information provided, what strengths do you see?*

? *How would you work with him to identify other strengths?*

? *What are some of your own internal and external resources?*

ASK FOR CLARIFICATION

If you don't fully understand what a client is saying, and are unable to record the information accurately, ask! Sometimes CHWs feel shy about interrupting a client or admitting that they did not understand what a client said. However, it is much worse to pretend to understand when you don't, to miss the opportunity to document important information, or to record misinformation. You might say something like: "I'm not sure that I fully understood what you told me about Christa's symptoms. Could you tell me again?" or "I want to make sure I fully understand what you are saying about the mold in your apartment. Did you say that it was there when you moved in?"

SUMMARIZE WHAT YOU HAVE HEARD

Depending on the nature of the interview, you may want to review some of what you learned in order to be certain that you are accurately documenting what the client shared with you. For example, you might say something like: "I just want to make sure that I have documented everything correctly. Your daughter Molly is doing better with her new inhaler, but continues to have difficulty breathing at night. You are going to remove the carpet in her room to see if that makes a difference. Did I get that right?"

DOES THE CLIENT HAVE QUESTIONS OR CONCERNS?

Check in regularly to see if your clients have questions or concerns, particularly if you sense that they may be confused or upset. Taking the time to address their questions as you go along aids in building trust. Talking about their questions or concerns may also provide you with important information about their lives, health issues, and situations so you can assist them to access relevant programs and services.

ASKING QUESTIONS: SOME EFFECTIVE TECHNIQUES

The key to a good client interview depends not only on the type of question you ask, but also on the ease of the conversation between you and the family member. You want to create a smooth conversation rather than an interrogation. Using a combination of open-ended and closed-ended questions can assist you to accomplish this goal.

Closed-Ended Questions   **Closed-ended questions** can be answered with a few words, like *yes* or *no*. They are used when you want to focus the conversation and get specific information. Closed-ended questions often start with *is* or *do*.

> "Do you have your asthma medication?"
> "Is your Medicaid enrollment up to date?"

Open-Ended Questions   An **open-ended question** invites the client to respond with more than a *yes* or *no* answer. It encourages people to talk and may facilitate dialogue. Typically, open-ended questions use words such as *what, how, when,* or *would*.

> "What brings you here today?"
> "What happened next?"
> "How did you feel when?"
> "When did that happen?"
> "Would you tell me more about that?"

Questions at the Beginning of the Interview   Asking a broad open-ended question, such as "What brings you into the clinic today?" or "How have things been since we last talked?" or "What would you like to talk about today?" opens up discussion and leaves plenty of room for dialogue. If you start the interview with a closed-ended question, you are setting the direction of the interview and may miss important information that is critical to understanding the situation of the person or family you are interviewing.

The following are two examples of an interview: 1) starting the interview with a closed-ended question, and 2) starting the interview with an open-ended question. The interview is with the Sanchez family and their five-year-old daughter, Christa, who has asthma. Christa's asthma has been under control, and they are here at the clinic for a checkup.

Starting an Interview with a Closed-Ended Question

CHW: "Hi, are you here for a checkup?"

Mrs. Sanchez: "Yes, for a checkup."

CHW: "Great. Has Christa had any problems with her asthma?"

Mrs. Sanchez: "Nope. She's been taking her medicines every day, and there hasn't been a flare-up."

CHW: "So is Christa's asthma under control?"

Mrs. Sanchez: "Yes, it is."

CHW: "Good. So I'll see you in four months for a follow-up."

Starting an Interview with an Open-Ended Question

CHW: "Hi, how is everyone today?"

Mrs. Sanchez: "We're okay, I guess. We're here for a checkup."

CHW: "Great. How have you and Christa been doing since we last talked?"

Mrs. Sanchez: "It's been busy. Christa is starting kindergarten next month, so we're here for her school exam."

CHW: "Wow. Starting kindergarten, that's exciting! We should probably get an extra spacer for Christa to bring to school and a copy of the asthma action plan for the school nurse."

Mrs. Sanchez: "Oh, I didn't think of that."

CHW: "After we talk, I'll get you another spacer and action plan. How have Christa's symptoms been?"

Can you see how starting the interview with an open-ended question enabled the family to disclose information important for Christa's asthma care?

Questions for Gathering Additional Information   There are times when clients will share information that is vague, such as: "Things could be better," or "I wasn't feeling well." To get a more accurate assessment of the issue or problem, you will need to ask an open-ended question.

"Can you tell me more about . . . ?"
"How do you feel when that happens . . . ?"
"What else is on your mind . . . ?"
"Could you give me an example of . . . ?"

If clients are being vague, there might be other reasons for this. If you press for more information and they are still resistant, check in and make sure you're not making them uncomfortable. For example: "Would you prefer to move on with the rest of the interview and we can come back to the subject later?"

Questions for a More Accurate Assessment   During initial interviews, you will gather information and assess what will motivate clients to better manage their health. The *who, what, when, where, how,* and *why* series of questions can serve as a guide to aid you in asking questions for a more accurate assessment.

WHO: "Who works with Christa to manage her medications?"

WHAT: "What happened next? What can assist Christa to manage her asthma? What is it that you are most worried about? What else do you think the family can do to aid in preventing Christa's asthma attacks?"

WHEN: "When did the asthma episode occur? When did it begin?"

WHERE: "Where does Christa tend to have the greatest difficulty breathing? Where does Christa seem to do best in terms of her breathing?"

HOW: "How did Christa learn to use her inhaler?" (If the child is older than four years or so, ask him or her directly how he/she felt.) "How does Christa's asthma impact the rest of the family?"

WHY: "Why do you think that it happened?"

Don't Interrogate!   Avoid the interrogation style of interviewing or asking a series of blunt questions at a relatively fast pace.

"What's your name?"
"Your address?"
"Your nationality"
"Your date of birth?"
"Why are you here?"

Asking too many questions too quickly like that can make clients feel uneasy and defensive.

Don't Ask More Than One Question at a Time   Asking several questions at once can be confusing. "When did your daughter first show signs of asthma? Was it before or after the episode on the playground at school? Did your family physician ever notice symptoms or speak to you about asthma?" Ask one question at a time.

Pace Yourself   Building a positive relationship with the client is more important than finishing your intake interview or assessment form. You don't need to ask every question during one interview. When we asked experienced CHWs what is important for new CHWs to understand about client interviewing, they said: "Relax. Make sure the families know that you are there for them, not the forms." They also mentioned to pace the speed of the interview. Slow things down so that families can think about questions before answering. You might say something like: "Take your time answering these questions." Or, as appropriate: "Let's put this interview form aside for a few minutes. Would you like to talk further about (whatever the issue is that seems to be a priority for the client)?"

AN INTERVIEW WITH THE PAN FAMILY THAT DIDN'T GO TOO WELL

In the following interview, Greg is a CHW at a neighborhood health center. He is interviewing the Pan family. Their child has chronic asthma.

Greg: "Come in and take a seat." [points to two chairs on the other side of desk]

Pan family: [sits down]

Greg: "Let's start with the forms, shall we?"

Pan family: "Okay." [phone rings]

Greg: [interrupts] "Hold on a second. Let me get my phone." [turns away, speaking quietly into phone] "Hello . . ." [has a short conversation with another colleague] "I have someone in my office. I'll get back to you later." [turning back to the Pan family] "Okay, now where were we? Yes, the forms. We need to fill out these forms before you see the doctor."

Pan family: [silence]

Greg: "Okay. Parents' first and last name?"

Pan family (mother): "Luanne and Charlie Pan."

Greg: "Your child's name and age?"

Pan family (mother): "Mark—he's seven years old."

Greg: "So Mark had a bad asthma attack last week?"

Pan family: "It wasn't that bad, but it scared us."

Greg: [writing in chart] *According to parents, asthma attack was not severe.*

Pan family: "How long do you think this appointment will take? We need to get Mark back to school, and we need to get back to work."

Greg: "We can give you a work and school slip, but I need to complete this form for my job."

There are several problems with the interview that Greg conducts with the Pan family:

⚙ Greg never welcomes the Pans or introduces himself.
⚙ Greg doesn't clearly explain the purpose of the interview, or ask the Pan family how much time they can take for the interview.

✪ Greg takes a phone call during the interview.
> Don't take calls during a session with a client unless it is truly an emergency. Remember that their time is just as valuable as yours.

✪ Greg documents in Mark's chart that, "According to his parents, Mark's asthma attack wasn't severe."
> Greg didn't ask appropriate open-ended questions to learn detailed information about Mark's attack. He doesn't know what type of asthma attack the Pan family considers to be severe. This is important information to document accurately.

✪ Finally, Greg dismisses the Pan family's concern about school and work, and tells them that they have to stay and complete the paperwork. He tells them that he needs to complete the forms as part of his job.
> Greg's work duties are not as important as the needs of the clients. This is the Pan family's interview, and their needs should come first.

?   *How would you conduct this interview differently?*

9.4 THE END OF THE INTERVIEW PROCESS

Don't rush the end of the interview process: this is a time to review questions, concerns, or decisions that the client has made. You don't want to undermine a good interview by rushing the client out the door or leaving the person confused about where to go next.

TIME MANAGEMENT

Toward the end of the interview, check the time remaining to see if it will be possible to complete the interview. You may need to allow time to schedule a follow-up appointment. If you need more time, you may be able to continue the interview for an extra ten or fifteen minutes. Ask the client if this will be possible: "Arnold, I want to be respectful of your time, and I'd like to finish the interview form. Would you able to stay for an extra fifteen minutes today, or would it be better to schedule a follow-up appointment?"

If you routinely find that you need extra time to complete initial client interviews, in spite of effective time management, you may wish to talk with your agency to see if it is possible to schedule longer appointments.

REVIEW DECISIONS MADE AND NEXT STEPS

The interview may or may not have clarified the client's eligibility and interest in participating in a particular program or service. If decisions have been made, be sure to review them together. If the client has decided to participate in follow-up meetings or services, be sure to provide a written copy of this plan, including when and where to access services, who their contact person or service provider will be, and how best to contact that person.

"Okay, Arnold, you clearly qualify for our hypertension management program, and I'm glad that you have decided to enroll. You have an appointment with Samuel tomorrow at 3 PM in this same building, and he'll hook you up with all of the services."

PROVIDE REFERRALS

In some cases, you will offer referrals to clients who have expressed an interest in additional services, such as transitional housing or legal assistance. Review what the referral is for, and provide them with clear information about where to go and who to contact.

"Arnold, you said you might be interested in the organization I mentioned, Joining Together. It is a group run by and for formerly incarcerated people. Here is their card. They do advocacy on behalf of formerly incarcerated communities, and they help connect people to educational opportunities, job training programs, and employment. They are located right on Market near 6th Street. I wrote down the name of Sally B. here. I really respect her and the work that she does. Do you have any questions about the referral? Do you think you might check them out?"

For more information regarding how to make an effective referral, please see Chapter Eleven.

ASK CLIENTS IF THEY HAVE ANY REMAINING QUESTIONS OR CONCERNS

Check in one last time to see whether clients have any outstanding questions or concerns that they would like to talk about. Even if the answer is no, asking the question communicates your concern for their welfare.

THANK THE CLIENT

Regardless of how the interview went, and whether or not the client ultimately decided to enroll in a particular program or service, the person invested significant time and effort talking with you. Thank them and leave them with an encouraging word. For example:

"Arnold, I am really impressed with your motivation to . . ."

"Arnold, I really appreciate all that you shared with me today. I will be keeping you mind, and I hope that you are able to reconnect with your family in the ways that you talked about."

"I hope you will enjoy the support group we talked about. I know the other participants will benefit a lot from what you have to share. If you can, please let me know how it goes."

PROVIDE YOUR CONTACT INFORMATION

If it is appropriate for clients to contact you in the future, give them your business card and contact information.

"Arnold, here is my card. You can always reach me at this number. Don't hesitate to call me if you think I can be helpful. I won't always be able to get back to you right away, but I promise I'll always call back."

9.5 DOCUMENTING CLIENT INTERVIEWS

Many CHWs dread the task of documenting their work. They may feel that they spend too much time filling out paperwork, that the forms take their attention and time away from clients. We want you to appreciate why documentation is such an important part of your work.

Filling out forms is an opportunity for CHWs and clients to work together.

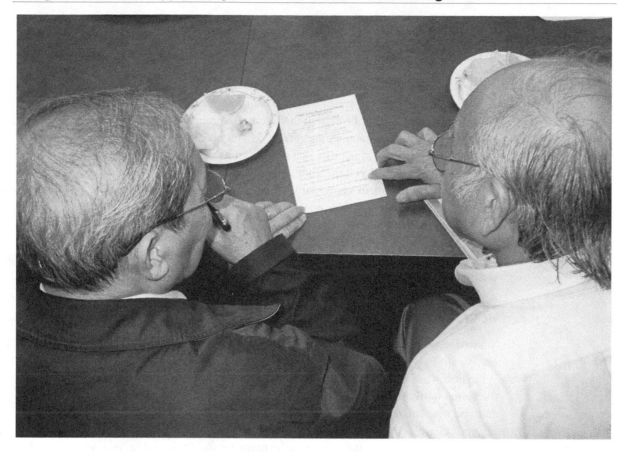

The primary purpose is to provide information that will be used to guide the delivery of care and services for clients. The information you document may also be used to evaluate services and programs, again with the purpose of improving the quality of services that clients receive. If you can't provide timely, clear, and accurate documentation of the services you provide, including initial client interviews, this could be harmful to the client and to your career.

BECOME FAMILIAR WITH THE FORMS YOU WILL USE

The forms you will use will vary depending on the nature of the interviews you conduct and the program and agency you work for. A good starting point is to carefully review all the forms that your program uses, not just the ones you are responsible for completing. Next, take all the forms you are responsible for completing and review each and every question. You should understand all of the terms used, why each question is being asked, how to document a variety of common responses, how the information you document will be used, and how it may impact the health of the client. Talk with a colleague or supervisor to clarify anything that you don't fully understand and couldn't explain to a client. The more familiar you are with the forms, the better you will be able to focus on talking with and listening to clients during an interview without constantly referring to the paperwork.

EXPLAIN THE FORMS TO CLIENTS

Tell your clients that you will be writing down the information they share with you on forms provided by your agency. Depending on the nature of the interview and the literacy level of your clients, you may ask them to fill out part of the form on their own and review it with them later. You might also provide clients with a copy of the form as you conduct the interview.

Take time to clearly explain why you are using forms to document the interview, and how the information will be used in the future. Be prepared for clients to stop you during an interview to ask something like: "Why do you need to know that?" For example, clients may be concerned about why you need to know their Social Security number, or what may happen if they tell you that they are experiencing domestic violence at home. Learn to view these moments as opportunities for deeper engagement with a client. Affirm their right not to answer a particular question. It may or may not be essential for determining their eligibility and participation in services, and you may be able to return to these issues in the future, once trust has been established. Most important, be prepared to honestly and accurately respond to their questions. If you aren't sure, say so, and if possible, find someone who can answer their questions.

HOW AND WHEN TO FILL OUT THE FORMS

Sometimes, CHWs think they will be able to interview a client and to document it later on. We strongly encourage you to fill out the documentation as you talk with clients. This is the best way to ensure that the information you record is accurate. If you wait to fill out the forms until after the interview, you may not remember all that they shared with you, and you may misrepresent important information. You may end up unintentionally harming your clients.

As you document the interview, explain to the client what you are doing. For example: "Arnold, I'm going to take some notes as we talk. I want to make sure that I keep an accurate record of the information you share with me. Is that all right?" Documentation doesn't need to get in the way of conducting an effective interview. The more familiar you are with the forms, and the more experience you have, the easier it will become.

T G: I made mistakes in the past by delaying writing up client notes, thinking that I would remember it all. Now I always document client information while we talk. I explain what I'm doing and why I'm doing it. It has never been a problem with a client.

Most forms ask for specific information: name, address, phone number, medical history, and so on. Some forms, especially those used during home visits, will ask for more descriptive information, such as about conditions in the home. This is where your observation skills will be essential. Some agencies use SOAP notes. SOAP stands for: Subjective, Objective, Assessment, and Plan. Whether or not your agency or clinic uses SOAP notes, it is a good format to use while taking notes. You will learn how to take SOAP notes in Chapter Eleven, "Case Management."

IF THE FORMS ARE A PROBLEM

We hope you will work with programs that have already developed culturally sensitive forms that guide you in conducting client-centered interviews and reporting accurate client information. However, some of you will be working with forms that are problematic in different ways. They may not have places to document your client's identity (if they are Arabic, multiracial, lesbian and in a committed relationship, transgender, and so on), or they may have places to document your clients' health-related risks, but not their resources or strengths. Sometimes, forms can be changed, and your input as a CHW will aid in improving them. This isn't always possible, however, particularly when working with standard forms used by city, county, state, or federal government programs. You may, however, be able to write down additional information in the margins of the forms, or create an addendum (additional piece of paper) that can become part of the client's file. If the forms you use pose problems, speak to your colleagues and supervisor to see if you can develop some practical solutions.

CHAPTER REVIEW

Imagine that you are a CHW at The Good Health Center and are scheduled to meet with Arnold—the fifty-two-year-old client described at the beginning of this chapter—to conduct an initial client interview. You have reviewed the form he filled out, and understand that he is interested in participating in programs and services (such as primary health care, health education, support groups) that will assist him to better control his hypertension (high blood pressure). Based on what you have learned, *and in your own words:*

- How will you welcome Arnold?
- How will you explain the purpose of the interview to him?
- How will you explain confidentiality?
- How will you obtain informed consent from Arnold?

- How will you document the information that Arnold tells you, and how will you explain this process to him?
- What will you do and say to keep the interview client-centered?
- How will you assess Arnold's external and internal resources?
- What open-ended questions might you ask Arnold?
- What will you say when he tells you that he just got out of prison?
- What will you say when he tells you that, more than anything, he wants to rebuild a relationship with his family?
- What types of referrals might you provide to Arnold?
- What will you say to end your interview session with Arnold?

ADDITIONAL RESOURCES

Community Health Works. 2005. *Managing Children's Asthma: A Community-Focused, Team Approach. Volume 3:* *Community Health Worker Manual.* Accessed on March 27, 2009: http://www.communityhealthworks.org

10

Client-Centered Counseling
for Behavior Change

Tim Berthold • Darouny Somsanith

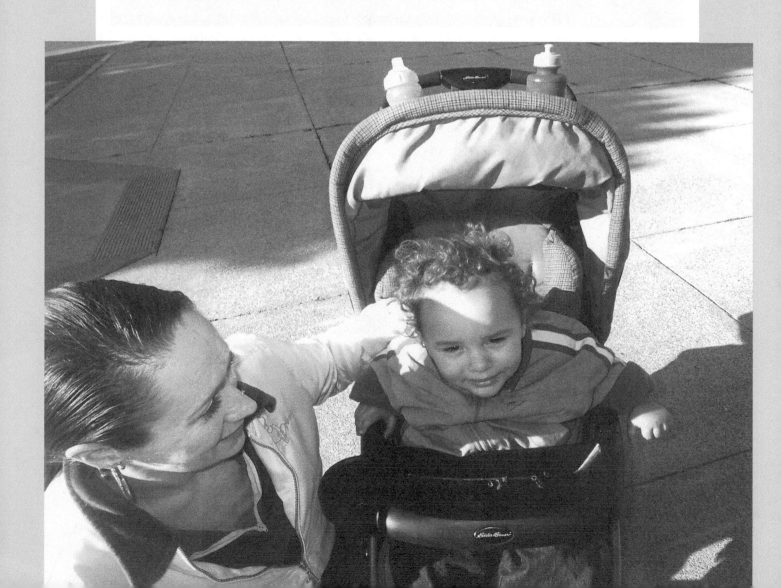

CASE STUDY: MEI

Mei is sixteen years old and recently started having sex. She met Joe three months ago. He is seventeen years old, Mei's first boyfriend, and her first sexual partner. Mei heard that she can get free birth control at the community health center. She wants to go, but is scared that her parents will find out about her visit. She brings her friend Sandee with her. They go upstairs to the drop-in program for youths. Mei fills out a form. After about twenty minutes, a CHW calls Mei's name and brings her to a private counseling room.

CHW: "Hi, I'm _____. I'm a counselor here. What brings you to the health center today?"

Mei: "Well, I want to get some birth control because I really don't want to get pregnant. My friend said I can get the pill for free, and you won't tell my parents?"

CHW: "Yes, that's right. We can assist you in figuring out what kind of birth control you want to use, and our services are confidential. That means that we can't tell you parents or anyone else about your visit or the decision you make about birth control. I'm really glad that you came in to talk about all of this—I know it can be a difficult thing to do."

Mei: "Yeah, I started to come twice before, but I just couldn't.... My friend Sandee came with me today, though. She's out there [*points back toward the reception area*]."

[The CHW goes on to explain the health center's policies, including the limitations to confidentiality, and to obtain informed consent as discussed in Chapters Eight and Nine.]

CHW: "Mei, there are lots of different birth control methods that can aid you in preventing pregnancy, including the pill. Part of my job is to share information with you about all the different methods you can choose from, and to assist you in deciding which is the best for you. How does that sound?"

Mei: "Okay. How long is this going to take?"

CHW: "Well, I'd like to spend about thirty minutes with you, if that's okay. And depending on what type of method you choose, you may also need to meet with one of our nurse practitioners. Will that work for you?"

Mei: "Yeah, I guess. I really want to get something ..."

CHW: "All right. Before we talk about birth control, I'd like to learn more about your situation. Can you tell me how long you've been having sex?"

If you were the CHW working with Mei:

✪ How would you support her to change behaviors and reduce risks of pregnancy and STIs?
✪ What concepts would guide your work?
✪ What counseling skills would you use? What questions would you ask her?
✪ What personal experiences, values, or beliefs might influence your work with Mei?

INTRODUCTION

CHWs support individual clients to change behaviors in order to reduce health risks and promote wellness. This chapter will address the process and challenges of changing behavior, and the skills that CHWs use to provide client-centered counseling to support clients to

Mei: "Well, me and Joe just started going out three months ago. We had sex a couple of times without anything, but then we talked about it because no way do I want to get pregnant. So we've been doing other things—like just messing around—and oral."

CHW: "Mei, I always want to check this out—is it your own decision to be sexually active? Is this something that you want and feel ready for?"

Mei: "Yeah. He's my first boyfriend, and I really like him. And I like doing it with him . . . having sex."

CHW: "Okay, so I hear that it is your choice to be sexually active with Joe. You are having oral and vaginal sex, and you haven't used any protection so far, is that right?"

Mei: "Yeah, but not anymore. I mean—you know, not for the sex, sex—vaginal—we're not doing it until I get some birth control."

CHW: "So your main worry is about getting pregnant. [*Mei nods.*] Are you also worried about sexually transmitted infections or STIs like chlamydia, genital warts, or HIV? You know, you can get STIs from vaginal or oral sex. Have you and Joe talked about this together?"

Mei: [*shakes her head*] "Not really. I mean, we talked about pregnancy, but we didn't talk about AIDS or anything."

CHW: "Mei, I'd like you to know how common STIs are in young women, and to encourage you to think about what you can do to prevent getting infected. What do you already know about STIs?"

Mei: "Well, I mean, I guess I don't really know so much about that chlamydia thing? But I know that HIV can turn into AIDS and you can't do anything about it. But I didn't really think it was a big problem for girls like me . . . "

CHW: "In general, STIs are most common in young women, and the rates of HIV are growing faster among young people and women than among any other groups. HIV and other STIs can have a really serious impact on your health and your future. Would it be all right for me to share some basic information with you about STIs?"

Mei: "Yeah, okay. I don't want to get HIV or any other of those infections, you know what I mean?"

[The CHW provides basic health information about STIs.]

change behaviors. It builds on information provided about the behavior change process in Chapter Eight. Please review this information before continuing with this chapter.

WHAT YOU WILL LEARN

By studying the information in this chapter, you will be able to:

- Discuss basic counseling concepts, including principles of counseling and characteristics of successful counselors
- Explain and apply basic concepts of client-centered counseling to facilitate behavior change, including the stages of change theory, harm reduction, and motivational interviewing
- Explain why self-awareness is essential for CHWs

✪ Evaluate your own performance as a counselor
✪ Develop your own professional development plan to enhance your counseling knowledge and skills

WORDS TO KNOW

Harm Reduction   Risk-Reduction Counseling   Ambivalence

10. 1 OVERVIEW OF CLIENT-CENTERED COUNSELING FOR BEHAVIOR CHANGE

This chapter will focus on the counseling skills that CHWs use when working with individual clients to change behaviors in order to improve their health. This chapter builds on concepts and skills already introduced in Chapters Three, Seven, Eight, and Nine, including the ecological model; cultural humility; ethics and scope of practice; client-centered practice; welcoming and orienting clients; and assessing clients' risks, needs, and strengths.

CHWs provide client-centered behavior change counseling with community-based organizations, hospitals, clinics, local health departments, and a wide range of other employers. Regardless of where you are working, the community of clients you serve, the health issues you address, and the types of behaviors that clients want to change, the way you approach facilitating behavior change is guided by similar client-centered concepts and skills.

While we will refer to this work as client-centered counseling or behavior change counseling, others may refer to it as risk-reduction counseling, health education, health advising, informal counseling, or peer counseling. Some people and organizations object to the use of term *counseling* to describe this work and argue that CHWs are not qualified to be counselors. As we acknowledged in Chapter Eight, other professionals often try to limit the scope of practice of CHWs. However, a review of the public health literature, and of the policies and programs of state and federal agencies such as the Centers for Disease Control and Prevention, makes it abundantly clear that CHWs do indeed perform a counseling role.

10. 2 OVERVIEW OF COUNSELING CONCEPTS

Counseling is provided by people with a wide range of training. Some counselors are also mental health clinicians with extensive education, clinical training, and licensure, such as psychologists and licensed clinical social workers. These therapists have the expertise to address the most challenging issues that clients will present. Other counselors, such as CHWs, are not licensed, but have been trained—and sometimes certified—to provide specific services. This includes, for example, HIV counselors, behavior change counselors, drug and alcohol counselors, and sexual assault and domestic violence counselors. Sometimes the term *peer counselor* is used to refer to those without advanced educational training, certification, or licensure.

Regardless of your educational background and whether you are certified, we encourage you to seek out opportunities to enhance your counseling skills. Opportunities may exist in the city or county where you live to receive free training, generally in exchange for volunteering, in areas such as reproductive health counseling and HIV antibody test counseling.

Suicide prevention/crisis intervention, domestic violence, and rape crisis centers are also outstanding resources. You will not only receive training in vital areas, and in some cases certification, but will have a chance to practice your skills as a volunteer and receive supervision. Other community-based organizations and community colleges also provide affordable workshops and classes that will enhance your counseling knowledge and skills.

? *What training have you already received in counseling skills?*

? *What educational and training opportunities exist in the area where you live?*

The following information has been adapted from a curriculum developed to train CHWs to provide behavior change counseling in Zimbabwe (International Training and Education Center on HIV, 2004).

COUNSELING OUTCOMES

Clients should be encouraged to talk about what they want to achieve from counseling. The client's counseling goals may change over the course of your work together and may be revisited many times. In general, however, when counseling has been successful, clients often experience the following outcomes:

Greater awareness of strengths, challenges and issues: Clients will begin to develop a deeper understanding of the issues, problems, or challenges that stand in the way of a healthy and meaningful life, as well as their own contributions to these challenges. Clients will also begin to identify their own internal resources or strengths for handling these issues and creating the kind of life and relationships they desire.

New responses to old issues: Clients not only develop new or enhanced understanding of themselves, but also new skills to address existing problems or challenges.

More effective relationships: Clients often learn how to develop and sustain healthier and more satisfying relationships with themselves and with others.

Reduced harm to self and others: Clients learn how to make decisions and take actions that will reduce potential harm to themselves and to others.

Increased self-esteem: Clients increase their ability to see and to value their own personality, strengths, skills, and accomplishments.

Greater confidence and independence: Clients increase their confidence in managing life challenges on their own, taking action to promote their own health and well-being, as well as the well-being of those around them.

? *Can you think of other counseling outcomes?*

? *If you have participated in formal or informal counseling, what were the outcomes for you?*

? *What outcomes might you seek from future counseling?*

CHARACTERISTICS OF SUCCESSFUL COUNSELORS

Your work with clients will be guided by concepts and skills of client-centered counseling. It will also be influenced by the personal qualities that you bring to the professional relationship. Successful counselors often share the following qualities and characteristics:

- Belief in the wisdom of their clients
- The desire to learn something new from each client and counseling session
- The ability to set aside personal issues, concerns, and beliefs when working with clients
- Cultural humility
- The ability to honor the life experience, feelings, opinions, and values of the client
- Acceptance of their own limitations and mistakes
- A deep commitment not to discriminate against clients on the basis of their identity, beliefs, behavior, or any other reason
- Acceptance of a client's ambivalence to change
- Understanding that resistance to change is natural and common
- The expression of empathy in a visible and authentic manner

? *What qualities or characteristics would you add to this list?*

10. 3 DEVELOPING A BEHAVIOR CHANGE PLAN

A key task of client-centered counseling is for the client to develop an individualized risk-reduction or behavior change plan. The plan clearly identifies the client's health goals, and outlines a set of specific and realistic actions for reducing risks and promoting health. The first step to developing a plan is to support the client in identifying their current challenges, risks, and needs. Together, you will prioritize these needs to create immediate goals. You will also support the client in assessing their strengths and identifying their internal and external resources (see Chapters Nine and Fourteen).

Sometimes, you will conduct client-centered counseling with a client who has been referred to your program to address a specific health risk or issue such as prostate cancer, smoking, or pregnancy. At other times, the issues that the client is most concerned about will emerge during the assessment. In the case study, for example, Mei comes to the clinic with the goal of preventing pregnancy. As she talks with the CHW, a second goal of preventing STIs also emerges. The priorities and goals of a behavior change plan are revisited often, and they can always be revised according to the wishes and needs of the client.

Each agency you work for is likely to have a slightly different form and structure for developing the behavior change plan (this may be called by different names such as a risk-reduction plan, treatment plan, action plan, health plan, and so forth). Ideally, the form will have a place to clearly document:

- Basic client information (including name, address, date of birth, sex/gender identity, primary language, and so on)
- Primary health risks
- Resource needs, such as mental health counseling, housing, or child care
- Strengths or internal and external resources
- Goals, such as to prevent pregnancy, reduce asthma symptoms, or prevent the further progression of HIV disease

⊛   Actions or steps to reach the goal, such as consistent use of contraception, reducing asthma triggers—such as dust or animal dander—in the home, or taking antiretroviral medications regularly and eating a balanced diet

⊛   Notes or comments about the counseling session (see how to take SOAP notes in Chapter Eleven)

⊛   Follow-up appointments and referrals

The behavior change plan form may be completed at the beginning of a session, but typically, the client's needs, strengths, and goals are identified over the course of one or more sessions.

T G :   You might think you are going to sit down and do this all at once in some logical order—assess risks and resources, come up with goals and a plan. But that isn't how it usually goes, at least for me. Especially when I first meet with clients, I want to follow their lead about what is most important to talk about. I know that if the client decides that they want to keep working with me—that we will develop this plan together, and I will write it down. Like everything, it's a process, and the plan keeps developing. That's a good thing, because new goals or priorities come up, or the client realizes that some of their action steps are just too unrealistic.

CASE STUDY: MEI (*Continued*)

Mei comes to the health center with a clear goal: to prevent pregnancy. She already has elements of a plan worked out as well: she wants to start using birth control pills and to stop having vaginal sex until the pill takes effect.

In talking with the CHW, another goal also emerges: to prevent STIs. Using the client-centered counseling skills presented below, the CHW supports Mei to explore her relationship with Joe, her concerns about STIs, and what she is ready to do to prevent infection. The CHW also talks with Mei about strengths and needs, including her relationship with her parents and friends, and her other life goals.

The following is a sample behavior change plan that could be developed with Mei:

THE COMMUNITY HEALTH CENTER
BEHAVIOR CHANGE PLAN

CLIENT'S NAME   CLIENT'S CASE NUMBER

DEMOGRAPHIC INFORMATION
(SUCH AS DATE OF BIRTH, ADDRESS, GENDER IDENTITY, ETHNICITY, PRIMARY LANGUAGE)

(Continued)

HEALTH GOALS	• To prevent pregnancy and STIs
HEALTH RISKS	• Having unprotected vaginal sex and oral sex • Never used condoms before • Hesitant to negotiate condom use with partner • Partner says he doesn't like condoms • Cannot talk with parents about sexual activity • Other: _____
INTERNAL RESOURCES	• Wants to prevent pregancy • Came to clinic, is willing to talk openly about her health issues and concerns • Is doing well in high school—wants to go to college • Other: _____
EXTERNAL RESOURCES	• Has friends she can talk with, including Sandee • Is enrolled in high school • Other: _____

HEALTH PROMOTION
ACTION PLAN
	• Start using the birth control pill as of today (06/12)
	• Stop having vaginal sex until pill is effective
	• Will carry condoms and lubricant with her
	• Will try to talk with Joe about condoms and
	  getting tested for STI
	• Will consider asking Joe to come to the health center
	  to talk with the counselor together.
	• Other: _____

COMMENTS	_____

FOLLOW-UP MEETING SCHEDULED

✔ Yes _____ No   When? June 17, 3:30 PM

REFERRALS PROVIDED   _____

COMMENTS: 16-year old girl in first sexual relationship. Nervous at first, but talked openly about her sexual behaviors, relationship and concerns. Primary concern is pregnancy. Not thnking about STIs when she came to the clinic. Now states she wants to prevent STIs, but is worried that her boyfriend won't use condoms. She is also worried that the relationship will be over if she insists on using condoms. She will talk with her best friend, and try to talk with Joe (boyfriend) about condoms. Have scheduled an appointment for next week. She may invite her boyfriend to come with her.

FOLLOW-UP MEETING SCHEDULED

_____ Yes _____ No   When? _____

REFERRALS PROVIDED   Mei met Nurse Practitioner at the Center for a prescription for birth control pills.

The client and the counselor will revisit the behavior change plan many times over the course of their work together. Goals and actions may be revised according to the progress and needs of the client.

USING A BUBBLE CHART

Bubble charts are a resource to assist a client to identify options for reducing risks and promoting health. The bubbles may be left completely blank for the client to identify, or may be presented with some options already filled in. The tasks are to identify a wide range of actions that the client can take, and for the client to decide which of these options are best to begin with (Bodenheimer, 2007).

In the example, the CHW is counseling a client with diabetes (see Figures 10.1 and 10.2). The CHW fills in some of the bubbles and leaves others blank for the client to fill in:

CHW: "Okay, let's talk about what you feel ready to do to better control your diabetes. I have a chart here [*shows chart in Figure 10.1 to client*] that shows some of the actions you might want to take to promote your health, such as checking your blood sugar regularly, exercising, and eating a healthier diet. Can you think of other things that you can do to aid in controlling your diabetes?"

Client: "Well, I guess one thing is to keep coming here and working with you. Another thing is—for me to really change my diet—I'm going to have to talk with my family about it. We all eat together, and I don't know if they want to change what they eat."

Figure 10.1 Bubble Chart from CHW.

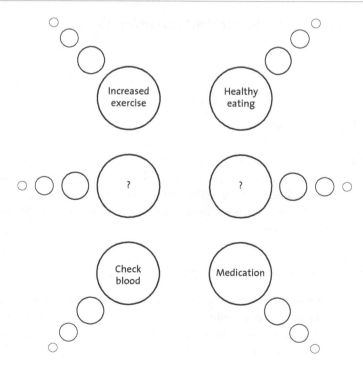

Source: Adapted from Bodenheimer, 2007.

Figure 10.2   Bubble Chart for Client to Complete.

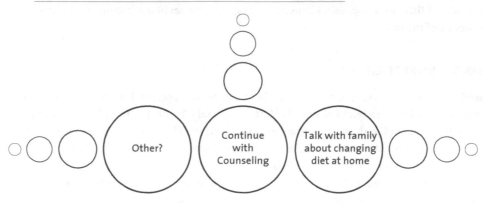

CHW: "Okay, let's add those to the chart." [*writes them in the blank bubbles in Figure 10.2.*]

CHW: "Which of these options do you want to start talking about? Which seems like the most realistic action for you to start with?"

Client: "Diet is going to be hardest. Well, they're all going to be hard, but . . . can we start with the exercise? But I want to totally honest—I don't really do *any* exercise now."

CHW: "I really appreciate your honesty. That is what this is all about—starting where you are today, and seeing what feels manageable for you to try to do to make a change. So you say that you don't do any exercise now—what about walking? How much do you walk in a day or a week?"

? *What do you think of the bubble chart?*

? *Would you use it when you are doing client-centered counseling?*

? *How could the CHW use the bubble chart in working with Mei?*

10. 4 KNOWLEDGE AND SKILLS FOR CLIENT-CENTERED BEHAVIOR CHANGE COUNSELING

The skills you will use as a counselor will depend on the issues you are addressing, the agency or program you work for, and your own level of knowledge and experience. With time, you may refine and adapt these skills and develop your own *implicit theories* of behavior change (see Chapter Eight). Please refer to the resources provided at the end of this chapter for further study.

HARM-REDUCTION AND RISK-REDUCTION COUNSELING

Harm-reduction and risk-reduction counseling offer useful strategies for client-centered work. **Harm reduction** is a philosophy about life and health, as well as an approach to behavior change that was started by a community of people who inject drugs. This community objected to the "abstinence-only" philosophy and approach that usually guides health and social service providers. The goal of abstinence-based programs and counseling is to support clients to stop using drugs as quickly as possible. Because abstinence-only programs focus only on supporting people to stop using drugs entirely, they offer little or nothing to clients who may not, or may not yet, be ready to quit using.

Harm reduction essentially views any action that will reduce harm to ourselves and to others as positive. Not everyone will quit smoking, stop eating sweet or fried foods, or stop drinking alcohol completely. However, if they change or reduce their use in some way, they can significantly reduce their health risks. For example, if someone who eats fast food six to ten times a week reduces this to two to four times a week, they can reduce risks for heart disease, diabetes, and other chronic conditions. Injection drug users may reduce their use, start to use in other ways, or stop sharing syringes and works (depending on the drug, this may include cottons and cookers, for example) with others. All of these actions can significantly reduce their risks for HIV and other disease-causing agents (such as bacteria) that may be carried in human blood.

Harm reduction is a highly pragmatic or practical approach to preventing risks and promoting health. It recognizes how difficult it can be to stop using drugs and alcohol, and that not everyone who uses wants to or is going to stop using immediately or at all. It recognizes people's autonomy, and understands that people will make these decisions for themselves.

Harm reduction remains a controversial philosophy and practice in the United States, particularly in relation to drug use. In countries such as Canada and the United Kingdom, however, governments have developed drug treatment policies guided by harm reduction. Local governments provide injection drug users with clean syringes and, in some cases, with uncontaminated drugs, such as heroin, along with counseling, including employment counseling and other social services. These policies and programs have been shown to dramatically reduce the harms associated with injection drug use, including rates of HIV infection, unemployment, and loss of family and home (Drug Policy Alliance Network, 2005).

The harm-reduction philosophy and approach can be applied to any number of health-related issues, not just to issues of substance use. For example, it can be used to support clients to reduce their risks for diabetes, pneumonia, malaria, sexually transmitted diseases, bicycle and driving injuries, and breast cancer.

? *What do you think about harm reduction?*

? *How does harm reduction apply in your life: what actions do you take that assist you in reducing health risks?*

Risk-reduction counseling is a form of behavior change counseling based on harm reduction. Clients identify behaviors that place their health at risk, such as unprotected sex. The CHW then assists a client to identity options for reducing these risks by changing behaviors, such as practicing less sex, using condoms, or using other safer sex strategies. This is the predominant client-centered approach to HIV prevention throughout the world (Centers for Disease Control and Prevention, 2001; World Health Organization, 2006; International Training and Education Center on HIV, 2004).

Increasingly, harm-reduction and risk-reduction counseling are used along with the Stages of Change theory and motivational interviewing.

CASE STUDY: MEI (*Continued*)

Mei could use harm-reduction or risk-reduction strategies in several ways. For example, the most effective way to prevent pregnancy is not to have vaginal sex. However, if Mei decides to continue to have vaginal sex, a range of options will help to reduce this ongoing risk. These options include contraception, including barrier methods (condom, sponge, and diaphragm) and hormonal methods (birth control pill, Depo-Provera, and so on). Mei's task is to determine the level of risk that she is comfortable living with and to choose the risk-reduction method that best fits her goals, life style, and comfort level. The task of the counselor is to help her explore these options, understand her level of risk or safety with each method, and make an informed decision.

When Lee Jackson started working with MR, he was really sick with HIV disease. He had lost a lot of weight and didn't have much hope for the future.

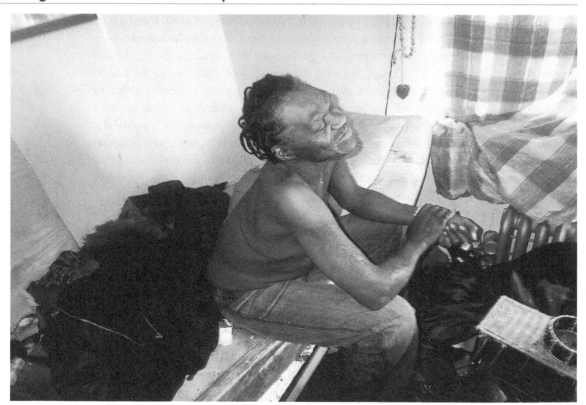

STAGES OF CHANGE THEORY

The Stages of Change theory provides a framework for understanding how people may change their behavior (Prochaska, Norcross, and DiClemente, 1999). The model is widely used and describes behavior change as a process that usually involves many steps rather than a single event. The model has been used to understand behavior change related to substance use, HIV/AIDS, nutrition, diabetes, and other chronic conditions.

The Stages of Change theory (Table 10.1) is often used with motivational interviewing and other counseling skills and techniques.

Table 10.1.   The Stages of Change.

Stage of Change	Definition	Behavioral Description	Role of the CHW
Precontemplation	The individual is not thinking about the health risks of their current behaviors (such as the risks of unprotected vaginal sex).	The individual is not planning to change within the next six months.	To encourage the client to begin thinking about their risks and possible behavior change.
Contemplation	The individual is thinking about change in the near future (such as trying condoms).	The individual is planning to change within the next six months.	To support the client to begin actively planning steps for changing their behavior.
Preparation	The individual is ready and making a plan to change (for example, has purchased condoms and lube and has planned for how to use them).	The individual is actively preparing to make changes within the next month.	To support the client to develop an individualized and realistic plan for behavior change.
Action	The individual has started making changes (for example, is talking with partners and using condoms and lube for vaginal sex).	The individual has made the change for more than one day and less than six months.	To encourage and support the client to take actions and change behaviors in accordance with their plan.
Maintenance	The individual has committed to the change long term (is practicing safer sex regularly, including use of condoms and lube for vaginal sex).	The individual has maintained this change for more than six months.	To acknowledge and congratulate the client for their success, to support them in maintaining new behaviors, and to prevent relapse to the previous risk behaviors.
Relapse	Individual has "relapsed" to previous patterns and risk behaviors (has had vaginal sex again without using a condom).	Individual found it hard to maintain new behaviors or faced challenges that made it hard to be consistent with the new behavior. May have relapsed due to relationships, trauma, loss, doubt, or any number of factors.	Not to judge the client and to assist them in accepting that relapse is often a normal and anticipated part of the behavior change process. To assist the client identify what influenced their relapse, what they have learned, and what they want to do now. To revisit and revise the client's behavior change plan.
Return to precontemplation or action	Behavior change is a complicated process, and people frequently have to keep trying before they are able to maintain new behaviors (uses condoms during next sexual encounter).	As above.	As above, CHWs support clients to continue to think about and take actions to reduce health risks.

T G: Stages of Change—yeah, its useful because the whole belief of harm-reduction and client-centered counseling is that you have to meet the client where they are. And Stages help me to understand where they are so that we can build from there.

CASE STUDY: MEI (*Continued*)

Mei is at the Preparation stage in terms of preventing an unplanned pregnancy. She is concerned about getting pregnant, thinking about it, and comes to the health center to ask about using the birth control pill.

However, when the Mei came to the health center, she wasn't even thinking about STIs (Precontemplation). Once the CHW began to talk with her about STIs, Mei moved to the Contemplation stage. She began to think about and to talk about her risks for STIs. She agreed to talk more about STIs and stated: "I really don't want to get HIV or any other of those infections, you know what I mean?"

? *What do you think about the Stages of Change?*

? *Does it seem like an accurate description of your own experiences with behavior change?*

? *Is there a behavior you are currently trying to change?*

? *Where are you on the Stages of Change?*

PROVIDING HEALTH INFORMATION

While a key principle of client-centered counseling is for the client to do most of the talking, there are times when CHWs will also provide essential information to clients. This might include information about topics such as parenting, immunizations, diabetes management, nutrition, or safer sex. It is important to clarify, however, that the purpose of providing information is to assist the client in making informed choices, not to tell them what to do. The information should be provided in a manner that increases the chances that the client will fully understand it:

- Start by asking what the client already knows about the topic.
- Take your time. Slow down. Break the information into manageable chunks or sizes.
- Clarify any new words or terms that you might use.
- Check in with clients to see that they understand.
- You might ask clients from time to time if they understand the information. The best way, however, to be confident that they understand is to ask them to tell you or show you what they have learned.

- Ask clients if they have questions or concerns.
- Use diagrams, photos, or other visual aids.
- Provide written materials in the proper language and literacy levels.
- Provide clients with an opportunity to learn by doing (see the example, below).

?   *What else would aid in making new health information accessible to clients?*

?   *What assists you to understand and learn new information?*

CASE STUDY: MEI (*Continued*)

In working with Mei, the CHW stops from time to time to provide information about topics such as contraceptive methods, sexually transmitted infections, safer sex, and condom use. Each time, the CHW will start by asking Mei to share what she already knows about the topic. The following exchange is about condom use:

CHW: "All right. Now, we talked about some of the methods for preventing pregnancy—there are lots of those. But there aren't as many great methods for preventing STIs. The best, of course, is not having sex. But if you are sexually active, using condoms and lubricant is what we recommend. What do you know about using condoms?"

[*The CHW takes out some condoms and lubricant.*]

Mei: "Well . . . " [*She starts to laugh, and looks embarrassed.*]

CHW: "These are regular condoms. We also have Reality condoms [*holds up a Reality condom*]—have you ever seen one of these? [*Mei shakes her head.*] Okay, I can show you about the Reality condom after, if you want. But let's start with regular condoms. Do you know how to use them? Have you ever put a condom on someone before?"

Mei: "I opened one to look at it, but that was it."

CHW: "Do you want me to show you how to put it on correctly?"

Mei: [*Laughs again, and then says*] "All right."

[*CHW proceeds to take out a plastic penis model and some condoms and shows Mei how to put one on. She also tells her about the types of condoms that are available and lubricants that are appropriate for them.*]

CHW: "Mei, would you like to try it yourself? Like most things, practice can really help."

[*Mei puts a condom on the plastic model, using lubricant.*]

CHW: "Perfect, you did great. How was that for you?"

Mei: "It's pretty easy . . . But the lube stuff is messy."

CHW: "Do you think you would feel comfortable using the condom with Joe?"

Mei: "Yeah, I'd be comfortable . . . but I don't know if Joe is."

In this example, the CHW presented information about condom use in several ways. She explained how to use condoms, showed Mei how to put them on, and gave Mei the chance to practice herself. She asked lots of questions along the way to assess what Mei already knew, and what she was comfortable learning.

MOTIVATIONAL INTERVIEWING

Motivational interviewing is widely used to conduct behavior change counseling and is defined as a "directive, client-centered counseling style for eliciting behavior change by assisting clients to explore and resolve ambivalence. . . . The examination and resolution of ambivalence is its central purpose, and the counselor is intentionally directive in pursuing this goal" (Rollnick and Miller, 1995). In other words, in motivational interviewing, the counselor gets the clients to talk about the contradictory feelings (**ambivalence**) they may have about making change, and aids them in working through and resolving those doubts and contradictions.

Motivation is an important factor in determining successful behavior change. Counselors who use motivational interviewing also understand that ambivalence about behavior change and resistance to behavior change are common. Behavior change implies giving up something that we have become used to and that may be important to us. It is natural that people feel ambivalent about or resistant to changing familiar patterns of living, eating, exercising, having sex, parenting, expressing anger, and using alcohol, tobacco, and drugs. This is a kind of loss, even if it may benefit and enhance our health in the long term. (See Figure 10.3.)

T G: I worked for a long time in the gay community, and I think we made some mistakes early on in the AIDS epidemic. We kind of pushed safer sex and condom use, and we didn't stop to acknowledge what a big change this was. I mean, sexual freedom and sexual pleasure are really important to most of the community. Motivational interviewing is a great resource for me to use when I counsel gay men, because it is a way to focus on what makes it so hard to change, how they feel about it, what they really want in their lives.

? **What behaviors have you tried to change over the course of your life?**

? **Did you ever feel ambivalent or have doubts about changing these behaviors?**

? **Did you ever resist changing these behaviors?**

? **What did you have to give up in order to make these changes?**

Motivation changes with time and circumstances. It is influenced by relationships, including interactions between clients and counselors. Motivational interviewing was developed from an understanding that the approach that counselors take, the skills they use, and the choices they make can undermine or enhance a client's motivation for change. In other words, what you say and do when working with clients can make a *big difference* in whether they move beyond their ambivalence and decide to work on making changes, or not.

? **What else might CHWs do to diminish or reduce a client's motivation?**

? **What else might CHWs do to enhance a client's motivation to change?**

Figure 10.3   Attitudes and Behaviors Used in Motivational Interviewing.

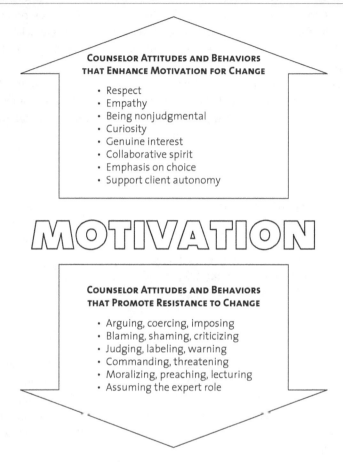

Source: "YES WE CAN Toolkit: Community Health Worker Manual" by Community Health Works.

Behavior change counselors should not pressure or persuade clients about what to do, think, or feel. Motivational interviewing, however, does encourage counselors to confront clients about harmful behavior as well as their ambivalence and resistance to change, but in a respectful and gentle manner (Rollnick and Miller, 1995). The counselor uses the skills described below to present clients with opportunities to identify and reflect on what is getting in the way of changing their behaviors. Through this dialogue, clients are supported to clarify what changes they can and want to make.

T G: Motivational interviewing is a lot different from the kind of counseling I got when I was going through recovery [from drug use]. In those days, they used a much more aggressive strategy to kind of break you down—to make you see and admit that you needed to change. But motivational interviewing doesn't force anything on the client, and I like that. I still have to challenge the client about what is keeping them from making the changes that they want to make. But they can talk about it with me or not. And motivational interviewing gives me the tools to do this in a better way.

OARS   Motivational interviewing draws upon a collection of counseling skills that are referred to as OARS: **O**pen-ended questions, **A**ffirmations, **R**eflective listening, and **S**ummarizing.

Open-Ended Questions   Open- and closed-ended questions were discussed in detail in Chapter Nine. Closed-ended questions generally prompt yes, no, or one-word answers from clients. They may be used to gather or verify information, but when they are used too often in the context of behavior change counseling, they tend to shut down dialogue rather than open it up.

In the Case Study, the CHW asks Mei several closed-ended questions: "Have you and Joe talked about this together?" and "Have you ever put a condom on someone before?"

Open-ended questions encourage a client to reflect and talk in a detailed way about their life experiences and their values, feelings, and beliefs.

CASE STUDY: MEI (*Continued*)

The CHW asks Mei several open-ended questions:

* What brings you to the health center today?
* What do you already know about STIs?
* What do you know about using condoms?

Open-ended questions are used to encourage a client to talk about their health risks, their readiness to change behaviors, and any ambivalence or resistance they may have about these changes. Providing space for dialogue without judgment also builds trust. It allows CHWs to form the necessary connection to talk about sensitive health topics, while honoring the opinions of the clients and acknowledging that they have the ultimate say in their own health. As always, the client must drive the behavior change process, and the solutions by which behavior change can happen must come from them. Without a client's buy-in, the process will not be a success.

Examples of other open-ended questions include:

- What do you think about that?
- What motivates you to think about changing this?
- What do you feel now—what is it like for you talk about these issues?
- What would you like to do about that?
- Can you tell me more about that?
- What else? Such as? How so? What happened then? What did you do then?
- What happened the last time that you _____?
- What would it be like for you to try _____? How might you begin? What might you say?
- What is it that most gets in the way of making these changes?
- What allowed you to accomplish this? What skills and resources did you bring to this situation?
- What is different now?

?   *Can you think of other examples of open-ended questions that you might ask when you are doing client-centered counseling?*

?   *What are some of your favorite open-ended questions to ask clients?*

? *What is it about these questions that is helpful to clients?*

T G: My favorite questions are simple ones like: "What's going on?" or "Do you want to tell me about that?" or "What was that like?"

Affirming **Statements** As discussed in Chapters Eight and Nine, many of the clients that you will work with rarely receive an acknowledgement of their strengths, internal resources, and accomplishments. Sometimes, when clients work with service providers, the focus is on what isn't working in their lives (rising blood pressure, a cancer diagnosis, a domestic violence situation), the "mistakes" they may have made, the risks they are facing, and their outstanding needs. Motivational interviewing places an emphasis on recognizing and affirming people's positive qualities, intentions, and accomplishments and the right to make their own decisions about how to pursue health in their own lives.

Affirming statements provide clients with direct and immediate positive feedback for their efforts and accomplishments, and encourage them to continue along the Stages of Change in reflecting about, planning for, and taking steps to change behavior. Providing affirmations should be done at the appropriate time—when clients have done or said something that is a positive contribution to their health—and in an authentic manner, using your own language and style.

CASE STUDY: MEI (*Continued*)

The CHW makes the following affirming statement to Mei: "I'm really glad that you came in to talk about this. I know that it isn't always easy," and "You did great!"

Other examples of affirming statements include:

- ✪ I respect how open you are to thinking about what you might want to change.
- ✪ It sounds like it took a lot of _____ (courage, strength, will power, and so on) to _____ (do that, talk with him, go to the meeting, and so forth).
- ✪ Great job. I know that talking to your partner about condoms was a hard thing for you to do.
- ✪ I know things didn't turn out like you expected, but you took a big chance and did your best in a difficult situation.
- ✪ You've survived some really difficult things in the past, and I trust that you can figure this out too.
- ✪ That was a really generous thing to do.

? *Can you think of other examples of affirming statements?*

? *Can you think of an affirming statement that you received in the last week?*

? *Are affirmative statements important to you and for your own attempts to change behaviors?*

Reflective Listening   Reflective listening is the art and the skill of reflecting back to clients what they have shared with you about their experiences, beliefs, feelings, behavior, and intentions. By reflecting back what they hear, CHWs:

- Clarify what clients have said, preventing wrong assumptions and miscommunications
- Let clients know that they are being heard and understood
- Give clients an opportunity to hear and reflect on their own statements
- Provide an opportunity to deepen the conversation

Reflective listening isn't easy to do: it requires commitment, concentration, patience, and cultural humility. There are different types of reflections that a CHW may share with a client, including those that attempt to echo back precisely or similarly what the client has said, and reflections that may add an interpretation or emphasis that permit the client to reflect and respond.

Reflective statements may include:

a. *Repeating:* Repeating back as precisely as possible words or phrases that the client has said.

For example, in the Case Study, Mei says: "Joe doesn't really like to use them (condoms)." The CHW might repeat this statement: "Joe doesn't really like to use condoms."

b. *Rephrasing:* Using different words to try to express the same meaning that the client expressed.

Such as: "So Joe won't use condoms when you have sex because he doesn't like them."

c. *Paraphrasing:* This is a step beyond rephrasing. The CHW attempts to interpret what the speaker means and to summarize it using the CHW's own words. The purpose is to assist the client to better understand their own experience, feelings, and meaning.

Such as: "So even though you told Joe that you were scared of getting pregnant, he wouldn't use a condom because it didn't feel as good as going without."

d. *Reflection of emotions:* The CHW will attempt to assess what the client may be feeling and to ask the client about it. The emphasis on emotions comes from an understanding that they are powerful resources for guiding our behavior.

Such as: "You are worried about not using condoms," or "Are you shy about talking about this stuff with Joe?" or "I'm wondering if you are scared about what might happen if you don't use condoms."

You don't have to get the emotion "right." Right or wrong, you present clients with an opportunity to clarify for themselves what they are feeling. You may intentionally amplify an emotion to assist clients to clarify what they are feeling. For example, a client might say: "I guess I feel a bit nervous about talking with my partner about condoms. I don't want to mess up the relationship." The CHW might reflect back: "Are you scared that just talking about condoms could make your partner start to question your relationship?"

T G: Sometimes when I use the OARS and I reflect back something that a client said, it helps them to really hear their own words, the feeling and meaning of what they said. Even when I get it wrong it can help because if the client says, "No, that's not what I said!"—then I have an opportunity to show that I want to listen, I want to understand.

e. *Reframing:* Reframing means to take information given by the client and reflect it back with a different emphasis or interpretation. The goal is to suggest a different way of viewing or thinking about an experience or an issue—one that may be more affirming or supportive to their behavior change efforts. Reframing can be particularly useful in terms of changing patterns of negative thinking that undermine a client's efforts. As always, the client is free to accept, to reject, or to change any suggestion you offer for how to reframe an experience (see Table 10.2).

? *What benefit do you see to reflective listening and sharing reflective statements with clients?*

? *In what situations might you make these statements?*

Summarizing Summarizing is a way to reflect back the main concerns, feelings, or decisions that a client shares. It is another way to demonstrate that you are listening deeply and that you have understood the most important information the client shared with you. It can be used to transition from one main idea or stage of change to another, to reflect the client's natural ambivalence about and resistance to change, and to clarify key decisions that the client has made. For example, the CHW might say to Mei:

✪ "I understand that you don't want to get pregnant. You want birth control, and you are worried that you parents will find out that you are using it. Is that right?"
✪ "You and Joe are worried about pregnancy, but you haven't talked about STIs, right?"

Other examples of summaries may include:

✪ "To summarize, you are not ready to stop using meth, but you do think that you can stop sharing syringes with friends. Is that right? What will assist you in putting this plan into action?"

Table 10.2.   Examples of the Use of Reframing in Behavior Change Counseling.

Client Says:	CHW Reflects and Reframes as:
I just don't know what to do anymore . . .	You say that you don't know what to do. But I see that you *are* doing something—you came here to talk with me and to ask for support.
I know I should start exercising, but I just can't fit it in. After work, taking care of kids, making dinner, I'm just too exhausted. I just don't have the motivation.	You feel like you don't have any motivation. But you must have a lot of motivation to work and raise a family. What motivates you to do these things so well?
I don't want to put myself at risk anymore, but I don't want to lose Joe either.	You care about Joe and want to keep your relationship, but you don't want to be vulnerable for STIs either. Maybe you feel like you will have to sacrifice one or the other. What would it be like to have them both?"
I keep dieting and I lose weight, but then I gain back even more, and I think I'm making it even worse. I just can't control what I eat.	How might you reframe this?
Your example here: _____	Your example here: _____

✪ "So, to summarize, you want to change your diet, but you are worried about giving up your favorite foods, is that right?"

✪ "Okay, let me see if I have heard you correctly: you really want to bring your blood pressure down, and you'd like to be able to manage it without using drugs. But you aren't sure what changes you can realistically make to do that. Should we talk about that next?"

MOTIVATION SCALE

A resource that is sometimes used to support motivational interviewing and other forms of client-centered counseling is a simple scale from 0–10 (Figure 10.4). The scale can be used to assess how important it is to clients to change their behavior, how ready they are to make a change, and how confident they are that they will succeed in making changes.

Figure 10.4 A Simple Scale.

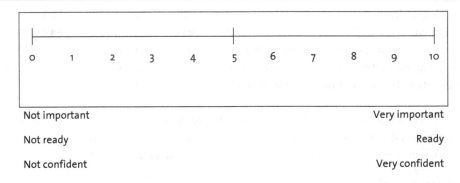

CASE STUDY: MEI (*Continued*)

The CHW working with Mei might show her the 0–10 scale and ask her:

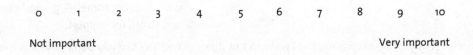

CHW: "Mei, on this scale from 0 to 10, how important is it for you to prevent pregnancy?"

Mei: "Like a 50! I'm not ready to get pregnant at all, and besides, my parents would kill me."

CHW: "Okay. Before we move on, I'm wondering how you're feeling now about preventing STIs. Using this same scale from 0 to 10, how important is it to you to prevent getting an STI like chlamydia or HIV?"

Mei: "I don't know . . . I guess maybe a 7, but if its HIV that's definitely a 10 because . . . I mean, I don't want to have AIDS."

CHW: "So it is very important for you to prevent HIV, but not other STIs."

Mei: "Yeah, I mean, you hear more about AIDS maybe, so you know you don't want to get that."

CHW: "It seems like you are less certain about the other STIs we talked about. What would be the difference for you between a 7 and, say, a 9 or a 10 in terms of how important it is to prevent getting other STIs?"

Mei: "Well, I guess really knowing more about what it would do to me . . ."

CHW: "Can we talk more about that now? Do you have time?"

Mei: "Yeah, I think I need to understand it better."

[*The CHW provides more information about the health consequences of STIs.*]

The following guidelines come from Thomas Bodenheimer, a physician, researcher, and advocate of new primary health care models that feature a central role for CHWs. He has promoted the use of the 0–10 scale in working with clients or patients with diabetes and other chronic conditions (Bodenheimer, 2007).

The 0 to 10 scale may be used to assess how important a particular issue is to the client. If the level of importance to the client is relatively high (a 7 or higher), the CHW can move on to explore risk-reduction steps and the client's confidence in putting them into action. But if the level of importance is low, the CHW may take time to talk about the issue further, providing the client with information about the risks that the issue may pose to the client's health.

When clients develop behavior change plans, the scale may be used to assess how confident they are in putting the plan into action. If the client's confidence level is relatively low, such as a 4, the CHW might ask the client why they rate their confidence at a 4 rather than a 1. This can aid in identifying what the client *is* confident about changing. The CHW might also ask the client what would make it possible for the person to move up the scale in confidence from a lower score, such as a 4, to a higher score, such as a 7 or 8. This may assist the client to reflect further about behavior change, what is getting in the way, and what the client may need to keep moving forward.

If there is a high enough level of importance and confidence to make the behavior change, the CHW should suggest discussing an action plan. The action plan should be tailored to the importance and confidence level of the client.

CASE STUDY: MEI (*Continued*)

The CHW working with Mei might ask her:

CHW: "Okay, based on what you know now, and using the same scale of 0 to 10, how confident are you now of using condoms when you have sex?"

0	1	2	3	4	5	6	7	8	9	10

Not confident   Very confident

(Continued)

Mei: "I'd say a 5 or a 6, but maybe more. I mean, I have to talk with Joe."

CHW: "Why a 5 or 6 when you chose a 9 for the importance of preventing STIs?"

Mei: "Because—what if we don't have one, and even if we do . . . Joe doesn't really like to use them."

Rolling with Resistance   Anticipate that clients will express ambivalence and resistance to change, and use your OARS in that moment to keep the dialogue and reflection moving along. Instead of meeting resistance with further resistance, motivational interviewing asks CHWs to try rolling with it. A client says: "I tried to stop partying, but if I totally stop using meth (methamphetamine) that would mean giving up all my friends, and I'm not ready to do that." In this moment, instead of trying convince the client to stop using meth, try reflecting this statement back to the client and giving the person time to think about it. For example, you might say: "I hear that you aren't sure you want to give up meth if it means giving up friendships, too."

This honors the client's right to self-determination and offers a safer place to explore difficult emotions, relationships, and choices. If CHWs push back in the moment when clients are expressing resistance to change, they may risk pushing clients away altogether and diminishing their ability to trust you or other service providers in the future.

T G: Sometimes, when a client is resistant to change—and haven't we all been resistant to change?—a counselor kind of digs in there, or the client and counselor can become kind of stuck. The counselor might think their job is to help to convince a client to change anyway, but some clients—most of my clients—that will only make them even more resistant. So the rolling thing is just acknowledging that the client is having a hard time making these changes, or is having second thoughts, and just kind of normalizing that. I feel like talking about it in this way kind of takes some of the power or the energy away and makes it easier to talk about whatever the client is facing.

CASE STUDY: MEI (*Continued*)

Mei and the CHW have been talking about using a condom to prevent STIs. Mei expressed both ambivalence and resistance to making this change. The CHW continues to rely on her OARS and to roll with resistance to address these issues.

CHW: "So, not having condoms and the objection of your boyfriend are the two things that are preventing you from using condoms. Is that right?"

Mei: "Yeah, pretty much."

CHW: "Can you tell me a little more about why you think Joe doesn't want to use condoms?

Mei: "I don't know . . . He just said that he tried them before, but he stopped because it . . . I guess they don't feel so good for the guy."

CHW: "So that means he's been with someone else? Do you know if he had sex with other girls without a condom? [*Mei nods.*] How do you feel about that?"

Mei: "I don't know . . . Nervous, I guess. Like if she had something—and Joe got it—he could give it to me, right?"

CHW: "Yes, that's how STIs get passed along. Do you know if Joe has been tested for STIs?"

Mei: "He said he was, right before we met, and he's clean, and I trust him about it. I mean, he told me about the other girls and everything."

CHW: "At some point you still might want to think about getting tested together, at the same time, just to be as confident as possible about your health status. We offer the tests here, and there are other places to get them done, too."

Mei: "Umm, hmm . . . I don't know." [*Mei looks down.*]

CHW: "We don't need to talk about testing right now. [*Mei nods.*] Okay. Can I ask you more about condoms? [*Mei looks up and nods.*] Mei, if Joe was all right with using condoms, would you want to use them?"

Mei: "Yes, that would be . . . I think I'd feel relieved. I wouldn't have to worry so much."

CHW: "You would feel a lot better if Joe agreed to use condoms."

Mei: "Yes—that would make me feel much better about being with Joe, and about having sex."

CHW: "Mei, I know that Joe doesn't like to use condoms. They do reduce some of the pleasure, but lots of guys use them, have satisfying sex, and preventing STIs at the same time. What would it be like for you talk with Joe about this?"

Mei: "That makes me nervous too. He's the first guy I've been with, and I really like him. I don't want to mess it up, you know what I'm saying?"

CHW: "I hear that you don't want to mess up your relationship with Joe, and you are worried about not using condoms."

Mei: "Yes . . . and I don't know what to do about it."

CHW: "You aren't sure what to do."

Mei: "Yeah, if I try to make him use condoms with me, maybe he'll just dump me . . ."

CHW: "What would that be like for you—if the relationship ended?"

Mei: "That would totally . . . [*tears come to her eyes*] . . . I'd feel so . . . I'd really miss him."

CHW: "I can see that you care a lot about your relationship with Joe."

Mei: "I do . . . It's been totally great."

CHW: "Mei, what if your friend Sandee had a boyfriend, and he dumped her because she asked him to use condoms. What would you think?"

Mei: "Oh, man . . . I'd think he was a jerk. But, I mean, I didn't really think about it like that. I guess if he did that, Joe would be choosing sex without a condom over me. That's pretty . . . That would make me pretty pissed off."

ADDITIONAL TECHNIQUES FOR BEHAVIOR CHANGE COUNSELING

In addition to the OARS skills used to guide motivational interviewing, a wide range of additional techniques exist that CHWs may use when providing behavior change counseling. The following examples are adapted from a curriculum for training CHWs in Zimbabwe (International Training and Education Center on HIV, 2004).

The Use of Silence   Silence is a natural part of our learning and communication process. Silence often allows the client to reflect on the question or issue at hand, to identify their thoughts and feelings, and to find the words to express them. Some counselors become unsettled by silence and rush to fill it with words. In these moments, learn to stop, breath, observe, and if necessary, count to ten before you say something. Give the client space and time. If the silence continues, you might comment on the process (see below) and then seek clarification. For example, you might say something like: "You're very quiet. Do you want more time to think about the question I asked, or would you like to move on to another topic?"

After working with Lee Jackson for nearly a year, MR was taking HIV medications regularly, had gained weight, and was making plans for his future.

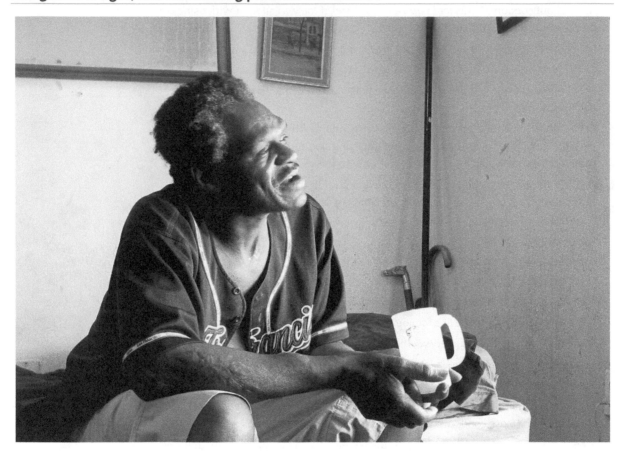

Commenting on the Process Commenting on the process draws the client's attention to what is happening *right then* in the counseling session. By commenting on the process, you create an opportunity to bring clients into the here and now and to focus on what they are doing, thinking, and feeling in the moment. Learning to be aware of their current thoughts and emotions and to express them in counseling may make things easier for them to learn how to do this more effectively elsewhere in their lives.

For example, if you sense a client's change of mood when a particular topic is raised, or a discrepancy between the client's verbal and nonverbal communication, it may be of value to comment on the process. For example: "I notice that each time we talk about your husband, your voice drops to a whisper." Or, "You say that everything is fine at home, but when you talk about it your eyes fill with tears. I wonder what you are feeling right now."

Commenting on the process can also be done as a way of acknowledging what the client has been through, while at the same time highlighting her strengths: "I am really impressed that you have been able to cope on your own for so long. How have you managed to do it?"

Finally, commenting can also highlight aspects of your interaction with the client: "I notice that you are trying to shift our conversation and to ask me questions about my life."

Widening the System

When people are facing challenges, they often forget that others may be able to assist. "Widening the system" refers to reminding clients to think about their external resources, including friends, family, and others who may be able to provide meaningful support. For example:

- ✪ "Have you shared this with anyone else?"
- ✪ "Who do you usually turn to for support or to talk about issues like this?"
- ✪ "What would it be like to talk with a family member or friend about what you are going through?"
- ✪ "What additional support would be helpful to you right now?"

Enactment or Role-Playing and the Empty Chair

Enactment and role-playing can be powerful resources for behavior change counseling, but they are not for everyone. Instead of continuing to talk about a situation or challenge, consider asking the client to act it out in some way. This technique can assist clients to think through and prepare for challenging situations and to practice skills that will support their behavior change.

The Empty Chair technique is a form of role-playing or enactment. Sometimes a counselor might use an empty chair to represent another person in the client's life. The counselor might ask the client to imagine that this other person (a parent, partner, child, service provider, or other significant person in their life) is sitting in the chair and ask them what they would like to say to them: "If your husband was sitting in this chair, what would you like to say to him?" This may assist a client to rehearse difficult conversations and to practice effective communication skills in a safer environment.

Not only might the client practice addressing someone else in the empty chair, but they may also try sitting in the chair to role-play the responses of the other person. For example, the CHW might say: "I wonder if you would consider sitting in the chair for a moment and playing the role of your husband. I'm curious what you think he might say about the situation. Is this something you would like to try?"

Role-playing is not for everyone, and these techniques must always be offered as a suggestion to the client. If you want to learn more about this technique, we suggest that you talk with colleagues and your supervisor about how to use it. Try practicing with colleagues before you introduce the technique to clients.

When done correctly, role-playing and enactment assist a client to "get in touch" with certain experiences, thoughts, and emotions that may otherwise be hard for them to identify or talk about. It can provoke insights that give clients an avenue to clarify complex issues and decide what they are ready to do to change their behaviors.

CASE STUDY: MEI (*Continued*)

CHW: "I hear that you don't want to mess up your relationship with Joe, and you are worried about not using condoms."

Mei: "Yes . . . and I don't know what to do about it."

CHW: "Mei, why do these two things have to be in conflict? What if you could use condoms and stay with Joe?"

Mei: "That would be perfect, but how could I . . . I don't know what I'd say."

(Continued)

CHW: "I have an idea—but let me know what you think about it. Imagine that Joe is here right now. What would you say to him about using condoms?"

Mei: "You mean like *right now?*" [*CHW nods.*] "I don't know. I guess, I'd say, 'Joe . . . I really want to talk to you about condoms. I know you don't like them and everything, but I'm really worried about us getting one of those diseases that are out there like herpes because you can't ever get rid of them. So I'm wondering—will you try using a condom with me?' "

CHW: "How did that feel?"

Mei: "It felt good . . . I'm surprised I could even figure out what to say . . . That was pretty good, huh?"

CHW: "*Really* good. You were so clear and direct. What would it be like to actually say this to Joe?"

Mei: "I don't know. I have to pick the right time. I will try, but—I just don't know if I'll be able to do it."

? *Which of the techniques described above have you used before?*

? *How do you feel about role-playing?*

? *What other counseling, communication, or active listening skills might you use when conducting behavior change counseling?*

10.5 COMMON CHALLENGES TO CLIENT-CENTERED COUNSELING

Because behavior change counseling asks clients to address highly personal issues, it can be challenging at times. Not only will clients naturally express ambivalence and resistance to change, but other challenges will also come up.

ANGER, AGGRESSION, AND CONFLICT

As we have discussed in other chapters, there are many legitimate reasons why clients feel angry. They may sometimes express anger or other emotions in ways that seem aggressive, threatening, or disrespectful. Being angry is natural, and learning to express it can be a powerful and positive resource for self-knowledge and behavior change. Yelling at or threatening a counselor, however, is not. When this happens, the challenge to the CHW becomes how to de-escalate the conflict and assist the client to learn to express it in ways that are acceptable. If you are unable to de-escalate a situation, end the session as quickly as possible. Your work should never come at the expense of your own safety needs. To read more about handling anger and conflict, please read Chapter Thirteen.

MAKING MISTAKES

Students who are training to become CHWs often say, "I just don't want to make a mistake!" They don't want to do something that may be hurtful, disrespectful, or harmful to a client's health. Despite your knowledge, skill, ethics, and best intentions, you *will* make mistakes: all of us do. Listen and observe your client carefully for signs that you have done this.

Hopefully the client will tell you by saying something like: "That is *not* what I meant: don't put words in my mouth!" When this happens, don't become defensive. As always, put your own issues and reactions aside for the moment, and focus on your client's experience. Learn the art of offering an authentic apology. Saying you are sorry or apologizing can restore your connection with the client and in many cases it can even deepen it. A sincere apology can create a foundation for deeper work (see Chapter Thirteen).

NOT UNDERSTANDING THE CLIENT

Sometimes CHWs feel embarrassed to admit that they haven't understood something that a client says. If you don't stop to clarify what was said, you risk misunderstanding something important and continuing to work with a false assumption. When you don't understand something, *ask*. For example, if a client talks with you about sexual or drug-use behaviors that you are unfamiliar with, ask for an explanation: "I'm not familiar with _____. Could you tell me more about it?" When you ask in this way, you are also expressing your interest in your client and your desire to learn about their life.

NOT KNOWING WHAT TO DO

You will face moments as a counselor when you are not sure what to say or do. With time and experience, this will happen much less frequently. There may also be times when you don't feel—for any number of reasons—that you are the appropriate counselor to be working with a specific client. Remember to reach out for support and to talk with colleagues and your supervisor about these situations. Ask for guidance and suggestions for what to do. In some situations you may determine, in consultation with your supervisor, that you are not the appropriate counselor for a client, and will refer the person to someone who you feel confident will be able to make a stronger connection and provide more effective services.

CRISIS

Sometimes your clients will be in crisis. They may relapse into heavy drug use, stop using the medications they need, become homeless, or become the victims of domestic violence. These are the moments to remember your scope of practice, turn to supervisors for consultation, or make an immediate referral. Over the course of your career, seek out opportunities for additional training on working with clients in crisis.

Reporting   As discussed in Chapter Eight, there are limits to client confidentiality, and you have a legal and ethical duty to report certain kinds of behaviors and events. If you learn that a client is harming or threatening harm to themselves or others, you must immediately report this to your supervisor and to appropriate law enforcement authorities. These events and behaviors include physical or sexual abuse of a minor, assault or threats of assault on others, and serious attempts or intentions to kill oneself. Don't be alone in these moments. Immediately contact your supervisor.

Have you experienced these types of challenges with clients?

Can you think of other types of challenges that you may face as a counselor?

Which of these challenges do you feel least prepared to handle?

Where can you go to access additional information and to enhance your skills for handling these challenges?

10.6 DOCUMENTING YOUR WORK

Other chapters in this book address the importance of documentation (Chapters Nine, Eleven, Eighteen, and Nineteen). Please refer to the guidelines presented there, and document each session as it happens or immediately afterwards. If you wait too long, you will forget some of the essential details from your meeting.

10.7 WORKING WITH SUPERVISORS

Working with supervisors is addressed throughout this textbook, including in Chapters Eight, Eighteen, and Nineteen. If you are doing client-centered counseling, you should meet regularly with a supervisor to talk about your work and to receive guidance and support. The person who provides supervision will ideally be an experienced counselor or mental health provider. Supervision is an opportunity to support you to provide quality client-centered counseling by addressing issues such as:

- Ethics
- Scope of practice
- Practicing cultural humility
- Challenges with documentation
- Personal issues that arise during or after counseling
- Understanding and resolving counseling challenges
- Counseling goals and developing risk-reduction or behavior change plans
- Counseling skills and techniques such as the use of motivational interviewing

You have an ethical duty to accurately reflect your counseling work to your supervisor. Don't waste this valuable time by avoiding difficult issues. If you are confused, uncertain, or struggling in your work with a particular client or bothered by personal issues, memories, or emotions, talk about these topics. The purpose of supervision is to support your continued professional development and your health and well-being so that you can provide culturally competent and client-centered counseling services that will promote the health of your clients.

10.8 SELF-AWARENESS

The essence of counseling, and client-centered practice in particular, is to focus on the client with unconditional regard and without judgment. Yet counseling others will naturally touch on your own life experiences, values, feelings, and beliefs. You have an obligation to ensure that your own issues do not get in the way of your work with clients. If your own cultural assumptions and beliefs, values, or emotional needs start to guide your work, you risk doing harm to your clients. If you become aware that this is happening, seek consultation immediately.

Signs that your own issues may be getting in the way of your work may include:

- A strong need to talk about your own ideas or experiences
- Finding it difficult to listen to the client
- Becoming overwhelmed or distracted by difficult memories and emotions
- The desire to tell the client what to do
- Strong discomfort working with particular types of clients

- Providing less counseling, or poorer-quality counseling, to certain clients (discriminatory treatment)
- Difficulty listening to particular types of issues (such as sexual issues)
- Difficulty providing affirmations to a client
- Becoming defensive with a client
- Treating a client with anger, disrespect, or contempt

? *Can you think of other ways that our own issues may get in the way of our ability to provide effective client-centered counseling?*

All counselors are challenged to keep their own issues from interfering with their work with clients. Good supervision, as discussed above, should focus not only on the challenges and needs that your client faces, but also on your own practice and specifically on the personal issues that arise during counseling. If, for example, you are working with a client who is the victim of domestic violence, and you grew up in a home characterized by domestic violence, talk about this with your supervisor, another colleague, a therapist, or a friend. Don't talk about it with your client. For further discussion of these issues and guidelines for self-disclosure (if or when to share personal information with a client), please see Chapter Twenty.

? *What issues may be particularly difficult for you to discuss with a client?*

? *Are you comfortable talking about sexual behaviors?*

? *Are there particular client behaviors or choices that it may be difficult for you to accept?*

? *Are there communities that you know less about and which may be challenging for you to work with successfully?*

10.9 SELF-ASSESSMENT

In addition to the supervision that you receive, and the evaluation of your counseling work by others (clients, peer observers, and supervisors), we recommend that you regularly stop to evaluate your own work as a behavior change counselor. The checklist in Table 10.3 can assist you to assess your own work.

? *When and how might you use this self-assessment?*

? *What else would you add to the checklist?*

10.10 CREATING A PROFESSIONAL DEVELOPMENT PLAN

As long as you provide behavior change counseling, you will continue to learn and to enhance your skills. Figure 10.5 shows a sample that can be used for tracking your goals and progress. Opportunities and strategies for continuing to grow and improve as a behavior change counselor including the following:

- Research and read about behavior change counseling and related issues including books, articles, and online resources

Table 10.3. Self-Assessment for Client-Centered Counseling.

Counseling Skill	Yes	No	Comments and What I Need to Work On:
1. Did the client identify their own health goals and risks?	——	——	_____
2. Did we assess the client's strengths or internal and external resources?	——	——	_____
3. Did the client determine a behavior change plan?	——	——	_____
4. Did we use a harm-reduction approach?	——	——	_____
5. Did I use open-ended questions?	——	——	_____
6. Did I provide the client with affirmations?	——	——	_____
7. Did I practice reflective listening?	——	——	_____
8. Did I summarize appropriately?	——	——	_____
9. Did I roll with resistance?	——	——	_____
10. Did the client speak as much or more than I did?	——	——	_____
11. Did my own agenda, values, or beliefs get in the way of client-centered practice?	——	——	_____
12. Did I identify personal issues that I should address in supervision?	——	——	_____
13. Did I share appropriate referrals?	——	——	_____
14. Did I document this counseling session for the client and the program?	——	——	_____
15. Other?	——	——	_____

- ✪ Attend conferences and trainings, including free trainings
- ✪ Participate in case conferences (see Chapter Eleven for more information)
- ✪ Shadow another counselor
  - Ask to sit in and observe an experienced counselor at work. The client must give permission for you to observe before you join the session.
- ✪ Self-reflection
  - Reflect on your own work. Keep a journal if that is helpful. Talk with family and friends about your work, your accomplishments, and the challenges you face. Use the self-assessment provided in Table 10.3.
- ✪ Debrief with colleagues
  - Talk with a trusted colleague about your work, particularly the challenges you face and the personal issues that may get in the way of client-centered practice.
- ✪ Participate in supervision
  - Participate in ongoing supervision with an experienced behavior change counselor or therapist.
- ✪ Learn from clients
  - This may be the most valuable way to continue to enhance your skills. Listen to the feedback that your clients provide about your approach, style, and skills. Pay particular attention to any critical feedback that you receive. Try not to be defensive, but to reflect on what you may want to change about the way you work.

?   *Which of these do you already do?*

?   *Can you think of other strategies and opportunities for professional development?*

Figure 10.5 Professional Development Plan.

Professional Development Plan

Name: _____

1. Identify one or more health topics that you would like to learn more about:	
2. Identify one or more communities that you would like to learn more about:	
What I will do to enhance my counseling skills:	When I will do it:

CHAPTER REVIEW

Jerome is fifty-eight years old. He has been smoking cigarettes since he was twenty-three. He smokes between a half and a full pack of cigarettes a day. Jerome's wife and children have been trying to persuade him to stop smoking for many years. Recently, his good friend and neighbor died of lung cancer, and Jerome is newly motivated to stop. He has tried several times over the years to stop smoking on his own, but never lasted longer than a month. He says: "Smoking has been a part of my life for so long, I don't know what I'd do without it. It helps me to relax. Its what I do."

You are a CHW working with Jerome. He shares the following information with you:

- ✪ "I just don't want to let my family down, particularly my wife. I know she's scared that I could get it (cancer)."
- ✪ "You think I'm bad now. I tell you, back when I was working at _____, we used to smoke all day long—up to two packs a day. They were a lot cheaper then, though."
- ✪ "You know, I wasn't gonna tell you, but I used to drink too much too. Almost ruined my marriage. My wife, she kicked me out at one point. Said she wouldn't take me back if I kept it up. And I did it. I quit, and I haven't drunk again. Thirty-five years now. What do you think of that?"

✪ "Is it gonna make any difference now—quitting? I've probably done enough damage already. Sometimes I lie awake at night and I worry that cancer is already there."

✪ "I don't know if I can quit. I used to think I'd give it up by the time I was thirty-five or fifty . . . but I just never did. It shames me, but I don't know if I've got what it takes to do this. When I stopped, all I thought about was smoking."

Answer the following questions about how you will do your work:

1. Where is Jerome on the Stages of Change in relation to stopping smoking?
2. What is an example of a harm-reduction strategy or approach that Jerome might take?
3. Use your OARS. Based on the information provided above, provide at least two examples of each of the following that you would ask or share with Jerome:
   ● Open-ended questions
   ● Affirming statements
   ● Reflective statements
   ● Summaries

4. Explain two different ways that you could use a 0–10 scale when working with Jerome:

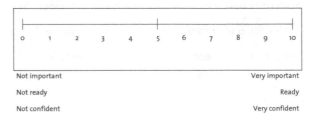

5. Jerome says to you: "I just don't know if I can do it anymore. It's been too long." How would you respond in a way that demonstrates *rolling with resistance?*
6. What personal emotions, thoughts, and behaviors will you pay attention to as you counsel Jerome? What will you do if you become aware that your own issues are interfering with your ability to provide client-centered counseling?
7. Identify at least three things that you will do to continue to enhance your skills as a behavior change counselor, and when you will do them.

REFERENCES

Bodenheimer, T. 2007. Self Management Support Tools.

Centers for Disease Control and Prevention. 2001. Revised Guidelines for HIV Counseling, Testing, and Referral. *Morbidity and Mortality Weekly* 50(RR19): 1–58. Accessed on March 27, 2009: http://www.cdc.gov/mmwr/preview/mmwrhtml/rr5019a1.htm

Drug Policy Alliance Network. 2005. Accessed on March 27, 2009: http://www.drugpolicy.org/news/062105naomitrials.cfm

International Training and Education Center on HIV (I-TECH) and the Ministry of Health and Child Welfare, Zimbabwe. 2004. *Integrated Counselling for HIV and AIDS Prevention and Care*: *Training for HIV Primary Care Counsellors.*

Prochaska, J., Norcross, J., and DiClemente, C. 1999. *Changing for Good: A Revolutionary Six-Stage Program for Overcoming Bad Habits and Moving Your Life Positively Forward.* New York: Avon Books.

Rollnick, S., and Miller, W. R. 1995. What is motivational interviewing? *Behavioral and Cognitive Psychotherapy, 23,* 325–334.

World Health Organization. 2006. *Prevention and Control of Sexually Transmitted Infection: Draft Global Strategy. Report by the Secretariat.* Accessed on March 27, 2009: http://www.raiseinitiative.org/library/pdf/A59_11-en.pdf

ADDITIONAL RESOURCES

Karen, G., Rimer, B. K., and Lewis, F. M. (Eds.). 2002. *Health Behavior and Health Education Theory, Research, and Practice.* San Francisco: Jossey-Bass.

Miller, W. R., and Rollnick, S. 2002. *Motivational Interviewing.* New York: Guilford Press.

Runkle, C., and others. 2000. Brief Negotiation Program for Promoting Behavior Change: The Kaiser Permanente Approach to Continuing Professional Development. *Education for Health 13*(3): 377–386.

11

Case Management

Tim Berthold • Craig Wenzl

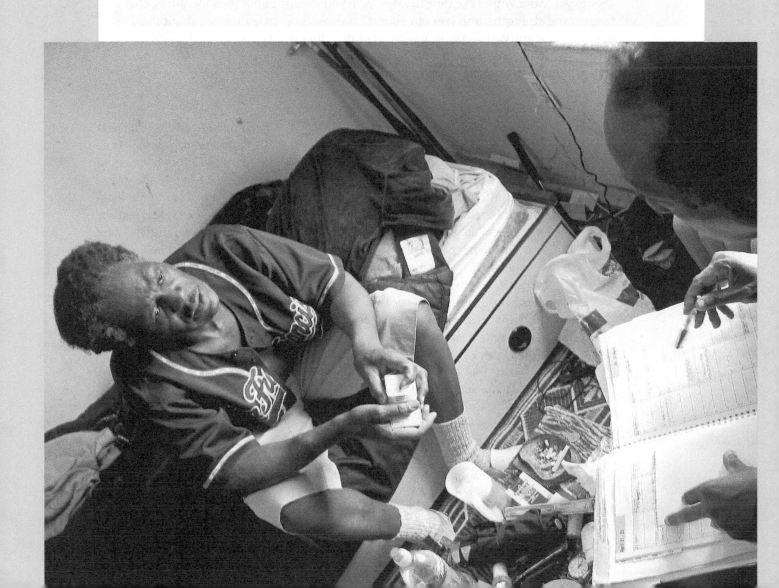

CASE STUDY: SIMONE

Simone is a thirty-four-year-old transgender woman who was recently kicked out of a residential drug recovery program for getting into arguments with other clients. She grew up in a small town, earned a bachelor's degree in business from a local university, and had a good job at a local bank. When Simone told people that she was going to start living as a woman and was changing her name (from James), she was rejected by her family and her church and fired from her job.

GENDER IDENTITY

There is growing recognition in the fields of medicine and public health of a diverse range of gender identities. People may identify as female, male, transgender, male-to-female, female-to-male, gender queer, none-of-the-above, or a growing number of other identities. What is most important for CHWs is to practice cultural humility: don't make assumptions or judgments about the gender identity of the clients you work with. Take time to learn from your clients about their identities, challenges, and strengths, and seek out educational resources to learn more about the communities you will be working with. Resources for learning more about gender identity are included at the end of this chapter.

Simone has been living in the city of _____ for almost two years. She thought things might be easier for her in a big city, but she faces constant harassment from people who stare at her and call her names. She has worked on and off in a variety of service sector jobs, but has quit or been fired from each one. At her last job, she started yelling at a customer who kept calling her "Mr." and "Sir." She has a hard time looking for work because she is worried that people will discriminate against her, and she doesn't tell them about her educational qualifications or past work experience because it is connected to her past identify and legal name of James. She has lived on the street and in shelters.

She feels deep pain about the loss of her family, especially her younger brother, whom she helped raise, and of her faith community.

You provide case management services to homeless adults. You meet Simone on the street outside a soup kitchen. One of your clients introduces you to her. The three of you spend some time talking. You make an immediate connection and are impressed with her charm and great sense of humor. When you tell her about the work that you do, she makes an appointment.

- ✪ What can you offer to Simone in your role as a case manager?
- ✪ What strengths and resources does she possess?
- ✪ What risks and challenges is she facing?
- ✪ What resources might promote her health and well-being?
- ✪ What types of referrals might you provide?

INTRODUCTION

This chapter provides an introduction to basic knowledge and skills for providing case management services. As a case manager, you will support clients in creating a realistic plan to promote their own health and well-being and to take action to implement that plan. You will link clients to resources and services that will enhance their health and safety.

WHAT YOU WILL LEARN

By studying the information in this chapter you will be able to:

- Define case management
- Explain your scope of practice as a case manager
- Work with clients from a strength-based perspective to identify both strengths and needs
- Support clients to develop detailed case management plans designed to promote their health and well-being
- Identify and provide meaningful referrals to community resources
- Organize your work and manage your case files
- Clearly document cases

WORDS TO KNOW

Caseload

11.1 DEFINING CASE MANAGEMENT

Because we live in a world characterized by unequal access to basic resources, rights, and opportunities, many of our clients face significant barriers to health. Case managers work with clients to identify the resources they already have and those that they would like to access. Based on this assessment, clients develop a plan to improve their health, and take realistic actions to implement this plan. As a case manager, you will develop an in-depth knowledge of local health, educational, and social service programs and work to link your clients to these essential resources. Occasionally, case managers also take a more active role in advocating with local agencies to provide services to clients in need. The challenge for CHWs is to provide case management services in a way that is client-centered and that supports the autonomy and empowerment of the client.

The following definitions of case management are from The Center for Human Resources at Brandeis University (Hahn, Aaron, and Kingsley, 1993):

> At the client level, case management may be defined as a client-centered, goal-oriented process for assessing the need of an individual for particular services and obtaining those services.
>
> At the systems level, case management may be defined as a strategy for coordinating the provision of services to clients within that system . . . to ensure continuity of services and to overcome systems rigidity, fragmented services, misutilization of certain facilities, and inaccessibility.

This is another way of saying that case management is needed because, as you learned in Chapter Six, our health care and social services systems don't work very well. People often have a hard time, on their own, planning for and getting access to the care, services, and resources they need in order to stay healthy.

PREVENTION CASE MANAGEMENT

Prevention case management is a relatively new concept that has been used extensively in the HIV/AIDS field and related areas. The focus of prevention case management is on *preventing* illness, disability, or other health-related problems such as HIV other sexually transmitted infections (STIs), hepatitis C, or relapse to injection drug use. Prevention case management is frequently provided by CHWs. The Centers for Disease Control and Prevention define prevention case management as:

> A hybrid of HIV risk-reduction counseling and traditional case management, PCM [prevention case management] provides intensive, on-going, individualized prevention counseling, support and service brokerage. This HIV prevention activity addressed the relationship between HIV risk and other issues such as substance abuse, STD treatment, mental health, and social and cultural factors. (Centers for Disease Control and Prevention, 2006)

Prevention case managers may provide more counseling services than other case managers, but this will depend largely on the policies and protocols of the agency and program you work for.

Some people object to the term *case management* because it may be interpreted to suggest that clients are the "cases" who need to be "managed." That view of people would clearly undermine the client-centered practice of CHWs, who work to support the autonomy and self-determination of clients. We view the "case" that requires management as the social context that creates health inequalities and deprives low-income and other vulnerable clients and communities from access to the basic resources that will promote their health.

CHW case managers work for a wide variety of public and private sector agencies, including local health departments, community-based nonprofit health and social services agencies, hospitals, and clinics. They work for programs addressing a wide range of health issues such as homelessness, mental health, domestic violence, maternal and child health, infectious diseases such as tuberculosis or HIV/AIDS, and chronic conditions such as diabetes or asthma.

Case management services are generally provided on an ongoing basis. It takes time to develop and implement a health plan and to successfully link clients to new services. Case managers may work with clients from two to three months to a year or more.

Your **caseload**, or number of clients you work with at one time, can range widely from a dozen or so to fifty or more, depending on the nature of the program you work for, relevant policies, and how frequently you have contact with clients.

Case management services are provided in a wide range of locations, including your office, a client's home, in the hospital, in a homeless shelter, soup kitchen, residential drug recovery program, or on the streets.

Т G: At my agency, we are supposed to work with clients for about six months, but some of my clients need more time, and sometimes I don't see them for a while and then I start working with them again. One of my clients, we've been working together for eighteen months. He just got out of jail and then went into the hospital, and he called me from there. I'm just glad that he keeps calling and reaching out to me, and even if he doesn't always succeed, I know that he wants a better life.

One of the challenges with the concept of case management is that it seems to imply that the services that clients need to access actually exist in local communities. The reality, however, is that many communities lack important resources such as transitional or affordable housing options, food assistance programs, mental health services, legal services, educational opportunities, or employment opportunities. This significantly complicates the work of CHW case managers, who may feel a deep frustration about the lack of services available to their clients.

ALVARO MORALES: I was working for a program serving people who were homeless. I tried to link clients to the resources they needed, like housing or jobs or family therapy. Sometimes, no matter how hard I tried, those services just didn't exist, or there weren't any spaces right then, or my client didn't fit the eligibility rules. Often, the best I could do was to offer a guaranteed place in a shelter, but a lot of our clients don't like shelters. I usually opened the drop-in center early in the morning, and some clients had slept outside in the doorway. When I went home at night to my family, I knew that most of our clients were sleeping on the streets. I often felt angry and frustrated because the situation is just so overwhelming and unfair and totally preventable.

IS CASE MANAGEMENT WITHIN THE SCOPE OF PRACTICE OF CHWs?

Some professionals question whether CHWs can or should provide case management services. Some have argued that case management should only be provided by professionals with more advanced education, certification, or licensure, such as social workers or nurses. We believe that CHWs are uniquely qualified to provide case management services because of their knowledge of local communities and resources, and their skills in client-centered education, counseling, and cultural humility. The reality is that CHWs provide case management services throughout the United States and the world. The federal Department of Health and Human Services, the Centers for Disease Prevention and Control, state governments, other national governments, and the World Health Organization all document the role of CHWs as case managers (see the resources provided at the end of this chapter).

11.2 BASIC CASE MANAGEMENT CONCEPTS

The approach to case management provided in this chapter draws on the concepts of client-centered practice discussed in Chapters Eight, Nine, and Ten. Basic elements of case management include:

- Work from a strength-based perspective that emphasizes a client's internal and external resources
- Support clients in developing their own health plans that include clear goals, priorities, and realistic actions to achieve these goals
- Practice cultural humility: don't make assumptions about the knowledge, behaviors, or values of your clients or impose your own cultural norms
- Provide client-centered education and counseling, as necessary, about the health issues or conditions relevant to the client
- Understand the three phases of case management and when to end services
- Develop an in-depth understanding of available basic resources and services and maintain ongoing professional relationships with these service providers
- Provide clients with referrals to resources, including clear guidance about why and how to access these resources
- Set boundaries and stay within your scope of practice
- Manage your case files and stay organized
- Document your work accurately
- Present your cases to the health care team or your program coordinator or supervisor

A note about strength-based case management: Some case managers focus exclusively or to a large extent on the problems or challenges that clients face and the resources they lack. Clearly, assessing a client's needs and challenges is essential to identifying basic resources that will promote their health. However, focusing primarily on what is lacking in a person's life can reinforce low self-esteem and the sense that they themselves are somehow lacking. Many clients, especially those who have been homeless, incarcerated, subjected to violence, or addicted to drugs or alcohol, have received these messages too many times already. This approach also overlooks the client's strengths, talents, and achievements. For all of these reasons, and with all clients, we ask you to use a strength-based approach in your work.

THE CASE MANAGEMENT PLAN

The focus of case management is to develop a client-centered case management plan documenting the strengths, needs, clear goals, and actions that will be taken to promote the client's health and well-being. Depending on where you are working, this document may be called a care plan, treatment plan, care coordination plan, service plan, case management plan, self-care plan or any number of other terms. The agency you work for will determine what the plan is called and what forms are used to document and monitor progress. For the purposes of this chapter, we will refer to it as a case management plan.

SCOPE OF PRACTICE AND WORKING AS PART OF A TEAM

As a case manager, you will always be working as part of a team. It may be a team of two, consisting of the client and yourself, or it may be a larger team and include other professionals such as social workers, nurses, or physicians. If you are working as part of a larger team, take time to clarify and understand the roles and scope of practice of each team member (review Chapter Eight for more on scope of practice). Ideally, you will have a chance to meet together regularly to discuss your work, the client's progress, and how best to work together to assist the client to implement the plan. The agency and program you work for should provide you with clear written policies and protocols to guide your work as a member of a team. These generally include participating in case conferences, described at the end of this chapter.

One way to define your scope of practice is to look at how the responsibilities are often shared among the members of the case management team:

Client Responsibilities   Clients often take responsibility to:

- Decide to participate in case management
- Decide whom to work with and provide informed consent to work together
- Provide accurate information in a confidential setting
- Identify strengths and needs
- Identify goals and develop a realistic plan of actions to meet those goals
- Communicate regularly with other members of the case management team, and attend appointments or call in advance to cancel if necessary
- Decide which other providers, if any, the case management team can share confidential information with
- Ask questions and raise concerns related to case management services
- Strive to learn new information and skills to enhance their health and well-being
- Identify additional services they are interested in accessing, and speak up if they are reluctant to access a particular service
- Follow prescribed treatments and use of medications and communicate with the team if challenges or concerns arise
- Actively participate in deciding when and how to end case management

? *Have we left out any important responsibilities?*

? *What else might a client do to contribute to the success of case management?*

CHW Case Manager Responsibilities   CHW case managers often take responsibility to:

- Conduct an initial assessment with clients; orient individuals or families to the program, services, and policies, including confidentiality
- Obtained informed consent to provide services
- Honor principles of client-centered practice, including the client's right to self-determination
- Work with the client to assess their strengths or internal and external resources, their health risks and priorities, and services that they would like to access
- Work with the client to develop a written case management plan and monitor progress in meeting identified goals and priorities
- Maintain proper documentation of all services provided and the challenges and progress made in the implementation of the case management plan
- Provide clients with referrals and resources to additional services
- Maintain client confidentiality as required by law and agency policy

- Ask for and obtain the client's permission before releasing information to other providers
- Reinforce health education knowledge and skills
- Maintain contact with clients and monitor and document their progress
- Conduct home visits if appropriate
- Advocate for client needs and priorities
- Participate in case conferences
- Participate in regular supervision sessions, clearly identifying challenges, concerns, and questions that arise in your work with clients
- Advise others working with your clients about changes within the community that might impact the clinic or program

? *Can you think of other responsibilities for case managers?*

Some CHWs will work as part of a team that includes other service providers such as social workers, psychologists, attorneys, nutritionists, occupational therapists, nurses, or physicians. In this case, the roles and responsibilities of all team members should be clearly defined. The team should also develop a process for working together, for identifying and resolving differing opinions or conflicts, and providing appropriate referrals.

If you work as part of a team that includes a health care provider, their responsibilities *may* include the following:

- Provide clinical care, including diagnosis of illness and prescription of treatments in accordance with established protocols
- Establish and maintain communication systems with other team members, departments, hospitals, and community organizations and agencies so that referral systems function smoothly and promote continuity of care
- Work with others to develop referral protocols, entry/exclusion/exit criteria, and clinical management protocols
- Obtain informed consent and necessary releases to share information with other health care providers
- Coordinate medical care services, including referrals for lab work and to specialists, as appropriate
- Maintain appropriate documentation of clinical services
- Participate in case conferences
- Provide program updates and share outcome data, maintaining client confidentiality

Sometimes you will question whether a certain aspect of care is your responsibility or if it should be handled by another member of the team. Remember to talk about these issues with your team and your supervisor.

COMMON STAGES OF CASE MANAGEMENT

Case management happens over time. The length of time that you work with an individual client (the number of meetings or sessions or the number of months) may be clearly limited by your agency or the institution that funds your agency. Regardless of the length of time you may work with clients, case management generally consists of several distinct stages including:

- The initial assessment of strengths, needs, and priorities
- The development of clear goals and steps to achieve those goals

- Implementation of the case management plan and monitoring of progress
- The end or completion of case management (sometimes referred to as discharge or termination)

11.3 DEVELOPING THE CASE MANAGEMENT PLAN

Every case management plan will use slightly different forms and slightly different language. Some plans will focus on particular issues more than others, such as mental health concerns, or housing, or pregnancy and parenting. Some case management plans are elaborate and may require ten to fifteen pages or more of documentation, including an extensive assessment. Others are more focused and require fewer details. Again, this will depend on the agency and the program you work for, the primary topic or health issue the program is concerned with (such as HIV/AIDS or mental health), and the population you serve. Despite these differences, most case management plans will include the following:

- An assessment of the client's strengths and existing resources
- An assessment of the client's risks and need for additional resources
- The development of one or more goals or objectives to improve the quality of the client's life
- The development of a detailed action plan outlining steps designed to reach identified goals or objectives
- Documentation of who is responsible for putting each step into action (client, case manager, or other professional)
- Documentation of referrals provided and accessed, and outcomes
- Progress notes
- Documentation of the end of case management services (also known as discharge or termination)

A case management plan is a working document to keep everyone focused on desired goals and how to achieve them. After the plan is developed, it is usually signed by the client or family, the case manager, and sometimes by another member of a team who you may be working with, such as a nurse or social worker. The client keeps a copy of the plan, and another copy goes into the file. As a working document, the plan can and is likely to be revised and updated over time, based on the experience and needs of the client.

THE FIRST MEETING BETWEEN CLIENT AND CASE MANAGER

Before starting to conduct an assessment or to develop a case management plan, apply the skills you learned in Chapter Nine to:

- Welcome the client and assist the person to feel comfortable in your agency
- Build rapport and a trusting relationship with the client
- Explain the nature and the extent of the services that you can provide as a case manager
- Describe any program restrictions and costs
- Clearly explain the limits of client confidentiality and other essential program policies
- Answer the client's questions and concerns
- Obtain informed consent to proceed with the assessment process

Take time to clearly explain your role as case manager, the types of questions you will ask as part of the assessment, and the purpose of asking such questions, as in the example that follows.

> ### CASE STUDY: SIMONE (*Continued*)
>
> Simone, I'd like to start our assessment today. If you agree, we'll talk about some of the resources that you already have, some of the challenges you currently face, and resources and services that you hope to access. This information will guide us in coming up with a plan to improve the quality of your life and your health in the ways that you care about most. My role is to help you develop and implement this plan. Some of the questions I'll ask—you can see them here on the case management form—are very personal, and I just want to be clear that you are the one who decides what we talk about together. If I ask you something about your life and you don't want to talk about it with me, or talk about it right then, just let me know, and I'll respect that, okay?

CONDUCTING AN ASSESSMENT

The purpose of an assessment is to establish a clear common understanding of the client's primary concerns, strengths, and needs. This information is then used to guide the development of a case management plan designed to address the client's concerns and promote their health.

Assessments take place in a variety of places, including the case manager's office or at other agencies or locations such as a hospital or juvenile hall. Sometimes case managers may conduct home visits (see Chapter Twelve) to develop a deeper understanding of their clients' home lives and the resources and risks affecting their health and their goals.

The assessment typically consists of gathering three types of information from clients:

- ✪ Basic demographic information
- ✪ Their strengths (or internal and external resources)
- ✪ Their current risks and needs (including needs for additional resources)

In Chapter Nine we discussed how asking for demographic information—the client's date of birth, address, family status, gender, ethnicity, and so forth—can create an uncomfortable distance between you and a client at the very moment when you are trying to establish a positive professional connection. For this reason, we suggest that you don't begin the assessment by gathering all the required demographic data. Instead, start with questions that are more likely to put clients at ease and may be most important to them, such as: "What do you hope to get out of case management?"

WHEN FORMS DON'T RECOGNIZE PEOPLE'S IDENTITIES

Review the forms at your agency. Are they inclusive of all people? Do they provide options other than single, married, and divorced to document relationship status? Do the forms recognize gender identities other than female and male? Do they recognize multiracial identities or instead force people to identify with just one ethnic category? If the questions we ask and the forms we use to document information aren't inclusive of the diverse identities of the clients we serve, we risk offending them and undermining our ability to work together successfully.

CASE STUDY: SIMONE (*Continued*)

In working with Simone, gathering demographic information may be challenging. Don't make assumptions about Simone's identity: she may identify as a woman, as a transgender woman, as gender queer, or none of the above. Do the forms at your agency recognize more than two forms of gender identity? Questions about name, income, address, and phone number may be difficult for her to answer, particularly if she does not have a stable address and if Simone is not her legally recognized name.

We recommend that you don't begin your assessment with Simone by asking for detailed demographic information. You may want to gather this data over two or more meetings, once you have established a positive connection. You may also want to talk about this with her directly, at the end of your first session. You might say something like: "Simone, here is a copy of the case management form to fill out as we continue to work together. As you can see, it asks for lots of personal information, including name, ethnicity, age, income, gender, and relationship status. I'd like to gather as much of this as possible, but as always, you decide what we talk about here and what you want to tell me. Can we start to fill out part of this together?"

ASSESSING THE CLIENT'S STRENGTHS AND AVAILABLE RESOURCES

As we have discussed here and in earlier chapters, client-centered practice emphasizes the importance of assessing, valuing, and building on a client's strengths. Starting from client strengths means that you recognize, and assist clients to recognize, what they have, rather than what they don't have; what they can do, rather than what they can't do; and what they've accomplished, rather than their perceived failures. Focusing on strengths allows you and your clients to identify *all* of the resources available to them and aids in buiding their confidence, capacity, and autonomy.

Assessment typically doesn't happen all at once during one interview in an office setting. Rather, you will learn more about the client's strengths as you establish your working relationship.

T G: I don't always start with a big assessment. I'll ask a few questions, but come back to the rest later as I get to know the client. Generally, I want to listen first to what is on their mind. They almost always have an idea of something they want, or want to change, or some resource that they need. If I can start by learning about that, and working to help them out—like helping them find a good doc (doctor) or some clean clothes or something to eat—then they're more likely to open up and answer all the questions I have to ask.

We encourage you to use a combination of open-ended and closed-ended questions to conduct your assessment of both strengths and needs, as explained in Chapter Nine. The program you work for and the policies, protocols, and forms they ask you to use will provide a certain degree of guidance about how to conduct your assessment and how to identify the client's strengths. In addition, please review the lists of common internal and external resources provided in Chapter Fourteen.

Over time, you will gain a deeper understanding of the client's strengths. One of the pleasures of case management is that you will often have the opportunity to witness clients developing new strengths along the way.

ASSESSING THE CLIENT'S RISKS AND NEED FOR ADDITIONAL RESOURCES

The case manager also asks questions to guide the client in identifying current life challenges, risks, and the need for additional resources.

The case manager will assess whether the client needs access to resources such as housing, interpretation services, drug treatment, employment, legal assistance, and health care.

Specific risks may also be assessed. For example, if you are conducting HIV prevention case management, you will be asked to assess the following types of risks:

- Current substance use
- Risks for exposure during injection drug use (sharing needles or works)
- Current sexual behaviors and risks for unprotected vaginal or anal sex
- Infection with hepatitis C or tuberculosis
- Not being under the care of a physician with advanced training in HIV/AIDS (for client who are HIV positive)
- Difficulty adhering to treatment guidelines, including medications

Open-ended questions are particularly helpful because they provide the client with an opportunity to identify needs that you may not ask about. Open-ended questions might include: "What are you most concerned about right now?" "What is the biggest challenge that you face right now?" "What do you most want to change about your life?" "What resources do you most need in your life?" "What are the biggest risks to your health right now?" "What places you at risk for HIV transmission?"

Finally, the client is asked to prioritize the risks and needs identified during the assessment. The case manager asks which of these issues or problems the client is most concerned about and what resources the person most wants to access. For example, Simone might say that a steady job and safe place to live are her highest priorities. She might also talk about her desire for community and a sense of belonging.

IDENTIFYING CASE MANAGEMENT GOALS

Based on the assessment, you will support the client in identifying one or more specific goals for the case management plan. While it is often meaningful for clients to talk about their ultimate life goals (working as a counselor, reuniting with and living near children or grandchildren, owning their own home, finding a sense of peace), the purpose of case management is to address more immediate concerns. The goals should come from the client, not the case manager, and should be specific and realistic. For example, while a client may not be able to purchase their own home in the next six to twelve months, the client may be able to find stable housing or a place in a transitional housing program. If goals are too unrealistic, this may set the client up for disappointment or a sense of failure. A key task of the case manager is to guide and support clients to develop goals that they can realistically work toward in a reasonable time frame. Other goals may include, for example: securing a part-time or full-time job; reducing risks for sexual transmission of HIV and other STIs; getting school clothes for their children; reducing blood pressure; or working to reestablish contact with family members.

CASE STUDY: SIMONE (*Continued*)

As a case manager, you might ask Simone: "What is your first priority for your case management plan? What do you most want to accomplish or change?"
Simone's goals might include:

* Finding a safe and stable place to live
* Connecting with a spiritual community
* Developing a support network of people who aren't using drugs
* Getting treatment for depression
* Reducing drug use
* Developing new friendships within and outside of the transgender community
* Working with a job counselor to identify career and employment options

Visiting a client in the hospital.

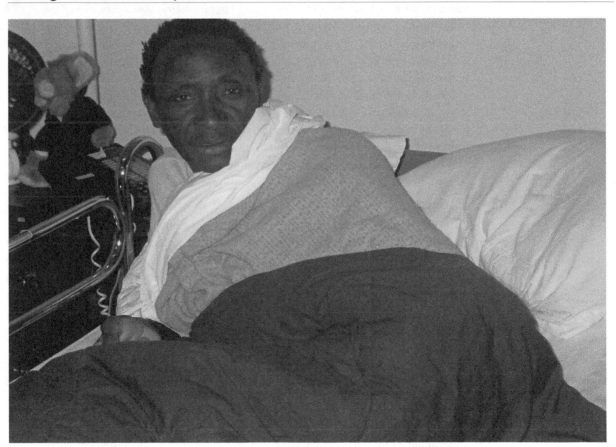

ESTABLISHING CASE MANAGEMENT PRIORITIES

When you provide case management services and work with a client to develop and implement a case management plan, you will establish priority issues or goals to work on. The issues that you as a case manager may view as priorities may be different from those of the client. Keep in mind that this is *the client's plan*, not yours, and the client is the one who should establish the priorities. At the same time, you will provide information, referrals, and guidance regarding priorities and actions for enhancing their health and well-being. As always, the client will decide whether to accept or reject this guidance.

You will often be employed to focus on specific health outcomes. For example, you may be working for a perinatal program with the goal of promoting the safe delivery and health of infants and mothers. You may want to focus on your client being able to have access to regular and ongoing prenatal care and to arrange for trained professionals, such as nurses, midwives, and dulas (labor coaches), during the delivery. While the health of her children will be a priority for the client, she may be struggling with other life challenges that pose significant obstacles to her health and ability to access perinatal care. She may be homeless or lack money for food or rent. She may be in a relationship characterized by domestic violence or have immigrations concerns. These issues may be her top concerns.

SERGIO MATOS: Part of the problem is that CHWs often have to work for programs, and the program goals are not in sync with the family's goals. Programs impose themselves on communities and often have different priorities. So you may go into a family's home to talk about asthma. But asthma might not be their real problem, even if they have asthma. They might be hungry or they might be experiencing violence or they might be worried about losing their home or unemployment or living underground with all this immigration hysteria. So asthma might not be at the front of their consciousness right now. But these programs impose these very rigid deliverables and actions that CHWs have to take. On the first visit, you have to talk about this, this, and this. And the second visit, you've gotta complete these five forms. And the third visit, programs can get very rigid and not respectful of what a family is experiencing or wanting. But the CHW is not at liberty to ignore the family's needs and wants, and so they have to negotiate that tension, that conflict. They have to find a way to serve the family to the best of their ability, sometimes in spite of the program they work for.

It is essential to respect the client's priorities. If a mother is most worried about getting school clothes for her children, finding a solution to this problem is the best place to begin your work together. Addressing one issue at a time, and accomplishing some sort of meaningful change—such as finding a place for free or low-cost school clothes for their children—will make it that much easier to establish trust and to move forward to address the next priority issue. Keep harm reduction in mind: anything that the client accomplishes that reduces risks for themselves and their family is a good thing. Make sure to acknowledge and celebrate the progress that your clients make.

T G: My clients wouldn't need case management if everything was working out for them. But they are dealing with big problems like HIV disease and on top of that maybe they're homeless, or they lost their job, or they relapsed and starting using drugs again, or their boyfriend beats them up and sometimes all of this combined together. And sometimes what I'm paid to do—like get them to follow through with their antiretroviral therapy—may not be a big concern to them. They almost always have other priorities—like being safe, or getting something to eat, or finding a place to stay. If I don't listen to what they want, then why should they listen to me? And if I'm not listening in the first place, then why am I working as a CHW?

DEVELOPING AN ACTION PLAN

The next step is to work together to develop a detailed action plan to reach the client's case management goal or goals. The plan will identify who is responsible for each action and will provide a timeline for completing these actions.

Case managers are generally responsible for the following types of actions: researching referral resources, preparing release forms at the client's request so that the service providers she works with can exchange information, providing health education or client-centered counseling services (such as risk-reduction counseling related to HIV disease), and advocating on behalf of clients (with their permission) with another service provider.

Clients may be responsible for the following types of actions: attempting to negotiate condom use; not using drugs before going to work; not sharing syringes or works to inject drugs; walking more and using public transportation less in order to exercise; carrying AIDS medications with them throughout the day to make it easier to take them on time; attending support groups; going to narcotics anonymous meetings; making appointments with employment counselors; or calling or writing letters to their mothers, granddaughters, nephews, or sisters.

The time frame for each intervention will depend on the issues, how difficult the steps in the action plan are, and the individual or family's strengths and risks. Include some action items that are scheduled for the next few days, week, and month. If the timeline is too long, it increases the likelihood that the actions won't be accomplished. Start with steps that are less intimidating and seem most possible.

CASE STUDY: SIMONE (*Continued*)

Actions that Simone may take include:

* Drop by the office of the employment counseling agency, pick up a brochure, and look at some of the job listings by the end of the week.
* Make an appointment to meet with a job counselor by next Tuesday.
* Start a list of her strengths, including difficult situations that she has handled in the past, before her next case management appointment.
* Walk by the Temple of Refuge, the church that she heard about, anytime during the week and possibly on Sunday.
* Ask her friend, Terry, about the transgender women's group she goes to.

Actions that the case manager may take include:

* Before the next appointment with Simone, research and identify local resources, including culturally competent mental health counselors, agencies, and services that focus on working with transgender and gender-variant clients.
* At the next appointment, talk with Simone about preparing a release of information to talk with other service providers about how best to coordinate efforts.
* Provide advocacy—if Simone agrees—with the agencies that Simone is referred to, to prevent further discrimination based on her gender identity.
* Identify opportunities to participate in additional trainings offered by members of the transgender community about issues related to gender identity, transgender health, and transphobia (prejudice and discrimination against transgender or gender-variant people). Sign up for a training.

Figure 11.1 is a sample case management plan from the Yes We Can Project (which aids families trying to manage their child's asthma). It is an example of one of many ways to create a case management plan.

Figure 11.1 Case Management Plan.

YES WE CAN: Family Action Plan

Date: _____

Family: _____ ID#: _____

CHW: _____

	Need	Resources	Goal	Plan	We did it!
	Describe the problem	Existing resources to use	What change will be made	The activities to get to the goal.	Date the goal will be reached
Basic needs: housing, food, etc.					Date: ❏ **goal met** ❏ **need more time** ❏ **no longer applicable**

	Need	Resources	Goal	Plan	We did it!
	Describe the problem	Existing resources to use	What change will be made	The activities to get to the goal.	Date the goal will be reached
Health/Social Care: Substance abuse counseling, mental health, etc.					Date: ❏ **goal met** ❏ **need more time** ❏ **no longer applicable**

	Need	Resources	Goal	Plan	We did it!
	Describe the problem	Existing resources to use	What change will be made	The activities to get to the goal.	Date the goal will be reached
Medi-Cal/ Health Families: (Eligibility for other government program).					Date: ❏ **goal met** ❏ **need more time** ❏ **no longer applicable**

COORDINATE WITH OTHER CASE MANAGEMENT TEAM MEMBERS

If you are working as part of a professional team, the case management plan should be developed collaboratively. The action plan will clearly detail which team member and service provider is responsible for which steps. All team members should attend regular meetings to monitor progress and any need to revise the case management plan.

PLANS CAN AND DO CHANGE

Sometimes clients will feel that some (or all) of the case management services are not working. Clients have the right to ask for changes to their case management plans and to withdraw from any services or programs that they feel are not working for them. Sometimes new needs will emerge that are more important to address than the issues identified in the original plan. For example, a client may become homeless or actively suicidal, be arrested, or relapse and start using drugs again. These circumstances will cause the immediate focus of case management to shift. When a client is not making progress with the plan, it is time to reassess. Perhaps the action plan or the goals should be revised. Perhaps the case manager should assume new responsibilities, such as advocating with other service providers on behalf of the client. On the one hand, you don't want a client to change the plan so often that no progress can be made (if this happens, it is important to assess why). And on the other hand, you don't want the case management plan to become so rigid that the client wastes times on actions that are not promoting the client's health or welfare.

PREPARING A RELEASE OF INFORMATION

You cannot divulge confidential client information to another provider unless they are part of the case management team or the client has given you permission to do so. It may be helpful for the case manager to talk with other service providers in order to better coordinate care and to learn more effective ways to support the client. For example, you might refer a client to a physician to treat their HIV disease, to a drug treatment program, or to an immigration attorney. If you and the client agree that it would be helpful for you as the case manager to be able to talk with the other service provider, you must all sign a release of information form. These forms will clearly identify the client, the service providers, the agency they work for, and the nature of the services that they provide. The form will state that the client authorizes these service providers to share information with each other and why. Most forms will detail what kinds of information can be shared between providers and give a timeline for when the agreement will expire or end. All parties must sign the form.

PROVIDING HEALTH EDUCATION AND CLIENT-CENTERED COUNSELING

Some case managers also provide health education and client-centered counseling (see Chapter Ten). For example, a case manager working with a client newly diagnosed with diabetes may assess the client's knowledge about their health condition. Depending on the assessment and the extent of the client's knowledge and interest, the case manager may provide additional health education and information to assist the client in better understanding the condition and knowing how to adhere to treatments, reduce symptoms, and enhance their overall health.

T G: I provide a lot of risk-reduction counseling to my clients. We talk about how to reduce risks for HIV and other STIs, or transmitting HIV to others. If clients are using drugs, then we talk about what they can and are willing to do to reduce their use or to change it so that they are less likely to be harmed—like going to the syringe exchange to get new syringes, and not sharing works with other people. To the extent that I can, I want to help clients look at what may be getting in the way of changing behavior and taking care of their health. Many clients have issues with self-esteem and depression or trauma experiences that get in the way. If they are willing to talk about any of that with me, that is a great opportunity. Of course, if I need to, I always make a referral—like I would try to link them up with a therapist if they are talking about really deep stuff that I know I'm not qualified to handle.

DOCUMENTING PROGRESS

Document or write down each contact you have with the client or other service provider who is working with the client. This will include in-person meetings with the client, phone and email conversations, and correspondence by mail. Document all relevant developments, including accomplishments and any further challenges to implementing the case management plan.

CASE STUDY: FROM SIMONE'S FILE

* 11/03/2008: Simone missed her appointment. Did not call. Don't have contact information for her. She may not have a phone or address.
* 11/11/08: Saw Simone at Raskins Park. Said hello. She ignored me. 30 minutes later she sat down beside me on a bench. She looked dirty and tired. No makeup. Bruised eye. Said she had heard from her brother. First time in 6 years. He was coming to town on business. He said he would meet her for coffee and would call back to schedule (she does have a cell phone), but never called again. He isn't returning her calls. She went out and "partied" with some guys she met on the street. Did crystal meth. Ended up getting in a fight and pushed down the stairs. She started to cry. Sat with her for 45 minutes. Gave her my business card again, a voucher to the grocery store, and made an appointment for tomorrow. She gave me her cell phone number: _____.
* 11/12/08: Simone was 15 minutes late, but she made it. Said: "I'm wearing my makeup today, so you better not make me cry!" Good to see her sense of humor back in action. She didn't want to talk about her brother today. She wants to start working on a plan. Said her priorities are to get a steady job so she can rent her own room in an apartment. She has been cleaning houses for money, and paying someone to sleep on their couch ("It's a dump, but it's better than staying in shelters or on the street.").
* Simone agreed to think about meeting a job counselor from Rise Up, but only if I talked with a counselor first to see if they would treat her with respect. She agreed for me to call Rise Up from the office, and she would listen in on the call.

I reached a counselor named Bev. Said I had a client that I wanted to send her for employment counseling. I told her that the client is transgender, has experienced a lot of discrimination, and wants to be sure that she will be treated with dignity. Thankfully, Bev was wonderful, and I could see that Simone sort of lit up—a big smile. I put Bev on hold and asked Simone if she wanted to talk with her, and she did. They made an appointment for Friday. Also talked with Simone about what she could do if she experienced discrimination on the job again, and if she might talk with me or Bev or someone else about learning new ways to respond so she wouldn't lose her job. She said she'd think about it.

* 11/20/08—office: (partial notes) Simone looked good. Has met with Bev at Rise Up twice. It is slower than she wants, but she is working on her resumé, and is going to a workshop on interviewing and to talk with someone about getting some professional clothes. Simone and I signed a release of information. She will bring it to Bev to sign so that we can talk.

T G: I can't live my client's life for them . . . but sometimes I fight the urge to tell them what to do. It gets so frustrating sometimes watching someone make the same mistake over and over again. When I start to feel this way, it is a sign that I need to take care of myself—and I usually talk with another CHW or my supervisor to get myself back on track. It also helps me to focus on the positive things, no matter how small they may seem. And every once in a while you get to focus on the truly big positive things. I was on the bus going home and this guy kept calling my name, and at first I couldn't tell who it was. It was a client from way back, someone I never thought would make it 'cause he was so caught up in using, and in and out of jail and prison, and really sick with AIDS. He looked so good. He had gained weight, his eyes were clear. He sat down and told me he was back in college studying to be a drug and alcohol counselor, and he had two years clean and sober. And when he was getting off the bus, he grabbed my shoulder and he said: "You never gave up on me, and that helped me to stop giving up on myself." I just sat there and cried—and I'm not someone who really cries—because nothing will ever feel as good as that moment. That's when I know that what I do is worth it.

SELF-ASSESSMENT

As a case manager, remember that your job is to support clients to develop clear goals and a plan to improve the quality of their lives and that of their families. Always keep in mind that *it is the client's plan, not yours.* To make sure that you are doing client-centered work, we recommend that you regularly ask yourself the following questions:

- ✪ Did the client actively establish the goals for the case management plan?
- ✪ Does this plan recognize the client's strengths and resources?
- ✪ Does it address their priority concerns?
- ✪ Did the client determine the list of actions to take to reach these goals?
- ✪ Does the client understand, and are they interested in, the referrals provided?
- ✪ Does the plan support the client's empowerment? Does it reinforce dependency on others?

ENDING CASE MANAGEMENT SERVICES

Ending case management services is also referred to as *discharge* or *termination*. Ideally, the decision about when to end case management will be made by both the client and the case manager, but clients can always decide whether or not to continue services. Ideally, case management will come to an end when clients have successfully implemented key elements of their action plans and enhanced their health or well-being. Case management also strives to assist clients in developing knowledge and skills that will aid them to stay independent and to successfully manage future challenges on their own.

Ending case management, like ending any professional relationship with a client, shouldn't happen suddenly, and should include making plans to support the transition and independence of the client. In preparation for completing case management, the team may talk about the following issues:

- What has been learned and accomplished through case management
- The client's internal and external resources
- Relapse prevention, if relevant:
  Supporting clients in learning skills to prevent relapsing to old behaviors or patterns they want to avoid, such as drug use or relationships characterized by domestic violence
- What the client can do when faced with challenges or crises in the future

As a case manager, be sure to thank clients for the opportunity of working with them, and congratulate them on the accomplishments that they have made.

Ending can be difficult for both the client and the case manager. If the work has been successful and the team has established a trusting professional relationship, it can be hard to say good-bye. If you find yourself hesitating in bringing your work to a close, reflect on what is happening and seek consultation with your supervisor. You want to be as certain as possible that you are neither prolonging nor rushing to end case management because of your own feelings and needs. Case management should be completed because it is in the best interest of the clients, when they have accomplished key aspects of their plans and gained confidence and skills in promoting their own health and well-being.

T G: I have terminated [ended] my work with some clients, but then started all over again if things got worse for them—like they relapse and start using drugs or go off their AIDS medications or whatever. Expect this to happen. On the one hand, it can get discouraging because a client who worked really hard to take care of themselves and get their life under control has slipped back—usually because something bad happened to them. On the other hand, I am always happy when a client reaches out to me and asks to work together again.

Sometimes clients terminate working with me. Sometimes they tell me why and sometimes they don't, and I just need to respect that. Sometimes they terminate me because they're mad at something I said, and then they come back and start working with me again. I had one client that must have fired me five or six times. I actually get more worried about the clients that don't want to terminate even when they've made good progress on their plan—it's like they get attached at the hip. I always worry—am I doing something to make them dependent on me?

11.4 OTHER SUGGESTIONS FOR EFFECTIVE CASE MANAGEMENT

KEEPING IN TOUCH WITH CLIENTS

Give your business card to clients, including your phone number and email address, and let them know the best way and time to reach you. Let people know how to leave a message for you and about how long, in general, it will take you to return the message.

Maintain professional boundaries, however, and don't give out your personal or home telephone number. This is a mistake that CHWs might be tempted to make with clients. It is rarely appropriate to extend your accessibility beyond the workplace, no matter how much you may want to provide aid to a client.

Ask clients what the best way is to contact them. If they don't have a phone, ask for the number of a neighbor or relative, or the number of the shelter where they're staying, or the number of the agency they are working with for housing. Write down the information and make sure it gets into their file.

Be as flexible as you can, and as your agency and safety require, in scheduling appointments. You may meet with clients at your agency, in their home, in jail or the hospital, or at a homeless shelter or other agency. If clients are uncomfortable or incapable of coming to you, see if you can go to them.

KEY TIMES TO OFFER GUIDANCE

One of the most important concepts of client-centered practice is to respect the clients' right to make their own decisions. However, this doesn't mean that you will or should always agree with or quietly accept the clients' ideas, plans, or actions. There are key moments when it is important to speak up, gently confront, or challenge your clients and to offer them guidance. These may include moments when:

- Clients establish unrealistic goals or expectations of themselves:
  Some clients develop case management plans that are overly ambitious. For example, a client who has always been heavy, with a long history of dieting and no history of sustained physical activity, may decide to work out for an hour every morning at a local gym. The concern is that they may be setting themselves up for failure, and if they don't follow through with their plans, they may feel bad about themselves, relapse to behaviors that put their health at risk, or drop out of case management. If you think this may be happening, say something. Assist your clients to remember that change usually happens incrementally—with small steps—rather than all at once. For example, you might say something like: "Kahlil, it is great to see you so motivated to start working out. But I'm concerned that this might be an overly ambitious plan. I've seen a lot of clients get really discouraged when they don't meet their goals. What about setting smaller goals at first, things that you can more easily accomplish and feel good about?" With further discussion, Kahlil may change his goal to start with something that is more realistic, such as meeting with a staff member at the gym to talk about options for starting to work out.

- Unrealistic expectations of you or others:
  Be wary of clients who put all their expectations or hopes on you or others to ensure that they succeed in their case management plan. Some clients may pin all their hopes on getting access to a particular resource: "When my Section 8 comes through and I have a permanent place again, then I'll be able to focus on getting a job." Some clients place high expectations on winning justice through the criminal

justice system: "Once this case is settled, and the judge gives me back custody of my children, then I can think about all this other stuff." Sometimes your role as a case manager is to work with clients to make plans for continuing to move forward in spite of big disappointments or setbacks: "Have you thought about what you will do if . . . (you don't get Section 8 housing, the courts don't award you custody of your daughter)? How will you continue to improve your life and your health, for yourself and for her?"

✪ Unsafe or harmful behaviors or choices:

If your client is considering harming or is actively harming themselves or another person, you will need to confront these behaviors and take action to prevent further harm. Let your client know that you have a responsibility to report potential harm to your supervisor or to legal authorities. For further discussion, please see Chapter Eight.

? *Have you had to confront clients before?*

? *What was this like for you?*

? *If you haven't done this yet, what are your concerns?*

? *Can you think of other moments when you would consider stepping in to offer more direct guidance to a client?*

WHEN TO ADVOCATE FOR A CLIENT

Sometimes clients are not successful in accessing the resources they have been referred to, and may benefit from some advocacy from you. For example, you might contact a drug treatment program, domestic violence shelter, or primary care physician and ask them to provide services for one of your clients.

However, the goal of case management is to support clients in managing their own lives and health, and in learning how to effectively advocate for themselves with service providers and others. If you step in too regularly to advocate on behalf of your clients, you are likely to increase their dependency on you and other caregivers and to undermine their own autonomy. To the extent possible, support your clients in developing the skills and the confidence to advocate for themselves. You might try making a call to a referral source together and asking the client to do most of the talking. If you decide to step in and talk with the other provider directly, debrief this afterward with the client: ask the client what this experience was like, and if they would like to do it differently the next time. If they make the contact on their own, follow up with them to find out how it went, if they were able to access services, and what their experience was like with the other agency or service provider. As with many aspects of your work as a CHW, the challenge here is to strike the proper balance between supporting the client's independence and autonomy and stepping in as needed to try to prevent unnecessary harm.

CASE STUDY: SIMONE (*Continued*)

As a transgender woman, Simone has experienced ongoing prejudice, harassment, and discrimination. While you can support her in learning new ways of responding when this occurs, you can also advocate for her—with her permission—to try to prevent further discrimination within your own agency and by the service providers you refer her to. This is a human rights issue: all people deserve to be treated fairly and with respect.

11.5 COMMON CASE MANAGEMENT CHALLENGES

CHALLENGING MOMENTS WITH CLIENTS

You will work with clients facing serious health problems on top of all the other challenges in their lives. They may be suspicious of your efforts to assist. They may not always be honest with you. They may complain about you to your supervisor. They may have diagnosed or undiagnosed mental health issues and may or may not be under treatment, have problems with drug use, or have difficulty communicating their needs.

A NOTE ON THE LANGUAGE WE USE

Some service providers use the phrase "difficult clients" to describe the challenges they face in working with clients. We don't like this language because it can be used to judge, stigmatize, and discriminate against people who are different from us, who we don't understand, and who may most need our compassion and case management skills.

Clients who are frustrated and angry often have good cause. They wouldn't require your assistance if everything were going well in their lives. Expect to encounter clients who are sometimes upset, angry, and argumentative. Don't take this behavior personally. With time, you may be able to support them in learning more effective ways of handling difficult emotions. Refer to Chapter Thirteen to review conflict resolution concepts and skills.

T G: Sometimes, when a client is acting out and making a scene or yelling or something, I just get so frustrated. I might have had a really hard day already, or maybe a client died recently or I had a fight with my boyfriend—whatever—and I worry that I'm going to lose it. Sometimes I just have to remind myself, "This isn't about me. This is their life, not mine." It's not like I don't know this, but sometimes I just have to remind myself so that I can take a step back and find a way to be patient and calm.

BEING HONEST AND SETTING BOUNDARIES

Be clear with clients from the beginning about what you can and cannot do to assist them in your role as case manager. Make sure the individual client or family understands your program's guidelines. For instance, as a CHW you may be able to assist a family to get groceries from a food bank and refer them to WIC or food stamp programs if they are not already enrolled, but you cannot lend them money for groceries.

LEE JACKSON: When it comes to loaning money to clients, no way. I explain my job to them and tell them that I have boundaries. Sometimes they'll ask you to lend them money and say they'll pay you back double or something like that. So I tell them: "No, I'm not a loan shark. I'm a health worker. I'm here to get you to your appointments and make sure you're okay and get you back on your feet, and if you need housing we'll help get you housing, but I can't loan you money."

Honesty and healthy boundaries enable your clients to trust you. Healthy boundaries protect your clients from unrealistic expectations and the disappointments that are inevitable when those expectations aren't met. Just as important, honesty and good boundaries protect you. Doing community health work can be very stressful. It can be draining to witness the hardships that your clients face. Nobody gains if you give clients unrealistic expectations that you can't meet. And nobody gains if you overextend yourself, burn out, and quit community health work altogether.

RAMONA BENSON: I worked with a young lady and visited her at her apartment. When she and her partner got high, he sometimes beat her up. She told me this when I did the initial intake. So, I went to her house several times, and I was trying to help her to leave and go into a safe women's shelter. It was a learning experience for me because I knew about the resource [the shelter] and I just thought all it took was to call them up and get a space and help the lady to move over there. But I needed to understand how much more complicated that kind of situation is and how hard it can be to leave. I didn't really think about or understand that there was danger there for me too, that I wasn't invincible to that danger, until her partner threatened me also. I just wanted to help her get away from the domestic violence. But rather than going back to the home to see if she was ready to leave, I gave her my number and I made a call to her, and later we met outside and she decided that she did want to go to the shelter. So, for me, it was a learning experience about danger, as well, and about how much I can take on—or what I can do for a client. But I'm still glad that this lady got out. Even for a while, it made her see and think differently about how her life could be.

A REMINDER ABOUT SELF-CARE

If you don't learn how to take care of yourself with the same dedication you show in working with your clients, you may harm your own health and your ability to provide high-quality, culturally competent services to others. For more information about self-care, see Chapter Fourteen.

11.6 IDENTIFYING COMMUNITY RESOURCES AND PROVIDING REFERRALS

A key part of your job as a case manager is to become familiar with the local resources that your clients may need, including housing, legal assistance, employment training and job counseling, education, child care, health care and mental health care, drug treatment resources, and more. In some cities and counties, local government or private agencies develop and regularly update a list of such resources. Increasingly, these detailed guides to local resources are available online.

If you don't have access to a comprehensive guide to local resources, you and your colleagues may need to develop one. This takes a lot of time, so make sure to talk with your supervisor and ask for support for this task. It will involve undertaking basic research to identify key resources. You can do this by conducting research on the Internet, going to the local library, reviewing local papers, including free papers, and talking with colleagues to create a list of the full range of resources that you want to assist your clients to access. Most important, don't forget to talk with your clients: they often have extensive knowledge about a wide range of available services, and strong opinions about which ones are the most and least beneficial.

We want to recognize that identifying resources is particularly challenging when you are working in rural areas or in a large county where services may be spread out geographically and difficult for your clients to reach, particularly if there isn't a good public transportation system.

DEVELOPING A GUIDE TO RESOURCES

If you need to develop your own resource guide, we recommend organizing it in a three-ring binder that will allow you to categorize different types of resources—such as housing resources—and to update them regularly by replacing outdated items with new information. For each agency, gather as much of the following information as possible:

- ✪ Name and address of the agency, and Web site if available
- ✪ A list of the services they provide (support groups, counseling, community organizing, legal or medical services, and so on)
- ✪ The cost of services
- ✪ Eligibility requirements (income limits, age limits, services for families without immigration papers, and so on)
- ✪ Phone number and best time to call
- ✪ Hours of operation
- ✪ How to get there: directions, public transportation, parking
- ✪ Can clients drop in, or do they need to make an appointment?
- ✪ Whom to ask for, if possible (you might want to include the business cards of individual service providers)
- ✪ What the client or family should bring to the first appointment

Your up-to-date list of referrals is one of the best ways you can guide clients to the care and assistance they need. However, not all referrals are good referrals. Many people have had the experience of receiving a referral and calling the number only to discover that the line has been disconnected, or they aren't eligible for services. Worse yet is when clients make the effort to go to the agency or program, only to find that the office is closed, that they should have brought certain identification or paperwork, or that they don't meet the eligibility guidelines. To avoid sending your clients or their families on a wild goose chase, provide up-to-date and thorough information about where you're sending them. Once you have gathered one or more resource guides for your area, call the numbers and find out from the agency how to refer clients. If it is a resource you will often refer clients to, build a relationship with a contact person(s) there. Get to know them by name, so that when you send someone there, you can call your contact person and let them know one of your clients is coming.

Be aware that some organizations that provide important services are funded by grants. When the grants end, the program or service may also end or change. Personnel at agencies and organizations also change along with phone numbers and addresses. In order to make sure you provide clients with good referrals, try to update your resource list every month or two. And, remember to reciprocate with other agencies. If your program experiences changes, get the word out to other agencies so that they can update their resource listings. This way, other agencies will also be able to make effective referrals to your program.

Whether a wonderful guide to local resources already exists or you have to create one, you should make time to network and establish professional relationships with local organizations and programs. In many cities there are regular meetings of service providers that you can attend. Bring your business card, and take time before and after the meeting, and during breaks, to introduce yourself to other providers, talk about your work, and learn about the services that they provide. Collect their business cards. If possible, make a time to visit the key resources that you most frequently recommend to clients. While you visit, pick up brochures and other information that will assist you in making effective referrals to the agency in the future. File them in your resource binder, if you keep one.

Lᴇᴇ Jᴀᴄᴋsᴏɴ: Since I've been doing this job, I've become friends with people in different agencies. If I need some help or a referral, I can just call these people and say, "Look, I have this client and they need to come in for detox. Do you have any beds?" Then they might say, "Well we have maybe two beds, but we'll hold one for your client."

The longer you work as a case manager, the more you will know about existing resources, the quality of services they provide, and the professionals who work there. Getting to know a competent provider at another organization is invaluable. When you can provide a client not only with a referral to a good organization that provides services they are interested in, but also with the name and phone number of a staff member whom you know and trust, you greatly increase the chance that your client will follow through with the referral and that they will be received and treated with the respect and attention they deserve. Remember that at the same time, you will become a trusted and valued resource for colleagues at other agencies. Receive the clients they refer to you in the same manner that you would like them to treat your clients.

Tɢ: The longer I do this work, the more I know about the resources that exist out there, even though they are always changing. And I have learned from experience what agencies I can trust to provide good service to my clients. Mostly, it is the same five to six resources that I refer my clients to: places to eat, decent shelters, mental health care, residential or day drug treatment programs, good primary health care—there is a great program at the public hospital, and legal assistance. It has been really hard to find good legal help about immigration issues. My clients have had some horrible experiences. Now I send them to a nonprofit center and let them provide the legal referrals because they are the experts in this area and I'm not. I go to a couple of meetings with different types of service providers so that I can get to know people. I like to know the person that I'm calling—or that my client is calling; it definitely makes a difference in terms of getting a quick response.

?   *What types of services have you or your family used in the past that you would refer clients to?*

? *What types of services do you think would be most important for clients from your own community?*

? *What types of services or resources do you think will be hardest to find in your community?*

PROVIDING EFFECTIVE REFERRALS

Providing an effective referral is harder than it sounds. Some providers assume that all they need to do is to pass on information to a client, and the client will quickly and successfully access this new service. But clients may face many obstacles. For example, the referral may or may not be a priority or relevant to the client. The client may or may not understand the nature of the referral and the services provided or be eligible for those services. The client may be hesitant to contact the agency, forget about the referral, or lose the business card or note you provided. The agency you refer them to may or may not provide services that are culturally or linguistically appropriate or accessible to the client.

T G: The thing I always hated when I was a client was when someone would hand me a slip of paper with the name of some organization I never asked them for and tell me that I should call up such-and-such agency and they could help me with such-and-such problem. Then they would just change the topic or leave and act as if they had done me some kind of favor. First of all, don't tell me to go somewhere without even asking me if I'm interested—that drives me crazy! Second, even if I was interested, do you think some paper with an address or a phone number or even a business card is gonna help me down the road if I don't really understand what the place is or what they do or who to talk to or anything? That's not a referral, that's an insult!

The goal of providing referrals is to successfully link clients with key resources that they are interested in and may receive services from. To fulfill this goal, we recommend the following:

- ✪ The referral should be to a service that is of strong interest to the client.
- ✪ Clearly explain the referral, including the name of the agency or provider, the services they provide, and how these may be relevant to the client's identified priorities and needs. To be absolutely certain that the client understands this information, ask the client to repeat it back to you ("Claire, I want to make sure that I am communicating clearly. Can you tell me what you understand about this program I am recommending and how it might benefit you?").
- ✪ Check the eligibility requirements of the agencies and their programs to be certain that they still exist and can indeed serve your clients (some programs have requirements based on income, gender, nationality, citizenship, age, language, disability, diagnosis with a specific health condition, length of time in recovery from drug or alcohol addiction, or other eligibility requirements).
- ✪ Provide clear and specific guidance about how, when, and where to access the agency or program. Where is it located? How can the client get there? When is it open? If you know and trust someone who works there a*nd may provide services to your clients, give them this professional's name. If you need to make a call to ask for further information, ask the client if she would like to make the call, or if she would like to make the call with you.

✪ If your client does not speak English, check to see whether the agency provides services in your client's primary language or will provide interpretation services.

✪ Remember to write down information about referrals for your clients so they can remember what you have told them. If you are working with clients who cannot read easily, it is still important to write the information down so that they can show it to family members or friends if they need assistance.

✪ Contact the referral agency to let them know that you have made the referral.

✪ Check in with your clients to see if they followed up with the referrals, if they accessed services, and what their experiences were like. Document this in the case files. Following up with your clients is particularly important. People frequently don't mention it if referrals don't work out, and they might not act on your future referrals if there were unresolved problems with the first one. Taking the initiative to find out what happened allows you to ensure that your clients actually get the services they need.

? *What has your experience been with referrals?*

? *Have you received helpful or unhelpful referrals?*

? *What else can CHWs do to provide effective referrals?*

SCARCE RESOURCES

It is often difficult to find resources for clients. Certain types of services may not exist in your community or nearby. Services may exclude your clients for one reason or another, such as their gender, gender identity, immigration or health insurance status, income, family size, or other factors. Health care, legal assistance, and housing are often among the most difficult types of referrals to locate for your clients. Keep building relationships and networking with other health and social services providers to learn about available resources. And be honest with your clients about the limited availability of certain resources.

11.7 ORGANIZING AND DOCUMENTING YOUR WORK

MAKE A SCHEDULE AND KEEP IT

Case management is a challenging job, and no two days are likely to be the same. There is no way to accurately predict the times when clients will experience crises or your caseload (number of clients) will increase. Create a schedule that shows the time and location of case management sessions, team meetings, case conferences, and other responsibilities each week. Be sure to include time to take a break, eat lunch, and to document the services you provide.

MANAGING CASE FILES

Documenting the services you provide and managing your case files is an ethical duty and part of your responsibility to clients and your agency. Forms are used to track the services your clients have received in order to evaluate the program and to provide reports to the institution that funds it. Accurate documentation and maintenance of case files are essential for ongoing funding.

Your clear records provide insight into the depth and quality of your work and assist supervisors to evaluate your performance. These records can also clear up misunderstandings that may arise.

Most important, these records are useful for understanding a client's progress and provide essential information for improving the quality of services that clients receive.

Basic guidelines for managing your case files include:

- Keep it confidential
- Alphabetize by client name
- Use appropriate forms
- Write clearly
- Keep forms in order
- Keep up-to-date

Keep All Files Confidential   Clients will share personal information with you. In order to maintain your clients' trust, you must protect that information. As a provider, you are also legally required to protect their confidentiality. Don't leave forms or folders lying around where other people might see them. Put files in a file cabinet or other location that you can lock at the end of the day. Treat the information with care and respect. Don't share personal information with other service providers unless you get the client's written permission first. Learn your program's confidentiality guidelines. If you have questions, ask your supervisor.

Alphabetize   Make a file folder for each client or family and keep the folders in alphabetical order by last name. Keep these files in safe place—such as a locked file cabinet or a file drawer in your desk.

Use Appropriate Forms   Use the forms that your agency provides to document client information and the delivery of services. It will be much easier to keep track of information and share it with other members of your team if everyone is using the same forms. If you don't like something about a form, talk to your supervisor. Perhaps the forms can be changed to improve the quality of your work.

Write Clearly   Write clearly when you complete forms and document progress notes. If your handwriting is hard for others to read, print. Write not only for yourself, but for others who will need to read your notes, including others who may work with this client in the future.

Keep Data in a Consistent Order   Keep all the information in each client's folder in the same order: this will make it easier to tell if anything is missing or incomplete. You might even want to use or make a checklist of what is supposed to be in the folder. You may come up with your own system to remind you of things you have promised to do for someone, but be sure that other people can understand it too.

Keep Up-to-Date   Update your active case folders periodically, such as every week or month, as appropriate to the program you work for. Jot down case notes every time you have completed a session with a client. Be sure to put down the date of the session, what was discussed, referrals you provided, and any agreements on future actions to be taken. Case notes are very important, but they only work for you if you can understand them when you read them later.

DOCUMENTING CASE MANAGEMENT SERVICES

L<small>EE</small> J<small>ACKSON</small>:   For documentation I have a client contact sheet, and each time I come into contact with a client, I document it. I make time every day just to do my notes, or I'd never be able to keep up. There's definitely a lot of paperwork with this job. I write down how much time I spend with the client, and the case management and health education plans we develop, and their progress. At the end of the month, I have to tally up all of my contacts, and we fax a report to the state health department.

TAKING SOAP NOTES

SOAP notes should be:

✪   *Brief, to the point*
✪   *Based on observations, not judgments*
✪   *Strength-based*

There are many different systems for documenting case management and other client or patient services. SOAP notes is one documentation system that is widely used by CHWs and other providers. They may or may not be used by the agency you work for. SOAP stands for: **S**ubjective, **O**bjective, **A**ssessment, and **P**lan. Below is an example of SOAP notes based on an interview with a family about the management of their child's asthma.

Subjective   The subjective part of the notes includes *what clients report to you* regarding their knowledge, feelings, attitudes, and behaviors. For example, this might include what a client tells you about their child's asthma, including what they say they do to aid in managing it, things that happened in the past, how they understand the issue, and how they feel about it. Subjective notes provide a picture of the client's experience and perspective. To gather this information, you will need to ask a number of specific questions designed to draw out specific details.

CASE STUDY: CHRISTA

Christa's mom reports that her asthma has been under good control. Last week, on her second day of kindergarten, Christa had her first flare-up in months. Christa says she got wheezy on the playground. Her mother thinks the episode may have been brought on by exercise. The teacher did have a copy of Christa's asthma action plan and sent her to the office for medication. Christa says she felt fine after that, but her mother is worried that there may be asthma triggers in the school.

Objective   The objective information that you document includes *what you directly observe and hear during your meetings and conversations with clients.* These notes will simply describe who did what and who said what, without any interpretation, judgment, or analysis from you.

CASE STUDY: CHRISTA (*Continued*)

When I visited the apartment on June 6, 2008, I saw that Christa's asthma action plan was taped to the refrigerator and her medications were in her medication box in the bathroom. The neighbor's cat came into the back kitchen while we were talking and rubbed against the furniture. Christa petted the cat. Her mother said: "I told you not to touch him!" The cat wandered down the hall into their apartment. Christa's mother told me that nobody smokes in the house. I saw an ashtray with more than two cigarette butts on the kitchen counter by the back door.

Assessment   The assessment is the place where you can document *your own thoughts, interpretations, and analysis (subjective opinion) about what you observed and heard* from the clients (objective information). You want to be careful about making judgments that the objective evidence does not support, particularly allegations that could potentially harm the client. Remember that you may be asked to explain or to defend any assessments that you make regarding your clients. When writing an assessment, be as detailed and as clear as possible about the situation you are describing.

CASE STUDY: CHRISTA (*Continued*)

Mrs. Lee seems to be more focused on Christa's asthma symptoms at school and in other environments outside the home. She does a good job keeping track of Christa's action plan and medications. She did not seem as worried about trying to control Christa's exposure to asthma triggers at home, such as smoke and the neighbor's cat.

Plan   This is the place to document *what you and the client plan to do in the future.* You will want to include actions that the client plans to take, any special requests the client may make, services you will provide, referrals, and reminders for the next home visit or appointment.

CASE STUDY: CHRISTA (*Continued*)

Mrs. Lee says she will make notes if Christa has another episode at school. She will also call the school nurse to ask for more information. I will check on Christa's asthma medications at the next visit, and talk with Mrs. Lee about smoking in the house. Will try to determine who is smoking and how to stop or reduce smoking in the apartment. Will bring Mrs. Lee a pamphlet on the risks of secondhand smoke, and some referrals for free smoking cessation programs. Will ask more questions about the neighbor's cat: Does Christa have symptoms when the cat is around? Has she been tested for allergies to cats (there is no note in the file)?

11.8 PARTICIPATING IN CASE CONFERENCES

Case conferences bring together members of a team who work with common clients, or colleagues who work with similar clients. The purpose of case conferences is to:

- Improve the quality of services provided to clients
- Improve coordination between service providers and service teams
- Enhance the professional skills of service providers

During a case conference, one team member may be asked to present information about a particular client or case. If the meeting is taking place only among team members who have permission from the client to share confidential information with each other, then any of this information may be discussed. If not, then the case is discussed in more general terms, keeping the identity of the client confidential.

Often priority is given to a CHW or other colleague who is working with a client in crisis or who is facing one or more challenges in their work. The CHW provides background information (maintaining confidentiality), including the client's case management goals and progress made thus far, and describes current challenges, questions, or concerns. The group discusses the case with the goal of identifying strategies for working with the client and referrals that may promote the client's progress and well-being. Sometimes another colleague will have information about the client that can shed light on the situation. In this way, participants share information and skills with each other, enhancing their own. Most important, clients benefit from new insights and suggestions that may arise.

If you have been asked to present at a case conference, make sure to prepare by updating and reviewing the case files, including the client's goals, strengths, accomplishments, and outstanding risks, needs, or concerns. What are your questions or concerns? Do you have questions about available resources for the client? What do you want to ask your colleagues? How might they be supportive of your work? What important information about the client should you share with the team, to enable them to provide the best possible care?

Strive to provide your colleagues with the same type of support that you would most benefit from. Let them know about the referrals that have been most beneficial to your clients. Share any suggestions that you might have based on your own experiences working with similar clients and challenges.

CHAPTER REVIEW

You have been working at your agency for six months and are in charge of coordinating care for clients who are homeless or marginally housed in your urban community. Today, a young man named Jorge visits you on a drop-in basis. Jorge is nineteen and has been homeless for about a year, living on the streets and getting by however he can. He was kicked out of his home when he was seventeen by his stepfather, and hasn't been in touch with his family for the past year. The other day someone on the street stole all of Jorge's possessions—a backpack with a few dollars, his I.D., some photographs, and other miscellaneous items. Increasingly, Jorge is using drugs and alcohol and says that it is the only thing that enables him to chill out from the stress of living on the streets. Jorge is not currently connected to any agencies that provide health care, counseling, advocacy, advice, or assistance in finding housing. Jorge is angry about the theft and says he is tired of living on the streets. An outreach worker from your agency gave him a card the other day, and that is how he found out about your agency's services. Jorge has come to you today—a very big step for him—to seek assistance to, as he put it, "get my life back on track."

Based on the information provided above, do your best to answer the following questions:

- What are some of Jorge's strengths (internal and external resources)?
- What may be some of his outstanding risks and needs?
- What specific strengths, risks, and needs would you want to assess? What questions will you ask Jorge in order to assess these?
- What types of referrals might you want to suggest to Jorge?
- What challenges might you face in working with Jorge?
- How might you evaluate whether or not you are providing client-centered case management?

- When and how will you document case management services?
- What questions might you pose to the group if you were presenting your work with Jorge at a case conference? What types of suggestions or support might assist you to provide more effective case management services to Jorge?

REFERENCES

Centers for Disease Control and Prevention. 2006. Defining Prevention Case Management. Accessed on March 27, 2009: http://www.cdc.gov/hiv/topics/prev_prog/CRCS/resources/PCMG/2–1.htm

Hahn, A., Aaron, P., Kingsley, C. 1993. *A Guide to Case Management with At-Risk Youth.* Waltham, MA: The Center for Human Resources, Brandeis University. Accessed on March 27, 2009: http://smhp.psych.ucla.edu/qf/case_mgmt_qt/Case_Management_with_At-risk_Youth.pdf

ADDITIONAL RESOURCES

Center for Housing Policy. 2007. *The Housing Landscape of America's Working Families.* Accessed on April 9, 2009: http://www.nhc.org/

Centers for Disease Control and Prevention. 2006. *Implementing a PCM Program.* Accessed on April 9, 2009: http://www.cdc.gov/hiv/topics/prev_prog/CRCS/resources/PCMG/4–2.htm

Housing California. Accessed on April 9, 2009: http://www.housingca.org/

Marsh, D. R., and others. 2008. Community Case Management of Pneumonia: At a Tipping Point? *Bulletin of the World Health Organization 86*(5), 321–416. Accessed on April 9, 2009: http://www.scielosp.org/scielo.php?script=sci_arttext&pid=S0042–96862008000500016&lng=pt&nrm=iso&tlng=en

Mesfin, M. M., et al. 2005. Community Health Workers: Their Knowledge on Pulmonary Tuberculosis and Willingness to Be Treatment Supervisors. *Ethiopian Journal of Health Development* 56. Accessed on April 9, 2009: http://www.ajol.info/viewarticle.phpo?id=24723

U.S. Department of Health and Human Services. 2007. *Community Health Workers National Workforce Study.* Accessed on April 9, 2009: http://bhpr.hrsa.gov/healthworkforce/chw/

Zeitz, P. S., Harrison, L. H., López, M., Cornale, G. 1993. Community Health Worker Competency in Managing Acute Respiratory Infections of Childhood in Bolivia. *Bulletin of the Pan American Health Organization* 27(2): 109–119. Accessed on March 24, 2009: http://www.ncbi.nlm.nih.gov/pubmed/8339109

SELECTED RESOURCES ON GENDER IDENTITY

Intersex Society of North America. Accessed on April 9, 2009: http://www.isna.org

National Center for Transgender Equality. Accessed on April 9, 2009: http://www.nctequality.org

The Transgender Law and Policy Institute. Accessed on April 9, 2009: http://www.transgenderlaw.org

Transyouth.com. Accessed on April 9, 2009: http://www.lydiasausa.com/Resources.htm

World Professional Association for Transgender Health. Accessed on April 9, 2009: http://www.wpath.org/

12

Home Visiting

Craig Wenzl • Tim Berthold

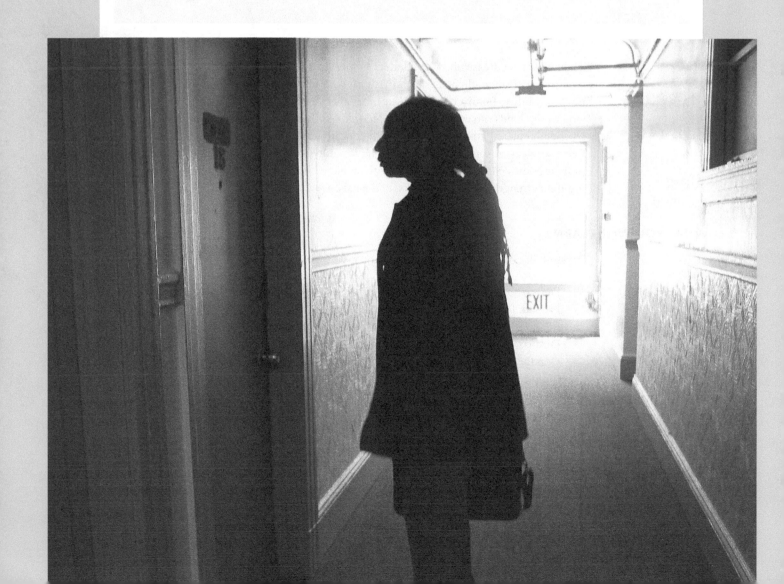

CASE STUDY: ROGER

Roger is forty-four-years-old and living with HIV and hepatitis C. You provide him with prevention case management services. Recently, Roger missed two appointments with his doctor. He has not been to your agency for over a month. You called Roger this morning and were able to get him on the phone. He sounds very weak and very ill. You set up a time to visit him this afternoon. You want to see how he's doing, if he's taking his meds, if he is eating, if he is willing to go to the clinic. When you arrive at Roger's trailer, he does not answer the door, but calls to you to "come in." The place is a mess: there are empty vodka bottles, glasses, syringes, spoons, and other drug gear scattered around. Roger is lying on the couch. When he sees you, he smiles: he is happy that you are there.

- How will you prepare for the home visit?
- What concerns might you have about the home visit and for Roger?
- What goals will you set for the visit?
- What type of assessment can you make, and how?
- What will you do to preserve Roger's privacy?

INTRODUCTION

This chapter addresses how to conduct home visits to clients. Home visits are a valuable way to reach some clients, especially those who find it difficult to leave home due to illness, disability, family responsibilities, or other reasons. Home visits are often an extension of the kinds of services that you provide in other settings—such as case management or client-centered counseling and health education. The key difference is that you provide these services in someone's home and have a duty to respect that setting. Meeting clients in their homes can also provide you with an increased understanding of their lives, including their strengths, resources, risks, and needs.

WHAT YOU WILL LEARN

By studying the information in this chapter, you will be able to:

- Define home visiting and provide examples of when and why they are conducted
- Prepare for home visits
- Identify key safety concerns and plan for ways to address them
- Discuss what to do (and what not to do) when you arrive at a client's home
- Conduct a subtle assessment of the home environment, and explain why this is important
- Identify and respond to common challenges related to home visiting

12.1 AN OVERVIEW OF HOME VISITING

Home visiting, as the name suggests, involves meeting with clients where they live. This may be an apartment, home, trailer, single-room occupancy (SRO) hotel, a shelter, jail, homeless encampment, on the streets, in the park—any number of possibilities. Home visiting is one of the most direct and personal ways to work with clients.

You will conduct home visits to clients who find it difficult, for one reason or another, to meet with you elsewhere, or because visiting clients at home will be helpful in terms of promoting their health. For example, visiting a client with asthma or a newborn infant can provide you with an opportunity to assess the home environment and to explore options for reducing health risks.

You may visit people you have never met before to encourage them to come to your agency for testing, health screening, counseling, or other services. You may follow up with an existing client who is unable to come to your office because of severe disability, injury, major health concerns, fear, or other barriers. Whether you have met the clients before or not, visiting them in their homes can assist you to better understand the context they live in and certain health risks, needs, and strengths. But visiting clients in their homes requires the utmost respect from you. They are inviting you into their spaces, their lives, and sometimes their families. Remember that you are a guest, and be as respectful as you would want a visitor to your home to be.

T G: I worked with clients in all kinds of places, including SROs [single-room occupancy hotels], apartments, shelters, group homes, tents in the park—you name it. No matter what kind of place I was visiting, I always remember that this is where the client lives, this is their space, and I respect that. And I always get a better understanding of my client, of how they live and what they may be up against. Also, I think because I am on their turf and not in my office—sometimes we are able to have the most personal or the deepest conversations. They might talk about experiences and feelings they never shared before.

WHY MAKE HOME VISITS?

There are many reasons why CHWs conduct home visits, including:

- To visit clients who are unable to come to your office or easily leave their homes
- To follow up with clients who recently received services from your program
- To contact clients who have not stayed in touch, to see whether they are all right and interested in participating in services again
- To see clients who have recently experienced a decline in health
- Because family members or friends of a client contact you out of concern for the client and ask you to visit that person
- To encourage clients to come to your agency for important services that cannot be delivered at their homes
- To support new parents or guardians
- To enable clients to assess their home environments and possible health risks, such as exposure to mold, dust, or other allergens that cause asthma
- To provide support and guidance to clients regarding how to take medications properly
- To notify clients that they may have been exposed to infectious diseases and to encourage them to be screened
- To meet with clients who are in the hospital, jail, or other institutions

?   *Can you think of other reasons to conduct home visits?*

ALVARO MORALES: I did partner notification for the health department. When people tested positive for HIV, we asked them if they would like us to contact people—anonymously—who could have been exposed by having unprotected sex or using needles with them. Not everybody wanted us to do this, but some did. My job was to visit these partners, to tell them that they might have been exposed to HIV, offer information and counseling, and ask them if they would like to be tested for HIV antibodies. I never knew what to expect. I called them first to see if we had the right contact information for them, to see if they were at home, and to ask them to meet with me. I'd say that I was calling from the health department, and I had some news to tell them, but I needed to tell them in person. It was awkward, but that was the policy. Talking with them on the phone gave me an idea of what kind of visit it might be. On the way to their home, I reviewed what I was going to say and prepared for the kinds of questions they might ask. I wanted to be prepared, and not to do anything that would make a difficult situation any worse. I was kind of surprised, but most people actually took time to talk with me, and some of them asked me to test them for HIV antibodies. I drew their blood—that was back when we still drew blood—and I would follow up to give them their results at their home or at one of our clinics—I let them decide.

THE CHALLENGES OF HOME VISITING

Home visits may be difficult for a number of reasons:

- ✪ Clients may not want you to visit or may not want to talk with you right then.
- ✪ Clients may be embarrassed about their living conditions.
- ✪ Clients may be concerned about their privacy.
- ✪ Clients may worry that you will judge them if they live in nontraditional families, or they may have other cultural concerns.
- ✪ They may worry that you will learn about or expose their immigration status, or worry that they could lose certain health, housing, or social benefits.
- ✪ Clients may have had bad experiences with home visits from child welfare, social workers, the police, or other authorities.
- ✪ You may witness or learn about drug use, neglect, or abuse.
- ✪ You may face risks to your personal safety.
- ✪ Your clients may be very ill or facing death.

? *Can you think of other challenges that you may face when conducting home visits?*

RAMONA BENSON: I've gone on home visits to new clients—and they won't open the door 'cause they don't really know me yet. I have clients who for whatever reason think "Oh, no. She's gonna judge me when she come in here." So until they get to know me and know that I'm not gonna judge them, the doors are gonna stay shut. But if I do my job right, down the road, they'll open up for me. I just need to be patient.

12.2 PREPARING TO CONDUCT A HOME VISIT

The nature of a home visit will be determined by the type of agency and program you work for and the context or situation in which the client lives. Careful preparation will assist you in providing quality services once you reach the client.

PLACE YOURSELF IN THE CLIENT'S SHOES

Imagine that you have been living with a life-threatening health condition for several years, and a CHW from a local agency is going to be visiting you for the first time. How might it feel to have a stranger come to your home? What concerns might you have about the visit? What would you want from the CHW? How would you want them to behave? What would you *not* want them to do, see, or ask?

RESPECTING A CLIENT'S RIGHT TO PRIVACY—DISCREET HOME VISITS

Some clients will have understandable concerns about privacy or confidentiality. They may not want others to know that they are working with you or your agency, or that they have a certain health issue such as HIV, cancer, or depression. How do you protect their privacy during home visits?

CRAIG WENZL: Several years ago, I was working with an HIV/AIDS service organization in the central United States. There was a lot of stigma affecting people who were living with AIDS. When conducting home visits, I noticed how some of the neighbors would look out their windows or look over from their yards to see who was visiting. Fortunately, I tucked all of my documents and materials into a backpack. I made sure that there was nothing on the backpack, my car, or my clothing that would indicate the agency I worked for. I learned to be as discreet as possible.

If you schedule the home visit in advance, ask the client how you can best preserve privacy. For example, if others are present, how should you introduce yourself? Will others be present with whom the client *does* want you to speak? Has the client disclosed the health condition to others?

If you don't arrange the visit in advance, be careful not to do or say anything that will disclose your client's private information to others. For example, don't introduce yourself by saying: "Hi, I'm Tranh, and I work for the AIDS Support Center." If you aren't sure what you can and cannot say in front of others, don't say it! If others are present when you arrive at your client's home, you might say something like: "Hey Bernadette, good to see you today. Is this a good time for a visit?" Or, if possible, speak with the client in private to ask whether you should continue with the visit or reschedule.

TG: Yeah, I've worked with clients who didn't share their HIV status with the people they lived with, like their parents, or children, or sometimes their lovers. I need to be careful not to say something that will break this confidentiality. In private, of course, I will ask the client about this. And if they are shooting drugs or having sex with someone, I'll talk to them about taking precautions or disclosing their status. But it is their health, their decision. If I pressure them, or break their trust, my chance to help them is pretty much over.

GET OFF TO A GOOD START—SHADOW ANOTHER CHW

If you haven't conducted home visits before, we strongly recommend that you spend time learning from an experienced CHW. Ask your supervisor if it is possible for you to accompany or shadow another CHW who works for your program or agency, or another program, on one or more home visits. If the CHW agrees for you to shadow them, closely observe what they do and how they interact with clients and their families. After the visits, ask questions about anything you want to learn more about. Incorporate what you have learned into your own work as you begin to conduct home visits.

Review and Prepare Client Files   Remember that your client has set aside time for the home visit. Being well prepared demonstrates respect. If you are going to be visiting a client whom you have already met or are already working with, review the client's file and key strengths, risks, needs, and health condition. The file may include a case management plan and goals (see Chapters Ten and Eleven). Check to see if referrals were provided. Is the client working with other service providers? Does the file include permissions to release information (or to share information about the client) with other providers? Bring copies of blank release forms in case you need them.

If the client does not have a file at your agency, create a blank one and complete any forms that can be done in advance of your visit. Bring blank copies of any additional forms you may need, such as informed consent forms, referral forms, and home visit assessment forms.

Organize and Pack Resources to Bring on the Visit   Pack everything you may need during the home visit, and review it carefully to be sure that you haven't forgotten anything. Develop a standardized checklist of materials (your agency may already have one) to guide you in preparing these resources. Some of the resources you might include are:

- Your identification badge and business card
- Written information (in the appropriate language or languages) about your agency, your program, and key policies and protocols, including confidentiality and its limits, and any costs
- Client files, blank new client files, and other forms
- Copies of any test results that you are authorized to review with the client
- Any medications or tests that you are authorized to bring and administer, such as daily observed therapy (DOT) for clients with tuberculosis or HIV antibody tests
- Educational materials to use to explain something more clearly (videos, pamphlets, booklets, and so forth)
- Risk-reduction or other health materials such as condoms, lubricants, hygiene kits, nutritional supplements, food or transportation vouchers, phone cares, and so on
- A list of other resources that you may want share with the client, such as resources for food, housing, health care and mental health services, or legal assistance
- A map, in case you get lost while trying to find the client's home
- A flashlight, in case you are visiting the client after dark
- A communication device (cell phone or two-way radio in case of emergency or in case you can't locate the client) and a list of emergency numbers

Can you think of anything else that might be important for you to bring with you on the visit?

Organize all of these items into some sort of bag or case to take with you on the visit, such as a backpack, duffle bag, or large briefcase. A backpack with several compartments works well, with places for files and different types of resources.

PLAN HOW TO GET TO THE CLIENT'S HOME

Review your contact information for the client. Do you have the proper address? If possible, verify this by calling the client. You'll want to know *exactly* where you will be going. Look at a map if you're unfamiliar with the area, to locate the following information:

- Client's address
- Landmarks nearby. You might try looking the location up online using Web sites such as MapQuest, Google, or Yahoo Maps.
- Parking availability or public transportation
- Anything you might need to know for your safety (see the section on safety below)

If you have an appointment and can talk with the client in advance, try to determine:

- If there is a house, apartment, or room number clearly marked
- If the client has a dog or other pets
- If there is a gate or intercom at the home or building and what you will need to do to get in
- Any possible problems you may encounter, getting to or entering the home

Make sure you have the client's phone number with you (if the client has one), in case you get lost or have trouble getting into the building.

IDENTIFY KEY OBJECTIVES

Write down what you hope to accomplish during the home visit. Be as specific as possible. For example, are you visiting to determine whether families are eligible and interested in enrolling in an SCHIP program (low-cost health insurance for children in low-income families)? Do you want to check in with a client with asthma to see if the person is experiencing symptoms and taking the medication properly? Don't set too many goals for a single visit. While it is important to identify the purpose of your visit, you also need to stay flexible. Talk with the client to learn about the person's current health status, needs, and priorities.

PREPARING TO CONDUCT A FIRST VISIT TO A NEW CLIENT

If you are visiting someone you have not met before, please review Chapter Nine: it provides basic concepts and skills for introducing yourself and the services that you provide, and obtaining informed consent from a prospective client. You must obtain informed consent before you conduct an initial assessment.

Your primary goal for a first visit will be to establish a positive connection with the client, to assess the client's resources and needs, and to determine whether the person is interested in the services that you can provide and would like to begin to work together.

PREPARING FOR FOLLOW-UP VISITS

You will also visit clients with whom you are already working. You may visit clients whom you usually see at the office or clinic because their health has deteriorated or they are unable to leave their homes. Try to prepare yourself for what you may see and learn. It is always difficult to witness a client who is in crisis, whose health is deteriorating, or may be facing death. Yet these are the very the times when clients need you most, particularly if they don't have strong family or other social support.

Even if you have worked with the client before, and are visiting to follow up on a specific issue that you have discussed in the past, don't expect that you will both have the same memory of what occurred in the past. For any number of reasons, including depression, deteriorating health, or other life challenges, the client may not remember the nature of your work together, including previous conversations and agreements, or care very much about it in the moment. As always, be patient and compassionate, and be prepared to take time to reintroduce yourself, to review your previous work together, and sometimes to start all over at the beginning. The essence of client-centered work is meeting clients where they are—don't assume that you know where they will "be" when you conduct a follow-up home visit.

Possible goals for follow-up visits may include to:

- ✪ Reintroduce yourself and the purpose of your visit
- ✪ Review your program's services and key policies, including confidentiality
- ✪ Answer the client's questions and concerns
- ✪ Obtain informed consent, again, to continue with your visit and to provide services
- ✪ Ask what the client remembers about your previous work
- ✪ Review any decisions, agreements, or accomplishments that the client previously made
- ✪ Assess their current concerns, needs, and priorities—what do they want to accomplish?
- ✪ Establish new goals that the client wants to work on, and let these guide your work
- ✪ Provide health education, client-centered counseling, and referrals, as appropriate
- ✪ Provide additional supplies as needed (for example, nutritional supplements, safer sex supplies, bandages, bedding, or clothing, and so forth).
- ✪ Set a date and time for your next visit

? *What other goals might you have for these home visits?*

12.3 COMMON COURTESIES AND GUIDELINES

RESPECT THE CLIENT'S TIME

If the client is expecting you, it is important to show up on time. If something unforeseen happens and you are running late, call the client and apologize. If you make a practice of being late, you risk losing the client's trust and respect: the client's time is just as valuable as your own.

If you schedule a home visit in advance, discuss how much time you both have for the visit. If you really need an hour, ask for it, but respect the client's limits and needs: "I'd like to visit for about an hour, will that work for you?" When you arrive, ask the client if it is still a good time to visit, and how much time the person will be able to spend with you. Stay aware, throughout the visit, of signs that the client may want the visit to end. Perhaps a family member is calling the client to go somewhere, or the client has to make a call, or go to the store, or rest. Be respectful: it is the client's home, the client's time, and the client's life. If you don't accomplish all of your goals during this visit, schedule a follow-up appointment in the home, at your agency, or at another location that works for both you and the client.

ANNOUNCE YOURSELF

When you arrive at the client's home—wherever it is—announce yourself. Use your name, but not the name of your agency in order to protect the client's privacy. You might say something like: "Hello, Sam? It's Sunil Gupta. We spoke earlier about meeting today. Is this still a good time?"

INTRODUCE YOURSELF

Once you're inside the home, introduce yourself again: "Hello, Sam. I'm Sunil Gupta. We spoke on the phone earlier. It's nice to meet you." Be sure you have proper identification with you when you arrive, and show it to the client or family if requested.

If you provide services related to sensitive and highly personal issues, and you are not confident that you are alone with the client, be careful about saying the name of your organization or the issue you are working for. If other people are around, follow the client's lead. If you aren't sure how to proceed, ask the client: "Sam, is this a good time to talk or would you rather reschedule our appointment?"

IF THE CLIENT IS NOT AT HOME

If no one answers, follow up with the client later. If someone other than the client answers, and the client isn't home, leave a simple message that preserves the client's confidentiality such as: "Could you tell him that Sunil dropped by to say hello? I'll call [if the client has a phone] again later."

DRESS FOR THE OCCASION

Make sure that what you are wearing is appropriate for the setting. Consider comfort, what is culturally appropriate and respectful to the community you are visiting, as well as the safety guidelines discussed below. Some situations call for slightly more professional clothing, and others for more casual wear. If you're visiting someone who is incarcerated, be sure to find out beforehand what the dress code is for visitors to the institution. If you are visiting a family with young children, wear comfortable clothes that will allow you to engage with the children. Ask your colleagues, particularly other CHWs who conduct outreach and home visits, what they would wear, and use your own best judgment.

DEMONSTRATE RESPECT AND ESTABLISH A POSITIVE CONNECTION

Whenever you are providing a home visit, you are entering a client's private space. Observe common courtesies when you are in the home: introduce yourself to others, ask people how they are doing, and thank them for inviting you into their home. Many of the clients you visit won't have much money and may live in housing of very poor quality, with many family members or roommates living in a small space. Your clients are likely to be struggling with other challenges as well, such as chronic illness, mental illness, addiction, disability, and interpersonal conflicts.

RAMONA BENSON: Sometimes the client's family had bad home visits in the past, and based on that experience, they ask me: "Why you wanna come to my house?" So I always say to people, "I don't have to come to your house. I'll meet you anywhere you want me to meet you at." I don't push myself on anybody—that's not going to do anyone any good. Sometimes they want to have the home visit at a McDonald's because home life is not fine, you know? Or they might want to have the home visit at the doctor's office, and so we meet there, but any public place where I'm meeting, I have to make sure that what are we saying is not being heard 'cause of confidentiality.

Your warmth, honesty, and kindness will assist in making the visits a success. Let your work be guided by respect for your clients' identities, cultures, and right to self-determination.

LEE JACKSON: Sometimes I go out to check on a client to see if they are okay. Some people you have to treat very delicately because a lot of them are living right on the edge. I always build rapport with clients, and this takes time. But by taking time to know them, and letting them know me, we establish a basis for our work together. I always acknowledge them when I see them in the community, and treat them as human beings. That way they don't look at me only as their health worker, but as a human being as well. It goes both ways.

PRACTICE CULTURAL HUMILITY

Home visits are a critical time to practice cultural humility (see Chapter Seven). The cultures, values, and traditions of the clients and families you visit will be reflected in their homes. The furnishings and art, the foods and smells in the homes, the religious symbols or lack of them, the makeup of the families, and their customs may be different from what you are familiar with. View this as an opportunity to learn more about the cultures of others. Abide by the rules in place in their homes, as you would expect in yours, and ask questions if you are unsure about what to do.

WHAT MAKES A FAMILY?

As you visit people in their homes, remember that there are many different kinds of families. Some families include people who are not related by blood. Don't assume that a family with children is comprised of a mother and a father. Children may have one or more parents or guardians, and this could include aunts, grandparents, a mom and a dad, two moms or two dads. In some families, many people take an active role in raising the children. Put your assumptions aside, be respectful, and learn about the family you are visiting.

SPEAK CLEARLY, SLOWLY, AND NOT TOO LOUDLY

People often talk quickly and loudly when they are nervous. Your calm voice can serve to relax others as well as yourself. If people are living on the streets, in shelters, at the hospital, in SROs or apartments with thin walls or a large family, your voice may be overheard. Speak loudly enough for the client or clients to hear you, but not so loudly that you broadcast private information to others. If you can't hear or understand what a client tells you, ask them to say it again: you don't want to miss important information.

Not everyone you work with will have a conventional home.

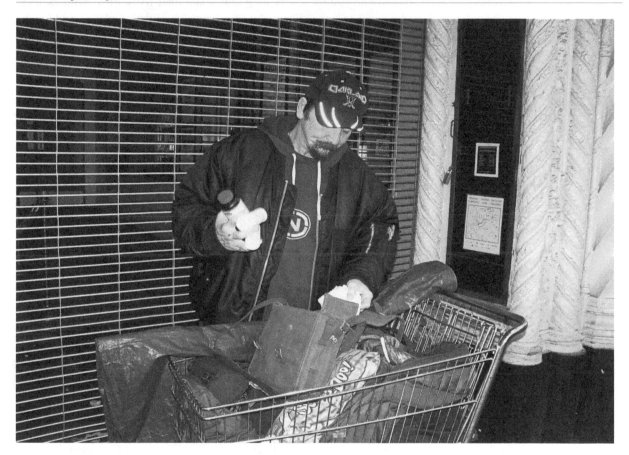

MAINTAIN HEALTHY BOUNDARIES

To aid in preventing potentially dangerous or harmful situations, maintain healthy boundaries with clients. Be cautious about disclosing personal information (home or cell phone number or address) or private details about your life. If a client asks you personal questions that you do not feel comfortable answering, be ready to explain and clarify your role as a CHW and why you won't answer these questions. You might say something like, "My role is to be here for *you,* to support you to improve your health. I don't talk about my private life when I'm at work, because that will distract us—this is *your time.*" Be clear and kind as you assert these boundaries. If a client starts to say things that are not acceptable (such as sexual innuendos), interrupt or stop the conversation. If the client continues, you may have to leave. For more information about boundary setting, see Chapters Eight and Twenty.

STAY ON-TOPIC

Plan for how you will disengage from conversations that are taking too much time and attention away from the primary purpose of your visit. At the same time, be prepared to do some casual visiting. This is a customary part of most visits to another person's home. The client may show you personal belongings, such as family photographs, or want to introduce you to family members who will engage you in discussions about a range of issues, from politics to the latest ball game.

While you hope that clients will feel comfortable enough to open up and talk with you about the personal issues that are influencing their health and well-being, some clients will want to talk with you for a very long time about their lives, their families, their hopes, and their dreams. For some clients, this may be a sign of their isolation and loneliness, or of fears related to their health and mortality. Develop your own kind and polite way to interrupt clients and remind them of the time and main purpose for the visit.

CRAIG WENZL: When I first began providing home visits, I discovered that some clients hadn't had another visitor in their home for a long time. They were lonely and starving for companionship. At first, I didn't know what to do when a client began telling me everything about their life. I didn't want to be rude or hurtful by cutting off the conversation, so I found myself in situations where a client would talk to me for a long time and I would run out of time to do other home visits. With experience, I became better at gently expressing that my time was limited. I also learned how to express to a client that the conversation was getting out of hand or too long. I might say something like: "Marty —here we go again, talking about other interesting things. I wish I had the time to talk about this today, but I don't. Let's get back to talking about the case management plan—all right?"

Whenever you are working with a client who likes to talk excessively, figure out a way to calm the person down or slow down the discussion. A lot of times, a client who is talking nonstop is actually doing so because of a combination of nervousness, loneliness, and other feelings. Be mindful of these feelings when you try to curtail excessive talking. And still be prepared to talk a little bit about things that may be off topic—this is often part of the process of building rapport with clients and showing them respect in their homes.

OVERCOMING DISTRACTIONS

You will encounter a wide range of distractions that may keep you and your client from communicating and working well together. The telephone may ring. People may be sharing a meal, watching television, or playing video games. Other people or pets may make it difficult to focus on the purpose of the visit. This goes with the territory when you conduct home visits—unexpected things will happen. As you become more accustomed to doing home visits, you will learn how to handle different experiences. Allow yourself time to adjust and learn.

To handle distractions such as the telephone, television, radio, or video games, ask the client if it would possible to turn these off or down in order to give all your attention to them. Be patient and polite. Always keep in mind that this is the client's home, not your office, and the client will make these decisions.

If there is a pet such as large dog that makes you uncomfortable, ask if it would possible to put it in another room. Describe this as your need. Explain that it would allow you to focus on the task at hand. But keep in mind that for many people, pets are family: they may not understand your request, or may be most at ease with the animal beside them.

If other people prove to be a distraction, find an opportunity to ask the primary client if it would be possible to talk privately. Perhaps you can move into another room or onto a porch to talk about confidential matters.

Drug and Alcohol Use   You may visit a client who is drinking or using drugs. Clarify your agency's policy about this. Some programs may limit your ability to work with people who are currently high on drugs or alcohol. A key concern is the ability of someone who is high to give informed consent. However, you may work with clients who are chronically high, and it won't be realistic to wait until they are sober. Do your best to talk with the client, to provide the services you are authorized to provide, and to be sensitive to informed consent issues, and don't ask a client to make big life-changing decisions when high. Evaluate if, how, and when you may be able to meet with the client when the person is not using. If the client has a history of being abusive or violent while high, don't attempt to work under these circumstances: this is a safety issue for you and the client, and leaving is probably the best policy.

?   *What are some other distractions that you might encounter?*

?   *Which types of distractions may be most challenging for you?*

12.4 SAFETY GUIDELINES FOR HOME VISITS

Whenever you are meeting people in the community—especially when you are entering their homes—pay attention to safety. Many of our clients live in poverty and in neighborhoods with disproportionately high rates of crime that may include theft, assault, domestic violence, drug sales, gang activity, and gun violence. You need to balance your commitment to serving the client with the need to protect your own safety.

Safety concerns for home visiting may include witnessing violence and other illegal activity; observing signs of neglect or abuse; the need to report harmful or abusive conduct; damage to your car (if you drive); unintentional involvement in police actions; witnessing arguments or domestic violence; threats and assault; or encountering an angry, aggressive, or threatening person.

Sometimes our own prejudices influence our assessment of safety issues. Try to be aware of the tendency for this to happen, and guard against discriminating against clients or communities who have already been harmed in this way. Remember that safety issues are present in any work setting and with clients of all backgrounds.

Some members of the community may see you as an outsider or intruder, and may view you with suspicion or fear. This is one of many reasons that it is so essential to take time to get to know the community you will be working in, and to forge respectful relationships with key opinion leaders. Knowing as much as possible about the neighborhoods and areas where you do home visits allows you to be prepared, and to keep yourself safe.

Listen to your instincts. When you arrive at the location for the home visit, evaluate the current situation. Is there anything unusual going on at this time? Your instincts will develop over time. Pay attention to them when you feel particularly ill at ease, anxious, or unsafe—they may be tipping you off to a dangerous situation. If you are concerned that the situation is not safe, consider calling or talking to your client about rescheduling the visit for another time.

LEE JACKSON: You're going into the trenches. Think about how to mentally prepare for your visits. You may not run into any problems, but be prepared in case you do. Be aware of what you're wearing. You want to be sure to wear slacks or jeans and comfortable shoes. Don't wear anything too expensive like nice jewelry or a watch— someone there might really need a fix that day.

SAFETY TIPS

Many of the following tips also apply to conducting health outreach, which you will learn about in Chapter Eighteen. Additional tips specific to street outreach will be covered in that chapter.

Be Prepared

- Find out as much information as you can about the clients you will visit (for example, have they reported domestic violence, do they live alone, do they have any pets that might be dangerous?).
- Find out what type of housing the clients live in and where.
- Find out detailed information about the locations you will be visiting, including the reputations of the areas and recent events such as homicides, assaults, and burglaries.
- If you are working in areas that the community itself considers risky, have a plan and be prepared. Consider working with a partner. Talk with your supervisor about the situation and what you can do to minimize risks to yourself and your clients.
- Let your supervisor know whom you will be visiting, where you will be going, and when.
- Dress appropriately.
- Avoid agency logos or signage on your car, clothing, or anywhere else that might draw attention.
- If you have a cell phone, bring it with you in case you encounter a safety concern or an emergency. If you do not have a cell phone and will be doing home visits, ask if your agency can provide one for safety purposes.
- If you are going to be visiting clients after dark, be sure to carry a flashlight with you.

Pay Attention, and Be Discreet

- Be discreet when visiting a new location. Try not to draw attention to yourself.
- Carry yourself with secure body language.
- The risks to women are different than for men. Be aware of these risks, and make decisions that preserve your safety.
- Be aware of your surroundings at all times.
- Be ready to think on your feet—to make quick evaluations and decisions about situations that are developing.

If Conflict or Danger Arises

✪ If possible, de-escalate the situation and work to calm the person involved: see Chapter Thirteen to learn skills for handling conflict effectively. Keep your own voice calm when interacting with someone who is angry.

✪ Apologize. You may have unintentionally done something that provoked the person's anger.

✪ *Leave* if you don't feel safe and don't feel confident that you can de-escalate the conflict.

✪ If you witness violence or other reportable incidents related to your clients, report them to your supervisor immediately, and document them in your field notes. Debrief the incidents with someone you trust.

✪ *Only call the police if it is absolutely required.* Most situations do not require such a drastic measure. If you feel you *must* contact the police in order to preserve your safety, then do so. However, consider the effect this might have on your work with this community. Be cautious about calling the police into a community that has a history of tensions with the law; you might lose the community's trust and respect, and hence your ability to continue to work with the community.

? *Can you think of other safety tips?*

? *What are your biggest safety concerns?*

? *How will you address them and keep yourself safe as you work in the community?*

12.5 HOW TO CONDUCT A HOME VISIT

Once you have introduced yourself and been invited into the home, confirm that you are talking to the client, or the primary caregiver in case of a child. You may have already met the client at your agency, on the street or elsewhere, or spoken with them by phone. If you have never met the client in person before, you might say something such as: "Hi, I'm Sunil Gupta, are you Mrs. Ramirez?"

If other people such as family members are present, be friendly and patient. Once you are talking with the client or primary caregiver, explain again why you have come and see if the two of you can find a quiet spot to work. Say something like: "Mrs. Ramirez, it's a pleasure to meet you. I'm Sunil Gupta from the Community Center Project. Is this still a good time for us to visit? Is there a private place where we can sit down together to talk?"

Clearly explain why you are conducting the home visit, and ask what the client would like to accomplish.

LaTonya Rogers: On my first home visit, I tell the families, I'm here to help you get what you need to handle your child's asthma. What would you like to talk about today?

CONDUCT AN ASSESSMENT

During each home visit you will conduct some type of an assessment. This will range from an assessment of:

⊗ A client's knowledge about and interest in a particular service

⊗ A client's strengths, risks, and needs in order to develop a case management or risk-reduction plan

⊗ A client's current health status and needs for additional services

⊗ Adherence to specific treatments such as taking daily medications for tuberculosis or HIV disease

⊗ A client's progress with a risk-reduction or case management plan

⊗ Exposure to environmental health risks

CHWs often conduct home visits to clients who are living with chronic illnesses. In these circumstances the assessment may also address:

⊗ The client's current understanding of the health condition. For example, does the client understand the risks of high blood pressure and strategies to reduce it?

⊗ Current signs and symptoms. While CHWs are not clinicians and must not work outside of their scope of practice (see Chapter Eight), they are often trained and authorized to check and report on specific symptoms and to communicate their findings to clinicians. This may include current asthma symptoms or complications from HIV disease.

⊗ Recent test results. Occasionally CHWs will be trained, certified, and authorized to perform certain tests, such as HIV antibody tests, or to teach clients how to understand the meaning of recent tests, such as blood pressure readings.

⊗ Adherence to health treatments, such as the proper use of medications, exercise, or special diets documented in the case management plan.

⊗ Scheduling and reminders about upcoming appointments, such as well-baby exams, and showing clients how to plan to keep the appointment.

JASON STANFORD: I also do in-home case management [with the Black Infant Health Program], which means that if a client is pregnant, I visit them at home. I provide referrals but also educational information about pregnancy. I focus on talking to the dad about parenting practices. But not just that, it's also helping him with issues that may be stopping him from being the best dad he can be. It may be a legal issue, it may be education, it may be getting a job, or changing some of his behaviors. It may be domestic violence, it may be anger management issues, just a whole host of things that I try to assist him with.

CONDUCTING AN ENVIRONMENTAL ASSESSMENT

During your visit, you will observe the home environment. What you observe may provide you with a better understanding of the client's strengths, risks, and needs. For example, you may observe:

⊗ The client's level of stress at home

⊗ Basic living conditions, including access to clean sheets, clothing, and resources for hygiene (toilet paper, running water, soap, shampoo, toothpaste, and so on)

- ✪ Availability of food
- ✪ Environmental risks such as mold, dust, animals, or safety hazards for young children
- ✪ The presence or absence of friends, family, roommates, and the quality of those relationships (Do they seem close? Attentive? Are they arguing?)
- ✪ Possible abuse or neglect

What else might you observe during a home visit that could inform you about your client's health and well-being?

Occasionally, you will be asked to conduct a more thorough environmental assessment during a home visit—with the client's participation and permission. For example, if you are working with a client living with diabetes, heart disease, cancer, or HIV disease, you may assess:

- ✪ Needs for immediate assistance or referral to a medical provider
- ✪ The status of medications. Are they up-to-date? Does the client have enough medications for the next few days, week, or month? Is the client taking the medications? Are the medications clearly labeled and organized? If the client takes multiple medications in a day, is there a schedule or system to remind the person to do this?
- ✪ Exposure to environmental factors that may trigger illness. In the case of asthma, this might include assessing exposure to excessive dust, mold, animals, secondhand smoke, and diesel emissions from a nearby street or highway.
- ✪ Access to food. Is there food in the house? Is it nutritious and in keeping with the diet prescribed by the person's health care provider? What did the client eat this morning or last night?
- ✪ Access to clean sheets and clothes, or a laundry
- ✪ Exposure to safety risks such as physical threats or abuse
- ✪ Signs of alcohol and drug use. Do they understand how street drugs and alcohol may interact with their medications and impact their health condition?

You can conduct an environmental assessment by observing what is in sight and asking the client's permission to look at other parts of the home. For example, you might ask: "Roger, where do you keep your medications? Do you mind if I check to see that they are up-to-date?" or "Do you mind if I look in the kitchen to see what you have to eat?" *Never* start to look around a client's home without the person's knowledge or permission. Be sensitive in the way that you ask, the way that you look, and the comments you make as you learn more about the home: this type of assessment can be difficult for clients who may be acutely embarrassed by the current state of their living conditions.

T G: I had a client who always wanted me to help him check up on his medications. He took so many that it was confusing and difficult to manage. I'd do what I could to help him organize them—and sometimes this would take us twenty or thirty minutes. But he never wanted me to look in his fridge or cabinets. He used to own his own home, but after he got sick, he lost everything: he lived in one small room. I think he was really embarrassed. I always respected his wishes, and his pride. But I also brought grocery vouchers or a bag of groceries from the food bank with me if I could.

Your goal is always to assist clients to identify any barriers or risks to their health, and to work with them to identify changes that they can and want to make to their environment that will reduce these risks. This may mean assisting clients to organize their medications, to report mold to the landlord or housing authority, or to make changes in the types of food that they prepare and eat at home.

PROVIDING CASE MANAGEMENT, CLIENT-CENTERED COUNSELING, AND HEALTH EDUCATION

Depending on the client's needs, your skills, and your existing relationship, you may provide additional services such as client-centered counseling, health education, or case management. You may continue to work with the client at their home, your office, or in other locations.

For example, you may provide health education about a specific condition—hypertension or heart disease—to clients who are at risk and interested. This may include assessing their levels of knowledge, providing information, and supporting them in thinking about relevant behavior changes such as changes to diet or patterns of exercise. You may also provide client-centered counseling (see Chapter Ten) about any number of issues, including parenting, domestic violence, or depression, and support clients in identifying their own risks and developing personalized risk-reduction plans.

EXPLAIN THE NEXT STEPS

Take time to clarify and to document what the next steps will be for you and the client. This plan should address each of the concerns and priorities that the client discussed with you. Confirm the date and location of your next appointment. Write down the plan and leave it for the client. If the client can't read, ask if there is someone who can review the plan with them.

GOOD-BYE AND THANK-YOU

Tell the client (and other family members) good-bye. Thank them again for their time and hospitality. If you need directions or assistance getting out of the building, ask before you leave.

12.6 AFTER THE VISIT

Depending on your program and your relationship with the client you just visited, you will have several things to do after your visit:

- Complete paperwork documenting the visit, any assessment you conducted, information you learned, services provided, and agreements made. The longer you wait to document your work, the less you will remember.
- Write down future appointments or visits in your day planner.
- Find out information you needed during your visit but did not have, such as the name of an agency that provides hot meals to shut-ins.
- Check in with the client by phone, with a follow-up visit, or with an appointment at another location. Check to see if the client has followed through or faced challenges in completing the action steps that you discussed together, such as a plan to see the doctor.
- Talk with your supervisor or another colleague about any remaining questions or concerns that you may have.

? *What else would you want to do to follow up on a home visit?*

12.7 COMMON CHALLENGES

VISITS TO PEOPLE WITHOUT HOMES

When you conduct a home visit to someone who is homeless, it may take place on the street, in a doorway, under the overpass, or in the park or parking lot where they spend time or sleep. Be as respectful of this space as you would any other home. All the same rules apply. If clients express that they don't want you there through words or actions, leave. Do your utmost to keep your communication confidential. Keep your voice low. If others are nearby and may be listening, don't discuss confidential matters, and follow your client's lead.

LEE JACKSON: To work with clients who are homeless, I'll ask them for three locations where they tend to hang out. This is a big help when I am trying to check in with them later on.

WHEN CLIENTS ARE ANGRY

Expect to work with clients who are in a "bad" mood, frustrated, or angry at times. You would probably experience the same emotions if you were walking in their shoes. While sometimes their anger will be about you—something you or someone else from your agency said or did—generally it is about other issues they are confronting, such as experiences of discrimination, violence, or incarceration; the loss of jobs, homes, or families; a relapse to drug use; the deterioration of their health; or confronting the possibility of their own death.

As discussed in Chapter Thirteen, keep your cool. Be patient. Keep in mind that you don't want to do anything that will harm the client or your professional relationship and reputation. Stay respectful, professional, and polite. However, if the client is acting in ways that are threatening or physically aggressive, and you are unable to de-escalate their anger, leave the situation immediately.

LEE JACKSON: Lots of times a client will be upset. Sometimes they'll be verbally aggressive. If you treat everyone like a human being and don't act judgmental, they'll usually come around. Always remember it's not personal. I will talk with them calmly and see if that helps. I might explain: "I'm here today to escort you to your appointment. If we need to, we can schedule you for a different time." If the client refuses to go, then rescheduling is a good way to go. If they can, maybe we go for coffee or a pastry. If I can't calm them down, I leave. I don't argue.

WORKING WITH CLIENTS WHO ARE INCARCERATED

Your program may work with clients who are incarcerated, or one of your ongoing clients may be sent to the local jail or juvenile hall. There are several things to consider when working in corrections facilities. You will need to gain a security clearance: contact the jail or prison in advance to apply for one. The facility will provide you with guidelines for your visit, including what to wear.

Even if you are uncomfortable working in a corrections facility, do your utmost to establish and maintain positive and professional relationships with the staff. Doing so will enable you to continue to have access to your clients.

Most clients will deeply appreciate your visit and understand that you had to jump through some hoops to see them. They may also be in a mood to reflect and talk about their lives and to make plans for when they are released. This may be especially true for clients who are caught up in street life and drug use. If possible, assist them in making plans for what to do in the very first hours and days when they are released. Clients with substance use issues are at risk of using as soon as they are released. If they want to make changes, assist them to figure out what they can do that will reduce their risks of using. You might ask them to call you when they know that they will be released or after they have been released, to schedule a time to meet as soon as possible. As always, these choices are up to the client.

T G: The clients who I visit in jail are usually really glad to see me, and in a mood to talk. They are motivated to make changes, because they never want to go back. They are missing their family and their freedom. I try to help them make a realistic plan for the near future—not something that sounds more like a dream. I try to talk to them about what they might face when they get out. Like if I know that they have been in and out of jail and prison, and they usually go right back to using as soon as they are released, I'll say: "You know, you told me that the last time you got out of jail, you fixed right away. What will help you to do it differently this time?" And I also let them know that if they don't follow through, I still want to hear from them: "Whatever happens, you know I'll still be there for you, right?"

CHAPTER REVIEW

Review the case study presented at the beginning of this chapter. You will conduct a home visit to Roger, who is living with HIV and hepatitis C. Please answer the following questions:

⚙   What are your goals for the home visit?
⚙   What challenges might you face?
⚙   What safety concerns might you have, and how will you address these?
⚙   How will you greet Roger?

⚙   What do you want to assess during the home visits? What questions will you ask?
⚙   How might you conduct an environmental assessment? What might you learn that would be helpful in guiding your work with Roger?
⚙   How will you follow up with Roger about his case management plan and actions that he can take to improve his health?
⚙   What referrals will you provide?

The Center for Home Visiting. Accessed on March 27, 2009: http://www.unc.edu/~uncchv/

Center for Occupational and Environmental Health at Hunter College of the City University of New York. 2008. Community Health Worker Asthma Education Project. Accessed on March 27, 2009: http://www.hunter.cuny.edu/health/coeh/index_files/page0013.htm

Department of Family and Community Medicine, Family Health Outcomes Project. 2006. Findings from the MCAH Action Home Visiting Priority Workgroup Survey: Home Visiting for Pregnant Women, Newborn Infants, and /or High-Risk Families. Accessed on March 20, 2009: http://familymedicine.medschool.ucsf.edu/fhop/docs/pdf/pubs/home%20Visiting%20Report%202006.pdf

Home Visiting and Child Maltreatment Prevention Programs at the CDC. Accessed on March 27, 2009: http://www.ncsl.org/programs/cyf/lutzker/

13

Conflict Resolution Skills

Darlene Weide • Tim Berthold • Joani Marinoff

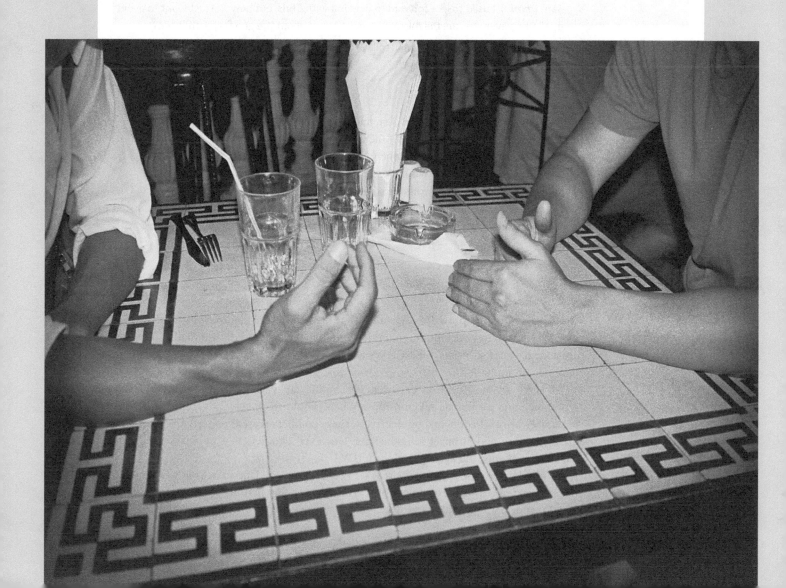

CASE STUDY: SAM AND CHRIS

Sam and Chris are CHWs and coworkers at a program that conducts health outreach to homeless youths. At first, Sam and Chris enjoyed working together and developed a friendship outside of work. Recently, the work relationship has deteriorated. They were scheduled to meet at 8 PM at their agency before leaving to do street outreach. Chris was there on time, but Sam was late: he arrived at 8:30.

Chris (*thinks*): I can't believe you kept me waiting again! You know I told Vince we'd meet him by the QuickMart at 8:30!

Chris (says): "You're late again!"

Sam (*thinks*): Stop riding me.

Sam (says): "Relax. Look, I brought you a coffee."

Chris (*thinks*): As if the coffee makes up for being late! Aren't you even going to apologize? This is the second time you've been late this month. You show me no respect: my time is important too. You're making me look like a fool who can't keep a promise to a client.

Chris (says): You were *there* when I told Vince that I would meet him tonight at 8:30. He said he might be willing to get tested tonight, and the mobile van is only gonna be out there until 9:00."

Sam (*thinks*): I used to look forward to working with Chris, but now . . . I just want to avoid it. All Chris ever sees are the mistakes I make. What about the good work that I do?

Sam (says): "Look, let's just go. I'll talk with Clarice (the person who runs the van) and see if she can fit Vince in tonight."

- ✪ What is the conflict between Sam and Chris really about?
- ✪ How might this conflict impact them and their work?
- ✪ What conflict styles are Sam and Chris using?
- ✪ If you were Chris, how would you deal with the issue of Sam's lateness?
- ✪ If you were Sam, how would you respond?
- ✪ Can you think of ways they each could have handled this that would have assisted to resolve the conflict, rather than aggravating it?

INTRODUCTION

CHWs are often employed by agencies that lack sufficient financial resources and provide services to low-income communities with long histories of discrimination. Given this context, it is not surprising that CHWs are likely to encounter conflict over the course of their career, including conflicts with coworkers, supervisors, and clients.

CHWs are not alone in experiencing conflict at work: it is part of every healthy workplace and all human relationships. When people work closely together, differences inevitably arise. If addressed productively, these conflicts present opportunities for greater understanding and stronger relationships. However, conflicts that go unresolved can be harmful to clients, the agency, and the CHW.

This chapter is designed to assist you to better understand the sources of workplace conflicts, to increase awareness of your own styles of engaging in or responding to conflict, and to aid you in learning skills to resolve conflicts and enhance your working relationships.

This is an introductory chapter, and we encourage you to look for classes and trainings in conflict resolution and assertive communication and more hands-on practice with these skill sets. Resources for learning more about conflict resolution are provided at the end of this chapter.

WHAT YOU WILL LEARN

By studying the material in this chapter, you should be able to:

✪ Define the terms *conflict* and *conflict resolution*.
✪ Identify common sources of conflict in the workplace
✪ Discuss the importance of understanding personal and cultural conflict styles and become more familiar with your own conflict style
✪ Discuss how power and anger can affect conflict resolution
✪ Negotiate a common framework and process for resolving conflict and explain why this is so important
✪ Apply active listening skills during conflict, and discuss their importance for conflict resolution
✪ Implement steps to take to handle your own anger professionally and to deescalate the anger of others

WORDS TO KNOW

Mediation   Active Listening

13.1 CONFLICT RESOLUTION SKILLS ARE ESSENTIAL FOR CHWs

Saul Alinsky (1969) says, "Life is conflict and in conflict you're alive." For CHWs, learning how to manage and respond to conflict is an essential job qualification: a survey conducted in the San Francisco Bay Area with employers of CHWs identified communication and conflict resolution skills as one of the most important qualifications for employment (Cowans, 2005). Why is it so important to have conflict management skills? Let's face it, being a CHW is a stressful job and work-based conflicts are bound to happen. CHWs often work with people who have experienced racism, poverty, exposure to violence, and a lack of access to safe housing or healthy food. Research has shown that when communities are under stress, more conflict is likely to occur (Cohen, Davis, and Aboelata, 1998). If CHWs do not learn how to effectively resolve conflicts, they are likely to miss out on opportunities for career advancement and promotion and may lose their job altogether.

Few CHWs have received training in the skills and techniques for successfully managing conflicts. Role models for productive communication, teamwork, and effective negotiation are often few and far between. As a result, CHWs may find that their work environment is one of quick fixes, hot tempers, avoidance tactics, and at times, deep frustration.

The good news is that conflict prevention and resolution skills can be learned. Resolving conflict requires courage, commitment, and compassion—traits that CHWs have in abundance. The goal is not to eliminate conflict, but to find ways to enhance its positive contributions to the workplace. When approached constructively, conflicts lead to insights and opportunities that might not have been seen otherwise. By developing conflict resolution skills, CHWs and their organizations can deepen their capacity for collaboration and creativity.

? *What words, feelings, and images come to mind when you think of conflict?*

? *As a child, how were you taught to deal with conflict? In your experience, what contributes to successful conflict resolution?*

13.2 UNDERSTANDING CONFLICT

There are many ways to define conflict. The Office of Human Resource Development (OHRD) at the University of Wisconsin defines *conflict* as "a disagreement through which the parties involved perceive a threat to their needs, interests or concerns" (Academic Leadership Support: Office of Quality Improvement, 2007).

Let's look closely at this definition. For conflict to exist there must be a disagreement, which is some kind of difference in the position of two or more people. Often the people involved in a conflict have very different perceptions about the cause or nature of the disagreement. When people experience a disagreement, they are responding to their own perception of a threat or demand.

Our first thoughts about a disagreement don't always go to the heart of what the conflict is about. Workplace conflicts are often very emotional and complicated. Learning to understand the core issues of a conflict is key to resolving it.

In addition, there is often a basic disagreement about who is involved in a conflict. A supervisor may be surprised to learn that everyone on her team is upset about a new policy. One coworker may express feeling burned out only to learn that others feel the same way. A coworker may be oblivious to the fact that his actions have upset another. An office mate may take sides without knowing the whole picture. Clients may be outraged that they don't qualify for services and take their anger out on staff members. When conflicts occur at work, it is necessary to take time to figure out who is involved in the conflict and who needs to be a part of the resolution process. Sometimes, two parties initially meet to discuss the issue. As the core issues are explored, it may be necessary to invite coworkers or a work team to discuss the issues and find solutions.

Conflicts are inevitable and may be both productive and destructive in the work environment (University of Mississippi, 2007).

Destructive Conflict   Conflict is destructive when it:

- ✪ Diverts energy from more important issues and tasks
- ✪ Deepens differences in values
- ✪ Polarizes groups so that cooperation is reduced
- ✪ Results in bias or discrimination
- ✪ Destroys the morale of people or reinforces poor self-concepts
- ✪ Harms the quality of services provided to clients and communities

Constructive Conflict   Conflict is constructive when it:

- ✪ Promotes new understandings of self, others, and working relationships
- ✪ Creates possibilities for positive change and transformation
- ✪ Enhances working relationships and the cohesiveness of work teams
- ✪ Reduces stress
- ✪ Results in better-quality services for clients and communities

? *Can you think of other ways that conflict may be destructive or constructive?*

13.3 COMMON SOURCES OF WORKPLACE CONFLICT

The first step in learning how to resolve conflicts is to understand common sources of conflict, as well as your own reactions to and feelings about conflict. Conflicts between employees can spring from a variety of sources. They may have a single cause or multiple causes. If left unaddressed, workplace conflicts can escalate from small annoyances to more serious issues.

Common sources of conflicts that occur at work may include (adapted from Gaitlin, Wysocki, and Kepner, 2007):

1. Insufficient Resources   Everyone requires sufficient resources to do their job well. Yet workers often compete for scarce resources. CHWs often feel frustrated about the lack of supplies, supervision time, space, adequate pay and benefits, administrative and technical support, and resources to share with clients. Funding from year to year may be tentative. When teams or individuals have less than they require, especially if they perceive others as having more, conflicts are quick to arise.

2. Conflicting Personalities and Work Styles   Personality clashes occur in all work environments. People have different work styles: one coworker may prefer to chat and talk loudly throughout the day, while another may need a closed-door setting. When these differences are brushed aside, over time, people's tempers can flare.

3. Delegation of Power and Authority   Some organizational leaders welcome input into decision making, while others are very hierarchical and place the power in the hands of a few. People in higher-status positions may be more free to engage in conflict and less likely to avoid confrontation. People new to the job or in lower-status or lower-paid positions may feel uncomfortable questioning authority and leadership decisions for fear of being fired.

4. Conflicting Values   It is common for workers in the public health and nonprofit sectors to share similar values such as commitment to diversity, social justice, equality, and community ownership of programming. Indeed, these values are often what motivates us to work in the field of public health in the first place. At the same time, when differences in values emerge, staff may feel tremendous tensions that can lead to conflict.

5. Lack of Acknowledgment for One's Contributions   Everyone wants to be acknowledged for one's hard work and contributions. Yet, not everyone needs the same type of acknowledgement. Some people like to be praised publicly, while others prefer a special lunch out with their boss, a bouquet of flowers, or time off. When a supervisor fails to acknowledge someone's work, or fails to acknowledge everyone in the same way, she may create frustration. For volunteer CHWs who are contributing their time and talent without getting paid, lack of acknowledgment for their work can be especially frustrating.

6. Disagreements over Roles and Responsibilities   Coworkers may disagree about who should do what and how things should be done. Some employees may be unaware or misinformed about the job duties of others. When new programs are developed, or when there is staff turnover or downsizing, questions about roles need to be reviewed.

Unrealistic work expectations or different perceptions about how the work should be done can easily result in conflict between individuals and between teams and leadership.

7. Intercultural Misunderstandings   People from different cultural backgrounds may have different expectations, verbal and nonverbal habits, assumptions, and beliefs. Workplace conflicts between parties from different cultural backgrounds can often be traced to cultural miscommunication, stereotypes, prejudices, or lack of understanding.

8. Poor Communication   Without clear procedures for handling conflict, workers may end up talking about their challenges in unproductive ways, such as venting problems behind people's backs. This type of indirect communication almost always increases tensions. Workers who gossip often lack skills to take more productive actions.

9. Poor Leadership and Unpredictable Policies   When employees feel that the leadership is not responding to the changing needs of an organization or team, staff can feel demoralized and frustrated. When low performance is allowed for some people and not others, the staff feel frustrated. When leadership values one department over another, resentments intensify. When leadership, at any level, avoids conflict, employees experience low morale. In the absence of clear workplace policies, uncertainty and conflict may arise (Hart, 2002).

10. Conflicting Pressures   Conflicting pressures occur when two or more staff members are responsible for completing different tasks with the same deadline. In this situation, the deadline of the person with more authority often takes precedence, putting pressure on other workers. For example, a program director needs to finish a report for a funder and needs some information from a CHW. The program director interrupts the CHW when she is busy organizing supplies for the night's work. The CHW feels upset that she is asked to stop what she needs to get done to provide information for the report.

11. Perceived Threat to One's Identity   The Harvard Negotiation Project emphasizes how conflicts may threaten our identity. For example, conflicts may provoke concern about whether we are valued, trusted, respected, and perceived to be intelligent, competent, hardworking, or ethical. When conflicts touch on these core concepts and feelings about our identity and worth, they are likely to trigger strong emotions and may be particularly challenging to address (Stone, Patton, and Heen, 1999).

Keep in mind that conflicts and disputes seldom have a simple cause and are typically influenced by a number of factors.

CASE STUDY: DENALI AND WALTER

Take a moment to brainstorm the underlying causes of conflict in the following scenario.

Denali is a CHW at a center for homeless youths. Because her department has not recruited enough clients to meet funding requirements, Denali's supervisor asked her to create a new workshop that will reach eighty more youths by the end of the quarter. Denali is proud of her efforts to create a new program called Chew and Chat—a discussion group for homeless girls that will meet in a neighborhood pizza restaurant. After developing trust with the girls, Denali hopes they will come to the center for other support services. Denali is feeling upset that Walter, the communications manager, has not produced the fliers she needs to promote Chew and Chat. She provided all the information Walter needed to produce the fliers well in advance, and now time is running out to promote her group. Walter told her that that the fliers will be on her desk as soon as he can do it. He is feeling annoyed by Denali's persistent requests. Denali feels that her needs are being discounted and minimized, while other programs are being prioritized and supported. She feels frustrated and stressed that she won't be able to get this extra work done.

? *What are the main sources of conflict that need to be addressed?*
Refer to the list of Common Sources of Workplace Conflict.

With their attention on the core sources of the conflict, let's see how Denali and Walter communicate about it.

On reflection, Denali realizes that the reasons for the conflict are probably not personal. She decides to talk to Walter about her concerns. Before meeting with him, Denali wonders if whether her conflict with Walter stems from a *lack of sufficient resources*—maybe Walter can't handle all the requests he receives for promotional materials. Perhaps the conflict is also due to *conflicting pressures* and the stress that Denali's supervisor is feeling because of funding requirements. She recognizes that being asked to develop and implement a new program at the last minute added a burden to her already full job description. Denali also realizes that part of her frustration is due to the *lack of acknowledgment* for her hard work. By thinking this way, she feels more equipped to enter into a conversation that is amicable rather than accusatory. She requests a meeting with Walter that works for both of their schedules.

During their meeting, Walter tells Denali that he is also frustrated with the *amount of work on his plate* and wishes that he had more time to get to her request. He appreciates that she told him what happened with her supervisor. He had thought she was being pushy and rude, but now he understands why she was so anxious about getting her materials. Together they decide that the real problem is that the *organization is contracted to do more work than they have staffing for.* What they really need is a volunteer to make the flier. They agree that they can work as allies and talk to their supervisor. Denali feels relieved that Walter is not ignoring her needs on purpose. She feels motivated to work with Walter and their supervisor to come up with a viable solution to both their concerns.

? *Think about a conflict you experienced at work. What were your initial perceptions of the cause of the conflict?*

? *Referring to the list above, what else may have contributed to the conflict?*

? *How could knowing about the causes of the conflict assist you in addressing it?*

SIGNS AND SYMPTOMS OF UNRESOLVED CONFLICT IN THE WORKPLACE

Common signs of conflict in the workplace include:

absenteeism	turnover	low productivity
accidents	poor teamwork	excessive competition
"us-them" attitudes	open bickering	gossip

(Continued)

aggression or hostility	blaming	high stress
sabotage	poor job satisfaction	low creativity
tardiness	alcoholism or substance use	prejudice, such as homophobia, sexism, or racism

Source: Sharon and Clark, 1989.

13.4   COMMON SOURCES OF CONFLICT FOR CLIENTS

CHWs often witness conflicts between clients and will also experience direct conflicts with clients themselves. The following list identifies some of the common sources for these conflicts (adapted from Sadalla, Henriquez, Holmberg, and Halligan, 1998).

1. Conflicts over Resources   These conflicts occur when two people want the same thing, and there is not enough to go around. These are often the easiest types of conflict to identify.

A client in a drop-in shelter for youths may be upset that there aren't enough beds in the shelter, enough food to eat, taxi vouchers, comfortable chairs or sofas to sit in, or enough time with a case manager. The client may act angry or aggressive. For example, he may yell at another client to get off the couch so he can sit down.

2. Conflicts over Psychological Needs   We all have the same needs for food, shelter, health care, friendship, love, belonging, accomplishment, safety, stability, and control. Clashes over these needs may be played out in conflicts about material things or seemingly trivial matters. Often, the real psychological motivations for conflict are harder to understand and to resolve: the client in the homeless shelter who starts a fight may be feeling powerless. If the underlying issue isn't attended to, these conflicts are likely to reoccur.

A homeless Japanese-American woman is hostile to the Caucasian staff at a women's shelter. She often says, "You're not the boss of me!" During a conversation, her case manager learns that as a child she was taken to an internment camp in Utah. Learning this allows her case manager to have a greater understanding of and compassion for her behavior.

3. Conflicts Involving Values and Identity   Values are the basis of our belief systems. Challenges to our values may also be experienced as challenges about our identity and worth, and may stimulate strong emotions and dramatic interactions. Keep in mind that for most people, and particularly people without a lot of material resources, our values and identities are our most important resources.

A transgender youth at a homeless drop-in center is continuing to engage in survival sex and is buying hormones on the street. A CHW raises concerns about the client's behavior and associated health risks. The client is used to people judging her identity and to adults trying to control her behavior. The client is frustrated and angry and says to the CHW: "You don't understand the first thing about what it is like to walk in my shoes!"

?   *Can you think of other common sources of conflict for clients?*

13.5 COMMON RESPONSES TO CONFLICT

How we perceive and react to conflict varies greatly from one person to another. It is often surprising to learn that coworkers feel differently about an important conflict. These differences are influenced by one's personal and cultural conflict styles.

Becoming aware of your own conflict style is an essential first step in learning how to successfully resolve conflict. An awareness of your own approach to conflict allows you to see what your strengths are as well as to see the areas in which you can improve. Awareness of what influences other people's approaches to conflict can assist you to create a common framework for resolving conflicts that arise.

Remember that none of us is born knowing how to resolve conflicts. These skills, like all social skills, are influenced by one's own temperament; family examples; past experiences; peer influences; social, economic, and political context and dynamics; and cultural factors such as gender roles and ethnic socialization (Figure 13.1). However, new skills for dealing with conflict can be learned and put into practice.

Figure 13.1 **Influences That Contribute to an Individual's Approach to Conflict.**

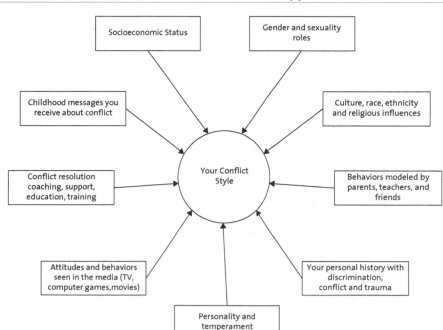

? *Can you think of other factors that influence the way you handle or respond to conflict?*

THE INFLUENCE OF CULTURE

Culture influences how we understand, communicate about, and react to conflict. For example, some cultures are more likely to value the needs of the group over the needs of the individual. These cultures may emphasize harmony and compromise in the face of conflict in contrast to cultures that encourage people to stand up for their individual rights (Ting-Toomey and Oetzel, 2001).

Continue to develop and practice cultural humility as you face conflict. Always keep in mind that *your way* of dealing with conflict, informed by your own culture or cultures, is just one way, not *The Way* of thinking about and responding to conflict. Don't make assumptions about the conflict styles of coworkers or clients. Use your active listening and client-centered counseling skills: ask open-ended questions, observe, and listen closely to learn how others understand and respond to conflicts.

? *Have you experienced conflicts that were influenced by cultural differences?*

? *How do your cultural identities influence your approach to conflict?*

PERSONAL CONFLICT STYLES

Your conflict style has been shaped not only by culture, but also by your personality and life experiences. Taking a conflict style inventory allows people to be aware of their own style of dealing with conflict and provides a resource for colleagues to talk about patterns of conflict resolution. Discussing one's style in a team or group setting can aid in developing a greater tolerance and patience for each other's styles.

Keep in mind that each of us probably uses several of these styles, depending on the context or type of conflict we face. Common ways that people deal with conflict are detailed in this section (Araiz-Iverson and others, 2006; *see also* Community Boards).

Avoiding   The person may simply ignore the conflict, pretend it does not exist, or decide that the risk of an argument is not worth any further effort on their part. The person withdraws and shuts down. When a conflict occurs, an avoider might say, "Leave well enough alone" or "It's someone else's responsibility." Because issues are not addressed, over time, this approach generally results in more conflict. There are times, however, when it may be the best approach.

Accommodating   The person sacrifices or compromises their own point of view by allowing the other party to have their way. Over time, the accommodator may become resentful of both the other party and of themselves for continually yielding their own interests.

Competing   This is the opposite of accommodating. The person works hard to get her own way at the expense of the other party's interests. The underlying interests of both sides are not clarified or addressed. A person with a competing style might think: "My way or the highway."

Compromising   The person works to find a mutually acceptable solution that partially satisfies all parties. Issues are addressed, although sometimes not fully or deeply. There is some mutual give and take that may result in "splitting the difference" or "finding the middle ground."

Collaborating   The person focuses on talking, listening, and working with the other party in an attempt to find solutions that satisfy all concerns. Spending time exploring, clarifying, and discussing the conflict often results in both parties' understanding each other's perceptions and finding creative solutions without feeling that anyone gave in or conceded their interests. A collaborator values the relationship with the conflicting parties and tries to produce a win/win, respected, trustworthy solution. You might hear a collaborator say, "Everyone can win if we work together."

Different situations require using different styles. From time to time, each of the styles identified here can be a valuable resource.

? *What are the pros and cons of each of these styles?*

? *Can you identify situations where it might be valuable to use these different styles?*

? *What problems can arise from using each style?*

? *What do you think is your dominant style?*

THE VALUE OF COMPROMISE

Many people approach conflicts with a win/lose mentality. They feel that they are mostly (or completely) in the right, and other parties are completely (or mostly) in the wrong. They seek a resolution to the conflict that will affirm their own position and compel the other party or parties to concede and make changes.

An unwillingness to compromise is problematic for many reasons, including:

1. Conflicts are rarely so simplistic that one party is 100 percent correct and the other party is 100 percent wrong.
2. Even if you are completely right, holding out for a "win/lose" solution where only the other party has to give in is likely to become a "lose/lose" solution in the long run. This mentality often leads to resentment and continued conflict that undermines your sense of comfort at work, and it is likely to create an environment that negatively affects clients and coworkers.
3. Being right is not the most important thing! Ultimately, it is much more important to find a way to work peacefully, professionally, and respectfully with coworkers and clients so that you can effectively promote community health.
4. Holding on to the need to be right is likely to create a lasting perception that you are rigid, controlling, or worse (insert your own adjective here!). It may undermine your career advancement.
5. It isn't good for your health. Always needing to be right is stressful and likely to be harmful to your physical and mental health. Learning to accept responsibility for your own contributions to conflict, and to compromise, can be deeply rewarding in

and of itself and promote your well-being. These skills are likely to be useful in your personal and family relationships as well, especially if you are a parent.

? *Have you ever interacted with someone who had a compelling need to be right?*

? *Did you enjoy this experience?*

? *Would you like to be in an ongoing professional relationship with someone like this?*

? *What gets in the way of your ability to compromise?*

? *What assists you in seeking a win/win solution to a conflict?*

IDENTIFY YOUR OWN CONFLICT STYLE

Try this activity on your own, with classmates, or with coworkers to learn more about your personal conflict styles. If you do this activity alone, place an X next to the statements you feel best describe your conflict style. If a facilitator is leading this exercise, have participants respond to each statement by raising their hands and stating, "That's me!" and voluntarily describe the circumstances when these statements apply.

THAT'S ME!

_____ I actively participate in conflict when it arises.
_____ I avoid conflicts and controversy at all costs.
_____ I always believe there is a middle ground.
_____ I feel very uncomfortable with conflict.
_____ I feel skilled at handling most conflict.
_____ I like to assist others when they are in conflict.
_____ Open discussion is the best way to address problems.
_____ I lose my cool when I experience conflict.
_____ I have to win at all costs when I am in conflict.
_____ I feel depressed or anxious when I am experiencing a conflict.
_____ It is better to keep friendships than get involved in conflicts.
_____ I'm afraid the other person will be mad at me, so I avoid conflict.
_____ I work for what I believe in.
_____ I enjoy coming up with new, creative solutions to conflicts.
_____ I had negative experiences with conflicts in the past and try to avoid them at all costs.
_____ I will give up some of my interests in order to win other more important interests.
_____ I take the lead in resolving conflicts.

Source: Adapted from Sharon and Clark, 1989.

13.6 THREE APPROACHES TO HANDLING CONFLICT ON THE JOB

There is no magic formula or method that can effectively resolve all conflicts. In conflict management, context is everything. There are many factors that influence a conflict and many situation-specific approaches to managing them. In this section we will look at a few different contexts and some new interventions for managing conflict. Three common approaches to conflict are: prevention, early intervention, and third-party intervention (often called mediation).

PREVENTION

Because conflicts are natural and inevitable, leadership in organizational settings should develop clear policies and protocols to address conflicts in their early stages. Supervision meetings where challenging issues are discussed, team meetings where staff talk about what is not working well, and conflict resolution trainings for staff are just a few examples of how organizations can work to prevent the development or escalation of conflicts. On a personal level, CHWs can begin to identify disagreements and misunderstandings in their early stages and address them using productive communication skills in a one-on-one or group setting. A CHW can approach a conflict by presenting their concerns specifically, clearly, and positively.

EARLY INTERVENTION

If the people engaged in conflict are still able to talk to each other, using a one-on-one approach is useful. A CHW may say, "I've been really affected by our lack of communication lately. It seems to be causing some serious problems between us. I'd really like it if we could sit down sometime soon and discuss what is at the root of our communication problems. It's getting in the way of my ability to focus on my work, and I imagine it's affecting you too. Would you be willing to talk with me so we can try to find a solution?" We will address skills for doing this later in this chapter.

THIRD-PARTY INTERVENTION

Sometimes, it isn't possible for two individuals or groups to resolve a conflict on their own. The issues may be too complex to be adequately identified by the people involved. Feelings may be too strong. In these situations, asking for assistance from someone with strong conflict resolution skills may be necessary. There are a number of well-tested third-party processes (Sadalla, Henriquez, Holmberg, and Halligan, 1998), including **mediation**. In mediation, a neutral person (someone who doesn't favor one side or the other) is asked to facilitate communication between the disputants as they express their feelings and needs and identify issues. After actively listening to both sides equally, the mediator assists the participants identify their own solutions to the conflict and come up with action steps. Sometimes, a mediator might facilitate the rebuilding or repair of the relationship between the participants.

The Influence of Power   What happens when the people in conflict don't have equal status or power? Over the course of your career, you are likely to experience conflict with a coworker who is your equal, with a supervisor who has power over you, and with a client whom you have power over. How will these differences in power affect your approach to conflict resolution?

Conflict with a supervisor can be particularly challenging. People often worry that addressing these conflicts will place their job at risk. Ideally, we want supervisors to invite and encourage us to speak freely about our concerns and challenges. However, supervisors often face competing pressures and may neither have the time nor the ability to listen or communicate well. If you are experiencing a conflict with a supervisor, reflect before you speak. Not all supervisors are skilled in conflict resolution. Sometimes silence and avoidance are prudent choices. Based on prior experience, do you trust that your supervisor will be able to work constructively and respectfully with you to resolve the conflict? If not, consider what the possible consequences of keeping silent or speaking up may be for yourself, your program, and your clients.

If you decide to address the conflict directly, be sure to follow your organization's "chain of command" and speak first to your supervisor rather than going above that person's head to speak to their supervisor. If your supervisor discovers that you have spoken to others about a mutual conflict before speaking directly with them, it may undermine your working relationship and your career at the agency. There are very few exceptions to this rule. However, if the conflict involves issues that are as serious as allegations of sexual harassment or corruption, it is often best to speak to someone who is higher up in the chain of command at the agency you work for.

It is helpful to know your workplace policies in advance, in case your conversation with your supervisor doesn't go well. Find out if your human resource manual outlines a grievance procedure. Do you have an employee assistance program in place that will allow you to talk to a counselor? Do you have a union representative who can advise you?

When you have a conflict with someone you have power over, whether that is someone you supervise, someone who volunteers with your program, or a client, you have responsibility to take leadership in resolving the conflict and in creating an environment in which the other party can honestly communicate their concerns. Recognize that by communicating about a conflict they have with you, they are taking a risk. Clients may be afraid to approach you about a conflict for fear of creating negative feelings or harming their ability to access services with you or your agency. You may need to take the lead in assuring your clients that you welcome input and appreciate their honesty in sharing concerns. Strive to model active communication skills.

13.7 COMMUNICATION SKILLS FOR CONFLICT RESOLUTION

CHANGING THE WAY WE VIEW CONFLICT

We want to emphasize three concepts from the Harvard Negotiation Project (Stone, Patton, and Heen, 1999), designed to shift the way we view conflict and promote resolution, outlined here.

Moving from Certainty to Curiosity   We have a tendency to make assumptions and judgments about conflicts, including what *really* happened and what the other parties did, thought, and felt. When we bring these assumptions to a conversation designed to resolve the conflict, we are likely to undermine our efforts and the outcome. Try shifting your perspective from one of certainty about the situation ("I know what really happened") to one of curiosity ("What happened? What was going on for _____ [the other party]?"). When you can set aside your prejudices and assumptions, you are likely to discover new ways of understanding yourself, the other party, the conflict itself, and possibilities for its successful resolution.

Disentangling Intent from Impact   During conflicts, we often make assumptions about the intentions of others. When we are hurt or harmed by the conflict, we may assume that the other party intended this result. Once again, these assumptions can keep us from seeing the true nature of the conflict and moving forward toward its resolution.

For example: Simon and Latanya get into a conflict. Simon says or does something that offends Latanya.

- Just because Latanya is offended, that does not mean that Simon intended to offend her.
- Just because Simon didn't intend to offend her doesn't mean that Latanya is not offended.

Give the benefit of the doubt to the other party. When we are able to separate the impact of actions from their intentions, we often diminish the emotional charge of the conflict and reduce its potential for escalation.

Distinguishing Blame from Contribution   It is easy for people in conflicts to become caught up in accusations and blame. Trying to prove who is to blame can easily derail us from being able to listen, to learn, to find solutions, and to build new working relationships and alliances.

Rather than focusing on what the other did wrong, focus on understanding the contributions that each party made to the conflict, *with an emphasis on trying to understand our own contributions first.* You are likely to find that both or all parties did or said something that contributed to the conflict. Understanding this can support you in identifying solutions and in preventing similar conflicts in the future.

The shift in focus from blame to contribution may seem subtle, but it can powerfully transform your efforts to resolve the conflict.

DEVELOPING A COMMON FRAMEWORK AND PROCESS FOR RESOLVING CONFLICT

We strongly recommend that you talk about the process you will use to resolve the conflict *before* you start to talk about the conflict itself. Many attempts to resolve conflicts are undermined because the parties don't take time to develop a common understanding of the process and ground rules that will guide their conversation. They may jump right in to the heart of the conflict, making accusations and stirring up strong emotions. This can escalate the conflict and make it more difficult for parties to communicate effectively in the future.

Consider the following guidelines for initiating a conversation designed to resolve a conflict:

1. Express your commitment to resolving the conflict.
2. Express your desire to establish a positive working relationship.
3. Acknowledge the value of the other party or parties. Find something positive to say about who they are, the work that they do, and a time when you worked well together.
4. Identify and acknowledge your common values, such as your commitment to providing quality services to clients or to advocating for social justice.

5. Be prepared to move from certainty to curiosity. Express your desire to listen and learn about their experience and perspective.

6. Negotiate common ground rules for your discussion that use the active listening skills described later on in this chapter. Ground rules may include, for example:

   a. Agree not to yell at each other, insult each other, use disrespectful words, or otherwise escalate the conflict.

   b. Use I-statements and emphasize your own experience rather than your assumptions or judgments about the other party.

   c. Take turns talking and listening to each other's personal experience of the conflict, using active listening skills. It is amazing how deeply listening, without making judgments, can often transform our understanding of the other party's intentions and feelings, and of the conflict itself.

7. Work to disentangle impact from intention.

8. Focus the discussion not on assigning blame (discovering who was wrong), but on understanding what contributed to the conflict and on identifying how you can transform your relationship to avoid similar problems in the future.

9. If you mean it, apologize and take responsibility for something you said or did that may have contributed to the conflict or been hurtful to the other party.

10. If things get heated and it seems as if the conflict might escalate, agree to take a break. Continuing to talk with each other when you are unable to control your emotions and statements may do lasting damage to the relationship, your career, and the important work that you do with clients and communities.

11. After you have talked about what contributed to the conflict, agree to focus on what you can do now to improve the situation and your ability to work well together in the future.

ACTIVE LISTENING SKILLS

The following set of skills will assist you to learn how to communicate so that both you and the other party experience the safety and support necessary to engage with the issues and feelings at the heart of the conflict.

Regardless of who is involved in a conflict, strong communication skills can enable the parties to move from tension to resolution. These communication skills include **active listening**, defined as listening with the intent to fully understand and to communicate your understanding of both the content and the feeling being expressed (Karp, 2008). Active listening demonstrates awareness of and respect for the other person's experiences, thoughts, and feelings and is an essential skill for CHWs; it is an example of client-centered counseling.

A person who is actively listening doesn't have to agree with the other party, but demonstrates that the other person deserves to be heard and understood. Active listening aids in breaking the cycle of conflict. When you show respect and empathy and reserve judgment, people are more likely to express themselves and to get to the heart of the conflict.

Active listening is difficult because it requires the listener to provide focused attention in situations that often involve strong opinions, emotions, and judgments. It requires respect for and attention to the other's values, needs, and feelings. And it requires you to express this respect and reflect what you hear. If all a speaker hears back from the party who is listening is silence or an occasional "uh-huh," they can't tell if they are successfully communicating about vulnerable feelings and issues. We don't want people in conflict to clam up. We want them to participate so that the conflicts can be resolved.

Lee Jackson negotiating with a client.

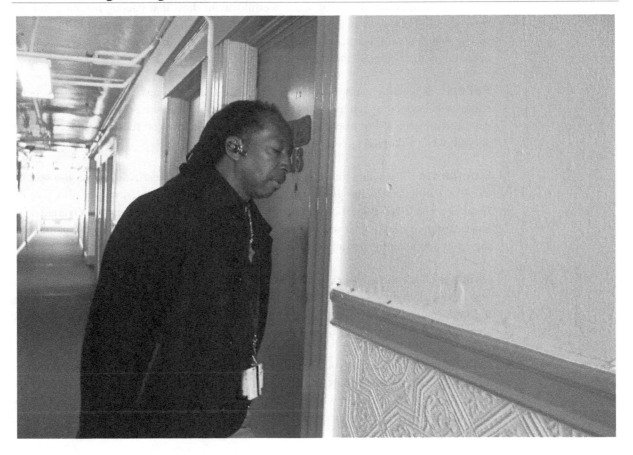

Here is a set of core active listening skills (Sadalla, Henriquez, Holmberg, and Halligan, 1998). Not everyone uses all of these techniques in each conversation, and how they are used varies from culture to culture. With practice, you discover which active listening skills work best for you. These skills are similar to and may be used to complement skills for client-centered counseling, including motivational interviewing, covered in Chapter Ten.

Encourage   This technique uses neutral words and open, culturally appropriate body language to convey interest and to encourage the speaker to continue talking. To be effective, encouragement must be based on the listener's genuine interest in hearing and understanding what is being said by others. For example, "I really want to learn about your experience and your point of view. Will you tell me more about it?"

Clarify   Clarifying involves the gathering of information in order to understand what the other party is saying. This is especially important when we find ourselves drawing swift conclusions about circumstances or other people based on our own experiences. Clarifying questions should be open-ended and phrased respectfully, so that people don't feel challenged or judged. For example, "Would you tell me more about what happened on the day of the incident?" or "I want to understand better. Did this happen before or after your meeting with Yana?"

Restate   Restating is to use your own words to express the main thoughts and ideas that the other party has communicated to you. This demonstrates that you have heard what is being shared, and allows you to check your understanding. People rarely feel understood in a conflict situation. Restating is a powerful way to show that you are listening. A common restating phrase may begin with: "Help me understand. If I hear you right, you are saying that you were frustrated during the training and felt like you weren't given enough opportunity to respond to the questions from the participants. Is that right?"

Reflect   Reflecting shows that you understand the feelings behind what is being expressed. Reflecting can assist the speaker to clarify what she is feeling and acknowledge these feelings. For example, "What I'm hearing is that you felt frustrated and disrespected when I showed up late to the training."

Summarize   By pulling all the information together, summarizing allows the speaker to know that he or she has given you all the information. Summarizing may also give the speaker a chance to correct or add some more information. For example, "Overall, what I'm hearing you say is that you weren't happy with the way that we worked together during the training, and you want to make sure that we do it differently next time."

Validate   A validation is a statement that acknowledges the speaker's worth, efforts, and feelings. When we validate, we show empathy toward the speaker by acknowledging the importance of their experiences. For example, "I appreciate that you took a risk and shared this with me" and "It sounds like it was a really frustrating experience for you."

"I" Messages   Whether you are doing the talking or the listening, there are a few other essential communication skills you'll need in your tool bag. When we are angry or upset, it is easy to blame others for what has happened, "You can't keep anything to yourself!" or "You never listen!" These types of messages blame the other person and rarely bring people

TURNING A YOU-MESSAGE INTO AN I-MESSAGE

Take a moment to practice turning these statements into I-messages.
Example:

> You-message: "You always avoid me when I'm in the room."
> I-message: "*I feel* ignored *when you* don't acknowledge me when we're in a room together *because* we used to work so well together. I wonder if you're upset with me about something."

"Once again, you are taking credit for my work and ideas."
I _____
"You always expect me to do more work than others on this team."
I _____
"You are just looking for ways to push your work off onto others."
I _____
You never carry through on the suggestions I offer you.
I _____
"You keep forgetting your commitments. These are your responsibility, not anyone else's!"
I _____

together to resolve the problem. With an I-message, however, the speaker describes her feelings about the other's behavior and how this behavior affected her. For example: Angela might say to Peter, "I felt angry when I heard that you had told John that I didn't think he was a good counselor. I don't feel like I can share my thoughts with you in the future."

I-messages focus on the speaker's wants, needs, or concerns. The listener is less likely to feel judged and more willing to listen. A formal I-message has three parts:

1. "I feel ... " State the feeling.
2. "When you ... " Describe the specific behavior.
3. "Because ... " Describe the effect of the other person's behavior on you.

Here are some examples: "I feel frustrated when you borrow my outreach bag and don't return it on time, because I can't get ready for my own shift." "I feel distracted when you turn on the radio so loudly, because I need to get a lot of work done and I work better when it's quiet."

Using I-messages take a lot of practice. Think of something that someone is doing at work, at school, or at home that is bothering you. How can you let them know what is on your mind using an I-message? Practice and see what happens.

THE POWER OF APOLOGY

None of us is perfect. We *all* make mistakes. We have all said or done something that contributed to a conflict and may have been be hurtful to others.

We strongly believe in the power of an apology to transform relationships. This is true with coworkers, supervisors, and clients. We view making an apology, like compromising, as a demonstration of generosity, humility, and strength of character. Be prepared to take responsibility for actions that may have contributed to the conflict and unintentionally hurt or harmed the situation or the other party.

Some examples are:

- "I hear that when I was late, it felt disrespectful to you. I want you to know that I really did try my best, and I am sorry that I was late."
- "I wish I had remembered to invite you to the meeting. I apologize. I'll make sure to put you on the email list serve as soon as I get back to the office."
- "I really didn't mean to insult you. I apologize. I truly respect you and enjoy working with you."

Unfortunately, some people seem to think that making an apology is the same thing as saying, "I am a bad person who is 100 percent wrong and deserves to be punished for the rest of my life!" However, if you can't learn to take responsibility for your own mistakes, and to provide an honest apology when appropriate, you will undermine the success of your career.

? *What are your thoughts and feelings about making an apology?*

? *Is it hard for you to apologize to others? If so, why?*

? *What would support you to provide an apology to a client, coworker, or supervisor?*

13.8 THE CHALLENGE OF ANGER

As we discussed above, conflicts in the workplace are often connected to important issues such as fairness, justice, respect, and values. Not surprisingly, such conflicts are often accompanied by strong emotions, including anger. We make a point of addressing the challenge of anger here because it is a difficult emotion for people to handle well, and it can significantly undermine the success of attempts to resolve conflicts.

Everyone experiences anger from time to time. It is a natural and powerful emotion with the potential to be both beneficial and harmful to our health and well-being. Anger can mobilize an individual, a team of workers, or a community to make positive change.

Anger becomes a problem when it is used in a way that is threatening, harmful, or insulting to oneself or others. Chronic anger may be turned inward toward the self, resulting in depression. When chronic anger is turned outward, it may be expressed as hostility. When you find yourself alienating those whom you need to work with, then you know that your approach to conflict is destructive and needs to be changed.

CASE STUDY: KEVIN

Kevin works for a nonprofit agency. When he perceives that his skills are being questioned, he is easily angered. He recognizes that he inappropriately vents his anger in the workplace, but he has a hard time changing his behavior. He just can't control getting angry. Kevin has the habit of shooting off angry emails when he feels upset. Several times, he has stormed into a coworker's office to make rude and insulting comments. Once he releases his anger, he feels better and gets back to work, and later apologizes. When he is not angry, most people on staff think Kevin is a nice, funny, creative, and hardworking guy. But, his rude and angry emails and name-calling episodes have upset most of the people he needs support from: his supervisor, most of his team members, and some of his volunteers. He has been written up for his behavior and has been given two warnings. He is on the edge of being fired.

Learning how to better manage your anger starts with being aware of what pushes your buttons and upsets you the most. There are many situations that can trigger someone's anger. It differs from person to person and from situation to situation.

HOW TO HANDLE YOUR ANGER PROFESSIONALLY

Knowing how to stay inbounds with your anger is an essential life skill and crucial for keeping your job. Here are some tips to stay inbounds with anger.

Be Aware   Become familiar with what triggers your anger. Do you get mad when someone questions your abilities or skills? When you feel excluded from a group, event, or committee? When you feel your autonomy or independence is threatened? When you feel your value as a person or coworker is questioned? What triggers your anger?

Stop   When you feel angry, *stop* and stay inbounds with your behavior. Take time away from the source of conflict. Breathe, write, walk, repeat a relaxing phrase such as "I can take it easy," or talk to a friend. Don't engage with others when you feel angry. Take time away to cool down. What works for you to interrupt your anger?

Think   Think about the consequences of taking action when you feel angry. Try to figure out what made you so upset. Try not to engage the person with whom you feel angry while you are still angry. Find an appropriate time to engage with the other person. How can you safely vent or express your emotion and return to the situation ready to take positive actions toward resolution?

Choose   Choose behaviors that stay inbounds, that are safe, and that do not hurt you or others. If you need assistance, talk to someone who can support you—a friend, coach, supervisor, or counselor. You are responsible for all the choices that you make.

Understand   Try to see the issue from the other person's point of view. Try to find a way to hold respect for the other person, even if you disagree with them or feel hurt by their actions.

Action   Do at least one thing that reduces the potential for harm and makes a positive contribution to improving the situation.

? *Think of a situation that made you really angry. What happened that led you to feel this way?*

? *How did you act or react in the moment?*

? *What result did it lead to?*

? *What would you like to do differently the next time?*

SUGGESTIONS FOR DE-ESCALATING THE ANGER OF OTHERS

ALVARO MORALES: I was called out to the front room at the drop-in center because there was this client there who was insulting employees. He had a long history of causing trouble at the center, so he was looking at a suspension [meaning that he couldn't return to the center for a period of time]. I was in charge of the suspensions, so I had to ask him to leave.

I started by reaching out to shake his hand and saying "Good afternoon, R_____ [calling the client by name]." I was talking with him as clearly and respectfully as I could, keeping my voice down. He kept raising his voice. I tried to calm him down. This was happening by the reception area in front of two other employees that I supervise, so I wasn't just dealing with the client, but also kind of teaching the staff how to deal with these situations. I felt the pressure, you know, that I really had to do it right. We have a plan for these situations at the center because it happens a lot. If the client gets more out of control and threatens anyone or does something physical, then one of the staff pushes a panic button and everyone comes to help out.

So I started talking with R_____, and he was insulting a staff person. I reminded him that it wasn't acceptable to call people names like that, and that he needed to leave the center. Then he started insulting me, too. I kept talking with him respectfully, but also more firmly. I just keep saying: " No, you have to leave now." We had to go through a hall full of clients to leave the agency, and he kept insulting me as we walked. I knew he was leaving, but he was still saying all these disrespectful things, and he wanted to stay because he knew that lunch was coming soon. So I just kept saying: "No, you have to leave and come back another day. We'll talk. Right now you're not able to talk calmly."

Then he spit on me. The whole room went "Ooooooh!" It isn't unusual for fights to break out at the drop-in center. Fights about things like somebody took my chair or somebody looked at me wrong, things like that. So for people to see somebody spitting on somebody—I am sure they thought we would start fighting. But I kept my cool, even though I was boiling inside. I escorted him outside, and other staff went to stand by the door. He left, cursing us, but he left. I just went into my office and kind of exploded internally. I didn't want to do it in front of the clients or my staff. On the bright side, R_____ returned to the center a week later and apologized, and we ate lunch together.

Alvaro handled this difficult situation calmly and professionally and took action to diminish the risks of harm to the clients, staff, and to himself.

Anger and aggression are often the products of feeling frustrated and powerless. Given the many challenges clients face in their lives, it is no wonder that they sometimes approach you or each other in anger. Before it is possible to work effectively to meet their needs, it will often be necessary to calm them first or defuse their anger. Remember that it is not always possible to calm an angry person. Taking actions to maintain safety may be necessary. When a client is really angry, the most important job you will have is to avoid escalation. Here are some recommendations for reducing anger in others while keeping yourself safe:

- *Listening skills are crucial to defusing anger.* The first element in defusing anger is to communicate your respect using nonaggressive body language and appropriate listening skills. Try to understand their concern. Avoid judging their behavior.
- *Offer reassurance and space for big emotions to settle.* Use a calm voice, ask them to take a deep breath, and acknowledge their emotions positively: "I can see that you are upset. Can you take a few minutes to catch your breath?"
- *Express your desire to understand the other party*, and encourage them to communicate with you in a way that will best make this possible. For example: "I'd like to hear about what is going on. Please take your time—and can you lower your voice? It's hard for me to listen and understand when you are speaking so loudly and quickly."
- *Asserting your own needs and agency policies is essential* for managing the potential crisis and will give your client a sense of boundaries and limits, too. Statements such as, "I am really glad that we can talk about this, but I want to remind you that we can't yell or disturb other clients. It's expected that everyone here, even when we're angry, will treat each other with respect. Are you able to follow these ground rules right now?" If the client does something that feels threatening, remember to use I-messages.
- *Everyone wants to feel understood and listened to.* Try not to interrupt or correct the person who is angry. When people are under stress, there is potential for miscommunication. Use active listening skills such as restating and paraphrasing, clarifying, validating, and gathering information. You don't have to agree with the person who is angry, but demonstrate that you are listening ("It sounds like you were really disappointed when your family didn't invite you . . ."). Show your curiosity. Use openended questions (for example, "Is there anything else that is going on in your life

that is contributing to this?" "What would you like to see happen now?" "What helps when you experience feelings like this?" "How can I be supportive?").

- ✪ *Reframing will allow you to redirect aggression into a nonthreatening discussion* of the person's underlying needs. Reframing changes direction and can clarify the positive attributes of the person in anger.
- ✪ *Safety should always be of utmost important to you and your organization.* Your workplace should have a prearranged safety plan. When escalation cannot be prevented, it is important to stay calm. Use a prearranged warning signal to alert others and to get backup. Talk slowly and calmly. At one clinic, the signal was to call out loudly for "Doctor Strong." When staff heard this, they came quickly to offer support.
- ✪ *Knowing when to disengage is essential.* If you feel yourself getting angry and unable to communicate professionally, it is time to disengage. Sometimes, a short break to get a drink of water or take a walk can allow the client to calm down. You can always recommend that you reconvene later when they have had some time to think over the situation. Perhaps someone else at the organization is better suited to this session. Let your client know this.

If you are unsuccessful in deescalating the situation and are still concerned about your own safety or the safety of others, disengagement may require you to leave the situation or to ask the other party to leave. If you ask the other party to leave, do so in a calm manner. If you feel safety is an issue, request assistance from a coworker or call 911 immediately. If the situation calls on you to leave, make an excuse, leave immediately, and get assistance.

When the situation has been resolved, debrief with coworkers. Discuss what you and your coworkers did well and how to improve the response to similar situations in the future.

? *Have you ever had to deescalate the anger of another?*

? *What did it feel like to face this challenge?*

? *What did you do in the situation, and what was the outcome?*

? *What recommendations do you have for others who face similar challenges?*

FOLLOW UP WITH OTHER PARTIES TO THE CONFLICT

Conflicts sometimes follow cyclical patterns, and even though you think it may be behind you, it may start up again in a similar way or take a new form. For this reason, we encourage you to check in with the parties to the conflict after you have resolved the issue to ensure that your professional relationship continues to go smoothly. It is particularly important for you to take responsibility for following up if the conflict was with someone whom you hold power over.

? *What would you do to follow up with R., the client who was so angry at the drop-in center?*

CHAPTER REVIEW

Apply conflict resolution knowledge and skills to the scenario between Sam and Chris that was introduced at the beginning of the chapter. Answer the following questions:

- What are some of the sources of this conflict?
- What may be some of the underlying issues?
- What conflict styles are the two parties using?

Imagine that you are Chris:

- How might you try to shift the way that you view this conflict, using the suggestions from the Harvard Negotiation Project?
- How would you talk with Sam to set up a process for communicating about your conflict?

- What would you want to communicate to Sam at the very start of your conversation?
- What ground rules would you want to negotiate?
- How would you express your experience of the conflict using I-message statements?
- How would you put active listening skills into practice (what would you do, say, and ask)?
- What type of compromise might you be willing to make?
- What will you do to follow through with Sam and the conflict between you?
- What other resources might be helpful to you in resolving this conflict?

REFERENCES

Academic Leadership Support: Office of Quality Improvement & Office of Human Resource Development. 2007. About Conflict. Madison: University of Wisconsin–Madison. Accessed on July 20, 2007: http://www.ohrd. wisc.edu/onlinetraining/resolution/index.asp

Alinsky, S. D. 1969. *Reveille for Radicals.* New York: Vintage.

Araiz-Iverson, R., Blagsvelt, K., Hoburg, M., Hopson, N., Lanctot, K., Lindbeck, L., Longfelder, M., Manning, B., McCracken, C., Piccagli, G., Proctor, B., Regal, C., Roberts, B., Rowe-Tinsley, T., Sadalla, G., Salazar, D., Stone, M., and Volante, H. 2006. *The Basics of Mediation: Community Boards' Mediation Training Guide.* San Francisco: Community Boards.

Cohen, L., Davis, R., and Aboelata, M. 1998. Conflict Resolution and Violence Prevention: From Misunderstanding to Understanding. *The Fourth R* 84: 3–8, 13–15.

Cowans, S. 2005. *Bay Area Community Health Worker Study.* [HED 892—Final Report]. San Francisco: San Francisco State University.

Gaitlin, J., Wysocki, A., and Kepner, K. 2007. Understanding Conflict in the Workplace. Gainesville, FL: University of Florida, Institute of Food and Agriculture Sciences Extension.Accessed on August 2, 2007: http://edis.ifas.ufl.edu/HR024

Hart, B. 2002. Conflict in the Workplace. Accessed on August 10, 2007: http://behavioralconsultants.com/Newsletters/conflict_in_the_workplace.htm

Karp, J. M. 2008. Teaching Assistants' Training Programme: Active Listening Workshop. Accessed on June 10, 2008: http://www.utoronto.ca/tatp/handouts/Listening_Workshop.pdf

Sadalla, G., Henriquez, M., Holmberg, M., and Halligan, J. 1998. *Conflict Resolution: A Middle and High School Curriculum.* San Francisco: Community Boards.

Sharon, R., and Clark, L. 1989. *Conflict: A Way to Peace—the AFDA Model: A Guidebook for Personal and Professional Development of Peaceful Conflict Resolution Skills.* Englewood, CO: AFDA Group.

Stone, D., Patton, B., and Heen, S.. 1999. *Difficult Conversations: How to Discuss What Matters Most.* New York: Penguin Books.

Ting-Toomey, S., and Oetzel, J. G. 2001. *Managing Intercultural Conflicts Effectively.* Thousand Oaks, CA: Sage Publications.

University of Mississippi, National Food Service Management Institute. 2002. Conflict and Challenge in the Workplace. Accessed on March 27, 2009: http://www.nfsmi.org

ADDITIONAL RESOURCES

Benun, I. 2006. *Stop Pushing Me Around! A Workplace Guide for the Timid, Shy, and Less Assertive.* Franklin Lakes, NJ: Career Press.

Bird, G. 1986. *William James.* London: Routledge and Kegan Paul.

Burton, J. 1990. *Conflict: Resolution and Prevention.* New York: St. Martin's Press.

Cloke, K. 2000. *Resolving Conflicts at Work: A Complete Guide for Everyone on the Job.* San Francisco: Jossey-Bass.

Dana, D. 2001. *Conflict Resolution: Mediation Tools for Everyday Worklife.* New York: McGraw-Hill.

Gopin, M. 2004. *Healing the Heart of Conflict: Eight Crucial Steps to Making Peace with Yourself and Others.* Emmaus, PA: Rodale Press.

Lippitt, G. 1969. *Organization Renewal: Achieving Viability in a Changing World.* New York: Appleton-Century-Crofts.

Maxon, R. 1999. Stress in the Workplace: A Costly Epidemic. Madison, NJ: Fairleigh Dickinson University. Accessed on March 31, 2009: http://www.fdu.edu/news-pubs/magazine/99su/stress.html

McClure, L. F. 2000. *Anger and Conflict in the Workplace: Spot the Signs, Avoid the Trauma.* Manassas Park, VA: Impact.

Salisbury, H. E. (Ed.). 1972. *The Eloquence of Protest: Voices of the 70s.* Boston: Houghton Mifflin.

Ury, W. 2007. *The Power of a Positive No: How to Say No and Still Get to Yes.* New York: Bantam Dell.

Community Boards

Based in San Francisco, Community Boards operates the longest-running, no-cost neighborhood mediation program in the United States. Community Boards is a local and national provider of training and training materials in dispute resolution, mediation, and facilitation and a national leader in youth-to-youth peer mediation through the Conflict Manager Program. Accessed on March 31, 2009: http://www.communityboards.org/

Web Sites

Association for Conflict Resolution. This is a professional organization dedicated to enhancing the practice and public understanding of conflict resolution. Accessed on March 31, 2009: http://www.acrnet.org/

CRInfo. This is a free service that maintains a keyword-coded catalog of over twenty thousand Web, print, organizational, and other conflict resolution–related resources. These core catalogs are supplemented with thousands of additional links to Web-based news stories, feature articles, cultural background information, documents describing ongoing conflicts, and government dispute resolution–related Web pages. Accessed on March 31, 2009: http://www.crinfo.org/

National Association for Community Mediation. Accessed on June 10, 2008: http://www.nafcm.org/

14

Stress Management and Self-Care

Tim Berthold • Joani Marinoff • Sal Núñez

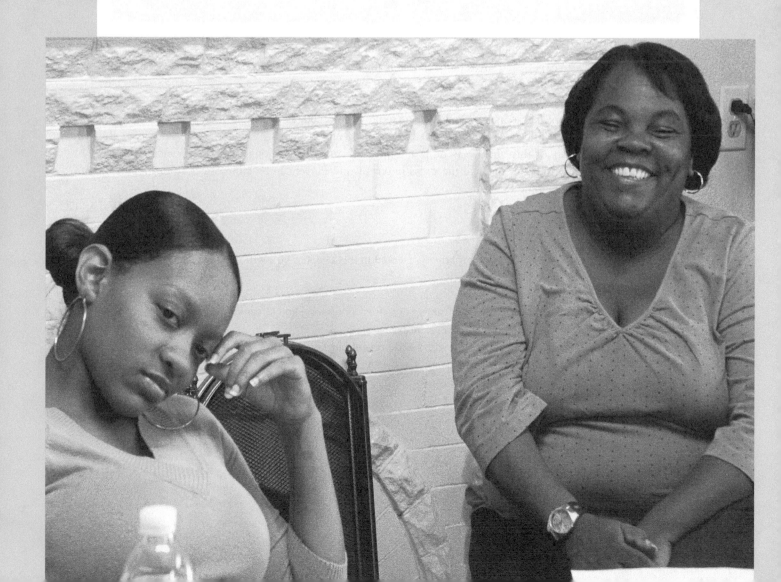

CASE STUDY: MAMPHELA

Mamphela's daughter is sick, and was dropped off at an aunt's house for the day. Mamphela was recently promoted to supervisor of a team of outreach workers, something she has been working towards for many years. She is happy about the promotion, but has inherited a team that does not work well together. Last night, one of the senior members of the team called Mamphela at home to say that she was thinking about quitting unless "You do something to get P.'s attitude under control. I can't work with P. anymore!" Between the conflicts at work and her daughter's illness, Mamphela didn't get much sleep last night.

- ✪ What do you feel as you read this scenario?
- ✪ Have you ever faced days like this?
- ✪ How do stressors like this—a sick family member, conflict at work, a new promotion, lack of sleep—affect you?
- ✪ What happens to you when you are feeling "stressed out?"
- ✪ What skills have you learned for coping with or managing stress?

INTRODUCTION

Everyone experiences stress; it is a natural and inevitable part of life. As a CHW, you will also experience stress on the job. It is important for both your professional success and your personal well-being to develop skills in managing the stress that comes with this work. This chapter is designed to assist you in identifying signs of stress and burnout in yourself and others, and to make a realistic plan to prevent burnout and promote your wellness.

While we recognize that CHWs also support clients in better managing stress, the focus of this chapter is on promoting self-care skills among caregivers. Once we learn how to better manage the stress in our own lives, we can be more effective in supporting others to do the same.

WHAT YOU WILL LEARN:

By studying the information presented in this chapter, you will be able to:

- ✪ Define *stress* and *burnout*
- ✪ Recognize common sources of stress (stressors) and stress responses
- ✪ Assess personal signs of stress
- ✪ Better manage your stress and prevent burnout
- ✪ Develop an action plan for self-care

WORDS TO KNOW

Stressor	Burnout	Post-Traumatic Stress
Secondary or Vicarious Trauma	Secondary or Vicarious Resilience	

14.1 DEFINING STRESS AND BURNOUT

What is stress? The term can be used to refer to different things. For our purposes, we will define *stress* as the way we respond to and are affected by events or situations that place a demand on our internal and external resources. The event or circumstance that places demands on us is called a **stressor**. As we will describe in greater detail below, stress may be characterized by physiological responses (responses in your body), including increased blood pressure, heart, and respiration rates, as well as by emotional, cognitive (thoughts and how the mind functions), behavioral, and spiritual responses.

STRESSORS

Stressors may include everyday events, such as juggling work and family responsibilities or driving in heavy traffic, as well as more dramatic events, such as the death of a loved one or exposure to war as a soldier or civilian. Stressors include events that may be characterized as positive, such as graduation from school or falling in love, or negative, such as separation from family, receiving a failing grade, illness, or death. Common stressors may include, for example:

- Moving
- Starting a new job
- Loss of a job
- Rushing to meet deadlines
- Planning a celebration
- Taking care of children
- Driving or taking public transportation during rush hour
- Financial difficulties
- Illness
- Joining a new community or social group
- Family conflicts
- Immigration
- Experiences of prejudice or discrimination

? *Are there other stressors you've experienced?*

? *What are common "positive" and "negative" stressors in your life?*

CHWs will also encounter stressors on the job. Some of these may include:

- A heavy caseload (too many clients to serve and not enough time to provide quality services to all of them)
- Working with a particularly challenging client (however you define this)
- Conflict with a coworker or supervisor
- Starting a new job or earning a promotion
- Supervising others
- Speaking before a large audience
- Lack of local resources for your clients such as housing, drug treatment, or health care
- Insufficient training and skills to perform a particular duty, such as facilitating a training or support group

- ✪ Ethical challenges
- ✪ Witnessing a client:
  - ● With declining health
  - ● Facing the end of life
  - ● Struggling with depression or suicidal thoughts
  - ● In an abusive relationship
  - ● Continuing to engage in harmful behaviors
  - ● Experiencing prejudice and discrimination based on their identity or history
- ✪ Insufficient pay or benefits
- ✪ Ending a successful professional relationship with an ongoing client
- ✪ Government policies reducing or eliminating access to essential services for your clients
- ✪ Lack of status and recognition for the role and contributions of CHWs
- ✪ Lack of stable funding for CHW positions or programs

? *Can you think of other on-the-job stressors?*

? *What types of client situations might be particularly stressful for you?*

14.2 INTERNAL AND EXTERNAL RESOURCES

Each of us is unique, and so are our responses to stressors. For example, two individuals who are exposed to the same event, such as an earthquake or hurricane, may be affected in very different ways. To a great extent, our response to stress depends on our access to internal and external resources—the same resources that we encourage our clients to identify and enhance.

Lᴇᴇ Jᴀᴄᴋsᴏɴ: I understand that there's a good possibility no matter how close I get to some of my clients with AIDS—that they're going to pass away. What I do is I make it as comfortable for them as possible and try to be there for them when they're alive. When they pass away, it's only human to grieve for them, but I realize and accept the fact that I can't get lost in the cause. You have to take care of yourself because if you don't, there's no way you can take care of your clients. You will get burned out.

INTERNAL RESOURCES

Internal resources lie within each of us and may include:

- ✪ A good sense of humor
- ✪ Patience
- ✪ The ability to put events in perspective
- ✪ Good health, particularly a healthy immune system
- ✪ The ability to achieve a calm and relaxed state of mind and body
- ✪ The ability to connect in meaningful ways with other people
- ✪ A sense of pride in your professional contributions
- ✪ An understanding that facing stress is a natural part of life

- ⊕ Healthy self-esteem (what you think and how you feel about yourself)
- ⊕ Confidence in your ability to face adversity
- ⊕ History of successfully coping with stressful life events
- ⊕ Knowledge of stress management techniques
- ⊕ Love of music, reading, writing, or other pastimes
- ⊕ Healthy eating habits
- ⊕ The ability to reach out and ask for support when you need it
- ⊕ Engaging in regular exercise
- ⊕ Faith, including religious or spiritual faith

RAMONA BENSON: One of the things that I love to do is to help women get empowered so they can eliminate barriers in their life and live a healthy lifestyle. Our program is eighteen months. I have seen a lot of ladies leave out of here like a blossomed flower, moving to environments that they never dreamed they could ever move into.

? *What are your most important internal resources?*

EXTERNAL RESOURCES:

External resources are located outside of us, and may include:

- ⊕ Close and supportive relationships with family
- ⊕ Strong friendships
- ⊕ A sense of belonging to a particular community or communities
- ⊕ Safety (including home, neighborhood, and society free from violence)
- ⊕ A strong sense of cultural identity
- ⊕ Supportive coworkers
- ⊕ Good, supportive supervision at work
- ⊕ Pets
- ⊕ Trust in and respect for a CHW, social worker, physician, teacher, or other helping professional
- ⊕ Access to quality education, stable housing, good nutrition
- ⊕ Access to parks and other recreational facilities
- ⊕ Employment benefits including health care, sick pay, and vacation leave
- ⊕ Government-provided disability benefits
- ⊕ Respect for and enforcement of your civil and human rights

? *What are your most important external resources?*

14.3 STRESS RESPONSES

Stress can result in physical, emotional, cognitive, behavioral, and spiritual responses. There is no way to predict how any individual will respond to a specific stressor. The following lists of common stress responses are not meant to be definitive: they do not include every possible response to stress. As you read the lists below, please think about what you might add.

The lists emphasize "negative" responses, as these tend to present the most difficult challenges. Remember that stressors can also include positive events, and that "negative" stressors, handled well, can sometimes result in positive experiences. Stress responses can compel us to new awareness and actions that create positive changes.

COMMON PHYSICAL RESPONSES

Stress is sometimes thought of as primarily a physiological (bodily) phenomenon. When confronted with a crisis or emergency, or significant new challenges or demands, our body responds by releasing hormones, such as adrenaline, which speed up our heart and respiration rates (breathing), blood pressure, and metabolism. These hormones deliver more oxygen and blood sugar to our large muscles, and dilate our pupils to improve vision. This physiological stress response is sometimes referred to as the "fight-or-flight" response, and it prepares us to take action during emergencies in order to avoid harm. Animals experience the same type of stress response in nature, which enables them, for example, to escape predators.

While this type of stress response prepares us to take action and to avoid harm during an emergency situation, in other situations, and over time, it can actually be harmful to our health. For example, when you experience this type of stress response as a consequence of a conflict at work, the release of hormones may leave you feeling jumpy, nervous, or overstimulated, and you may be less able to focus on the situation at hand and to take calm, measured, and effective action. When we are exposed to stressors on a more frequent or chronic basis, the stress response can also suppress our immune system and contribute to hypertension, heart disease, and stroke.

Other physical responses to acute (short-term) or chronic (ongoing) stress may include:

- Fatigue
- Changes in sleeping patterns, including insomnia and nightmares
- Chest pain, palpitations, or tightness
- Breathlessness
- Pain, including headaches, stomachaches, backaches
- Nausea, digestive tract problems, ulcers
- Changes in menstrual cycles
- Rashes
- Freezing or the inability to move or take physical action
- A surge of energy
- Quick reactions in moments of crisis

? *Can you think of other physical stress responses to add to the list?*

COMMON EMOTIONAL RESPONSES

- Frustration and anger, including anger directed at yourself
- Embarrassment or shame
- Guilt
- Anxiety or fear

- Sadness, sorrow, or despair
- Numbness or lack of emotion
- A feeling of hopelessness
- Elation, joy, satisfaction (particularly when we respond to crisis in effective ways)

COMMON COGNITIVE RESPONSES (THOUGHTS)

- Worrying (about the stressor)
- Thinking about the stressors or events over and over again
- Difficulty concentrating
- Trying to avoid thinking about the stressful situation
- Memories about other similar experiences
- Doubting your own abilities and value
- Thoughts about escaping your current situation by quitting your job, dropping out of school, ending a relationship, or moving
- Thoughts that life is no longer worth living, or thoughts of suicide
- Thoughts or fantasies of revenge
- Thoughts of gratitude for escaping harm

COMMON BEHAVIORAL RESPONSES

- Withdrawing from family, friends, or community
- Building community by working with others to confront common challenges or stressor.
- Avoiding locations or activities that are stressful, including work, school, and home
- Snapping at or yelling at others, including people who have not had a part in causing the stress
- Changing patterns of eating, drinking, smoking, drug use, hygiene, or dress
- Engaging in behaviors that may seem to relieve or escape the stress, but that are harmful, especially smoking, drinking alcohol, overspending, or using drugs
- Stopping behaviors that used to give you pleasure
- Developing behaviors that enable you to better manage stress, including exercise, meditation, talking with friends, reading or writing, going to support groups, spiritual practices, playing an instrument or making music

RAMONA BENSON: I was hearing things from my daughter and my husband, who were saying, "What's wrong with you?" I just wasn't acting like myself because of all the stress I was facing at work. It was a wake-up call for me to find a better way of handling it.

COMMON SPIRITUAL RESPONSES

- Loss or weakening of religious, spiritual, or metaphysical faith or beliefs
- Loss of a sense of meaning or purpose
- A sense of hopelessness or despair
- A sense of alienation from others
- Anger at god, creator, human kind, fate, or luck

✪ Finding or strengthening religious, spiritual, or metaphysical faith, beliefs, and practices
✪ A sense of connectedness to others, the world, god, or creator

BURNOUT

Burnout presents a very real risk for CHWs and others working in public health. A resource developed to train CHWs working in HIV/AIDS in Zimbabwe provides the following definition of **burnout**:

> Burnout is often difficult to conceptualize. It can be thought of as the point a person reaches when the demands made on her/him over an extended period of time are too great for the resources she or he possess[es]. Burnout has been described as a physical, emotional, psychological and spiritual phenomenon—an experience of personal fatigue, alienation and failure—or a progressive loss of idealism, energy and purpose sometimes experienced by people working in helping professions. (International Training and Education Center on HIV, 2005)

The I-TECH curriculum refers to the Stage Theory of Burnout. Under this framework:

First Stage: The initial stage includes physical warning signs, such as the inability to shake off a lingering cold or fever, frequent headaches, and sleeplessness. The thought of going to work loses its appeal.

Second Stage: The middle stage involves such emotional and behavioral signs as angry outbursts, obvious impatience or irritability, or treating people with contempt. An attitude of suspicion often intensifies at this stage.

Third Stage: The last stage is critical and severe, and it occurs when someone becomes sour on one's self, humanity, everybody. Intense feelings of loneliness and alienation are characteristic.

For CHWs, when the high level of commitment to clients and communities is combined with stress on the job and the lack of adequate professional support, it can lead to burnout. Situations that CHWs face can aggravate and increase the likelihood of burnout, such as:

✪ Witnessing widespread illness, violence, or death in the communities they serve. For example, in Zimbabwe approximately 24 percent of all adults have HIV disease. In the United States, many urban communities face an epidemic of gun-related violence and death.
✪ Witnessing clients relapse to previous behaviors that are harmful to their health (such as drug use).
✪ Inability to assist your client to access local resources such as shelter, safety, food, or health care. For example, in Zimbabwe, most patients with AIDS do not have access to medical treatments. In the United States, more than forty-seven million people are uninsured and do not have access to a regular source of primary health care.
✪ Lack of adequate training, supervision, and support necessary to providing quality services to clients and communities.

? *Can you think of other circumstances that could contribute to burnout among CHWs?*

Because burnout may happen gradually, or over a series of stages, it can be difficult to recognize it in ourselves or in others.

When we are burned out, we are often incapable of providing services well. In the worst circumstances, we can actually do harm to our clients. A CHW who is "burned out" may:

- Not show up to work on time or keep appointments with clients
- Fail to complete necessary paperwork accurately or in a timely fashion
- Fail to listen deeply to clients
- Act as if they don't particularly care about the client's situation
- Bring their own issues and feelings into their work with clients
- Act out their frustration on clients or coworkers
- Fail to pay attention to details and miss opportunities to make effective referrals that could prevent poor health outcomes for clients

? *Have you ever received services from a CHW, nurse, social worker, teacher, or other aid professional whom you think may have been burned out?*

? *What did you observe?*

? *What was this experience like for you?*

Have you ever experienced any of these stages of burnout? What signs did you experience and when did you recognize them?

POST-TRAUMATIC STRESS

Post-traumatic stress (PTS) is a special sort of stress response that may occur when people are exposed to war, torture, child abuse, sexual assault, incarceration, natural disasters, and other traumatic experiences characterized by intense fear, horror, or a sense of helplessness. These events often involve significant loss of control and a threat of death.

Traumatic experiences are sometimes considered to be rare or unusual occurrences. However, as Judith Herman writes, quite the reverse is true:

> Rape, battery, and other forms of sexual and domestic violence are so common a part of women's lives that they can hardly be described as outside the range of ordinary experience. And in the view of the number of people killed in war over the past century, military trauma, too, must be considered a common part of human experience: only the fortunate find it unusual. (Herman, 1997)

The impact of traumatic experience on survivors may be similar to the list of stress responses provided above. However, trauma responses are generally more severe and long-lasting. Because traumatic events are so common, it is likely that some of you, and many of your clients, will have been exposed to trauma and may have signs of PTS. *Please note:* If you are working with a client who informs you that they are a survivor of trauma, or who appears to be suffering from post-traumatic symptoms, we encourage you to provide the client with a referral to a local program or provider who specializes in working with survivors of trauma.

CHWs are also at risk for a phenomenon known as **secondary trauma** (also known as **vicarious trauma**). This refers to the effect on helping professionals who work with survivors of traumatic events including war, rape, and child abuse. Sometimes, as a result of their work, helping professionals may develop their own symptoms of traumatic stress. Developing strong skills in self-care is essential to preventing secondary trauma among CHWs.

Just as CHWs and other caregivers may experience secondary trauma, they may also experience **secondary or vicarious resilience**. This happens when caregivers who work with survivors of trauma are affected and inspired by the survivor's own resilience in the face of trauma, and the tremendous courage and other resources they bring to their own process of healing or recovery.

We encourage you to seek out additional opportunities for training on issues related to trauma. These may be available at local colleges or public health, mental health, or social services agencies. For example, many cities and counties have rape crisis centers, suicide prevention centers, and domestic violence agencies that provide outstanding training in exchange for a volunteer commitment. These trainings are an asset to your work as a CHW.

To learn more about post-traumatic stress, please see the resources listed at the end of this chapter under *Trauma*.

14.4 ASSESSING FOR STRESS AND BURNOUT

Sometimes we become so accustomed to stress in our personal lives and on the job that we lose sight of how it affects us. When this occurs, we may be at risk for burnout.

We can learn from senior CHWs who have worked in the field for decades without experiencing burnout. They have accomplished this by developing stress management skills and a regular practice of self-care. Ongoing self-care is only made possible, however, by developing self-awareness and skills in assessing your exposure to stressors and their impact in your life. To do so, consider the following:

1. *Reflect upon your exposure to stress and its impact in your life.* The following questions may assist to guide your reflection. Consider writing down your responses.

- What types of stressors are most difficult for you?
- What event or circumstance was particularly stressful for you today, this week, and in the past year?
- In general, how do you know when you are under stress?
- How does stress impact your body? Your thoughts? Your emotions? Your behavior? Your spirituality or beliefs?
- How do these stress responses impact your personal life, work, or experience in school?
- Are there things that you do when you are under stress that sometimes heighten your stress response or make the situation worse?
- What do you do to better manage when you are under stress?

2. *Sometimes we don't always have a clear picture of how stress affects us.* Consider asking someone you trust and who knows you well to share any observations they may have about how you are affected by stress. Be sure to ask for this feedback at a time when you are truly prepared to listen to whatever your friend, family member, or colleague may have to share with you. Be prepared to be surprised and to learn something new about yourself. Don't try to respond to what they say, or to defend yourself. Ask questions that will assist

you to clarify the feedback you receive (for example: "Can you share a couple of examples with me? Do you notice anything about the type of situation when I may be more likely to respond in this way?").

Continue to reflect on what you hear from others. What else would you like to know? How might this information be useful in your life?

3. *Take a stress self-assessment.* There are many stress self-assessment tools available on the Web and elsewhere. Many assessments will provide you with a "score" that is designed to tell you something about your stress responses and risk for burnout. As you will see below, we have decided not to quantify or score these self-assessments, because much of our experience and response to stressors is highly personal and subjective. We found it difficult to quantify or assign a numeric value to the range of our responses. Some people may be exposed to multiple stressors in a short period of time, but not experience strong or harmful stress responses. Others may experience profound stress responses after a single exposure. While some people find that physical stress responses are most problematic in their lives, others are more impacted by emotional or spiritual stress responses. Please use the assessment below to identify the stresses you might be facing, your access to resources for dealing with stress (internal and external), and your symptoms (stress responses).

We have included questions not only about recent exposure to stressors, but also about lifetime exposure to traumatic events and your risks for secondary trauma. We do this because exposure to traumatic events, and witnessing the trauma experiences of others, can affect us in profound and enduring ways that call out for support and recovery.

Take this self-assessment. Reflect on your answers. Feel free to use this self-assessment as a resource, share it with coworkers and clients, and revise or rewrite it.

STRESS SELF-ASSESSMENT

STRESS SELF-ASSESSMENT

1. EXPOSURE TO STRESSORS

Have you recently experienced the following stressors (Define *recently* for yourself. Many self-assessments use the timeframe of 6 months or a year):

Yes   No

___ ___ The death of a family member or close friend?

___ ___ A serious injury or illness?

___ ___ The end of a long-term relationship?

___ ___ The beginning of new relationship or marriage?

___ ___ Birth or adoption?

___ ___ Serious argument or conflict with family members or close friends?

___ ___ Financial or legal difficulties?

___ ___ Significant changes in your sleeping or eating patterns?

___ ___ Depression (lack of feeling or persistant and overwhelming sadness)?

___ ___ Violence or witnessing violence?

___ ___ Loss of housing or employment?

___ ___ Beginning school, a new job or moving to a new home?

___ ___ Jail or prison or incarceration of a close family member?

___ ___ Discrimination in school, employment, housing or other contexts based on your identity?

___ ___ Other (fill in events that you think are significant stressors)

___ ___ Other

___ ___ Other

(Continued)

Have you ever experienced the following types of traumatic events:

Yes No

___ ___ Incarceration
___ ___ Armed conflict or war
___ ___ Physical abuse or assault
___ ___ Intimate partner violence
___ ___ Sexual abuse
___ ___ Fleeing your country of origin
___ ___ Other
___ ___ Other
___ ___ Other

Work related stressors:

___ ___ Received a professional evaluation that you felt was not fair?
___ ___ Changed jobs or received a promotion or demotion?
___ ___ Missed work because you felt too stressed to go in?
___ ___ Conflict with a co-worker?
___ ___ Conflict with your supervisor?
___ ___ Witnessing the decline of a client's health or related circumstances?
___ ___ Worked closely with a client who shares their trauma experiences with you?
___ ___ Other
___ ___ Other
___ ___ Other

For the following questions, we suggest using a Likert Scale. Rank your response to each question on a scale from 0–5.

Strongly Disagree   Strongly Agree

0   1   2   3   4   5

My input is valued by my employer — 0 | 1 | 2 | 3 | 4 | 5
I can rely on guidance and support when I need it at work — 0 | 1 | 2 | 3 | 4 | 5
Workplace policies are implemented in a fair manner — 0 | 1 | 2 | 3 | 4 | 5
My contributions are recognized and valued — 0 | 1 | 2 | 3 | 4 | 5
I feel safe at all times on the job — 0 | 1 | 2 | 3 | 4 | 5
I am isolated in my job — 0 | 1 | 2 | 3 | 4 | 5
I receive the resources I need to perform my job — 0 | 1 | 2 | 3 | 4 | 5
I have at least one colleague at my workplace who I feel values and connects with me as a person and an individual — 0 | 1 | 2 | 3 | 4 | 5

2. STRESS RESPONSES

Please circle yes or no if you have recently experienced the following stress responses:

Yes No

___ ___ Difficulty sleeping
___ ___ Smoking or drinking more frequently/more than I want to.
___ ___ Being more irritable with family and friends
___ ___ Difficulty getting out of bed in the morning, going to work, keeping social commitments
___ ___ Withdrawal from valued family, friends, community, activities
___ ___ Muscle tension and chronic pain or nausea

___ ___ Increased blood pressure
___ ___ Difficulty sleeping, including insomnia and nightmares
___ ___ Significant changes in diet
___ ___ Difficulty breathing or panic attacks
___ ___ Increased symptoms of depression
___ ___ Critical thoughts about my own value, intelligence, or abilities
___ ___ Thoughts of not wanting to be alive or thoughts of suicide
___ ___ Significant changes in spiritual life or faith Yes/No
___ ___ Other

Have you experienced the following at work?

___ ___ Tuning out when listening to a client
___ ___ Talking more than your clients during sessions
___ ___ Increased anxiety about work
___ ___ Increased irritation with clients or colleagues
___ ___ Less satisfaction from professional contributions
___ ___ A lack of hope related to my work or the prospects of my clients.
___ ___ I take it personally when clients fail to progress and achieve their goals
___ ___ I spend a lot of time worrying about my clients or other aspects of my job when I am not working.
___ ___ I have difficulty creating a strong boundary between by work and the rest of my life.
___ ___ Other

3. INVENTORY OF INTERNAL AND EXTERNAL RESOURCES

For the following questions, we suggest using a Likert Scale. Rank your response to each question on a scale from 0–5.

Strongly Disagree   Strongly Agree

0   1   2   3   4   5

I exercise on a regular basis.	0 | 1 | 2 | 3 | 4 | 5
I regularly experience restful and uninterrupted sleep	0 | 1 | 2 | 3 | 4 | 5
I eat a healthy diet	0 | 1 | 2 | 3 | 4 | 5
I drink too much coffee	0 | 1 | 2 | 3 | 4 | 5
I smoke cigarettes	0 | 1 | 2 | 3 | 4 | 5
I rely on alcohol or drugs to help me relax	. 0 | 1 | 2 | 3 | 4 | 5
I do something fun on a regular basis	0 | 1 | 2 | 3 | 4 | 5
I have one or more close friendships	0 | 1 | 2 | 3 | 4 | 5
I enjoy close positive relationships with family	0 | 1 | 2 | 3 | 4 | 5
I have a faith, religion or set of beliefs that provide me with a sense of purpose and comfort	0 | 1 | 2 | 3 | 4 | 5
I am able to express my emotions, including feelings of frustration and anger	0 | 1 | 2 | 3 | 4 | 5
I do something that helps me relax when I am experiencing stress	0 | 1 | 2 | 3 | 4 | 5
I do not have a major health condition	0 | 1 | 2 | 3 | 4 | 5
I am able to pay my bills on time	0 | 1 | 2 | 3 | 4 | 5
Based on previous experiences, I am confident that I can handle most life challenges	0 | 1 | 2 | 3 | 4 | 5
I have stable housing and health benefits	0 | 1 | 2 | 3 | 4 | 5
I like my job	0 | 1 | 2 | 3 | 4 | 5

(Continued)

I respect my employer	0 | 1 | 2 | 3 | 4 | 5
I am a valued member of a work team	0 | 1 | 2 | 3 | 4 | 5
I know that I make a positive difference in the lives of the clients and communities I work with	0 | 1 | 2 | 3 | 4 | 5
I am prepared and confident in my ability to witness the trauma experiences of clients	0 | 1 | 2 | 3 | 4 | 5

ANALYZE YOUR RESPONSES:

Notice how many times you indicated that you are exposed to stressors or signs of stress responses.

What have you learned about your exposure to stressors?
What do you notice about your response to stress?
How do you assess your level of access to internal and external resources?
Are you prepared to enhance your skills in managing stress and preventing burnout?

14.5 PRACTICING SELF-CARE

SO, WHAT CAN WE DO ABOUT ALL THIS STRESS?

Don't become disheartened if you have a lot of stressors in your life. Most of us do.

The *good news* is that we can each cultivate positive, life-affirming, and health-sustaining activities. We can use these activities or practices to counter the stressors in our lives. Despite our neurological programming and the challenges inherent in our society and in our professional and personal lives, relaxation is possible. When we develop good skills and habits for caring for ourselves, we are better able to deal with the negative experiences we face and are more confident about our ability to handle positive challenges and opportunities.

LEE JACKSON: I meditate and relax, go to the gym, listen to jazz. Basically, I take care of myself.

HOW DO YOU RELAX?

Many of us already participate in practices that are relaxing and stress relieving. There are many simple activities that we use to alleviate stress, such as:

- Getting adequate rest and sleep
- Eating a well-balanced and nutritious diet
- Taking a hot bath
- Spending some quiet time alone
- Listening to or playing music
- Playing games
- Exercising
- Journaling, writing, poetry
- Painting, drawing, sculpting
- Cooking

What brings *you* joy in life?

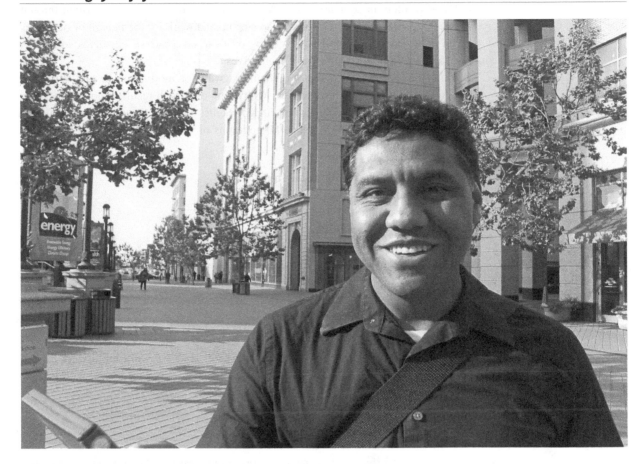

- ✪ Gardening
- ✪ Walking on the beach or in the woods, parks, or other natural settings
- ✪ Spending meaningful time with family, friends, and pets

? *What are you already doing to relax and refresh yourself and to alleviate stress?*

MOTIVATION

What about those of us who have a hard time making the activities that reduce stress a regular part of our lives? Sometimes, just trying to find the time to do stress-reduction activities can create even more stress. In addition, we often do things that may seem like stress reduction or taking care of ourselves in the moment, but over the long term they actual damage our health and well-being. Examples include smoking cigarettes; using drugs or alcohol; being lulled into a stupor by the television, Internet, or digital gadgets; and "shopping therapy" that overspends our budget.

How can we be motivated to participate in healthful stress-reduction practices? One definition of motivation is to impart courage, inspiration, or resolution. It takes courage to step back and take care of ourselves in skillful and health-promoting ways, in the midst of a consumer culture media frenzy that is trying to sell us so many ways to distract ourselves and escape.

This may be where courage and resolution come into play. CHWs are courageous, inspired, and resolute in so many ways. We work for the benefit of others, often through great obstacles and challenges. We must also step up and work for the benefit of ourselves. Our loved ones and our clients are depending on us to take care of ourselves so that we continue to assist them in taking care of themselves.

A friend once commented that we shouldn't wait for motivation to just happen in order to do something good for ourselves. Motivation often will result through experiencing the benefits of the practice. One of our colleagues keeps images that motivate him posted around his office. These include photographs of family, artwork made by clients, and posters of inspirational heroes.

- ✪ Where does your motivation come from?
- ✪ What does motivation mean to you?
- ✪ How can you sustain it?
- ✪ Why do you reward yourself?
- ✪ How do you choose what to use as your reward?
- ✪ How can self-care and respect be put into practice every day?

14.6 SELF-CARE

First, we'll look at some of the key areas for self-care. Then we will look in depth at one very easy and effective activity that some people engage in to reduce stress, with instructions for how to get started.

WHAT DO YOU EAT AND DRINK?

An elder once stated that food is medicine, providing you use the right ingredients and prepare it with love. This is true for many of us, and putting this into actual practice can in itself be a stress-busting activity. Food choices, recipes, and preparation vary from culture to culture. But information about how to eat "right" abounds, and it is often hard to figure out what *is* right for you and your family.

Proper nutrition is essential to good health, which can aid us in countering stressors we experience in everyday life. A useful nutritional guideline is to eat a variety of colors in your choices of fruits and vegetables daily, and to eat five to nine servings of fresh fruits and vegetables per day. Another useful guideline is to choose whole grains whenever possible and avoid processed foods that often include saturated and transfats, cholesterol, corn syrup or other added sugars, salts, or alcohol. It is also important to drink plenty of water and avoid soft drinks (often described as liquid candy), which have been recently identified as an important factor in the rise of childhood obesity and type 2 diabetes.

? *Can you make time to prepare and slowly enjoy a healthy meal this week?*

? *What will this meal consist of?*

EXERCISE

Exercise is another effective strategy to reduce stress. A regular program (in consultation with your health provider) of cardiovascular or aerobic exercise such as running, swimming, dancing, playing soccer, and many sports activities can have healthful benefits, including the alleviation of many of the physical and emotional symptoms of stress. Cardiovascular or aerobic exercise is basically vigorous exercise that gets your heart pumping. Walking or hiking can also be a great form of exercise. It is cheap and can be social, and is good exercise for people at all fitness levels. In some workplaces, people have begun holding walking meetings, or have created walking clubs that walk during the lunch hour or during breaks.

Tai Chi and yoga are examples of exercise programs that are becoming more widespread in the United States. Both are particularly good stress busters, because they include a focus on relaxation and peaceful concentration as part of the exercise itself. For both of these, initial instruction is recommended for beginners and can usually be found at your local community college, a neighborhood center, or private settings. With more advanced and ongoing instruction you may develop a deeper practice.

Tai Chi is a practice from China and is thousands of years old. The focus of Tai Chi is on concentration and simple flowing movements to balance the energy called Chi (pronounced "chee") in the body.

Yoga is a practice from India and is also thousands of years old. The focus is to encourage an individual feel whole. Yoga teachings include physical, mental, and spiritual dimensions. In the West, a yoga practice of physical poses or *asana* is the most common, and can strengthen muscles and increase flexibility, coordination, and balance. A central teaching is to simply be present and accepting of the action of the body in any given moment or pose. Yoga is not a competitive sport. A teacher once explained that progress is measured not by increasing strength or flexibility, but by the big heart of compassion for what is, right now.

?   *Do you engage in some form of exercise that allows you to relax?*

?   *How can you enhance your ability to exercise more?*

?   *Can you make time to exercise, even briefly, this week?*

PRAYER, FAITH, AND SPIRITUALITY

Although individually unique, these inner resources and practices have been shown to have a profound effect on health. Research indicates that the states of consciousness often produced by deep faith or prayer can provide permanent relief from worries and difficulties and lead to enduring physical, emotional, and mental change. Religious practices vary significantly from person to person. Some individuals attend a church, temple, mosque, or other center, while others prefer to practice independently, in community, or by communing with nature.

?   *Is prayer, faith, or spirituality an important resource in your life?*

?   *How can you enhance your ability to access these resources in ways that will serve to relieve stress?*

DEEP BREATHING AND MEDITATION

Deep Breathing   One of the most basic and effective relaxation methods is diaphragmatic breathing (deep breathing). The diaphragm is a dome-shaped muscle located between the lungs and abdominal cavity. Simply inhale deeply into the lungs while flexing the diaphragm, marked by the expansion of the abdomen rather than the chest. Usually individuals inhale slowly through the nose until the lungs are filled and follow by slowly exhaling through pursed lips to regulate the release of air. Practicing diaphragmatic breathing for five to ten minutes for three or four times a day may significantly reduce your level of stress.

Meditation   Meditation generally involves a state of concentrated attention or mindfulness, directed to a single focus. Often, meditation will use the breath as the point of focus. Whereas with diaphragmatic breathing, you control and direct your breathing in specific ways, in meditation you simply observe it.

There are different forms of meditation. Many, though not all, are associated with spiritual and religious practices. Almost all cultures have some set of practices that assist people to develop awareness of the present moment. In many traditions meditation can become a life-changing experience, going very deep. At the same time, learning to practice simple meditation techniques, and doing so for even five minutes a day, can aid in reducing stress on a day-to-day basis. Meditation is used to quiet the mind and calm the body. It eases some of the symptoms of stress, such as the racing heart or relentless thoughts about a stressful event. It creates some breathing room, some distance and perspective on the situation.

Research has now shown that meditation offers powerful benefits. It has been used effectively even with patients who are critically ill, and has aided in reducing their anxiety and the experience of suffering in their illnesses. Being mindfully aware, and focusing on present here-and-now experiences, says Daniel Siegel, M.D., codirector of the UCLA Mindful Awareness Research Center, results in demonstrated improvements in physiology, mental functions, and interpersonal relationships. Mindful awareness can promote healing and immune response, as well as a sense of general well-being. The effects of mindful awareness may even "directly shape the activity and growth of the parts of the brain responsible for our relationships, our emotional life, and our physiological response to stress" (Seigel, 2007). Dr. Siegel describes meditation, more poetically, as "a journey into the heart of our lives."

STRESS REDUCTION BY PROFESSIONALS

There are a wide range of professional services that are helpful in managing stress and preventing burnout. These include, for example:

Massage is the systematic and intentional manipulation of soft body tissue and may include joint movements and stretching. The goal is to assist the body to achieve well-being while alleviating distress and specific disease-related symptoms. Different systems of massage include Swedish, deep tissue, neuromuscular, Chinese, Indian, Thai, Japanese, Indigenous American, and Caribbean (such as *Sobadoras)*. Practitioners usually use their hands to apply fixed and movable pressure to the body.

Acupuncture works by correcting the balance of energy known as *Qi* (pronounced "chee"). It involves inserting hair-fine needles into specific anatomic points in the body to stimulate the flow of energy. Practitioners also apply pressure, suction, electromagnetic stimulation, or heat to the acupuncture points.

Coaching and psychotherapy are overlapping models. Coaching generally focuses on the here and now, problem solving, and assisting individuals in developing new skills to cope and adjust to present life situations. Psychotherapy focuses on evaluating, diagnosing, and treating emotional problems and severe psychological conditions. Although talking about your sense of distress with a friend, family member, or peer may be effective, seeking professional support is recommended if the level of stress becomes high and ongoing. Professional support is also particularly valuable if you are experiencing post-traumatic stress.

Sweat lodges and temexcales are sacred and spiritual healing spaces created and utilized by the indigenous peoples of North and South America, respectively. The lodge or *temexcal* is often seen as a womb that gives birth and life, and also serves for communing with the Creator. The sweat lodge ceremony is complex and traditionally led by an experienced elder. The etiquette varies according to the lodge leader and may include singing, chanting, and drumming, all of which is considered prayer. The lodge ceremony provides cleansing of the spirit, heart, mind, and body, and has been successful in treating certain conditions.

?   *Can you think of other professional services and traditions that may be helpful in reducing stress?*

14.7 A MEDITATION PRACTICE

Though meditation traditions use a variety of things as their focus for meditation, a good place to start is simply to focus on your breath. Breathing is always happening; our breath is always present and available to us as a point of concentration. It is always changing, allowing our attention to become ever more subtle to enable us to follow the tiny changes in sensation of the breath. This attention to sensations takes us away from the ever-present verbal chatter in the mind, our own internal dialog. Any time we notice we are distracted by thought, feelings, or emotions we can, simply and without any judgment, note what has distracted us, and gently allow our awareness to return to the breath.

Through this process of focusing the attention, meditation quiets the mind. And as we concentrate, we experience how our mind continually shifts from thought to thought, sensation to sensation, memory to memory, and plan to plan. Remember, our neurobiology is wired to notice what is around us and figure out if it represents a threat to our safety or survival. Thus, it takes a good deal of patience, commitment, and a heart full of loving kindness for yourself as you continue on this path of practice. An important way to be kind to yourself in developing a mediation practice is to start with what you can do consistently right now. Five minutes a day, every day is great. You can gradually increase your time in meditation as your interest and situation allow. By doing an Internet search for "meditation," you will be able to find many resources and local centers and teachers for support and community.

Here are instructions for a simple sitting meditation. If you choose to give it a try, set aside at least twenty minutes.

LEE JACKSON: I'm spiritually grounded. To me that's number one. That's the key in my life. I don't push it off on anyone else, but that's what works for me: a firm belief in a supreme being or a force greater than me that's a power unseen. That's God to me.

A SITTING MEDITATION

LET YOUR MIND SETTLE LIKE A CLEAR FOREST POOL

To begin this meditation, select a quiet time and place. Be on a cushion or chair, taking an upright yet relaxed posture. Let yourself sit with quiet dignity. Close your eyes gently and begin by bringing a full, present attention to whatever you feel within you and around you. Let your mind be spacious and your heart be kind and soft.

As you sit, feel the sensations of your body. Then notice what sounds and feelings, thoughts and expectations are present. Allow them all to come and go, rise and fall like the waves of the ocean. Be aware of the waves and rest seated in the midst of them. Allow yourself to become more and more still.

In the center of all these waves, feel your breathing, your life-breath. Let your attention feel the in-and-out breathing wherever you notice it, as coolness or tingling in the nose or throat, as a rising or falling of your chest or abdomen. Relax and softly rest your attention on each breath, feeling the movement in a steady easy way. Let the breath breathe itself in any rhythm, long or short, soft or deep. As you feel each breath, concentrate and settle into each movement. Let all other sounds and sensations, thoughts and feelings continue to come and go like waves in the background.

After a few breaths, your attention may be carried away by one of the waves of thoughts or memories, by body sensations or sounds. Whenever you notice you have been carried away for a time, acknowledge the wave that has done so by softly giving it a name such as "planning," "remembering," "itching," "restless." Then let it pass and gently return to the breath. Sometimes waves will take a long time to pass, others will be short. Certain thoughts or feelings will be painful, others will be pleasurable. Whatever they are, let them be.

At some sittings you will be able to return to your breath easily. At other times in your meditation you will mostly be aware of body sensations or of thoughts and plans. Either way is fine. No matter what you experience, be aware of it, let it come and go, and rest at ease in the midst of it all. After you have sat for twenty or thirty minutes in this way, open your eyes and look around before you get up. Then as you move try to allow the same spirit of awareness or mindfulness to go with you into the activities of your day.

The art of meditation is simple but not always easy. It thrives on practice and a kind and spacious heart. If you do this simple practice of sitting with mindfulness or awareness every day, you will gradually grow in centeredness and understanding.

Source: Kornfield, 1994. Additional meditations on walking, eating, loving-kindness, and forgiveness are also presented in this book

CHAPTER REVIEW

DEVELOP YOUR SELF-CARE ACTION PLAN

Please consider developing a simple plan for self-care. Write down your answers to the following questions and keep the page in a place where you can easily refer to it in the future.

1. Two ways that stress is currently affecting me that I want to change are:_____
2. The reasons why I want to address and handle this stress effectively include:_____
3. Three realistic actions or steps that I can take to help relieve stress and take better care of myself are:
   a. What I will do, when I will begin, and how frequently I will do it:_____
   b. What I will do, when I will begin, and how frequently I will do it:_____
   c. What I will do, when I will begin, and how frequently I will do it:_____

4. Internal resources (my personal qualities, strengths, knowledge, and skills) that will assist me to achieve my self-care action plan include:_____
5. External resources and sources of support that will assist me to achieve my self-care action plan include:_____
6. A professional colleague (such as a classmate or other CHW) whom I will talk with about my self-care action plan is: _____.
7. A meaningful source of motivation that will assist me to achieve my plan is:_____
8. Something productive and positive that I will do if I face challenges or set-backs in implementing my self-care action plan is:_____

Signature: _____

Date: _____

REFERENCES

Herman, J. 1997. *Trauma and Recovery: The Aftermath of Violence from Domestic Abuse to Political Terror.* New York: Basic Books.

International Training and Education Center on HIV (I-TECH) and the Ministry of Health and Child Welfare, Zimbabwe. 2005. Integrated Counselling for HIV and AIDS Prevention and Care: Training for

HIV Primary Care Counsellors. Unpublished training manual.

Kornfield, J. 1994. *Buddha's Little Instruction Book.* New York: Bantam Books.

Seigel, D. 2007. *The Mindful Brain: Reflection and Attunement in the Cultivation of Well-Being.* New York: W.W. Norton.

ADDITIONAL RESOURCES

City College of San Francisco. Trauma Prevention and Recovery Certificate, Interdisciplinary Studies Department. Accessed on April 9, 2009: http://www.ccsf.edu/departments

International Society for Traumatic Stress Studies. Accessed on April 9, 2009: http://www.istss.org/resources/index.cfm

Perry, B. 2003. *The Cost of Caring: Secondary Traumatic Stress and the Impact of Working with High-Risk Children and Families.* Booklet published by The Child Trauma Academy, for parents, teachers, and various professionals working with traumatized children.

Accessed on March 28, 2009: http://www.childtrauma.org/ctamaterials/SecTrma2_03_v2.pdf

Sidran Foundation: Traumatic Stress Education and Advocacy. Accessed on April 9, 2009: http://www.sidran.org/

University of California, Los Angeles, Mindful Awareness Research Center. Accessed on April 9, 2009: http://marc.ucla.edu/

Van Dernoot Lipsky, L., with Burk, C. 2007. *Trauma Stewardship: An Everyday Guide to Caring for Self While Caring for Others.* Seattle: Las Olas Press.

15

Professional Skills: Getting a Job, Keeping a Job, and Growing on the Job

Amber Straus • Rhonella C. Owens • Tim Berthold • Jeni Miller

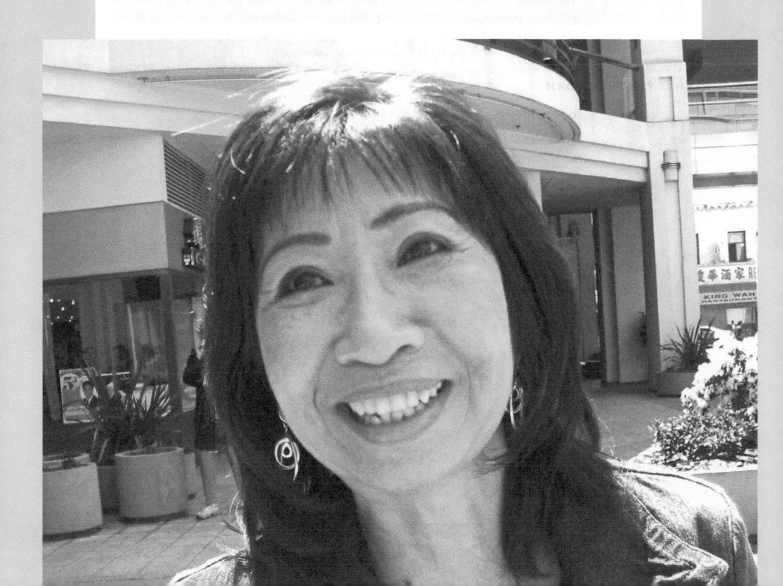

CASE STUDY: NORMA

Norma has worked for five years as a CHW at a large nonprofit agency that provides services to girls and women. Norma is highly respected by coworkers and by the clients and communities she serves. Six months ago, Norma was honored as Outreach Worker of the Year at an agency fundraiser.

Recently, Norma applied for a job at her agency as the supervisor of a team of six CHWs. Norma was not offered the position: a younger woman with much less experience and a college degree was hired. Norma met the other candidate on the day of their interviews. Norma was dressed as she does everyday to conduct outreach and brought flip-chart paper to make a presentation to the hiring committee. The woman who was hired wore a suit and brought a laptop computer to make a PowerPoint presentation.

When Norma asked the executive director why she wasn't promoted, she was told to work on her professional skills, including the way that she presents herself, and her written communication skills.

INTRODUCTION

This chapter addresses professional skills designed to better enable you to get a job or volunteer position as a CHW, to keep that position, and to advance in your career. These skills will also assist you to be more effective in your efforts to promote and to advocate for the health of the clients and communities you work with.

WHAT YOU WILL LEARN

By studying the information in this chapter, you will be able to:

- ✪ Discuss the meaning and challenges of code switching
- ✪ Develop a professional résumé
- ✪ Prepare for a job interview
- ✪ Identify dress codes at your internship site or workplace
- ✪ Discuss the challenge of establishing healthy professional boundaries and making sound choices regarding disclosure of personal information
- ✪ Identify and practice verbal and written communication skills relevant for CHWs, including giving and receiving feedback in a professional manner
- ✪ Apply time management skills to your life, study, and work
- ✪ Develop life and professional goals, including a plan for professional development

WORDS TO KNOW

Code Switching   Résumé   Supportive and Corrective Feedback

15.1 WHY THIS CHAPTER IS IMPORTANT FOR CHWs

All workplaces have written or unwritten codes of conduct that guide proper dress, time management, professional boundaries, written communication, and giving and receiving critical feedback. Adapting to the professional environment and codes of conduct at work can be challenging. This challenge is sometimes called **code switching** (or moving between one or more sets of expectations and guidelines for conduct or behavior). There are different codes of conduct—rules of the road—for different contexts, communities, cultures, and employment settings. The codes that we learn from our families and in our communities are sometimes different from what employers expect. When we move from the community to the workplace, we may not understand the new codes of conduct and why they matter. As a consequence, like Norma, we may miss out on opportunities for employment or promotion.

Most of us have had some experience with code switching, though we probably didn't think of it in these terms. We may act or speak differently with our family and friends, at school, at work, or in church or other spiritual places.

? *Can you think of places where you switch codes?*

? *Have you ever been in a new environment and not known what the codes of conduct or rules of the road were? What was this like?*

? *How did you begin to identify and adapt to the new codes of conduct?*

Professional codes are sometimes arbitrary, and may discriminate against people with different cultural or educational backgrounds, or who speak differently from those in authority. Some people find the very concept of code switching problematic: they don't feel that they should have to change the way they dress or speak or manage their time in order to be fully recognized and valued in the workplace. The decision about whether or not you will switch codes to adapt to a professional setting is up to you. We would rather that you had an opportunity to make an informed choice about code switching, however, instead of losing job opportunities for failing to meet a professional standard that you didn't know existed.

ALVARO MORALES: I had to learn that there were different ways for me to dress and to talk—different words to use—when I was conducting street outreach versus counseling in the clinic versus making a presentation to the City Council. Sometimes I dressed up—even though I'm not really all that used to wearing a suit or tie—so that my message would be better heard by a professional audience. And I would use different kinds of language to talk about the same things—like sexual behaviors—with my supervisor versus my clients, or adults versus youths. It is kind of a balancing act—switching between different cultures without losing who you are. As an immigrant to the United States, I'm used to that kind of balancing act—I have to do it all the time.

In some work settings, as you become a trusted and respected colleague, you may be able to advocate for a broader definition of professional dress or speech, one that honors the formality of a professional setting yet is more inclusive of cultural differences.

This may be a part of assisting your agency to practice cultural humility and enabling it to become a place that is more welcoming and comfortable for the diverse communities it serves.

Code switching is also important to your clients. They may not know about, want to, or be able to follow the codes of conduct at the various agencies and institutions they turn to for assistance with legal, medical, public benefits, housing, or social services. Unfortunately, the professionals in these agencies sometimes judge or discriminate against clients who do not adapt to their codes of conduct. We hope that as CHWs, you will always do your best to make clients feel welcomed and respected regardless of their identity, background, desire, or ability to "switch codes."

15.2 GETTING A JOB

Getting a job requires three key steps:

1. Finding out about available jobs
2. Applying for jobs
3. Interviewing for jobs

FINDING JOB OPPORTUNITIES

There are many ways to find out about jobs in your community:

- Search online job sites on your own or with the help of a career counselor (generally available for free at a community-based or community college career center)
- Look at the Web sites of employers in your community for job openings, including local health departments (or departments of public health)
- Visit or call up agencies that you are interested in working for to see if and when they may have job openings
- Ask CHWs or other public health providers if they are aware of any openings in their own or other organizations

A common practice in the professional world is the "informational interview." You can request an informational interview at an organization, even when they don't have a job listed. At an informational interview, you ask questions about the organization, the type of work they do, and the roles and work of the CHWs and others who work there. Informational interviews are good ways to get to know the agencies and organizations in your area, and to develop relationships with people who can keep you informed about jobs when they arise.

Once you hear of a job opening, request the job description and read it carefully to learn whether this is an opportunity you are truly interested in and qualified for. Job descriptions also provide information to guide you in writing your application, including which experience and skills to highlight.

? *If you were interested in the job as a CHW with the Maternity Care Coalition, which of your skills and work or life experiences would you highlight in your application?*

SAMPLE JOB DESCRIPTION

Community Health Worker position with the Cribs for Kids program to conduct community education and outreach to pregnant and parenting families with a focus on reducing risks for Sudden Infant Death Syndrome (SIDS). Duties include conducting home visits to promote safe sleep, and facilitating educational workshops in the community. Qualified candidates will have knowledge about community resources; an interest in maternal and child health; excellent communication, organizational, and computer skills; and the ability to work effectively with people from diverse backgrounds.

Additional Qualifications:

Spanish speaking preferred. High school diploma or GED required.

How to Apply:

Send cover letter, résumé, and the names and contact information of three professional references to Human Resources, Maternity Care Coalition, 3000 Hamilton St., Suite 505, Philadelphia, PA 19130. Email: hr@momscare.org. Fax: 215-982-8266.

APPLYING FOR JOBS: APPLICATIONS, COVER LETTERS, RÉSUMÉS, AND REFERENCES

Applications   For most jobs, you will be asked to fill out an application. The employer will review all applications received. You want yours to stand out in a positive way. If possible, type the application, or fill it out on a computer. If the application can only be filled out by hand, use a black or blue pen and fill out the application neatly. Check your résumé to correct any spelling or grammatical errors.

Some job applications ask you if you are a U.S. citizen and if you have ever been convicted of a crime. It is important to answer these questions truthfully. Citizenship or permanent resident status may not be a requirement, and the agency may distinguish between misdemeanor and felony convictions, between long-past and recent convictions, and understand concepts of recovery and rehabilitation.

Cover Letter   You should include a cover letter with every job application. The letter should be simple and include your contact information at the top, the date, the person to whom you are submitting the application (by name if possible), and a formal salutation (Dear Mr. Jones:). In a couple of brief sentences, identify the job you are applying for (its exact title and job number if there is one), how you learned about the job, and why you are qualified for the position.

Résumés   When you apply for a job, employers will usually ask to see a résumé, a formal document listing your work experience and education. The goal of a résumé is to engage a potential employer's interest at a glance.

Your résumé makes a first impression; it is key to getting the job you want. Your local library, community college, or employment development department may hold free résumé writing classes. You can also review sample résumés on the Internet and in books at your local library.

Résumés follow standard style guidelines, although there are a variety of accepted styles. Take a look at the sample résumé below. Notice the order of the words, the

SAMPLE COVER LETTER

Jane Q. Doe
P.O. Box 14567
Centerville, PA, 19876

February 9, 2009

Mr. John P. Jones
Human Resources
Maternity Care Coalition
3000 Hamilton St., Suite 505
Philadelphia, PA 19130

Dear Mr. Jones:

Attached please find my résumé and application for the job of Community Health Worker with the Cribs for Kids program, listed on the Coalition's Web site on January 31. I am a certified and bilingual (English/Spanish) child care worker with years of experience working with diverse children and families. This position would be an excellent opportunity for me to use my experience and skills to serve my community.

Thank you for your attention to my application. My résumé includes three references who can tell you about my qualifications.

Sincerely,

Jane Q. Doe

Attached: application; résumé

---

type of information the applicant provides, and how easy she makes it for potential employers to:

- Find the applicant's experiences
- Review the applicant's skills
- Know exactly where to call or e-mail the applicant to discuss the job

Writing a Résumé   There are a number of ways to organize a résumé, as you will see if you look for samples online, at the library, or in a career counselor's office. One example of a résumé is shown in Figure 15.1. However you organize your résumé, it should include the following information, on one to two pages, organized in a way that is easy to read at a glance.

Name and contact information: Your name and up-to-date contact information should be at the top of the résumé. Make sure that all of your contact information is current, including your mailing and e-mail address and phone number. If you do not have a reliable phone with voice mail, you may provide only an e-mail address. Make sure your e-mail address is appropriate to share with a potential employer.

Education: List your education and training, beginning with your current or most recent educational experiences. Be sure to list any certificates, degrees, scholarships, or honors.

Experience: Summarize your qualifications and work experience. List paid and unpaid work, including internships. Start with the most recent experience and go back in time. Include the name of the company or organization, the city where it is located, your job title, and the dates you worked. Don't use any acronyms in your résumé, such as the initials used

Figure 15.1 Sample Résumé.

Cassie Adanya
409 Landover St.
New Orleans, LA 70183
(614) 852-5555
cassieadanya@email.com

OBJECTIVE

Seeking a position as a Community Health Worker that will use my skills in working with diverse children and their families.

QUALIFICATIONS AND ACHIEVEMENTS

- Community Health Worker Certificate
- First Aid and CPR certified
- Volunteer, New Orleans Regional YMCA Youth Summer Camp
- Special Olympics Volunteer
- Food Pantry Volunteer, First Methodist Church

EXPERIENCE

New Orleans Safe House, New Orleans, LA

Counselor and Program Coordinator, June 2000 to Present

Work with developmentally disabled children ages 6–12. Facilitate small group activities and provide individual counseling as required. Coordinate the Safe House summer camp program. Organize daily activities, and supervise a staff of three.

Jubilee Camp, Elbert, LA

Assistant Teacher, August 1998 to June 2000

Provided daycare for infants and children ages 0 to 36 months. Responsible for creating and implementing a daily activity plan and facilitating small groups of three to six children.

EDUCATION

Carlton Community College, New Orleans, LA
Community Health Worker Certificate 1998
Ceader Cliff High School, New Orleans, LA
Graduated, 1996

REFERENCES

Cindy Young, Director, New Orleans Safe House
(123) 456-7890

Albert Williamson, Director, Jubilee Camp
(234) 567-8901

Lorena Martinez, Instructor, CHW Certificate Program, Carlton Community College
(345) 678-9012

for an agency or coalition instead of the full name of that agency or coalition. List your professional responsibilities, the skills you used on the job, and your key accomplishments. Use positive action words.

Always be 100 percent truthful about the information you include on your résumé. Any inaccurate statements may be cause for termination and could seriously damage your reputation in the community.

Action Words—When you list your experiences, use action words to explain your responsibilities and accomplishments. These words show an employer the skills you have to offer. Be sure to use the past tense for past experiences and the present tense for your current work. Describe briefly how you **led, demonstrated, coordinated, accomplished, created, managed, organized, repaired** . . . you get the idea.

"I don't have any work experience! What do I put on my résumé?"

Even if you have never had a 9 to 5 job, you have had life experiences and had an impact on the world around you. Focus on what you have learned by working in your community or family, and use action words to present your skills to employers.

References   On your résumé or in your cover letter, list at least three people who can tell a potential employer about your qualifications for the job. If your present employer knows you are looking for a job and can be expected to give you a good reference, that should be the first reference you list. Teachers, ministers, and other community leaders are also good references; family members are not. Ask potential reference candidates if they would be willing to provide a reference, and tell them about the job you are applying for so they can be as helpful as possible when they talk about your strengths and skills. You can also ask them if they will write you a letter of reference for CHW jobs. You can include copies of these letters of reference with your résumé and application, or bring them with you to interviews.

?   *Who will you ask to be your references?*

?   *Which of your skills, personal qualities, and experience will they be able to talk about with potential employers?*

?   *How are these relevant to employment as a CHW?*

INTERVIEWING FOR A JOB, INTERNSHIP, OR VOLUNTEER POSITION

You sent in your application with a cover letter and a résumé, and you've been called for an interview. Now what do you do? Relax; interviewing is a skill. It can be practiced and learned.

Job interviews are about finding out whether there is a good 'fit' between the interviewee, the job, and the agency. The interviewer asks questions to learn whether you would be the best employee for the position they are trying to fill. You can also ask questions to see whether this organization is one that you would like to work for. In other words, they are interviewing you, but you are also interviewing them. If you know how to conduct a good client interview, you can learn to do a good job interview.

Preparing for the Interview   *Know the agency.* Learn as much as you can about the agency you are applying to. You can often find out much of what you want to know from an organization's Web site:

- What is their mission statement?
- Which communities do they serve?
- What services do they provide?
- What have they accomplished?

Practice interviewing with a career counselor or friend. We encourage you to practice or rehearse what you will say in the interview. You might do this with a trusted friend or family member, a colleague or classmate, or a professional at a local employment or career counseling center.

Practice responding to common interview questions such as:

- Why are you interested in this position?
- Please describe your qualifications for this position.
- What experiences have prepared you for this position?
- Why are you considering changing jobs?
- Please describe your educational background and accomplishments.
- Why are you the best candidate for this position?
- What are your greatest accomplishments or successes?
- What are your greatest strengths? Your greatest weaknesses?

Ask for feedback from your friend or colleague, and consider how you might improve or clarify your responses to these interview questions. Be prepared to address or explain gaps in employment history and reasons for leaving previous jobs.

What to take with you to the interview:

- Copies of your résumé, a list of professional references or letters of recommendation
- Driver's license or other form of identification

Dressing for the interview. Dress in a professional manner, and more formally than you will on the job. A suit, or suit jacket over slacks or a skirt is almost always considered appropriate for an interview, even for places with a much more casual daily work culture. Don't wear jeans, T-shirts, shorts, or other casual clothes.

Greet all of the people who are interviewing you. Speak slowly and clearly, and look your interviewer in the eye often. Prepare questions to ask about the job and agency during the interview. Use the interview to find out how you could fit into the organization and as an opportunity to share your skills with a potential employer.

What Employers are Looking for

- Skills and abilities that fit the job
- Good communication skills and the ability to answer all questions satisfactorily
- Interest in the agency and the position
- Enthusiasm
- Confidence
- Neat and appropriate appearance

The Interview Itself   The interviewer will generally break the ice and make an introduction. He or she may ask for general information about you, your background, or your
goals, such as:

- ✪ "Tell me about yourself."
- ✪ "Why are you interested in our organization?"
- ✪ "What are your goals for the next year? Next five years?"
- ✪ "Why did you enter this field?"

Then the interviewer will probably share general information about the organization
and the job position before asking you specific questions.

Strategies for responding effectively to interview questions:

1. Listen carefully to the question and answer it as specifically as possible.
2. Ask clarifying questions when necessary.
3. Speak clearly, but don't talk too much, for too long. Try not to repeat yourself.
   Interviewers don't want candidates to take up too much of their time.
4. Focus on the job you are applying for.
5. Present yourself and your skills, abilities, and qualifications clearly and show how
   you are a match for the job.
6. Discuss your goals—immediate and future.
7. Focus on your accomplishments and successes.
8. Answer questions in a way that supports your strengths (don't answer with "yes" or
   "no" remarks, but state your strengths).
9. Clearly demonstrate your interest in the position.
10. Don't forget to be yourself!

When you get nervous, reduce stress through deep breathing. Engage the interviewer.
Instead of seeing the interview as an exam you must pass, try to view it as a conversation in which you have valuable information to share with the employer, and they have
valuable information about their organization to share with you. Ask your interviewer
questions: "Please describe a typical day in this position." "What communities does your
agency serve?" "What do you like best about working here?"

Closing   This is a time to ask any remaining questions that you may have but, again, be
conscious of time and don't ask too many. These questions might include, for example: "Is
there anything else I can tell you about my qualifications or experience?" "I have copies of
my letters of recommendation. May I leave them with you?" "When may I expect to hear
from you?"

Remember to thank the interviewer for the opportunity to meet with them.

After the Interview   Reflect upon and evaluate your performance. What did you do
well? How might you improve your performance in future interviews?

Thank the interviewer in a follow-up letter or e-mail:

- ✪ State your interest in the position again
- ✪ Summarize how you qualify for the position
- ✪ Include any additional pertinent information you may have forgotten to discuss during
  the interview

15.3 KEEPING THE JOB

Keeping your position as a CHW will depend to great extent on your interpersonal skills. The most important part of your job is how you interact with clients. You will also interact with peers in your workplace, with your supervisor, and with your colleagues in other agencies, clinics, or organizations, and with the general public—the community. And, depending on the work you are doing, you may interact with public officials and policymakers. In addition to the other skills you are learning, mastering the skills that follow will guide you in making the best impression and inspire trust and confidence from the people your agency serves.

DRESS CODE: WHAT YOU WEAR MATTERS

What people wear is like a language. It is often the first information that someone you meet in person has about who you are. The doctor's white coat, the mechanic's overalls, and the team uniform are obvious examples of clothing that communicate to others something important about who someone is or what they do. You dress up for a job interview as a signal to a potential employer that you understand the codes of the professional world. Codes are cultural, too: someone's ethnic, national, or religious background may influence what they wear and how they perceive what you wear. Before getting dressed for your interview or workday, ask yourself how others might see you.

Phuong An Doan Billings: For the Vietnamese community, our culture is very formal. I have to wear my best clothes when I go out to the community. To me it's very natural. That's the way we are. As a teacher in Vietnam, I had to stand in front of a few hundred students every day. Before I left the house, I always had to dress up, even going to the market, because I might meet my students there.

When you work with the community, you have to know how to present yourself. I don't dare to go out to do presentations if I don't have on good clothes. If I didn't dress formally, they wouldn't listen to me. I have to be formal and in a style appropriate to my age and my status.

If I have some staff that I feel do not dress appropriately, we talk about it. I say to them, "You know, this is how our community is. We are formal. That's the reality we have to accept."

The dress code at your job may be different from the dress codes in the community you are working with. When you work in the community, consider these questions about what you wear:

- Will it put my clients at ease? Will it put them off or alienate them?
- Will it show respect to the community I'm working with?
- Will it give people the confidence that I have the skills and knowledge to assist them?

In most of the situations you will face at work, a helpful guideline is to dress a half to one step above how your clients dress. Wearing jeans and T-shirts may not be appropriate, but if your clients typically dress in jeans and T-shirts, dressing a half to one step above their clothing may translate into you wearing khakis or cotton dress pants and a button-down

Some work situations require more formal dress. Lee Jackson prepares to attend a court hearing with a client.

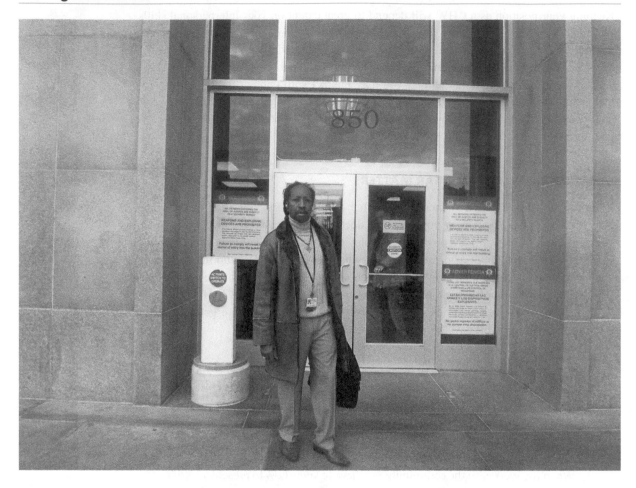

shirt, polo-style shirt, or a sweater. As we saw above, however, some communities may expect you to dress much more formally as a sign of respect or to gain their confidence.

As a CHW, how would you dress to meet with the following groups?

- ✪ Homeless youths
- ✪ Program managers and the board of directors
- ✪ The women's auxiliary at the local mosque

In order to for you and your work to be taken seriously, you may need to alter your appearance to fit the context (for example wearing a jacket, dress, or tie to talk with the local Health Commission). These adjustments may assist people to focus on your message, rather than getting distracted by what they think about your appearance.

VERBAL COMMUNICATION AND BODY LANGUAGE

How you present yourself verbally and through body language makes a difference in how people hear you.

Do you stay focused on the topic when others are speaking, asking clarifying questions? Is your voice friendly, assertive, and clear? Do you find yourself telling people what to do? How loudly are you speaking?

Do you stand or sit very close or far away from others? Do you fail to engage in eye contact or insist upon it? When others speak, do you cross your arms, frown, or roll your eyes? How might these or other types of body language be perceived by others?

Some types of communication are not welcome in the workplace:

○ Sexist, racist, or homophobic language is never appropriate. It is illegal and could get you fired.
○ Profane language. You should never use curse words under any circumstances. Some words might not be curse words, but are still rude or distasteful.
○ Talking or gossiping about your coworkers or supervisors negatively is unacceptable. Use the appropriate outlets to get your concerns heard constructively. See the section of giving and receiving critical feedback below.
○ Repeating the same information over and over, constantly interrupting others, or taking time away from a common agenda to talk about other topics can be perceived by others as rude or disrespectful.

Talking on the Telephone　　You will probably spend a lot of time on the phone, contacting clients about their appointments, talking with representatives from other agencies who can provide services for your clients, or contacting local businesses to ask for donations or support for events in your community.

Here are some tips for professional phone calls:

1. Start with a friendly, time-appropriate greeting such as "Good morning."
2. Identify yourself and your agency.
3. State the reason for your call, and ask whether it is a good time to talk, giving an indication of how long the call might be.
4. Write down any key information that other callers provide you, such as names and phone numbers, and read them back to make sure they are accurate.
5. If you will need to call again, say so and ask when you might do so.
6. End the call with "thank you" and "good-bye."

If you leave a message:

1. Begin with a greeting such as "Good morning" or "Good afternoon" followed by the person's name. Deliver these words in a friendly voice.
2. Follow the greeting by identifying yourself and your agency.
3. Briefly state the reason for your call.
4. Repeat your name and give your phone number again.
5. End the call with "thank you" and "good-bye."

Preserve confidentiality. Do not leave any sensitive or confidential information in a message.

Cell Phones and Other Digital Technology　　Receiving cell phone calls or text messages can be both distracting and inappropriate in the workplace. Be sure that your digital technology is turned off during meetings and do not check digital technology while talking to others (checking for text messages makes you seem distracted and uninterested).

Be aware of your surroundings. If you are working in the community and need to make a call concerning a client, find an appropriate place to speak quietly on the phone without disclosing confidential information in public.

CHWs do a lot of their work by phone.

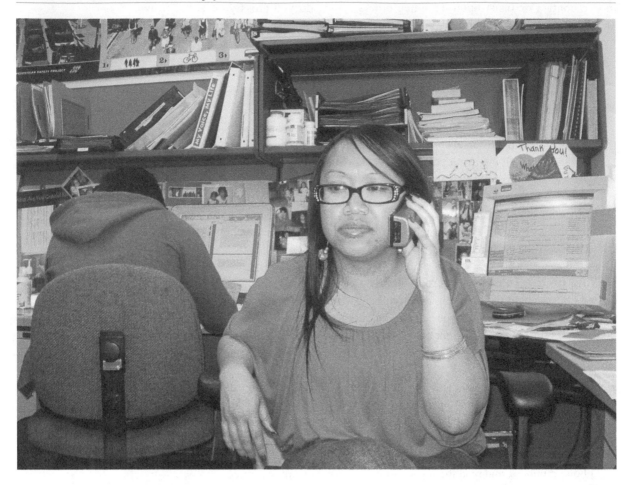

Written Communication   How well you write makes a lasting impression on the people who receive your written communications. Written communications pose particular code-switching challenges. The emphasis in school on spelling, punctuation, and grammar was basically teaching you a "professional" (white, middle-class, English-speaking) code. The way we were taught, and the way that we were judged, can leave us feeling inadequate and intimidated when we have to write letters, memos, e-mails, and reports.

If you know that written English is a particular challenge for you, consider an adult education class at your high school or community college. Here are some commonsense tips to make your written communications reflect your skills as a successful CHW.

Why are you writing? Depending upon the length and scope of what you write, you may want to jot down a brief outline of what you really want to say before writing. What are your main points? Think of questions your reader may have, and answer them.

Put yourself in your reader's place. Read your message aloud. How would you feel reading this letter or e-mail? Remember: once it has been sent, you cannot take it back. Is your message short, clear, and easy to read? Is there any slang that may not be understood by everyone or may not be appropriate? Is the information accurate? Did you double-check your facts? Is your tone professional and courteous?

Use a simple structure. Start with an introduction. Give the details. Summarize or conclude.

Use clear language. Don't use too many abbreviations, acronyms, or jargon used only at your agency or only in your profession. Keep the language simple and at a level you know all people will understand.

Spell-check is your friend. When you have completed the message, be sure to use spell-check on your computer before you send it.

E-mail   Increasingly, professional communication is conducted by e-mail. Because it is so easy to write and send, we can be tempted to think of e-mail as less formal or less important than mail that's printed out on paper. *E-mail is professional communication just like any other form of written communication.* Everything about written communication above applies to e-mail, and there are a few tips that apply to e-mail in particular.

Subject line. The subject line is like the headline of a news story. Be sure that what you write in the subject line is short and accurate. Some busy people will not open e-mail if the subject line doesn't grab their attention.

Replying. Sometimes you will get an e-mail that is addressed to an entire group of people. Be careful to reply only to the sender of the message; it is unprofessional to reply to everyone unless you have a clear reason for doing so.

Don't hit the send button when you're mad! We've all done it; someone sends you an e-mail message that upsets you, and you respond from your anger. If you're upset, don't send the e-mail: wait until you are in a calmer state and can think more clearly about the potential impact. You might want to check out some of the conflict resolution tips in Chapter Thirteen.

GIVING AND RECEIVING CRITICAL FEEDBACK

It isn't always easy to receive critical feedback from clients, peers, or supervisors calmly and professionally, or to provide critical feedback to others in a way that is most likely to aid them to improve their performance. Most professional settings will provide feedback in the form of an annual performance review or evaluation for employees. The inability to receive or provide critical feedback in a professional manner is one of the primary reasons that CHWs are disciplined, denied a promotion, or terminated (fired) from a job.

Feedback may be supportive or corrective. **Supportive feedback** reinforces current behavior by identifying what is being done well or right. **Corrective feedback** indicates desired changes in behavior, by explaining what didn't work, was wrong, went badly, or needs improvement. In both cases, the goal should be to improve performance and effectiveness.

We encourage you to consider feedback as a gift, even if it is hard to hear, because honest feedback and guidance from others can assist us in learning how to provide better services to the clients and communities we work with.

Guidelines for Giving and Receiving Feedback   We will share brief guidelines here for giving and receiving critical feedback. We also encourage you to seek out professional development opportunities to enhance your skills, and to learn from experienced and respected colleagues. The information provided in Chapter Thirteen on conflict resolution is also highly relevant.

Giving Feedback   When providing others with feedback, we recommend the "love sandwich" approach. Basically, this means sandwiching corrective feedback between substantive supportive feedback. In other words, start and end your conversation by sharing positive feedback with your colleague. Everyone we work with has strengths. Let them know you what you appreciate about their attitude, knowledge, skills, and contributions.

Other guidelines include:

- ⊛ Don't provide feedback when you are feeling angry or unable to focus on supporting your colleague.
- ⊛ Speak in a respectful tone of voice.
- ⊛ Provide detailed and specific feedback (what, where, when) about the person's behavior or conduct. What did they do—or not do—that you want to draw to their attention to?
- ⊛ Explain what you think the impact of these behaviors may be on others, including yourself and the clients.
- ⊛ Provide realistic suggestions for what your colleague could do differently the next time they face a similar situation. Refer to your agency or program standards, goals, or policies.
- ⊛ Don't hold back on important corrective feedback. When we do this, we deprive a colleague of the opportunity to learn how to enhance their skills and performance.
- ⊛ Feedback should be timely: share it in the moment it occurs or as soon afterward as possible.
- ⊛ Invite the person or group to ask questions to clarify the feedback you provide and to respond.
- ⊛ Invite your colleague to talk with you and to identify concrete steps they can take to improve their skills and performance.
- ⊛ Whether the person agrees or doesn't agree with the feedback you provide, express your appreciation for their listening to you.

? *What else would you want to do when providing critical feedback to a colleague?*

Receiving Feedback

- ⊛ Actively listen to the person's description of your behavior and recommendations, including suggested changes. Although it may sound easy, this takes practice.
- ⊛ Ask questions to clarify the feedback your colleague is providing: you want to understand what they are sharing with you. If the feedback is vague or unclear, ask them to provide you with specific examples.
- ⊛ Paraphrase or summarize the feedback to make sure you have heard it correctly.
- ⊛ Notice if you are feeling defensive. Don't react in the moment with anger, or try to defend yourself, especially if the person providing the feedback is a client, your supervisor, or another leader at your agency or in the community.
- ⊛ Listen and strive to understand. Trust that the intent of the feedback is to enable you to enhance your skills and performance as a CHW.
- ⊛ Ask for a break if you need one, and only return to the conversation when you are truly prepared to listen to what your colleague has to say. Vent any strong emotions later, away from the workplace. You can always respond to your colleague at a later date, when you are calm and prepared for a constructive conversation.
- ⊛ Honestly reflect on the feedback provided and decide if and how you will incorporate what you have learned into your future work.
- ⊛ Clearly and respectfully communicate any requests you have for the other party to make changes in their own behavior that would support you to change or improve your own.
- ⊛ Whether or not you intend to use the feedback, express appreciation to the other person for caring enough about the relationship to give you the feedback and request that he or she continue to do so.

? *What else would you want to do when receiving critical*
feedback from a colleague?

COMMUNICATING WITH YOUR SUPERVISOR

In an ideal work situation, communication with your supervisor(s) is clear, straightforward, and effortless. Unfortunately, most of us are likely to face some challenges in working with our supervisors. Some of these challenges will arise from unwritten codes raising their heads again: does your supervisor have certain expectations that they have not clearly explained? Do you get the feeling your supervisor doesn't want you to raise your concerns in staff meetings or at a case conference?

Supervisors want you and your program to succeed, and are looking for employees who are reliable and consistent and who can grow on the job. If you think there are problems between you and your supervisor, consider taking the initiative by asking to have a meeting to talk about your concerns. Be respectful and patient. Don't do or say anything in the heat of moment that might undermine your employment status or career. If you have difficulties with a supervisor that you cannot resolve, you may need to turn to your union or human resources department for assistance in mediating the communication.

BOUNDARY ISSUES AT WORK: DISCLOSURE OF PERSONAL INFORMATION

You will spend a lot of time with your coworkers. It's only reasonable that you may want to develop closer personal relationships with some coworkers, or to talk with them about personal issues.

You may find yourself trying to decide whether or not to disclose or share certain information about yourself on the job. For example, this might include your recovery from drug and alcohol use; living with a health condition such as cancer, diabetes, hepatitis C, or a mental health condition; your identity as a lesbian, gay, bisexual or transgender person; or a history of incarceration. Sharing this information may be perfectly natural and common at the agency where you work as a CHW. It is common, for example, for people living with chronic health conditions to be employed by programs addressing these issues, for people in recovery from drug and alcohol use to work with programs addressing these issues, and so on. But you don't have to share personal information, and we encourage you to consider the potential consequences before you do. Are you someone who is completely comfortable with other people knowing these details of your life? Do you have a good reason to trust that your employer and coworkers will understand and be supportive when you share this information? Are you working in a context where this information could be used to harass or discriminate against you?

On the other hand, some of your value to the community you serve may be as a role model. If you have gone through and overcome challenges that are similar to what your clients face, it may give them hope that they, too, will overcome it. As with disclosing personal information to clients (see Chapters Eight and Twenty), consider your motivation for sharing this information and the possible consequences before you speak up

GETTING IT DONE: MANAGING YOUR TIME

As a CHW, you will always have too much to do and competing demands on your time at work and at home. Time management can make the difference between success and failure at work and in life. It gives you the tools to make conscious decisions about how to address competing demands.

Some people resist the idea of time management because they like the idea of being spontaneous. But having a plan for each day can free you from the mental energy of remembering what to do and when, or being backed into a corner when you forgot to do something and the deadline is fast approaching. Managing your time also lets you spend more time doing the things you want to do.

Planning and Doing   If you don't have one already, purchase a portable calendar or planner. It may be paper or electronic. It will be a valuable tool for keeping track of your busy schedule.

Take a minute. Before you start planning, take a minute and imagine how you would spend a few hours or a day if it were completely up to you. This will allow you to plan some time for yourself in your busy week. No matter how full your life is, leave some time for quiet relaxation, time for the people you love, and time to have fun. Develop a weekly plan that includes these things. If you sacrifice personal priorities week after week in order to get your work and chores done, you will put yourself at risk of burning out. A sustainable schedule will give you more energy and can lead to peace of mind in the long run.

Next, in your calendar or planner, write the important events in your week: appointments, meetings, deadlines, family obligations and activities, and so forth.

Make a "to-do list" of all the other tasks you need to accomplish that don't have a specific date and time commitment. Mark those tasks that are the highest priority for the upcoming week.

Now write down the tasks you need to complete—including meetings and other commitments—in your calendar. Don't schedule every minute of each day: leave room for new demands on your time that will come up, and for ongoing activities that always take time, such completing case notes and other forms of documentation. Review your calendar and your to-do list to make sure that you have scheduled all key tasks and obligations.

The truth is that most of us have more things to do than we can actually accomplish. Part of managing your time involves making conscious decisions about what your priorities are—what you will do right now, what you will postpone, and what you won't do. There will be times when you have to say "No" to certain activities and responsibilities and stick to your original plan in order to accomplish your tasks. At work, your commitment to your clients should always be your number one priority. Don't fill up your calendar with other activities that make it difficult for you to fulfill your commitment to the community.

Finally, at the end of each day, take 10 to 15 minutes to review tomorrow's schedule. Identify one or two priorities, and make sure you have set aside enough time to complete them. Look at appointments you have, and think about whether you need to prepare anything in advance. Review your personal and family needs for the day, to see if you need to do errands on the way to or home from work, if you need to make phone calls, or do any urgent tasks at home. This one simple habit, if you do it each evening at the end of the work day, or at home before you go to bed, will help you feel prepared to manage your responsibilities at work and at home.

When you start managing your time, you may find yourself frustrated or feeling as though keeping a planner and maintaining a daily to-do list is taking up too much time. Don't give up! In the long run, this kind of planning will give you more control over your busy days. It will help you make sure you get the most important tasks done. And it will help you balance your work demands with taking care of yourself and your family.

15.4 PROFESSIONAL DEVELOPMENT AND CAREER ADVANCEMENT

Rᴀᴍᴏɴᴀ Bᴇɴsᴏɴ: I came from the community and my highest education was the twelfth grade. I had some life experiences that weren't so great, and because of those experiences, my confidence level wasn't high. So when I first became a CHW, I struggled with having the professional people see me as genuine or respect my suggestions or ideas, or just respect me. What helped me was the CHW certification program. It validated my knowledge and skills. I was able to do the work and that said to me, "You are college material." That helped boost my confidence. It also made me more comfortable interviewing for jobs and telling employers all the knowledge and skills that I would bring to their agency. I also decided to stay in school. This year I'm in Berkeley City College and if all goes well, which it will, at the end of the year I will have my associate's degree.

Imagine that you are working successfully as a CHW. You've settled into your current position and you're doing a great job. Now is the time to think about professional development—enhancing skills for your present job and to help you to advance to new positions with more responsibility (and better pay and benefits).

Continuing Education   Continuing education is seeking out opportunities to enhance your knowledge and skills in any key areas related to your work as a CHW. This might include, for example, knowledge about:

- Specific health issues such as depression or prostate cancer
- Local resources such as mental health services
- Statistics or epidemiology

It may also include skills in areas such as:

- Public speaking
- Crisis intervention
- Program planning and evaluation
- Research or community diagnosis
- Grant writing
- Media advocacy
- Conflict resolution
- Cultural humility
- Supervising and managing others
- Leadership

? *What other skills or knowledge do you think would assist you to advance in your career as a CHW?*

Continuing education opportunities include participating in free or low-cost trainings at a nonprofit agency or the local health department; enrolling in a class (including online classes); attending a lecture at a local college or university; conducting research; and reading articles and books or watching a documentary by yourself or with others.

Case Conferences   If you work in a team setting, you may have the opportunity to participate in case conferences (see Chapter Eleven) and to discuss your work with colleagues. This is a wonderful opportunity for professional development: you receive immediate feedback from peers and other professionals on an urgent problem such as working with a suicidal client or a pregnant thirteen-year-old. Whether you're getting the advice or assisting a colleague, case conferences can be a great opportunity for continuing education.

Support and Mentoring   Mentoring by an experienced CHW may be the best form of professional development you can hope for. You may work surrounded by doctors, nurses, or social workers who want to know, or think they know, what it takes to be a great CHW: but only an experienced CHW can really know this. Ask to meet regularly with an experienced CHW. Share your questions and concerns, and listen to their guidance. If you are fortunate enough to work near a CHW network, take advantage of it. If you are more isolated, you may find support through regional or national networks such as the American Association of Community Health Workers (www.aachw.org). And in ten years, you will be the experienced CHW who supports a new CHW in establishing their career.

CHAPTER REVIEW

Please practice and apply the information covered in this chapter by:

- ✪ Writing or revising your résumé
- ✪ Rehearsing what you might say in a job interview about your experience, knowledge, and skills as a CHW
- ✪ Create a prioritized to-do list—including professional and personal responsibilities—for next week, and schedule these activities in a planner
- ✪ In the next month, practice giving or receiving professional feedback. Reflect on your performance using the guidelines presented in this chapter.

- ✪ Identify two or more skills or areas of knowledge that you would like to learn or enhance that will assist in advancing your career. Identify professional development opportunities to enhance your knowledge and skills.

- ✪ Identify a peer support network or an experienced CHW who might serve as a mentor to you. How do you feel about contacting these resources? What type of support will you ask for? What questions do you have?

ADDITIONAL RESOURCES

Decker, D. C., Hoevemeyer, V. A., and Rowe-Dimas, M. 2006. *First-Job Survival Guide: How to Thrive and Advance in Your New Career.* Indianapolis, IN: JIST Works.

Grazly, J. 2008. Is That the Reason I Get Abused? Learn How to Create and Maintain Healthy Boundaries in Your Relationships. Accessed on March 31, 2009: http://www.asktheinternettherapist.com/is-that-the-reason-i-get-abused.html

Kissane, S. F. 1997. *Career Success for People with Physical Disabilities.* Chicago: VGM Career Horizons.

Owens, R. 2002. *The Journey of Your Life.* Washington, DC: Thompson Publishing.

Pardeck, J. T. 2005. An Analysis of the Americans with Disabilities Act (ADA) in the 21st Century. In J. W. Murphy and J. T. Pardeck (Eds.), *Disability Issues for Social Workers and Human Services Professionals in the Twenty-First Century* (pp. 121–151). Binghamton, NY: Haworth Social Work Practice Press.

Snyder, K. 2003. *Lavender Road to Success: The Career Guide for the Gay Community.* Berkeley, CA: Ten Speed Press.

RESOURCES ON WRITTEN COMMUNICATION

About.com. Accessed on April 9, 2009: http://email.about.com/od/emailnetiquette/Email_Netiquette_Proper_Usage_and_Email_Productivity.htm

emailreplies.com. Accessed on April 9, 2009: http://www.emailreplies.com/

The OWL at Purdue. Accessed on April 9, 2009: http://owl.english.purdue.edu/handouts/pw/p_emailett.html; http://owl.english.purdue.edu/handouts/pw/index.html

Yale University Library. Accessed on April 9, 2009: http://www.library.yale.edu/training/netiquette/

RESOURCES ON PLANNING, TIME MANAGEMENT, AND GOAL SETTING

MindTools. Accessed on April 9, 2009: http://www.mindtools.com

The Productivity Institute. Accessed on April 9, 2009: http://www.balancetime.com.

PART 3

CHW Skills and Core Competencies: Working in Your Community

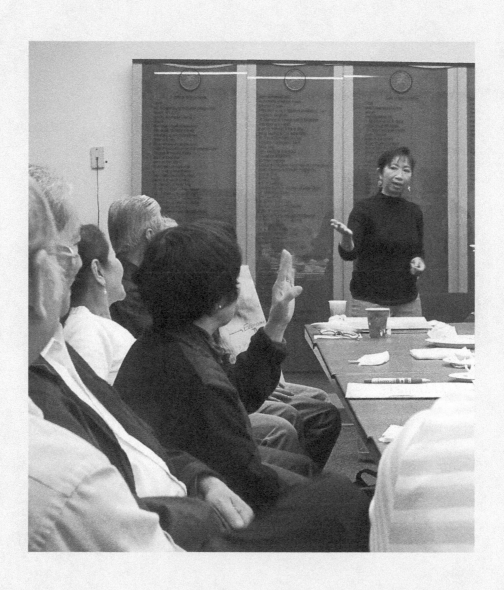

16

Working to Promote Health at the Community Level

Jeni Miller • Alma Avila-Esparza • Tim Berthold

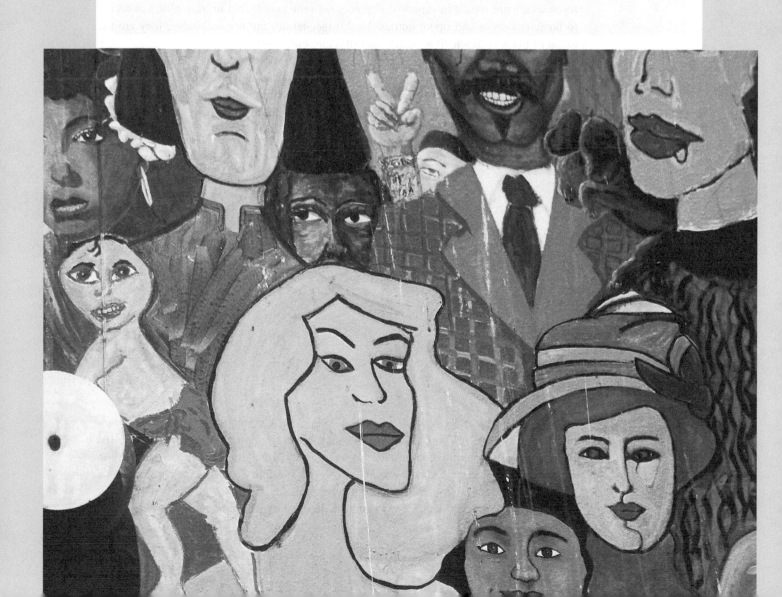

CHW SCENARIO

You work at a community health center, supporting low-income families in learning how to manage their children's asthma. You discover that a significant factor contributing to the high asthma rates in your community is the fact that the city doesn't enforce rules that require landlords to repair apartments and eliminate mold. Many of the children you work with live in apartments with mold and old carpeting that make their asthma worse, no matter how well the family manages their child's medications. The families you work with are frustrated and angry about these conditions. You think the families would be eager to organize and work to change these circumstances. *What can you do?*

INTRODUCTION

CHWs work at both an individual and a community level. In Part One of this book, you learned about ecological models for understanding the social, economic, and political forces that shape people's lives and their health. Our social context results in health inequalities—significant differences in health status for different communities. These differences are not rooted in genetic differences between people, but in inequalities in access to basic resources and opportunities. Health inequalities are not inevitable, they are the result of the way in which we create and structure our society.

Part Two introduced you to many of the skills that CHWs use when working to promote the health of individual clients in spite of a social context that is likely to make them ill.

In Part Three, you will learn to work with your community to *change that context* and to take action to promote community health and social justice.

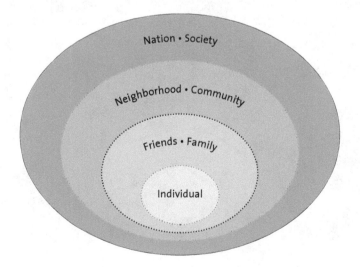

Working with individual clients and working at the community level are interconnected. Every time you support clients in taking action to improve their health, you assist in developing a potential community advocate. Every time you support a community in organizing, building support networks, or advocating for policy changes, you are creating a community that promotes the health of its individuals. In Part Three of this book you will gain the knowledge and skills for working with groups and at the community level.

WHAT YOU WILL LEARN

By studying the information in this chapter, you will be able to:

⊗ Describe how working at the community level builds upon core values and skills for working with individual clients
⊗ Explain how community-level action benefits local communities
⊗ Identify and describe some of the ways that CHWs can work at the community level
⊗ Analyze the role that CHWs play in supporting the participation and leadership of community members in community-level interventions

16.1 THE VALUE OF PROMOTING CHANGE AT THE COMMUNITY LEVEL

There are limitations to working with individual clients to assist them to improve their health. While this work can result in significant health improvements for individuals and families, it does not address or change the social determinants—such as the lack of housing, nutrition, human rights, safety, employment, or health care—that are so harmful to the overall health of communities.

Some CHWs work in partnership with communities to change the social conditions that harm their health. In Chapter Three, we introduced the spectrum of prevention, a resource for understanding the range of strategies that CHWs may use to promote the health of clients and communities. Levels 4 to 6 of the spectrum involve working at the community level:

4. *Fostering coalitions and networks:* Convening groups and individuals for broader goals and greater impact
5. *Changing organizational practices:* Adopting regulations and shaping norms to improve health and safety
6. *Influencing policy and legislation:* Developing strategies to change laws and policies to influence outcomes

Working at the community level to address and change social conditions is significant for several key reasons. It requires communities to unite and organize in order to take collective action. This process is inherently empowering, and provides the community with knowledge and skills to address other social problems in the future. Working at the community level can also result in changes that enhance the health of many people, a larger impact than is possible by working with individual clients.

16.2 HOW COMMUNITY-LEVEL CHANGE HAPPENS

? *Have you ever contributed to changes within your family, school, religious or faith community, neighborhood, or city?*

? *Have you ever spoken up for yourself when you felt you were being treated unfairly?*

? *Have you ever gotten together with others to address a common challenge?*

Many of us have participated in efforts to promote social change. While not all CHWs will be paid to work on community-level projects, there are many ways to participate in social change efforts, both professionally and personally. For example, you may facilitate a community organizing project with a local agency. You may participate in a protest or join a parent teacher association (PTA) to improve conditions at a local school. You may vote, write a letter to a newspaper or policymaker, or testify at a public hearing to influence or change policies that have an impact on the health of your community. You may support others in doing these things. All of these efforts are valuable, and each contributes to creating a healthier community.

As discussed in Chapter Five, a policy is a law or rule that governs the actions of individuals, organizations, or institutions. Government policies include federal and state laws, state propositions, city ordinances, state-mandated guidelines or restrictions, and the rules put forth by government agencies. Many government policies, such as laws and ordinances, are passed by being voted on by elected officials. Other types of government policies are decided within agencies, such as a local health department. Private institutions also establish policies. For example, banks make policies about where and how they invest money and whom they loan money to. All of these policies contribute to shaping and determining the social system within which people live, work, and strive to maintain good health. These policies, and their enforcement (or lack of enforcement), create the context for people's health choices, behaviors, and opportunities.

It may seem as if the forces that shape our society are beyond human control, but all policies are the result of decisions made by groups of people. Ultimately, what community organizing and advocacy boil down to is making the effort to have a voice in the decisions that shape the communities and society we live in.

Another way to think about this is to ask: What is the current balance of power in the community? Who is making the decisions that most profoundly affect community health and community life? Who is making the rules? Is it the people in the neighborhood? Is it the people in city hall? Is it the CEOs of multinational corporations who make money marketing and selling products to the community? What role are local communities taking in these decisions?

While it is true that corporations, elected officials, and big institutions have a lot of power, and money to back it up, by organizing a community to draw attention to an issue, you *can* shift the balance of power. Once that power begins to shift, a community can continue to influence the process of social change.

16.3 HOW WILL THE COMMUNITY BENEFIT?

Remember that the community itself always has the most to gain from any collective effort to make change. Working together to make change, community members can:

- Identify factors that harm their health
- Gain a clearer understanding of the circumstances that promote their health

- ✪ Articulate a common vision of a healthy future for their community
- ✪ Identify where the power lies now—who is making the decisions that affect the community
- ✪ Identify key allies who support their vision and proposed policies
- ✪ Learn to unite and work together for a common purpose
- ✪ Develop an action plan to advocate for policies that result in meaningful social change for their community
- ✪ Develop knowledge and skills in leadership, community planning, organizing, and advocacy
- ✪ Develop confidence in their own leadership skills
- ✪ Identify and resolve internal disagreements and conflicts that keep the community from moving forward together
- ✪ Change policies and improve access to the basic resources, rights, and opportunities that support their health and well-being

? *Can you think of other ways in which advocating for social change will benefit a community?*

Meeting together is a good first step.

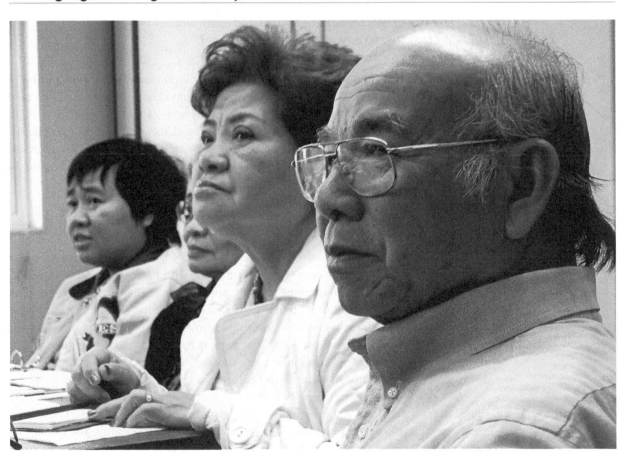

16.4 THE ROLE OF CHWs

CHWs contribute to community-level efforts to promote health in many different ways, including:

- Sharing knowledge and raising awareness about health issues affecting a community
- Sharing information about how public policies are created and changed
- Providing training in skills such as facilitating meetings, conducting a community diagnosis, and developing a policy position
- Bringing people together and facilitating discussions in which community members can identify problems and brainstorm solutions
- Assisting the community to identity local resources and needs
- Connecting the community with additional resources such as health information, services, policymakers, training and educational opportunities, and allies who may support their interests and efforts
- Supporting leadership from within the community
- Assisting community leaders to break down big goals into smaller steps and to stay on track in achieving their goals
- Assisting a community to recognize and celebrate their successes along the way

? *How else can CHWs contribute to assisting communities in working together to advocate for social change?*

There are many ways to participate in community-level change, and CHWs can play many roles in this process. Just as in your work with individual clients, you will be most successful if you find and develop your own authentic style. There is a place for people who are outgoing and can energize others. Just as important, there is a place for people who excel at quietly affirming other people's ideas and supporting others to take on leadership roles. Trust in your own personality and style, and look for the ways your talents can be used most effectively in this work.

THE CONNECTION BETWEEN CLIENT- AND COMMUNITY-CENTERED WORK

When you work at the community level, we encourage you to draw on and apply your skills for working with individual clients. Your work with individual clients should be client-centered, and focus on listening to and supporting the client's goals (not yours) for living a better and healthier life. Similarly, when working at the community level, your efforts should be community-centered. Your role is to listen to community members and to support them in identifying the issues that *they* are most concerned about; drawing on the strengths they already possess in order to address those issues; and connecting them to resources that will support their efforts to create change.

Just as you do when working with individual clients, you will ask the community open-ended questions and use active listening skills. By posing the right questions, you can get people to think about the root causes of the issues or concerns they identify. You can support them in developing a vision for how they want their community to be and an action plan to make this vision a reality.

When you work with individuals, you don't want to make your clients dependent on you and your constant intervention on their behalf. Your goal is to show them how to gain the knowledge, skills, and confidence to access resources on their own and to advocate for themselves, to maintain good health. The goal is similar when working at the community level. There may be times when you will take the lead—you may, for example, start a social or support group for people with diabetes or organize the first meetings to talk about the community's concerns about the violence they face every day. Ultimately, however, your role is to support the community in identifying and cultivating its own natural leaders, and in gaining skills and the capacity to continue to organize on its own behalf.

Sometimes a community has been oppressed for so long that they have temporarily forgotten how to imagine a better future. Communities may be deeply affected by generations of poverty and historical traumas such as the African American experience of slavery; the Native American, Jewish, Cambodian, or Sudanese experiences of genocide; or the traumas of fleeing war-torn homes to seek political asylum. Communities continue to face ongoing discrimination such as racial profiling, domestic violence, anti-immigration violence and hate crimes. They have also experienced more subtle disillusionment: businesses, agencies, and government representatives have come into the community making big promises, but failed to deliver something that is ultimately meaningful to those who live there. Sometimes, your role will be to believe, at a time when the community doesn't, that things can be better. Your role may be to hold on to hope when the community has lost it, just as you do in your work with individual clients.

It is vitally important that you are honest with you community about what you can and cannot do. *Don't ever promise what you can't deliver.* It can be much more meaningful to aid a community to identify and successfully reach a small goal than to tackle something big, and fail. Through these smaller successes, the trust they build, and your knowledge of the big changes that community organizing *has* achieved, you can support the community in identifying larger goals and taking action to make them a reality.

WHEN WORKING FOR SOCIAL CHANGE IS NOT PART OF YOUR JOB

Working at the community level to advocate for social justice has always been an important part of the work that CHWs do. Some grants or programs give CHWs support to do community organizing, but most do not. Some employers welcome your strong voice and advocacy on behalf of local communities both inside and outside of your agency, while others won't support this role or will ask you to tone it down.

If your employer doesn't support your participation in community organizing, consider the following options:

✪ Advocate within your organization. Raise awareness about the issues you would like to see addressed through community-level work. Though it may take time, you may witness meaningful changes in people's awareness and understanding. You are the eyes and ears of the organization in the community—you have a unique perspective.

✪ Investigate whether your agency could seek a grant to do community-level work.

✪ Talk with leaders in your agency about whether you could establish a volunteer program, patient advisory council, or support group. These groups could lead the agency in identifying the need for community-level work and advocacy efforts.

✪ Find out if there are groups in your area that are engaged in advocating for the concerns you have identified. Inform your clients about these organizations and their work: they may want to participate.

✪ Organize and advocate during nonwork hours. You may not be able to participate in community organizing and advocacy on the job, but no one can forbid you or take away your right to work with others to improve your community.

- Find out if there are jobs in your community with advocacy organizations. Your connections with the community, and your skills working with people, might be just what they are looking for.
- Meet with other CHWs and learn how they feel about participating in community organizing efforts.

You may be successful at changing your agency's perspective about engaging in community-level organizing and advocacy. However, advocating for big changes within your agency may also place your job at risk: it depends on where you are working. Remember to apply your CHW skills to this challenge, including your active listening and conflict resolution skills. These skills will guide you in creating alliances with colleagues and in communicating about new ideas in ways that people are most able to hear them.

16.5 THE QUEER YOUTH ACTION TEAM: A COMMUNITY-CENTERED MOVEMENT FOR SOCIAL CHANGE

Across the country, lesbian, gay, bisexual, and transgender (LGBT) youth face discrimination at school, including harassment and assault. The Center for Human Development (2006), a nonprofit agency serving youth and families in Contra Costa County, California, developed and managed a youth-led program to address these issues. They established the Queer Youth Action Team (QYAT), supporting LGBT youth from local high schools to advocate for safer school environments. Staff provided youth members with training in skills such as how to conduct a community diagnosis, advocacy, and public speaking. With training and support, the youth were able to take ownership of the project and to make all key decisions about their efforts to promote social change.

The QYAT members decided to advocate for local school districts to adopt and implement antidiscrimination policies to protect the rights and well-being of LGBT students. Their first campaign would focus on the West Contra Costa Unified School District (WCCUSD). The youth developed and submitted a resolution to the local school board; conducted outreach to garner support for the resolution; developed and sent out press releases; conducted interviews with print, radio, and television news agencies; and spoke at a school board meeting in February of 2001.

A description of their work—"Making It Real: The Queer Youth Action Team's Story"—can be found on the Web site of the Gay, Straight Alliance Network (2009). The article explains the QYAT's planning process:

> We developed a strategy chart outlining our long-term and short-term goals, and identifying our allies. . . . We also asked ourselves more personal questions such as what were our strengths and weaknesses as a group as well as what type of tactics we were going to use.

The QYAT members also organized a forum for LGBT and straight students to talk about their experiences in high school and the need for stronger antidiscrimination policies.

> On March 8, 2000, QYAT organized a youth forum called "Give Us the 411" at the Richmond Unity Church in West Contra Costa County, specifically for students in the district. The event was a major success, with youth both queer and straight showing up

from all over the district to tell us what they thought about homophobia in their schools. With some animated discussion, everyone came to the conclusion that there were some major problems that needed to be addressed in the district regarding homophobia. . . . Yet undoubtedly, the most unforgettable part of the forum was [were] the school climate surveys and personal stories the youth left. As we read each story, I felt something inside of me begin to stir. Why are we treated differently because we are queer? It seemed so unfair to me. . . . That was the moment we all became emotionally invested in this fight.

The QYAT developed a draft resolution and antidiscrimination policy for the school district to consider. After a lengthy struggle to get the resolution on the school board's agenda, QYAT members started to advocate on behalf of the policy:

> We went out into the community and collected over 200 signatures of WCCUSD constituents. We created QYAT postcards of support, hundreds of which were sent to different board members. Finally, we collected 40 letters of support from parents, teachers, PFLAG members, various religious organizations, PTA groups, as well as the teacher's union, all of which urged the board to pass our original version of the resolution.
>
> On February 7, 2001, a year after our efforts had first begun, came the day of the WCCUSD Board meeting where the fate of our resolution would be decided. . . . A few days prior to the event, QYAT sent out media advisories to local news agencies, and in response KQED, KPFA, KGO [radio stations], the San Francisco Chronicle, the Contra Costa Times, and Contra Costa Television showed up to witness this historic event. With the community out in full force and wearing hot pink stickers in support of QYAT, we began our presentation with legal information, statistics, and personal testimonies of students. Many students felt uncomfortable being seen at the meeting, so their stories were told by other youth, who pointed out the author's reluctance to be identified. There were more than 30 speakers in favor of QYAT's resolution.

As a result of their organizing and advocacy efforts, the WCCUSD became the first school district in Contra Costa County to pass a new policy prohibiting harassment and other forms of discrimination against LGBT youth.

> With a unanimous vote, the board passed the amendment, and the crowd simultaneously broke out in a roar of cheers. At that moment my eyes flooded with tears as I hugged my fellow QYAT members in celebration of our victory. It was the greatest feeling ever to watch the crowd of students and adults light up with hope and enthusiasm where once only fear and hopelessness existed.

Not only did this project result in new policies to protect students from discrimination, it also empowered youth leaders who learned how to successfully organize and advocate for social change and social justice.

CHAPTER REVIEW QUESTIONS

Think about what you have learned so far, and answer the following questions:

- For CHWs, how is working with communities similar to working with individual clients?
- What are some of the ways that CHWs can work at the community level?

- What are some of the benefits, for community members, of community-level health promotion efforts?
- What is the role of CHWs when facilitating community-level projects?

REFERENCES

The Center for Human Development. 2006. Queer Youth Action Team. Accessed on April 1, 2009: http://www.chd-prevention.org/qyat.htm

Gay, Straight Alliance Network. Making It Real: The Queer Youth Action Team's Story. Accessed on April 1, 2009: http://www.gsanetwork.org/ab537/action/success.html

17

Community Diagnosis

Susana Hennessey-Lavery • Mele Lau-Smith • Alma Avila-Esparza
• Jill Tregor • Tim Berthold

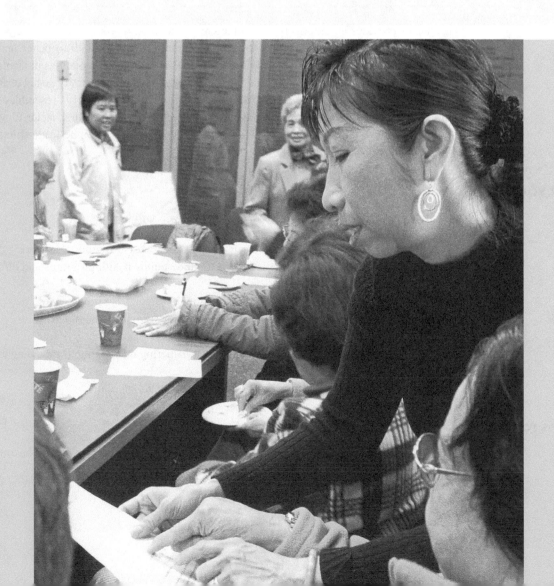

CHW SCENARIO

You work for a coalition of nonprofit agencies in a county with a large and diverse Native American population. Native communities are concerned about the high rates of low birth weight and infant mortality that their families experience. You've been asked to work with Native American communities to conduct a community diagnosis. Together, you will gather information to guide the development of an action plan to advocate for policies that will reduce low birth weight and infant mortality rates.

- ✪ How will you begin this community diagnosis?
- ✪ Who will participate in this diagnosis?
- ✪ As a CHW, what will your role be?
- ✪ What types of information do you want to gather?
- ✪ What types of research might you conduct?
- ✪ How will the information you gather be analyzed?
- ✪ How will this information be used to promote the health of the communities at risk?

INTRODUCTION

This chapter provides an introduction to community diagnosis, a process and a strategy for community members to identify important concerns and conduct research to better understand the root causes of these problems. The diagnosis also supports communities in identifying their own strengths and resources, and in developing a plan to advocate for social change that promotes their health and welfare. In some ways, community diagnosis resembles the client-centered process of developing a case management plan addressed in Chapter Eleven. As a CHW, your role in the community diagnosis process is to facilitate the leadership and self-determination of the communities you work with.

WHAT YOU WILL LEARN

By studying the information provided in this chapter, you will be able to:

- ✪ Define community diagnosis, and discuss key concepts used to guide this work
- ✪ Explain how community diagnosis is used to guide public health programs and efforts to advocate for social change
- ✪ Describe and apply seven key steps in a community diagnosis process
- ✪ Conduct a community-centered and strength-based community diagnosis
- ✪ Define the role of the CHW in community diagnosis
- ✪ Identify and develop effective research tools for gathering information for the diagnosis
- ✪ Summarize and analyze research findings
- ✪ Explain how research findings are used to develop an action plan

WORDS TO KNOW

Needs Assessment   Quantitative and Qualitative Data   Leading Questions

17.1 DEFINING COMMUNITY DIAGNOSIS

Community diagnosis is the art and the process of identifying community concerns or problems, uncovering their root causes, and developing a clear plan to overcome them. Many communities have experienced people coming in from the outside to conduct research that does not lead to any meaningful benefit or positive change. In contrast, a community diagnosis involves community members in all phases of research and planning, and supports them in making all key decisions along the way.

COMMUNITY DIAGNOSIS

Community diagnosis is known by many names:

*   Community-based participatory research (CBPR)
*   Participatory action research (PAR)
*   Action research
*   Participatory research

What these research methods have in common is that they are research conducted by the community rather than by outside experts.

COMMUNITY DIAGNOSIS IS STRENGTH-BASED

Traditionally, public health workers have done **needs assessments** on behalf of the community. These needs assessments can provide a false view of what's happening in the community because they frequently focus on the negative—the risks, problems, and lack of resources and skills. While all communities have problems, they also have strengths. When a CHW works with an individual client, the CHW supports the client in identifying the client's own strengths and resources. Working at the community level should be the same. The strengths of any community are numerous and may include their shared experience, culture, wisdom, skills, and history, including histories of resistance and past accomplishments. Resources may also include the ability and desire to work together; a vision for the future; commitment to justice and peace; formal and informal leaders; parks; faith-based, educational, health, and social services agencies; and existing employers with safe working conditions that pay a living wage. The positive elements evident in all communities should always be highlighted in a community diagnosis and used in planning for solutions (Kretzman and McKnight, 1993).

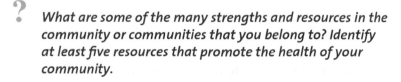

What are some of the many strengths and resources in the community or communities that you belong to? Identify at least five resources that promote the health of your community.

A FOCUS ON ROOT CAUSES

A community diagnosis must go beyond the surface, to conduct an in-depth analysis of the root causes of the issues and concerns a community identifies. Research that does not identify root causes is likely to result in a simplistic or superficial understanding of a problem or concern. This can lead to solutions that "blame the victim" or place responsibility for fixing the problem on the very people who have already been most harmed.

For example, consider the high rates of infant mortality within the Native American communities mentioned at the beginning of this chapter. An analysis of the causes of this problem that stays on the surface might identify factors such as low rates of participation in prenatal care and breast-feeding. An analysis that goes deeper—beneath the surface of the problem to consider its root causes—might identity factors such as institutionalized racism; unequal access to basic resources including quality housing, education, employment, health insurance, food, and safety; hazardous working conditions; living in poverty in neighborhoods characterized by high levels of crime and lack of safety; and the chronic stress that these inequalities produce (see Chapter Six). This type of analysis will guide the community in determining what actions they wish to take in order to reduce infant mortality rates.

An analysis of root causes assists the community to view their work as part of a larger movement. For example, in tobacco control, many of the smoke-free policies that exist today at the state level started at the local level in cities and towns. In San Francisco in the 1990s, a local youth agency diagnosed and compared tobacco advertising targeting different neighborhoods. The results of their community diagnosis influenced statewide and national efforts to restrict tobacco advertising. We now see restrictions on tobacco advertising as one of the key pillars of the international Framework Convention on Tobacco Control. These local policies shaped the need for statewide, national, and global policies and treaties to control the actions of transnational tobacco companies.

WHEN TO CONDUCT A COMMUNITY DIAGNOSIS

Community diagnosis serves many purposes and may be conducted at different times in the life cycle of a community program, project, or movement. Sometimes the community diagnosis will be initiated by the community itself, and sometimes by others such as the city council, mayor's office, or local department of public health.

Some groups come together to improve the general health of their community, but have not yet decided which particular issue or problem they want to tackle first. These groups might conduct a broad community diagnosis to clarify what issues the community is most concerned about and what types of change they want to prioritize.

Other groups have already identified the issue or problem they want to work on, such as infant mortality. These groups might conduct a community diagnosis because they need to gather data and information to guide and support the actions they will take to address the problem. Often, the diagnosis assists the community to further define the problem and their proposed solution or action.

Finally, many groups do both. They start with the broader diagnosis to prioritize an issue or concern, and then they conduct a more targeted diagnosis to further define potential solutions and actions to create change.

THE ROLE OF THE CHW

Regardless of the community or communities you belong to and the organization you work for, as a CHW, your role in a community diagnosis is to support and facilitate diverse leadership from the community. Your role is not to make key decisions about the diagnosis: the community must identify their own issues of concern, analyze the research data gathered, and develop their own action plan. As a CHW, you may assist in facilitating meetings (or not) and support the community in deciding what types of research tools to use and how to develop and implement them.

When you provide client-centered services to individual clients, one of your key roles is to ask simple open-ended questions designed to aid them in clarifying their strengths, risks, needs, goals, and steps to reach those goals. Similarly, when you assist in facilitating a community diagnosis, you will ask open-ended questions that will support the community in sharing their experience, knowledge, and proposed solutions. These questions might include, for example: "What do you want to know about the problem you have identified? Who else would you like to invite to participate in this community diagnosis? What does this information tell you about the problem of infant mortality? What factors seem to contribute to this problem? What are some of the most important strengths and resources in your community? What other strategies might assist you to promote greater equality and to reduce low birth weight and infant mortality?"

If you participate in a community diagnosis, ask yourself the following questions along the way to reflect on whether or not you are doing community-centered work:

- Who identified the issues, concerns, or problems that are the focus of the community diagnosis?
- Were all segments of the community invited to participate in the community diagnosis?
- Have you treated all community members with courtesy and respect?
- Did the community determine what type of research they wanted to conduct? Who developed the questions that were used in the surveys, focus groups, or other research tools?
- Who analyzed the research findings? How active was the community in this process?
- Were any key sectors of the community left out of the process? If so, why?
- Did the community develop their own action plan? Who participated in these decisions?
- Have you or your professional colleagues attempted to influence the outcome of any part of the community diagnosis?
- Were you able to comfortably accept decisions made by the community that were different from the decisions that you would have made?

WHEN RESEARCH IS NOT COMMUNITY-DRIVEN

Most research is quite different from a community diagnosis; it does not invite community members to participate in a meaningful way in its design, implementation, analysis, or dissemination (sharing of results). CHWs are often hired to work on public health research studies. As we discussed in Chapters Two and Three, research plays an important role in providing information to guide efforts to promote community health and eliminate health inequalities. However, not all research studies are equally valuable.

If you are considering a job with a research study, we encourage you to ask questions to determine how the research will benefit the community. These questions might include, for example:

- What issues or questions are the focus of this research? Are these topics and questions important to the community in which the research will be undertaken?
- To what extent will researchers involve local community members in the research process and project? Have community members been consulted about the research focus and methods? Will community members be hired to work on the study?

✪ How might the information gathered by research ultimately be used to promote the health and well-being of the community?

✪ How will the results of the study—including positive and negative results—be shared with the community and with the subjects of the research (the people who participate in surveys, questionnaires, and focus groups or who donate blood or other biological samples)?

✪ What is the past record of the lead researchers (sometimes called principal investigators): Have they made efforts in the past to share research findings with the communities they studied? Has their research been used to promote the welfare of the communities they studied?

Increasingly, researchers are changing the way they conduct their studies to be more responsive to community needs. For example, all research studies in the United States that involve gathering information from people must be approved by human subjects or institutional review boards (IRBs) to ensure that the research is ethical and does not harm participants. Historically, IRBs have been based in institutions—such as universities—that conduct research and have been composed of fellow researchers. Recently, community-based IRBs have been developed to evaluate the ethics of proposed research in communities. For example, the Native Hawaiian Health Care System (NHHCS) Institutional Review Board (IRB) was established to:

> maximize the benefits and minimize the risks of research in Native Hawaiian individuals and communities but additionally to educate researchers to build capacity within communities so that communities can participate in and partner with research that addresses existing community health concerns. (Papa Ola Lokahi, 2008)

KEY CONCEPTS OF COMMUNITY DIAGNOSIS

Community diagnosis is based on concepts of popular education and models from Africa, Latin America, and other parts of the Global South. It is greatly influenced by the work of Paulo Freire and Orlando Fals-Borda in Latin America, and Miles Horton of the Highlander Institute and Kurt Lewin in the United States (Minkler and Wallerstein, 2003). Popular education is discussed in more detail in Chapter Nineteen. Community diagnosis does the following:

✪ Educates and raises the consciousness of all participants, including community members and CHWs assisting with the research (Tsark, 2001)

✪ Values knowledge generated from the life experiences of the community (Tsark, 2001)

✪ Actively involves the language and cultural values of community members in both the design and implementation (Arble and Moberg, 2006)

✪ Prioritizes issues of gender, race, class, and culture in the design and analysis of the research (Minkler, 2003)

✪ Values collaboration, ensures that all partners are involved equally in the research process, and recognizes the strengths that they bring to the process (W. K. Kellogg Foundation, 2001)

✪ Begins with an issue of concern to the community with the aim of combining knowledge and action for social change to improve community health and eliminate health inequalities (W. K. Kellogg Foundation, 2001)

✪ Seeks the participation of all members in development of the research questions, as well as the design, data collection, analysis and dissemination of the results (Tsark, 2001)

⊗ Exposes and examines issues of power and power relations, and works to promote individual and community empowerment (Tsark, 2001)

⊗ Seeks political action, social change, or both (Tsark, 2001)

17.2 KEY STEPS IN CONDUCTING A COMMUNITY DIAGNOSIS

A community diagnosis usually consists of at least seven steps:

1. Define the community and bring them together
2. Choose a focus for the community diagnosis
   a. For example, infant mortality, gun violence, homelessness, or heart disease
3. Select research tools
   a. These may include, for example, conducting research at the library or on the Internet, researching existing policies, conducting qualitative interviews with or administering a survey to community members, facilitating a focus group, mapping community resources and risks and counting physical objectives, or developing other visual documentation such as photo voices.
4. Conduct research
5. Summarize the research findings
   a. Often the information and data that you gather will be large or technical (or both), and it must be summarized in a way that makes it understandable to the community.
6. Analyze the research findings
   a. Community members analyze the information that has been gathered to learn more about the root causes of their concerns strengths and risks, and to guide them in taking action.
7. Develop an action plan
   a. Community members determine—guided by the research findings—what they can do to create social change and promote their health and well-being, such as advocating for culturally competent services, transitional housing programs, closure of the incinerator, or stricter controls on emissions.

Chapter Twenty-Two will introduce you to the community action model, which builds on community diagnosis to implement an action plan and advocate for policy changes that promote social justice.

STEP 1: IDENTIFYING AND BRINGING THE COMMUNITY TOGETHER

A community may be defined and brought together to conduct a community diagnosis in different ways. As discussed in other chapters, the community or population may be defined by factors such as geography (neighborhood, city, county, and so on) or by other common characteristics, including ethnicity, nationality, language, risk factors, interests, gender, or sexual orientation. Remember, however, that all communities are diverse in some way. A truly meaningful community diagnosis will actively reach out and attempt to include all members of the community.

The community diagnosis process may begin with a series of meetings at accessible locations such as a community center, school, or social services agency. These meetings, and the community diagnosis process itself, should be advertised and promoted throughout the community. Enlisting the participation of formal and informal leaders or key stakeholders

Breaking out into small groups gives everyone a chance to participate.

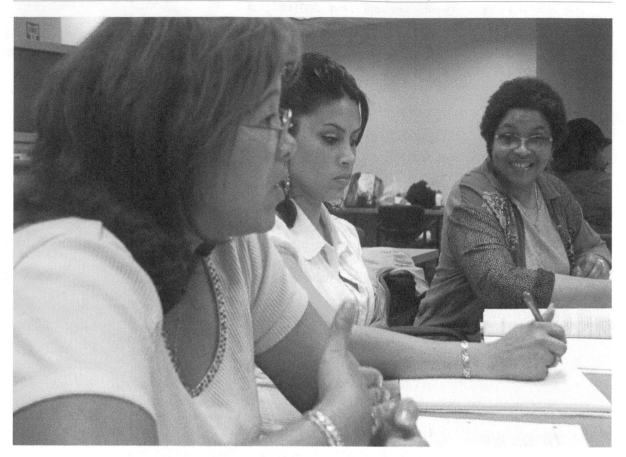

will aid in ensuring that the entire community learns about what is going on. This may include asking local media, schools, faith-based organizations, service organizations, businesses, unions, and activists to assist in getting the word out. For more information about how to identify and build relationships with formal and informal leaders in a community, see Chapter Eighteen.

? *How would let your community know about a community diagnosis that was about to begin?*

? *Who are some of the key stakeholders in your community?*

? *What parts of the community are sometimes left out of efforts like this?*

? *How would you reach out to invite them to participate?*

STEP 2: CHOOSING A FOCUS

The next step in the process is for the community to select a specific problem or concern that will be the central focus for the community diagnosis. Sometimes the focus has already been selected, and this is the reason that people have come together to conduct a community diagnosis. At other times, community diagnosis will lead the group to identify issues that the community is most concerned about and wants to change.

We recommend that the community use the following criteria to choose the issues or problem they will work on. The focus of the community diagnosis should be:

- *Meaningful:* Addressing this issue will make a real difference. It will result in a significant improvement in people's lives.
- *Public support:* It will be easy to get support from the public and community leaders to address the issue.
- *Reach:* Addressing this issue will impact many people.
- *High need:* There is an underserved population or geographic area that has a high need related to the issue.
- *Political will:* There is political will within the community to address the issue.
- *Practical:* The expertise, time, and resources are available to address the issue.
- *Clear target:* There is a clearly defined policymaking body (such as a city council or health commission, county board of supervisors or state legislature) that can influence the identified issue or concern.

The next step will be for community members to create a list of the questions to guide them in learning more about the issue they identified. The following questions can aid the community in coming up with their own list:

- What don't you know about the issue?
- How is the community hurt by the issue?
- What factors and forces are creating the issue or making it worse?
- Is there a law or policy that deals with your issue?
- Do other communities experience the same issue? What have they done to address this problem?

EXAMPLE: REDUCING TOBACCO ADVERTISING AND SPONSORSHIP

Questions to answer:

- How many people smoke in my community?
- What are the health hazards of tobacco use?
- How does tobacco use hurt our community?
- How do the tobacco companies target our community?
- How much money do the tobacco companies make on selling their product and how much do they give away?
- What local organizations and events take tobacco money?
- How do the tobacco companies benefit from giving money to these events?
- Who can decide not to take the tobacco money? What is the decision-making process?

STEP 3: SELECTING RESEARCH TOOLS

Once the list of questions has been developed, the community will decide which research tools are best to use to find answers. A research tool or method is what you use to gather information about the focus issue. Your community diagnosis may use one or many research tools depending on the type of information you want to gather. As a CHW, you play an important role in bringing resources to communities. You may have the opportunity to invite a consultant who is familiar with evaluation, epidemiology, or research to meet with your group and work with them to design the diagnosis. This person can give you advice about which types of research to conduct and how to do it.

You may use some or all of the following types of research (we'll talk about each one in the next section):

- ✪ Research at the library
- ✪ Research on the Internet
- ✪ Research at city hall, city departments, state and federal government
- ✪ Research to count physical objects
- ✪ Focus groups, community groups, community forums
- ✪ Surveys
- ✪ Community maps and diagrams
- ✪ Visual documentation such as Photovoice or video

DIFFERENT TYPES OF INFORMATION

Research tools will assist you to gather quantitative or qualitative data. Both are useful in better understanding the problem that the community has identified.

Quantitative data: This type of information lets you know how many times something is happening, how many people share the same experience or opinion, or anything else that can be measured numerically or by counting. Surveys, mapping, counting, and public health data records are all good ways to get quantitative data.

Qualitative data: This type of information gives you an in-depth or deeper understanding of how people feel about or experience an issue. Interviews, focus groups, and community forums are all good ways to get qualitative data about your issue.

Example:

> *Question:* How does smoking hurt our community?
>
> *Quantitative data:* The number of people who report that their health has been harmed by smoking, the number of tobacco billboards or ads in a community, or data from the local health department on the number of people in the community who smoke and the number of people with chronic diseases that are caused by smoking such as emphysema, lung cancer, and heart disease.
>
> *Qualitative data:* Real-life stories of how smoking hurts the community: the story of someone who died too young because they smoked; how a group of parents feels about tobacco advertising that targets their community; or how people feel about limiting smoking in public housing. You gather this information by conducting interviews, focus groups, or community forums.

WHEN TO USE DIFFERENT TYPES OF RESEARCH

Table 17.1 provides information to aid you in deciding when to use a specific research tool.

STEP 4: CONDUCTING RESEARCH

This step requires a lot of organization! It may mean making trips to the library or calling up agencies to ask them for information. You may need to design survey tools and train

Table 17.1.   Uses of Specific Research Tools.

Type of Diagnosis	Description	When to Use it	When Not To Use It
Library	Visit a local library and work with librarian and library computers to research your topic.	For access to local statistics, resources, and history that might not be available elsewhere.	If the information or data is available on the Internet.
Internet	Use search engines like "Google" or reputable health sites like "http://www.cdc.gov" to get data or to network.	To do a quick initial search; a broad search; to access records/data unavailable locally.	If the information does not come from a reliable source
Existing Policies, Regulations	Research at local, state, federal level whether there are existing policies relevant to your topic and whether they are being enforced.	This should be a standard part of your diagnosis!	This is always relevant!
Count Physical Objects	Visit sites and count actual items to assess their prevalence in the community (like # of alcohol ads, condom dispenser, etc).	Useful when you want to demonstrate how much something is occurring in your community.	This quantitative data always is more powerful if coupled with qualitative findings.
Community Forums	Organize evening or weekend community meetings to gather community input, feedback, perceptions and experiences.	When you want information from the community at large and want to raise awareness that an issue is being addressed.	If you do not have the resources available, as Community Forums are labor intensive
Focus Groups	Strategically choose 6-12 people representing a variety of views on your issue. Facilitate a discussion to get their perceptions and experiences.	When you want to get deep and in depth qualitative information about your issue. This information complements information from community surveys.	If you want to be able to talk about what the community thinks about an issue – you need to survey at least 300 members to get an idea of what the community thinks as a whole
Survey Individuals	Decide on the number of people you will survey. Come up with a survey or questionnaire to use to ask those people what their opinion's are on the health issue you are concerned about.	When you want a representative sample of the communities responses in an organized way. This information goes well with focus group information.	May not provide you with the qualitative "stories" you are looking for. Complements information from qualitative research.

(Continued)

Table 17.1.   *(Continued)*

Type of Diagnosis	Description	When to Use it	When Not To Use It
Survey Individuals (*Continued*)	Then come up with a survey design (decide how many to survey, where, etc.) and conduct the survey.	This information can also be counted such as the number and percentage of those surveyed who share similar experiences, risks, or opinions.	
Qualitative Interviews	Set up individual interviews to find out why people "feel the way they do."	When you want deep information such a "quotes," "stories," and detailed descriptions of people's experience, behavior, attitudes, feelings, and opinions.	Will not get you statistics or other quantitative data.
Community Map	Take a large piece of paper and "map" a place such as a neighborhood, inside a store etc. Plot important items you are looking for. Can also use "Google Maps"	When you want a visual representation of a place. For example, to show how many liquor stores or parks are in your neighborhood.	When it is difficult to define the community geographically.
Photo Voice	Use cameras to "document" or take pictures of issue you are working on.	When you want to show the media or policymakers what's happening in your community.	When you don't have the resources.

community members in how to use them to collect information. If you conduct focus groups or community forums, you will need to work with the community members to identify the questions you want to ask, and recruit people to participate in the groups or forums.

This is the action part of the research where community members really begin to feel as though they are working toward change. Be sure to provide training or skill-building sessions as necessary so that community members have the skills they need to do the job.

A WORD ABOUT BIAS

It is possible to conduct a community diagnosis so that you learn only what you want to hear. If you think that the community should start a campaign to close a nearby waste incinerator, you can set up the community diagnosis to increase the chances that this will be the final outcome. But this type of manipulation contradicts the true purpose of a community diagnosis: to gather information without prejudice and to let the community express their own concerns and their own ideas for change.

Common ways that bias can undermine a community diagnosis include:

- Determining who participates in the community diagnosis—such as including only people who already agree with a certain position.

- Asking **leading questions** or questions that lead people to the answers you want them to provide. An example of a leading question is: "Do you think that racism is one of the most important factors that contributes to high rates of infant mortality in the community?" An open-ended and unbiased question would be: "What do you think are some of the most important factors that contribute to high rates of infant mortality in the community?"
- Summarizing data to highlight information that supports your position, withholding data that does not, or presenting it in a confusing way.
- Guiding the analysis or trying to do the analysis for the community, and telling them what the data says.
- Guiding the development of the action plan, by calling on and supporting the voices of people who agree with you, or by asking questions that lead people to the type of action that you think is best.

As a CHW, allowing your own bias or that of your agency to influence the results of a community diagnosis is likely to undermine the community's trust in you. It may also weaken and damage, rather than strengthen, the community's own capacity. It is a violation of your ethical commitment to respect the right of communities to choose their own course of action.

LIBRARY RESEARCH

Library research can provide access to local data, history, and other resources that might not be available elsewhere. We recommend that you start by finding a librarian and asking him or her for a general orientation and guidance in researching your topic. Librarians are experts in conducting research and are there to provide training, guidance, and support. You can also use library computers to find local, statewide, national, or international information and resources. Ask the librarian for assistance with the computers and how to enter key words to find your information. Key words are those you enter into a computer or Internet search program that tell it what information to look for.

For example, a group of youth advocates in San Francisco was concerned about peers who smoked *bidis* (cigarettes hand rolled in South Asia, without filters). This became the focus of their diagnosis and their project. Neither the city health workers nor the youth advocates knew much about bidis, so they decided to go to the city library to research whether bidis contain tobacco or other harmful substances, and whether smoking bidis is harmful. Their search at the library revealed that bidis do contain tobacco and other unknown substances. They found out that smoking bidis can cause cancer, just like smoking other types of cigarettes. They also found out that bidis are often rolled by women and young children who work twelve to sixteen hours a day for little pay.

Library privileges are easy to get, usually requiring some proof of residence (drivers license, utility bill, and so on). Colleges and universities also have libraries and often allow community members to use them.

INTERNET RESEARCH

To research information on the Internet, go to a search engine such as "Google," "Google scholar," "Yahoo," or others, and type in key words, such as "bidis" or "bidi cigarettes" or "bidis and health." Be sure to try different key word combinations to do a broad enough search. Research on the Internet allows you to get the most updated research findings on your topic. It also assists you to connect with other organizations working on similar issues (so you can see what other groups are doing, what materials they are using, and what research they've done).

Be sure to look at sources of data from local governments, such as the local health department, and private organizations, including universities and foundations. Information that you may find on the Internet includes health statistics that can assist people to better understand the scope of the problem, its causes, and the consequences.

Note: It is important to verify sources when searching the Internet. Health information on the Web varies in quality . . . *anyone can post health information on the Web!*

Here are examples of reputable public health Web sites:

- The Centers for Disease Control and Prevention: www.cdc.gov
- Office of the Surgeon General, Reports and Publications: www.surgeongeneral.gov/library/reports.htm
- Healthy People 2010: www.health.gov/healthypeople
- Partners in Information Access for the Public Health Workforce: www.phpartners.org

? *What is the Web site for your local city or county health department?*

RESEARCH EXISTING LAWS AND POLICIES

A key component of any diagnosis involves researching existing laws. There are many laws, regulations, and policies that already exist at the city, state, or federal level that may influence the issue your group is working on. Within city government a number of city departments also have policies that may be relevant to your work. For example, many cities have laws that limit the amount of advertising in corner stores. A group of community advocates concerned about tobacco and alcohol advertising in neighborhood stores might find that their city limits outdoor advertising to no more than 10 percent of window space. They could identify stores that exceed this amount and work with city enforcement agencies to get unhealthy advertising reduced in their community.

You can begin the process by going to city hall or onto the city Web site to search for the city agency with jurisdiction over your issue. For example, if you want to find out about local laws regulating signs and advertising, you could start by getting on your city's Web site and searching using the key words "sign laws." You might be directed to the city planning department or the city municipal codes that include these laws. This type of research requires patience and persistence. Every system is organized differently, but the more you familiarize yourself with city, state, and federal systems, the easier it becomes. Sometimes the best you can do is find a phone number and start by calling and asking for assistance. Try a variety of methods to find the person or city agency responsible for addressing your issue. Don't give up!

COUNTING PHYSICAL OBJECTS

Counting physical objects can show how aspects of the physical environment positively or negatively affect the community. For example, if you wanted to show how often tobacco companies promote their products to children, you could come up with a checklist, visit all the stores in your neighborhood, and count how many times each store has tobacco ads located below three feet in height or near candy.

Things You Might Count:

- The number of grocery stores selling fresh produce (vegetables and fruit)
- The number of fast-food restaurants in the community
- The number of liquor stores and bars in the community

- The number of after-school recreation facilities or programs for school-aged children
- The number of clinics or physicians accepting Medi-Cal
- The number of colleges, adults schools, or employment training programs in the community

What else might you count as part of a your community diagnosis?

To conduct this type of research:

- Work with community members to design a standardized tool or checklist to document how often something (such as alcohol or tobacco advertising) occurs, where it occurs, and any other important information they want to gather.
- Work with community representatives to develop a research plan. Do they want to count objects in all stores in your neighborhood, or do they want to visit a sample of all stores citywide? What are the geographic boundaries of the neighborhood?

The youth advocates researching bidis worked with a researcher to develop a sample list of one hundred stores in their city. They took a map and plotted the stores on the map. They came up with a one-page survey tool and visited each store to see if the store sold bidis, what flavors they sold, if the store sold to underage youths, and if the bidis had warning labels. They documented their findings on a one-page research form.

SURVEYS

You can also find out what the community thinks by surveying a sample of individuals. You might survey youths, parents, teachers, agency leaders, or members of any group. Surveys can be completed in apartment buildings, on the street, at community events, and in waiting rooms. Sometimes surveys are done in two neighborhoods with different characteristics to compare and contrast. The important thing is to take the time to prepare your survey questions and set up a good survey design that will represent the community you are working with.

Developing an Effective Survey   Start by working with community members to identify the type of information they want to gather and how that information will enhance their understanding of the focus issue or concern. Next, create a list of questions to include in the survey that are designed to gather this information. Narrow the questions down to no more than two pages. Use straightforward language and don't use abbreviations. Finally, put your questions in a logical order (from the general to the more specific).

Start the survey with the questions that are the most interesting and least threatening. Save the more difficult questions for the end, and avoid leading questions ("Don't you think . . . ?").

As much as possible, use closed-ended questions for surveys rather than open-ended ones. This will allow you to collect data and analyze your findings. When including questions that ask people to compare or rate items, be sure that the scale includes options from both extremes. Keep this simple (for example, *poor, okay, great*). If you want to give respondents a list of answers or categories to choose from, try to keep it fairly short (no more than five choices). Questions that ask people to remember things from the past should focus on the near past in order to document accurate information.

Once you have your survey in draft form, pretest it with a few people representing the group you want to survey to ensure that all the questions are clear and prompt responses that are useful to the community diagnosis. Finally, come up with a brief memo to attach to the survey describing who you are, why you are doing the survey, and how you will use the information gathered. You will want to hand this out to everyone whom you ask to participate in the survey.

The survey in Figure 17.1 was developed and used by Literacy for Environmental Justice to assess community attitudes and feelings about tobacco advertising in the Bay View Hunter's Point neighborhood of San Francisco.

Figure 17.1 Tobacco Advertising Survey (Literacy for Environmental Justice).

With the following survey, we would like to find out from you how you feel about tobacco advertisements in your community at your community corner/liquor stores here in Bay View Hunters Point. We would appreciate your spending a few minutes to complete this survey. The results from this survey will be used to fight the placement of tobacco ads in our community.

First, we would love to learn more about you.

Age: ☐

Gender: Male ☐ **Female** ☐

Zip Code: ☐

What is the primary language you speak at home? ☐

What's your ethnicity? ☐

Do you or any family members smoke cigarettes? Yes ☐ **No** ☐

On average how many cigarettes do you/they smoke? _____

What brands do you/they smoke? _____

Where do you or your family members buy your cigarettes?

_____ **In the BVHP** _____ **Elsewhere: where?** _____

Did you know that the tobacco industry provides incentives to stores to advertise and promote tobacco?   Yes ○ **No** ○

Where do you see advertisements for tobacco?:

_____ **Outside of stores** _____ **Inside stores** _____ **Magazines** _____ **Movies** _____ **Other**

What brands of cigarettes do you see advertised the most? _____

Are you aware that there are tobacco advertisements in your community liquor stores?

Yes ☐ **No** ☐

Name one way that you think tobacco companies advertise tobacco: _____

Do you think that tobacco ads influence young people to smoke? Yes ☐ **No** ☐

What about tobacco ads do you think is influential: _____ **Pictures** _____ **Messages** _____ **Slogans** _____ **Other**

Do you think that the tobacco companies should compensate the city/public for the harm caused by tobacco advertising and use?   Yes ○ **No** ○

Would you support efforts to reduce advertising in the community?   Yes ☐ **No** ☐

If yes, what are some ways we might try to do this? Would you support:

- **Trying to get the tobacco companies to pay for city efforts (GN) to reduce exposure to tobacco promotion for youths and others   Yes ❏   No ❏**

- **Amending the Lee Law (that restricts ads in store windows) to reduce advertising?   Yes ❏   No ❏**

- **Getting programs to replace tobacco and alcohol ads with ads about healthy eating and healthy and sustainable communities?   Yes ❏   No ❏**

You can learn more about designing surveys online at Info Poll: www.accesswave. ca/~infopoll/tips.htm.

FACILITATE DISCUSSIONS WITH COMMUNITY MEMBERS

Other strategies to find out what the community is thinking include:

- ✪ Inviting the community to attend local forums or meetings
- ✪ Visiting community agencies and groups
- ✪ Facilitating focus groups

Community Forums   Invite community members to a large meeting or community forum to talk about the issue or concern you are investigating and to share their experiences, feelings, and opinions. A community member may introduce the forum or meeting and explain the community diagnosis process, what you are doing, the type of information you hope to gather, and how you intend to use it. Let the audience know that their knowledge and information will be used to guide efforts to promote the community's health. You may identify specific questions and facilitate a structured conversation in one large or several small groups. Or you may decide to use an open microphone and let community members speak up as they choose about the issue that you are addressing, such as low birth weights and high rates of infant mortality. Appoint two or more people to take notes in order to document the information shared during the meeting. Community forums can be effective ways to discover various perspectives on an issue and to generate a range of ideas about how to approach it.

Visits to Community Agencies, Associations, or Groups   Compile a comprehensive list of the agencies, associations, or groups in your community. Come up with a standardized survey or interview guide that outlines the questions you want to be sure to cover in your visits. Try to put the questions in order so that they flow from easier to more difficult and prepare them so you can group responses (do content analysis). Determine who you will talk to at the agency. This is an opportunity to build relationships and identity potential allies who will support the community diagnosis and advocacy for social change.

Facilitating Focus Groups   A focus group is essentially an interview conducted with a group of six to twelve people. Focus groups generally last one to two hours, address one main topic or issue, and ask five or six questions to guide a discussion. We devote more space to describing focus groups, because they are often a great research tool to learn more out about commonly held experiences, ideas, and feelings. However, not every community diagnosis will use focus groups, and not every kind of information you want to learn is best gathered by focus groups. Focus groups are a great tool to use when you want in-depth information about a specific topic.

RESOURCE FOR CONDUCTING FOCUS GROUPS

We can only provide the briefest introduction to the focus-group process here. Learning the skills required to facilitate a productive focus group takes time and experience. The best possible beginning would be to observe a focus group, or even to take part in one as a participant. There are many resources that can provide more information, including *The Focus Group Kit (*Morgan and Krueger, 1998). There are also many Web sites that offer free assistance with setting up focus groups, including the Free Management Library, an online resource for nonprofits (www.managementhelp.org/evaluatn/focusgrp.htm) and The Community Tool Box, a community health resource (www.ctb.ku.edu/tools//sub_section_main_1018.htm).

Why Use a Focus Group?   Like a community forum and qualitative interviews (see following sections), a focus group provides an opportunity to gather more in-depth and potentially surprising information. Focus groups also give people the opportunity to interact *with each other*, in addition to responding directly to a question. The conversation that participants have with each other is the richest part of any focus-group process.

How to Facilitate a Focus Group   Focus groups should not be facilitated by one person. You should always work with others to determine your focus-group goal(s) and questions. And in addition to the participants whom you invite to take part in the focus group, you will need someone to act as the moderator or facilitator, as well as someone to act as the recorder and to document what participants say.

1. Identify Your Goal   A clearly stated goal will better serve to keep you on track throughout the focus group. What is it that you want to learn? How will that information be helpful to the community diagnosis?

2. Formulate Your Questions   Your questions must be open-ended but inspire conversation. A question that is too open could leave participants confused or overwhelmed. It's smart to start simply, with questions that are easier for people to understand and answer, and build to more complex questions.

A sample set of questions might look like this:

a.   What do you like about living in the neighborhood?
b.   What are your concerns with safety in your neighborhood?
c.   How do these safety concerns affect the community?
d.   What needs to change to promote safety in the neighborhood?
e.   _____?
f.   _____?

3. Recruit Participants   Generally, you want to make sure there are enough people in the room to keep a good conversation going, but not so many that some participants won't have a chance to speak. Eight to ten people in the focus group is ideal. In planning the number of participants, anticipate that one or more individuals may not show up. Generally, if twelve people have confirmed that they will participate, ten will show up. If everyone shows up, it would still be a manageable size for a focus group, and if fewer than twelve show up, you will still have enough people to keep the conversation flowing.

Diversity of perspective: Often, having people who are similar in some way is useful—for example, having all the participants come from the same neighborhood, all be single parents, or all be of the same gender, age, or ethnicity. Other times, it's helpful to have more diversity. You might hold several focus groups on the same topic. Talk with your colleagues about what you think the right mix will be for the information you wish to learn.

Incentives for participation: If you have a budget for this, small gift cards or other incentives will be appreciated by the participants and encourage them to show up for the focus group.

4. Create the Right Environment   *Build rapport and trust:* Participants need reassurance that you and the other group members are trustworthy. Let people know what you are doing and why, and follow through on any commitments you make to the group.

Power dynamics: Will everyone in the room feel equally empowered to speak up? If a person's supervisor is present, they might not be comfortable talking about certain job-related concerns. In certain cultures, women are expected to defer to men, and are therefore less likely to speak up if men are present. Some power dynamics can be handled through good facilitation, however. If some people are more dominant participants than others, the facilitator can say, "I'd like to hear from some of the people who haven't spoken yet."

Consider the interests and strengths of the group you'll be convening: Different groups of people may require different strategies in your facilitation. For example, with young people, you might not get answers by asking straightforward questions.

CONDUCTING A FOCUS GROUP WITH HIGH SCHOOL STUDENTS

In a focus group with ninth-grade students for the purpose of identifying the after-school activities they most enjoyed, and the factors that encouraged or discouraged participation in these activities, the facilitator was aware that students could lose interest very quickly. The facilitator worked with several youth to develop the questions for the focus group. The facilitator also had the students draw a picture that showed the after-school activity they would offer if they were in charge and if resources were not a problem. The students were asked stand up and present their idea to the group. The facilitator could assess the enthusiasm that peers had for the idea as well as ask questions about any details that might be of interest. Asking them to write their name, age, gender, languages spoken at home, and languages spoken with friends also helped to increase participation and dialogue.

Facilitation: Don't try to control the conversation too much, but make sure that you get answers to your most important questions. Understand that people build ideas by talking to each other and asking each other questions. Let that happen!

Child care: Depending on the group you are bringing together, it is a good idea to have a plan for child care. Offering child care might enable some people to participate who would otherwise decline.

Refreshments: Providing healthy snacks and drinks is an important way to thank your participants, and to make sure they get the brain fuel they need to participate fully.

Languages spoken: Know the language needs of your participants, and arrange for interpretation, if necessary. You might consider holding more than one focus group if you have enough participants to hold, for example, an all-Russian language group as well as an all-Spanish language group.

Documentation: Documenting the focus group accurately is very important. Use a tape or digital recorder, and test all your equipment ahead of time. Bring plenty of extra batteries and blank tapes. Also plan to take your own notes. You want to keep track not just of what people say, but of how they say it. For example, people's body language is important to notice. Ideally, one member of your team will act only as the recorder and not do anything else. Be sure to inform participants that they are being recorded.

5. Making It Work   *Ground rules:* Setting basic ground rules allows everyone to know what to expect. You might suggest some, and then ask those in the group if they have any they want to add. Post them on flip-chart paper so everyone can keep them in mind. *Confidentiality* is important to discuss. You need to assure participants that what they say will be treated confidentially by you, and they in turn need to agree to keep what they hear and say confidential.

Agenda: Plan to spend between sixty and ninety minutes, and not more. You should have a clear agenda that you share with participants at the beginning of the session.

Facilitation suggestions: Make sure that everyone has the chance to speak. Let people know what you are going to do with the information they have provided.

6. Analysis   As soon after the session as possible, write down your thoughts and review your notes. Spend some time with your fellow facilitators and share your reflections. Identify strongly held views, major areas of agreement among participants, and surprising information. Generally, you will do a content analysis similar to what is explained in the next section related to conducting qualitative interviews. Content analysis is a way of identifying common themes that are shared by focus-group participants.

QUALITATIVE INTERVIEWS

Sometimes you want to gather in-depth information about people's experiences, feelings, and opinions expressed in their own words. You may be looking for insights into sensitive or controversial issues, or want to learn more about the history of the community. This kind of data is gained by qualitative interviews, or structured conversations with people. The insights of the CHWs quoted in this textbook were obtained from qualitative interviews.

Like focus groups, qualitative interviews can strengthen or provide a context for other data and statistics that you gather and may show *why* people feel the way they do. Qualitative interviews can provide quotes from community members that serve to attach meaning to the numbers or statistics you have gathered. Qualitative results also help community advocates evaluate how well projects were implemented and provide feedback from community members on the process involved in implementing social change efforts. Finally, qualitative interviews reveal unexpected positive or negative outcomes of your efforts.

Conducting Qualitative Interviews   Ideally, qualitative interviews should feel like a conversation. Ask people about themselves in relation to the issue at hand. ("When did you first become aware of the high infant mortality rate in your community?" "How does this problem affect you and the community?" "What do you think causes or contributes to this problem?" "What do you think should be done to reduce the problem of infant mortality?") In general, people like to be asked to share their opinions. Similar to surveys, start with nonthreatening questions. People may not want to answer very personal or difficult questions until they get comfortable with you and the process. Open-ended questions are best. As people begin to answer questions, use probing follow-up questions to get more information such as: "Can you tell me more about that?" or "Is there anything else you wanted to say about this issue?" Sometimes it is useful to stay silent and give the person you are interviewing time to reflect and respond. Use your client-centered counseling and motivational interviewing skills (see Chapter Ten).

You can encourage the person being interviewed (the respondent) with positive feedback and by paying attention to nonverbal cues and body language. Don't share your views on the subject in case this may influence what the respondent says. Finally, let the respondent know that you are taking notes to be sure to remember key points. If you are looking for material you can quote, use a recorder to make sure that you get it right. Let the person you are interviewing know you are recording the interview. They will be reassured that you will not distort what they say. It is unethical to record anyone without that person's knowledge and consent. If you think there is any reason to believe the person you are interviewing might get upset with your using the interview, clarify the situation by asking them to sign a release form giving you permission to use the interview for the specific purposes that you tell them. This can also reassure people that the interview will not be used for any other purposes.

RELEASE OF INFORMATION

I, _____, give _____ [name of interviewer] permission to use material from this interview only in material created by the Tobacco Free Project.

Signed and dated:

_____

Note: If the person you are interviewing is less than 18 years old, a parent or guardian must give permission.

The most important question:

After you have finished the interview, but before you turn off the recorder, always ask if there is anything else the person wants to tell you. Don't suggest what that might be. Wait for as long as it takes for the person to decide that they are done. Some of the most interesting insights come when people answer the question you didn't think to ask.

Content Analysis of Responses   There are different ways to analyze qualitative interviews. Transcribing the interview—writing it down word for word from a recording—often helps with this. To identify key themes from one interview or common themes

Table 17.2.   Summary of Qualitative Interviews Conducted in Z. Neighborhood.

Major Themes	Out of 20 Interviews, No. of People Who Mentioned the Theme:
Closing of shipyard	12
Poor quality of local schools	6
Racism	15

from more than one interview, do a content analysis of what was said. Do this by looking for categories or common themes in what people said, issues that come up again and again, or that the respondent gave particular importance to. A theme might be something like: lack of education or good schools; the closing of a big employer in the community; conflict between certain segments of the community; or racism. In your summary and analysis of the interviews, look not only for opinions and themes that were shared among the respondents, but also for particularly strong or powerful opinions. Write down insightful quotes to include as part of your analysis. To find out how common particular themes are, you can create a simple table (see Table 17.2) to identity the themes mentioned and to count how many people mentioned them.

COMMUNITY MAPPING

Mapping can be a powerful research strategy. Maps are used to provide a visual image of the risks and negative influences that impact a community, such as sources of environmental pollution, dangerous crosswalks or intersections, or very poor quality housing. Maps can show the distribution of illness and death in a community or region such as homicides, infant mortality, or other conditions. Maps can also show the strengths and resources in a community that promote well-being and health, such as quality housing, parks, schools, public transportation, health centers, and grocery stores.

A classic early example of a map that was used to guide public health work is the map that Dr. John Snow drew of cholera deaths in London in 1854 (see Figure 17.2). As you can see, the map revealed that a large number of deaths had occurred near the location of the Broad Street Water Pump. The map assisted Dr. Snow to convince policymakers to turn off the pump, which resulted in a dramatic decline in cholera cases and deaths. The map also lead to a new understanding of how cholera was transmitted from person to person, eventually resulting in new strategies for prevention (University of California, Los Angeles, 2008).

Mapping is increasingly used by local, national, and international health agencies to identify populations with the highest health risks and to better understand the factors that contribute to those risks. Mapping is often done using Geographic Information Systems (GIS) that rely on information gathered from satellites and other sources to create detailed electronic images. An example is provided in the documentary film series "Unnatural Causes," in which the Louisville Kentucky Health Department showed how race and income were associated with health inequalities and differences in life expectancy (Unnatural Causes, 2008). To read more about the GIS technologies, please see the resources at the end of this chapter from the Centers for Disease Control and the World Health Organization.

Figure 17.2 Map of cholera deaths in London, 1854. The X marks the location of the Broad Street water pump.

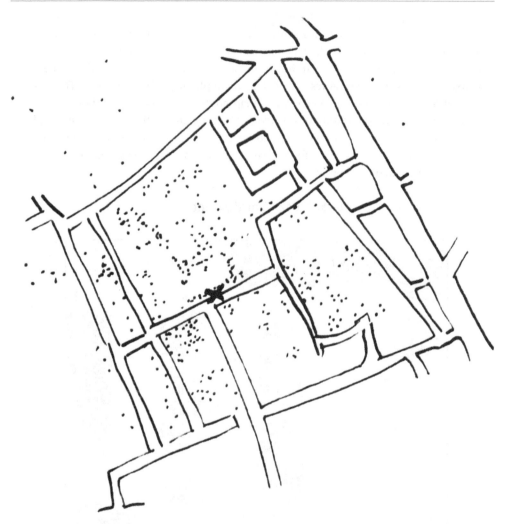

Mapping doesn't require advanced technology, however; it can be done by hand, with graph paper, on top of paper maps of your neighborhood or city, or through using Web resources such as "Google Maps" or "Google Earth" (maps.google.com or earth. google.com).

PHOTOVOICE

Another resource for conducting a community diagnosis involves using cameras to document what is happening in a community. This powerful tool is known as Photovoice. One example is the project conducted by Legal Services for Children described in Chapter Twenty-One. This project—"Invisible Punishment: Photovoice Challenges the Prison System"— gave cameras to people with family members who are in prison to record the impact of high rates of incarceration on communities. To read more about Photovoice, check out http://www.photovoice.com.

Community mapping and Photovoice produce compelling visual representations of what is happening in the community. Many CHWs and community advocates use photos,

LITERACY FOR ENVIRONMENTAL JUSTICE

A project supported by the Tobacco Free Project was carried out by Literacy for Environmental Justice (LEJ), a nonprofit agency, and a group of youth advocates. They were concerned about the lack of fresh and healthy foods in the corner stores in their community. They visited the eleven stores in their neighborhood and drew maps of the inside of the stores. They created simple maps for each store. The following diagram (Figure 17.3) recreates a map produced by the youth advocates for one of the eleven stores: Jimmy's Market. The map shows that 35 percent of all products sold at Jimmy's Market were nonfood items, 27 percent were alcohol and cigarettes, 24 percent packaged food, 10 percent all other beverages, and just 4 percent were meat and fresh produce.

Figure 17.3 Jimmy's Market, 6245 Third Street

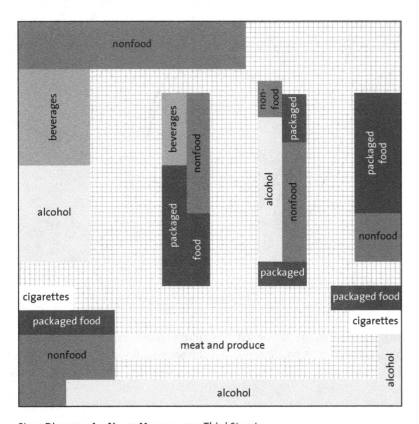

Store Diagram: **ALL NIGHT MARKET,** 5190 Third Street

35%	nonfood products
27%	alcohol and cigarettes
24%	packaged food
10%	all other beverages
4%	meat and produce

THE FOCUS PROJECT

Since 2005, the Tobacco Free Project (TFP), a program of the San Francisco Department of Public Health, has funded the FOCUS Project. FOCUS is a collaboration of the Chinese Progressive Association (CPA) and People Organizing to Demand Environmental and Economic Rights (PODER). The collaboration grew out of a desire to support the empowerment of working-class immigrant communities in Southeast San Francisco and to improve the dire environmental health conditions in those neighborhoods.

CPA/PODER conducted a community diagnosis to understand the scope of environmental impacts and health problems, and analyzed the role that the transnational tobacco industry plays within these working-class communities of color. They created a map to show the results of their community diagnosis. The resulting map of San Francisco showed that the greatest number and concentration of tobacco outlets were located in communities with the highest levels of poverty and the largest number of immigrants and people of color. These communities also had the highest rates of smoking. The maps were used to show that the number of tobacco retail outlets put the community at greater risk of tobacco-related health inequalities—greater rates of illness and death.

Ultimately, this research influenced decisions about local policy and how to prevent exposure to environmental health risks, including tobacco.

maps, and diagrams when presenting public testimony to local policymakers or when discussing their issue with the press.

STEP 5: SUMMARIZE YOUR RESEARCH FINDINGS

If you collected three hundred surveys, and want community members to come together to analyze them, would it be helpful or efficient to hand out all three hundred copies of the two-to-three-page surveys at a meeting? What would community members do with this information? How would they analyze it?

CHWs often work in partnership with community representatives to assist in summarizing the information gathered for a community diagnosis in a way that makes it possible for community members to understand. Qualitative data—information gathered by focus groups, community meetings, and interviews—is often harder to summarize. Perform a content analysis to look at the major themes that emerged. You may also want to highlight strong minority perspectives that do not agree with what most people tell you for the community to consider. If you haven't done a content analysis before, talk with your supervisor or ask an experienced colleague to assist you with this part of the work.

Quantitative data can be summarized numerically and is much easier to present to the community. However, not everyone will be comfortable analyzing numbers or statistics, so the way that you present this data can make a big difference. You don't want some members of the community to feel left out of the process of analyzing the findings of the community diagnosis simply because they have less training, experience, and comfort talking about statistics (we address this point in greater detail below, under Step 6).

Most important, work as a team, and reflect on whether your assumptions and prejudices are influencing the outcomes. Are you leaving any important findings out of the summary? Are you presenting the community with accurate information to guide them in their analysis and future work together?

STEP 6: ANALYZE YOUR RESEARCH FINDINGS

Now it is time to present the information or research findings to the community for them to analyze and interpret. This is a crucial step in the process. The analysis of the information will assist community members to identify a possible solution to their common concern. The analysis will also assist community members to identify the "startling statistics"—the information that will compel decision makers to do something about the issue.

As the community is reviewing the information gathered, you may use the following questions to guide their analysis:

- What does the information tell them about the issue they investigated?
- Who in the community is most affected by the problem?
- What percentage of people who participated in the research is highly concerned about the problem?
- What does the community think about the causes and consequences of the problem?
- What are their proposed solutions?
- Do different parts of the community have different experiences or opinions—for example, do women express different opinions from men, do youths express different opinions from elders? Are there any differences in opinion based on where people live in the community?

IMPORTANT THINGS TO REMEMBER:

1. Don't take the data at face value . . . there are different ways to interpret the same data.

For example, your data may show that there has been a decrease in the number of illegal tobacco and alcohol sales to minors. This could mean that: (1) fewer merchants are selling tobacco and alcohol to minors, or (2) less enforcement is taking place due to a lack of funding or some other reason. It is important to look deeper to show the whole story.

2. Information or data gathered cannot always tell the whole story.

For example, data that has been collected at the neighborhood level cannot be used to say what is happening in different neighborhoods or in all neighborhoods. Focus groups and interviews only give you information about the people you interviewed. When describing this type of data, always include language that notes that such as, "Of those people surveyed, 80 percent reported . . . " or "Survey respondents reported that . . . " or "Focus group participants felt . . . "

PREPARING YOUR FINDINGS IN A VISUALLY COMPELLING FORMAT

Once the community has analyzed and interpreted the data, we recommend that you develop a clear way to present the data to others. You will want to share this information with allies who will assist you to advocate for changes in the community and to policy-makers who have the power to make certain changes. How you present the data often can make all the difference in terms of whether or not people will understand it (also see Chapter Twenty).

The community group analyzing the data should try to identity the five top findings that will become their "startling statistics." What information is most compelling to the community? What information supports their final analysis? What information will be useful in assisting policymakers take action on the community's behalf?

Tip: You are looking for startling statistics that:

- Show how your community is adversely affected by the issue compared with other communities
- Show that your community is concerned about the issue and wants something done about it
- Show that your community understands the issue and has done their homework around it
- Show that policies already exist that address the issue
- Show that local solutions exist to address the issue

There are many ways to present your data, including:

- Tables
- Pie charts
- Bar or line graphs
- Photos
- Maps
- Pictures
- Case studies and quotes

? *What do you think of the way the information is presented using the pie chart?*

? *Is the information easy to understand?*

? *Can you think of other ways that you could present this information?*

LITERACY FOR ENVIRONMENTAL JUSTICE:

How One Group Presented Their Findings in a Visually Compelling Format

As described above, youth advocates working with Literacy for Environmental Justice (LEJ) were concerned about the lack of healthy food sold in their community, which had very high rates of diabetes and other chronic diseases. They were also concerned about the health problems caused by smoking and alcohol.

(Continued)

The youths drew a map of eleven local stores showing the products that they sold. From this information, they created a pie chart showing the types of products sold at the stores in their community. The pie chart shows, for example, that 26 percent of the items for sale in neighborhood stores were alcohol and cigarettes, and only 2 percent of the items for sale were produce (vegetables and fruit).

Information gathered with this survey:

> ### Literacy for Environmental Justice: Store Diagram Directions
> #### Completed by:
>
> 1) Walk into the store and look around noticing, as many details as you can.
>
> 2) Introduce yourself to the clerk:
>   *"Hello! My name is_____ and I am doing a geography project for summer school. Can you help me by allowing me to make a thematic map of your store? Thank you so much!"*
>
> 3) Walk the perimeter of the store, noticing the layout, shape, and size of the store.
>
> 4) Record the environment of the store below:
>
> Sounds: Clerks:
>
> Cleanlines: Feeling(s):
>
> Customers:
>
> Can you play the lottery?
> Does the store accept food stamps?
> Are there a lot of advertisements? For what?
>
> 5) Check a few expiration dates and record below:
>
> 6) Draw a diagram of the store. Be sure to include the following items:
>
> | | |
> |---|---|
> | Store entrance | Candy |
> | Windows | Alcohol |
> | Storage space | Beverages |
> | Backdoor | Chips |
> | Garbage | Frozen food |
> | Tobacco products | Produce |
> | Food products | Other |
>
> 7) Double-check your data. Make sure that you are accurate and diagram is proportional. Thank the store clerk and exit the store.

Became this chart:

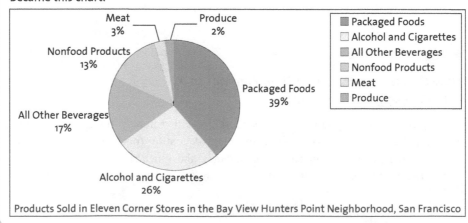

Products Sold in Eleven Corner Stores in the Bay View Hunters Point Neighborhood, San Francisco

STEP 7: DEVELOP AN ACTION PLAN

Based on the analysis of research findings, community members will come together to develop an action plan to address the concerns they identified and to create changes that will promote their health. An action plan lays out the steps the community will take to make or advocate for change. This process should be as inclusive as possible, providing an opportunity for all members of the community to participate if they choose. Getting this process right is more important than doing it quickly. If you rush and forget to include certain members of the community, you risk losing support for your action plan or creating a new conflict and problem in the community. Be as transparent or open and honest as possible about this process: let everyone know how and when they can participate.

You will learn how to develop an action plan in detail in Chapter Twenty-Two.

QUEER YOUTH ACTION TEAM

In Chapter Sixteen, we described the work of the Queer Youth Action Team (QYAT), a project of the Center for Community Development in Contra Costa County, California. The QYAT was a group of lesbian, gay, bisexual, and transgender (LGBT) high-school-aged youths who came together to address health concerns related to HIV, harassment, and discrimination. With support from CHWs and other staff at CHD, the youths conducted a community diagnosis to guide them in developing an action plan. This plan involved advocating for new policies at local school districts to prohibit harassment and other forms of discrimination against LGBT students.

? *What are some possible actions that the Native communities mentioned at the beginning of this chapter could take to reduce high rates of low birth weight and infant mortality?*

CHAPTER REVIEW QUESTIONS

YOUR COMMUNITY DIAGNOSIS

Think about a community you belong to or know well. Apply the information presented in this chapter to answer the following questions:

1. Define and describe the community that will undertake the diagnosis.
2. What is the focus of the community diagnosis? What issue will the community address?
3. What are you trying to find out about your focus or issue? What questions are you asking about your issue? List at least five questions here.
4. What research tools will you use to you find this out? How will you do your research?
5. How will you work with community members to analyze your findings and come up with "startling statistics." List three to five "startling statistics" here!
6. How will you prepare your findings for the community and policymakers (in charts, graphs, written form, with pictures, or in packets)?
7. What type of actions might the community take to address their priority concern and create positive changes?

REFERENCES

Arble, B., and Moberg, D. P. 2006. Participatory Research in Development of Public Health Interventions. *Translating Research into Policy and Practice* 1(6). Accessed on April 1, 2009: http://pophealth.wisc.edu/uwphi/

The Centers for Disease Control and Prevention. Accessed on April 1, 2009: http://www.cdc.gov/nchs/gis.htm

The Community Tool Box. Accessed on April 1, 2009: http://ctb.ku.edu/tools//sub_section_main_1018.htm

The Free Management Library. Accessed on April 1, 2009: http://www.managementhelp.org/evaluatn/focusgrp.htm

Info Poll. 1998. How to Write a Good Survey. Accessed on April 1, 2009: http://www.accesswave.ca/~infopoll/tips.htm

Kretzman, J. P., and McKnight, J. 1993. *Building Communities from the Inside Out.* Chicago: ACTA Publications.

Minkler, M., and Wallerstein, N. 2003. *Community-Based Participatory Research for Health.* San Francisco: Jossey-Bass.

Morgan, D. L., and Krueger, R. A. (Eds.). 1998. *The Focus Group Kit.* Thousand Oaks, CA: Sage Publications.

Papa Ola Lokahi. Accessed on April 1, 2009: http://papaolalokahi.org/hoe2/index.cfm?wwa_ID=93B99296-EF41–4D27–9ECEB62C082DD382&sub=yes

Tsark, J. A. 2001. A Participatory Research Approach to Address Data Needs in Tobacco Use Among Native Hawaiians. *Asian American Pacific Island Journal of Health* 9: 40–48.

University of California, Los Angeles. School of Public Health, Department of Epidemiology. Accessed on April 1, 2009: http://www.ph.ucla.edu/epi/snow.html

Unnatural Causes. Accessed on April 1, 2009: http://www.pbs.org/unnaturalcauses/assets/resources/louisvillemap.pdf

W. K. Kellogg Foundation, Community Health Scholars Program. 2001. Definition developed and adopted by the Community Health Scholars Program based on B. A. Israel, A. J. Schulz, E. Parker, A. B. Becker, In Review of Community-Based Research: Assessing Partnership Approaches to Improve Public Health. *Annual Review of Public Health* 1998, 19: 173–202.

The World Health Organization. GIS and Public Health Mapping. Accessed on April 1, 2009: http://www.who.int/health_mapping/gisandphm/en/print.html

18

Health Outreach

Craig Wenzl • Tim Berthold

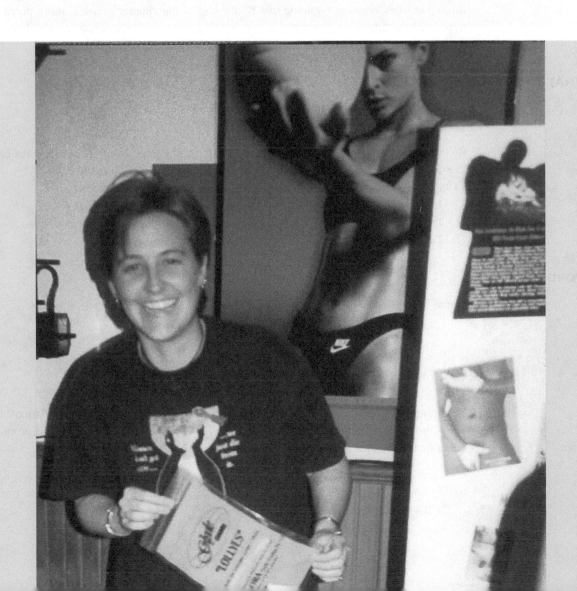

CHW SCENARIO

You have been hired by a local health department that is concerned about the increasing rates of an infectious disease in an immigrant community. Your job is to conduct outreach to this community, to provide them with information about the disease, and to support them in accessing local clinics for screening and treatment.

- ✪ How would you begin your outreach work?
- ✪ What do you want to know before you begin? What types of information will you gather?
- ✪ What types of resources would you rely on to guide your work?
- ✪ How would you know if your outreach program was successful?

INTRODUCTION

This chapter is an introduction to health outreach skills. Outreach links vulnerable communities to services that will promote their health. Some CHWs specialize in outreach services and may be called Community Health Outreach Workers or CHOWs. Even if they are not specialized outreach workers, most CHWs will participate in some level of outreach during their career. We will use the terms CHW and CHOW interchangeably throughout this chapter. We hope that by the end of the chapter you feel more prepared to answer the questions posed above and to bring your own experience, personality, and creativity to the task of conducting health outreach.

WHAT YOU WILL LEARN

By studying the information in this chapter, you will be able to:

- ✪ Define outreach
- ✪ Discuss the types of communities served and the health issues addressed through outreach
- ✪ Identify and provide examples of different outreach levels and methods
- ✪ Describe and apply strategies for approaching people you do not know
- ✪ Identify key safety concerns and strategies for outreach workers
- ✪ Document outreach services accurately and explain the importance of doing so
- ✪ Develop an outreach plan

WORDS TO KNOW

Social Marketing   Venue   Key Opinion Leaders

18.1 DEFINING COMMUNITY HEALTH OUTREACH

Community health outreach aims to identify, contact, and establish positive relationships with communities defined as "at risk" for specific health conditions in order to promote better health outcomes. Additional goals for health outreach may include to:

- ✪ Increase awareness about a particular health issue (such as breast cancer)
- ✪ Promote health knowledge and changes in health behaviors (such as regular breast self-exams and mammogram screenings)

- ✪ Recruit participants for research (such as research on the effectiveness of specific breast cancer treatment options)
- ✪ Establish links to and partnerships between existing communities and existing health programs (such as between a local church and a women's health clinic)
- ✪ Increase community participation in the design, implementation, and evaluation of health programs and policies (such as development of new outreach programs to assist women of color in gaining access to breast cancer screening and treatment services)
- ✪ Mobilize community members to participate in community organizing and advocacy efforts (such as expanded access to health care)

? *Can you think of other goals for conducting health outreach?*

18.2 QUALITIES OF SUCCESSFUL COMMUNITY HEALTH OUTREACH WORKERS

Outreach programs are often designed to work with communities who have experienced discrimination and who may face significant prejudice from the larger society, such as formerly incarcerated people. It is sometimes hard for an outsider to gain entry into the target community and to build the trust required to provide effective services. For these reasons, public health programs often recruit outreach workers from the communities to be served, with an emphasis on hiring culturally and linguistically competent CHOWs. For example, when a local health department was developing an outreach program to promote breast cancer screening among Hmong women, they hired a local Hmong woman to work as a CHOW.

S. did HIV prevention in the predominantly African American community where she grew up.

> **S.** Everyone around here knows me as the condom lady. I drive up in my car and pop the trunk, where I keep all my supplies, and everyone crowds around asking for stuff. After they've talked with me a few times, they call me over to talk about the personal things like getting tested or how their son died of AIDS or how they just tested positive. They trust me, but even though I grew up around here, I had to bust my butt to *earn* that trust!

Of course, not all outreach workers come from the communities they work with. Regardless of whether or not they are already familiar with the community, successful CHOWS tend to share the personal qualities outlined in Chapter One, including self-awareness, open-mindedness, and interpersonal warmth. In addition, because all CHOWs spend so much of their time building new relationships in the community, it is helpful to be:

- ✪ A "people person" who is good at talking with strangers as well as acquaintances
- ✪ *Extremely* patient
- ✪ Capable of earning the respect of all members of the community (and, sometimes even more important, someone who will not alienate particular subgroups within the community)
- ✪ Flexible and able to adapt to a variety of different working conditions
- ✪ Viewed as trustworthy by others; someone people feel comfortable talking to about personal issues

? *What other qualities do you think may be especially important for outreach workers?*

One of the biggest mistakes that new outreach workers make is to imitate the style and personality of more experienced CHOWs. However, the clients and communities you work with have a sixth sense for anything that is false or fake. Be your authentic self: if you pretend to be something or someone you are not, you will alienate the community and make it harder for them to trust you.

There are as many styles of outreach as there are outreach workers. There is room for all personality types in this profession. Be patient with yourself: with time and experience, you will develop your own unique approach to conducting outreach. Whether you are quiet, energetic, calm, or outgoing, your personality can inform and guide your work as a CHOW.

? *What skills do you already possess that make you a "natural" outreach worker?*

? *What skills do you need to cultivate?*

18.3 COMMUNITIES TO BE SERVED THROUGH OUTREACH

The communities served by outreach efforts are defined by a variety of factors, including epidemiologic and other public health data that document a clear risk for a specific disease or health condition. The communities are also defined by geographical boundaries that may be nationwide, statewide, or within the boundaries of a particular county, city, school district, ZIP code, or neighborhood. Other factors include age, ethnicity, nationality, immigration status, housing status (including homelessness), primary language, income, sexual orientation, gender, gender identity, behaviors (such as the use of injection drugs), and affiliations (such as membership in a particular labor union or religious organization).

Most communities served by outreach lack access to essential health resources and face significant barriers to health, such as poverty, lack of legal status, a history of discrimination, lack of access to educational programs or primary care services, geographic isolation, or homelessness.

Lᴇᴇ Jᴀᴄᴋsᴏɴ: I do HIV outreach where it's needed most, like in areas where there's a lot of drugs and sex work. If a lot of people are injecting drugs, and people are trading sex for drugs or money, and they don't always use condoms, there's gonna be a high rate of STDs (sexually transmitted diseases), especially HIV.

18.4 HEALTH ISSUES ADDRESSED BY OUTREACH

Outreach programs address a wide range of health issues including:

- Infectious diseases such as tuberculosis, HIV, malaria, schistosomiasis, syphilis, hepatitis, and the need for immunizations
- Chronic diseases such as cancer, diabetes, asthma, hypertension, and heart disease
- Mental health issues

- Accidents and injuries including automobile and pedestrian injuries
- Violence, including domestic violence and handgun violence
- Environmental and occupational health issues, including exposure to toxins and infectious agents where people live and work
- Enrollment in free and low-cost health insurance programs including Medicaid and SCHIP/Healthy Families programs
- Enrollment in research studies
- Community planning efforts related to local health concerns
- Organizing and advocacy efforts related to health issues

? *Can you think of other health-related issues to address through outreach?*

18.5 OUTREACH LEVELS

Outreach programs can operate on the level of the individual, group, institution, or population.

- *Individual level:* CHWs talk one-on-one with individuals, using client-centered practice. The CHW responds to the individual's questions and concerns, and provides health information, counseling, and referrals, as appropriate. CHWs may also provide testing or screening services such as HIV antibody test counseling.
- *Group level:* CHWs speak with a group from the target community, such as clients at a homeless shelter, a youth group at a local church, or mothers at a local Supplemental Nutrition Clinic for Women, Infants, and Children (WIC). The CHW provides health education and referrals and addresses the group's questions and concerns.
- *Institutional level:* CHWs work with representatives of a specific institution to reach their membership including, for example, schools, labor unions, employment sites, churches, mosques, or temples.
- *Population level:* Outreach efforts sometimes target a particular population within a city, county, state, or nation. This may include campaigns to reach youths, families with uninsured children, pregnant women, or smokers. Because these populations are large, the outreach methods usually include **social marketing** or the use of media such as television or radio to promote particular actions such as enrolling in Healthy Families, testing for HIV antibodies when pregnant, or the importance of regular exercise.

18.6 COMMON OUTREACH METHODS

CHWs use many outreach methods, depending on the characteristics of the target population, their preferred means of communication, the nature of the health issue to be addressed, and the type of health outcomes the program aims to promote. Outreach methods include:

STREET OUTREACH

Street outreach usually involves a team of two or more CHWs spending time in a neighborhood with the goal of locating and talking with members of a specific community, such as homeless youths. As we will discuss in the following section, what makes this approach effective (like all outreach efforts) is the ability of the CHWs to develop positive relationships with key members of the target community. CHWs approach clients and try to start a conversation. While the outreach workers may have one agenda, such as promoting condom use to prevent HIV infection, the clients often have different priorities. In order to build trust and ongoing relationships, CHWs need to listen first to the concerns and questions of prospective clients. CHWs usually carry outreach materials with them: brochures, lists of referrals, first aid kits, health resources such as condoms and lubricant, and other incentives such as hygiene kits (including soap, toothpaste and toothbrushes, and so on) for people who are trying to survive on the streets.

Far too many people are homeless in America. CHWs play a vital role in reaching out to those living on the streets.

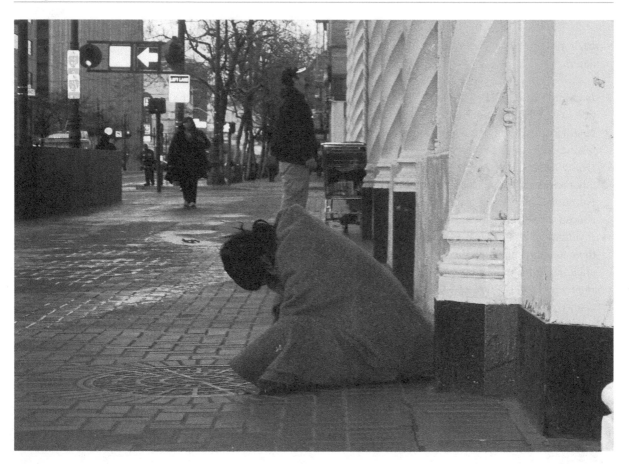

VENUE-BASED OUTREACH

In the public health field, the term *venue-based outreach* refers to outreach strategies that target particular places (a **venue** is a place) where the target community spends significant time. Venues may include schools, homeless encampments, public housing units, market places and cafes, public transportation stations, job sites, bars and clubs, sports events, parks, and churches, mosques, temples, and other places of worship.

PHUONG AN DOAN BILLINGS: At Asian Health Services we go out and try to connect the underserved populations to our clinic because one of the most important challenges for some communities is getting access to health care. The newcomers (or new immigrants) might be eligible for Healthy Families (health insurance for low-income families) or Medicare, but they don't know about these programs, and they are scared that they will have to pay, or their sponsors will have to pay, so they just stay home. That's why we need the outreach workers to be from the community. We go to English as Second Language (ESL) classes and nail salons and other places where the community is. For the Korean community, we go to small stores, like dry cleaning stores, markets, or churches. To reach the Vietnamese, we also go to the churches. And to temples, pagodas. We go to senior centers too.

? *Can you think of other venues or places to conduct outreach?*

Creating a venue. Sometimes CHWs need to *create* a venue at which to conduct outreach. For example, the Mpowerment Project developed by the Center for AIDS Prevention Studies at the University of California, San Francisco seeks to reach young (ages eighteen to twenty-four) men who have sex with men (MSM) to reduce risks for HIV disease. In many of the cities or regions where Mpowerment projects were developed, there were no well-established venues where young MSM congregated. Mpowerment groups created the venues where the target population could spend time together: drop-in centers, BBQs, dance parties, and movie nights. At these venues and events, CHWs conduct outreach and provide group and individual HIV prevention information, education, counseling, and referrals.

RECRUITMENT OF VOLUNTEER PEER EDUCATORS

Sometimes the best way to connect with a particularly hard-to-reach community is to recruit volunteer peer educators (VPE). CHWs identify **key opinion leaders** (people whom the community respects and looks to for guidance), build relationships, and ask the leaders to participate in the outreach effort on a volunteer basis. These VPEs may receive formal training in a workshop or informal training via conversations with CHWs. Depending on the nature of the outreach program, VPEs may pass out information or other resources (such as condoms), provide basic education, and make referrals to local services. VPEs can assist an outreach program to reach more members of the target community. While recruiting volunteers from the community can expand the reach of an outreach program, it is also time consuming and requires thoughtful recruitment, training, and supervision of VPEs.

WORKING WITH KEY OPINION LEADERS

CHWs were working in a Bay Area county with the goal of increasing condom use among local sex workers. They reached out to recruit key opinion leaders from the community, who in turn promoted the negotiation of safer sex and disseminated condoms, lubes, and referrals for additional services, including HIV test counseling, syringe exchange, and free and low-cost health care.

In Oakland, California, the Asian Health Center has organized Patient Leadership Councils to assist in reaching new immigrants.

PHUONG AN DOAN BILLINGS: We do outreach to recruit people to be part of the Patient Leadership Council. We try to recruit people from each community that we serve—people who we think have potential, and we train them. We train them in leadership skills and basic knowledge about the clinic and health issues that are big in the community, and they go out and do more outreach to spread the word about the clinic. They talk to their neighbors: "Hey I just came back from Asian Health Services today, and there is something so good about this place." They share this news and answer questions and encourage people to get health care if they need it. And they advise us about how we can do a better job serving their community.

INSTITUTIONAL OUTREACH

Many communities belong to or are represented by institutions that they trust and respect. Outreach programs can establish partnerships with these institutions to reach a specific community more efficiently. These institutions may include schools, ESL classes, churches, labor unions, clinics or health plans, or artistic, professional, political, or community membership groups.

PARTNERING WITH FAITH-BASED ORGANIZATIONS

CHOWs working in a San Francisco Bay Area county established partnerships with black churches to develop and implement outreach strategies to provide HIV prevention education to their congregations. With the support of religious leaders, CHOWs were able to conduct outreach to the African American community about a heavily stigmatized health issue. At several churches, ministers agreed to talk about HIV/AIDS as a part of their sermons, and CHOWs facilitated workshops and discussion groups after the services.

INTERNET OUTREACH

As access to computers and the Internet continues to expand, CHOWs have developed outreach strategies to take advantage of computer technology. Online outreach can take many forms:

⭐ Create a Web site that appeals to the target population, includes graphics and features to hold the interest of the audience, and is culturally appropriate. Include a blog (Web log or journal) to share updates about what has been happening with your program, events that you've held, volunteer opportunities, social marketing campaigns, and so on.

⭐ Add a Web page to your agency's existing Web site that focuses on your program and includes information that you want the audience to discover. Update it regularly.

- Create an electronic mailing list that can serve as an Internet forum. People can join the list on their own, or you can add them to it, and they can communicate by e-mail. Examples include Yahoo Groups, Google Groups, MSN Groups, and so on.

- Develop a list of community members who are able and willing to be contacted by e-mail. Send out news of interest, information, event announcements, and your outreach schedule so that they can visit your site. (This is different from an electronic mailing list because *you* are the only one who sends information out and participants can respond only to *you* and not to the entire list.)

- Create a social networking group (group of people with common interests) that people can view, join, and participate in. Examples include MySpace, Facebook, hi5, and so on.

- Add your program to the Links section of related Web sites, resource listings, and so forth. Make sure the word gets out about the services you're providing and how to reach you.

- Log into existing chat rooms (see the example below)

Benefits to using the Internet to conduct outreach include:

1. *Privacy*—much of your information can be provided on your Web site without the consumer having to expose any personal information.
2. *Cost-effectiveness*—you can reach a large number of people via the Internet for a small amount of money. You may be able to add a page to your agency's existing Web site, or you may be able to create a free Web page or other Internet resource (see Internet Resources at the end of this section).
3. *Reach*—your Web page(s) can be accessed by almost anyone at any time in any country all around the world.

Limitations to using the Internet to conduct outreach include:

1. Many people still do not have access to a computer because of the cost of equipment and Internet access.
2. Cultural competency issues. Many communities may not want to engage with you via the Internet and may prefer in-person opportunities for education, counseling, and relationship building.
3. Client concerns about the privacy of their communication and information online.

Target populations with whom Internet outreach can be very effective may include:

- Youths and young adults
- Communities with higher incomes
- Sexually active individuals or relationship seekers (for safer sex messages)
- Participants in social networking sites

Using Chat Rooms for Online Outreach   Chat rooms are interactive online discussions. Participants engage in live conversations with one another via the World Wide Web by typing in their comments and reading those of others. Many Web sites, social networking sites, agencies, and communities sponsor chat rooms. You might be able to find one or many chat rooms that you can enter to join the discussion. For example, AOL has hundreds of chat rooms that you can access. Each room is based on specific interests, demographics, geographic locations, or a combination of categories. In recent years, many agencies have experimented with and discovered effective ways to use chat rooms for outreach.

CRAIG WENZL: When I was working at the Monterey County AIDS Project, I experimented with entering AOL chat rooms geared toward men who were at high risk for acquiring HIV, to engage participants in discussion and provide them with information. I found that this worked for some people, but not for others. The key was to respect the community members in the chat room and not interrupt the flow of the conversation that was going on in the room when I entered it. I subtly mentioned that I was in the room and could answer any questions that participants had. Some people responded, and I was able to engage in some lengthy discussions about safer sex and substance use.

? *Can you think of a way that you could use the Internet to conduct outreach to your community?*

SOCIAL MARKETING

Social marketing uses the same methods that businesses use to sell products (such as soft drinks or cell phones) to promote specific health outcomes. Social marketing campaigns may seek to promote immunizations or screening for breast cancer, or to prevent smoking, domestic violence, or driving under the influence of alcohol. Social marketing techniques include the use of posters, billboards, pamphlets, and brochures as well as public service announcements (PSAs) on television, radio, the Internet, or cell phones. To be successful, social marketing campaigns need to analyze and understand their target market (the community), select a medium (such as television or radio) that is popular with the target market, and develop a persuasive and culturally relevant message. CHOWs sometimes participate in the development of social marketing campaigns, and they often work in accompaniment with social marketing to reach specific audiences.

One of the best-known social marketing campaigns is the truth©campaign, an antismoking campaign waged with TV ads. The campaign Web site (www.protectthetruth.org/truthcampaign.htm) says that 75 percent of all twelve to seventeen-year-olds in the United States can describe one or more of the ads.

Another example of a more targeted kind of social marketing is a photo novella (a booklet including photographs) about the health risks of exposure to pesticides developed by Californians for Pesticide Reform (www.pesticidereform.org) and titled *Cuando los Pesticidas Invaden su Hogar* ("When Pesticides Invade Your Home"). You can download a copy at www.migrantphotographyproject.org/Fotonovela1.pdf.

? *Have you recently seen or heard a social marketing campaign?*

? *Where did you encounter the campaign (TV, radio, the Internet, a poster, billboard, or pamphlet)?*

? *What health outcome did the campaign attempt to promote?*

?   *Are you a member of the "target" audience?*

?   *What do you think of the social marketing message?*

?   *Is it effective for you?*

?   *Have you ever conducted health outreach to a particular community as a CHOW or a volunteer?*

?   *Have you ever been approached by an outreach worker?*

?   *What have your experiences been like?*

?   *How do you like to be approached by an outreach worker?*

?   *How do you not want to be approached?*

?   *What are your thoughts and feelings about conducting outreach yourself as a CHW?*

18.7 PLANNING HEALTH OUTREACH

Careful planning and preparation will improve the quality of a health outreach program. At the end of this chapter, we will ask you to develop a preliminary health outreach plan for a community that you are familiar with. Remember, a plan is not static: it should change as you analyze your work and learn from the community you are serving.

Outreach workers are often hired to work for a program that has already been designed, hopefully with extensive planning. In these circumstances, the target community has already been determined, along with the health issue to be addressed, goals and objectives, and outreach methods. In other circumstances, CHWs will play an important role in developing the core elements of a health outreach plan.

Regardless of whether you are developing a new outreach program or working for an established one, it may be helpful to use some of the community diagnosis methods presented in Chapter Seventeen to inform your work. Your research should include reviewing existing documents and conducting qualitative interviews with community members. It's particularly important to learn the history and reputation that the agency you work for has in the community, as well as that of other projects that may have tried to use similar outreach methods or address similar health topics in the community. Identifying past successes and mistakes can allow you to avoid making errors and can assist you to build and sustain positive relationships.

Define the Community to Be Served by Outreach   To learn about the community you will be working with and its health status, review available literature and reports, including reports generated by state and local health departments. Seek out available epidemiological data that will provide you with an understanding of the prevalence of the health condition you are addressing. (How many people are affected? Which parts of the community are at greatest risk?) Read local papers to find out what is currently happening in the community. The most important research you will do, however, is in and with the community. Take your time getting to know members of the community and talking with them about the work you plan to do. If possible:

- ✪ *Identify key opinion leaders.* These are the natural leaders found in all communities. They do not necessarily hold positions of formal authority, but have earned the respect and confidence of the community (for more information, see the following section on Conducting Health Outreach).
- ✪ *Identify potential outreach sites* where the people you hope to reach spend time. If you will conduct outreach in the community (rather than via social marketing or the Internet), conduct research and talk with community members to determine the locations where you will focus your first outreach efforts (these may include parks, schools, bars, churches, hair and nail salons and barber shops, homeless encampments, syringe exchanges, drug treatment programs, or soup kitchens, depending on the population you wish to reach).
- ✪ *Visit local agencies* to find out about the services they provide: for example, health clinics, counseling programs, educational institutions, food pantries and soup kitchens, and shelters.

RAMONA BENSON: I do street outreach and we have a flyer that talks about our services at the Black Infant Health Program. I also go out and visit local businesses and organizations like nail and beauty salons and churches. I tell them who I am and, if they have time, I tell them about our program. I ask if I can post my flyer or if they may want to pass it out. I always get some ladies that come to our program saying that they saw the flyer in their church or at a nail shop, so I know that it works to get the word out about our services.

IDENTIFY THE HEALTH ISSUE AND THE HEALTH OUTCOMES YOU WILL PROMOTE

Most outreach programs are funded to address one or more health issues such as breast cancer, hepatitis C, or gang violence. Remember that the issues you are paid to focus on may not always be the greatest priority for the community you work with (we will address this in greater detail).

Your outreach efforts will be most effective if you are clear about the health outcomes you are trying to achieve. Is your goal to prevent further hepatitis C infections among injection drug users? Is it to promote testing for hepatitis C? To link people living with hepatitis C to treatment resources? All of the above? By defining your goals, and researching the health issue and the community, you can develop outreach strategies that are more likely to promote your desired outcomes. And, if some of your strategies aren't effective, you will be better prepared to adapt or develop new ones because you have a clear sense of what you want to accomplish.

Conduct Research About the Health Issue   Part of your job will be to offer accurate information to community members. You need to fully understand the health issue's *etiology* (causes), consequences, available treatments, and methods for prevention. Be sure to research previous programs and outreach campaigns, if any, that addressed the same health issue in the same community. What did these programs do? What was the outcome? How did the community perceive these programs? Try to identify both the successes and the mistakes that were made by other programs, and do your best not to repeat the mistakes.

As you conduct health outreach, you will inevitably learn more about the community, and this information will guide you in revising your plan to respond to local needs, culture, and suggestions.

Organize the Outreach Team   Take time to talk with your supervisor and colleagues in order to determine:

- The number of people you will need on your team (Are you going solo, or will you have a partner or two?)
- The materials you should bring to the site (written materials or pamphlets, business cards, safer health supplies, promotional materials, hygiene products, resource listings or directories, and so on)
- The referrals that you will provide
- The forms you will use to document your contacts with people and the services that you provide
- How will you dress when conducting outreach? (Casual clothing? Street clothes? Professional attire? An outreach shirt that identifies you as an outreach worker with your agency?) While this may seem like a trivial issue, how you dress often sends a message to the community. For more information about dress codes and code switching, please refer to Chapter Fifteen.

18.8 CONDUCTING HEALTH OUTREACH

This section discusses how to build relationships in the community, approach new clients, handle rejection, work as part of a team, manage outreach materials, and enhance your safety.

BUILDING RELATIONSHIPS IN THE COMMUNITY

When you are conducting health outreach, the community will closely observe what you do and say, how you treat people, and if you remain true to your word. You will need to work hard and be patient, giving the community time to get to know and accept you. While this is particularly challenging for CHWs who work in communities that they are not a part of, even when you come from the community you are serving, it may take time for your work to be understood and accepted.

When you are initiating a new health outreach project, begin by developing relationships with the community. Here are some suggestions for how to do this:

- If you come from or are already familiar with the community, *contact people you already know.* Tell them about your new role as a CHW and the agency you are working for. Let them know what services you plan to provide and how you think these will benefit the community. Ask for their assistance and advice about how to get your message and services out to the community.
- *Identify key opinion leaders in the community.* Don't assume that you already know who they are. Key opinion leaders are not always those with formal authority (such

as elected leaders), but are the people in every neighborhood and community whom others listen to, respect, and turn to for advice. If, for example, your job is to conduct outreach to homeless and runaway youths, observe and ask whom they most respect and turn to for guidance and support. Introduce yourself, explain the work you will be doing, and ask for their guidance about building relationships in the community. Take time getting to know these opinion leaders, and when the moment is right, ask them for their support and guidance regarding your outreach work: ask for their advice regarding how, when, and where to conduct health outreach in the community. Remember that relationships require constant nurturing: keep returning to visit these key opinion leaders and to continue this dialogue. Keep a confidential list of these key contacts and where to find them.

Please note: If some of your contacts are engaged in illegal activities, such as prostitution or drug use, always make sure to preserve their privacy. Don't include identifying information in your reports. If you break their confidentiality or in some way expose or threaten their activities, you may not be able to continue working in the community and are likely to have irrevocably harmed the reputation of the agency you work for.

- ✪ *Network with the community* at local events and meetings and let people know what services you offer. Bring business cards and be prepared to introduce yourself clearly and quickly and explain your role as a CHW. You will need to repeat this information many times before people begin to understand who you are and what you will be doing.
- ✪ *Identify community agencies* that share common goals. Introduce yourself, explain what you will be doing, and explore options for strategic partnership and collaboration. For example, you may refer clients to their agency. Other agencies, in turn, may invite you to conduct outreach to community groups that they work with.
- ✪ Work with key opinion leaders to *organize a community forum* to introduce yourself and your program. Invite as many people as you can. Make sure that you advertise the forum well. You can print flyers to announce the forum and carry these with you so that you can hand them out at every opportunity.
- ✪ *Encourage community involvement.* Let people know that their guidance and suggestions are welcome. Let them know how they might be able to volunteer or become more involved with your program and your outreach work. Invite them to come to your agency to find out more about your services.
- ✪ *Listen and observe.* Your first priority should be to get to know people. Remember the diagram of the client-centered CHW with big ears and big eyes: you shouldn't be doing most of the talking. Create a space for community members to share information, concerns, and opinions with you. Ask them what they know about the health problem you will be addressing, the key resources in the community, and whom they think you should be talking with.
- ✪ *Be patient.* Don't push your agenda. Your top priority should be to listen to what the community says is important.
- ✪ *Keep your promises.* If you say that you will show up at a certain location at a certain time—be there. Unfortunately, the communities you serve are likely to recall a long list of broken promises from health and social service providers—don't add to this list!

? *What else have you learned about how to build effective relationships in the community?*

ALVARO MORALES: For day laborers, I found out that doing outreach early in the morning wasn't a good time because this was when they were trying to find a job. The end of the day wasn't the best either, because some people were gone and those who are still there are frustrated about not finding work. So I found out the middle of the day was the best time to go. I also learned that I need to do outreach regularly so that people will get to know you and you can build trust. In the Latino community, if you find somebody who has already been working there and you can partner with them, then you will save a lot of time earning that trust. For day laborers, trust is also something that you have to maintain. Because if you stop coming, then it seems like you have to start rebuilding it all over again. That's what is so hard when you're working on a grant because the grant might end and you have to stop services. Then maybe the grant will be renewed, and you have to start up all over again.

How to Approach Potential Clients When you are approaching someone for the first time, do what comes naturally—introduce yourself. At most outreach locations, you will be able to make a full introduction. Speak clearly and with a friendly, welcoming tone. Let the person know your name, which agency you represent, and why you are at the outreach location.

> Hi, I'm Janet from the Center City Health Center. I work with a breast cancer prevention project, and I'm out here tonight to let people know about the services we can provide.

Depending on the circumstances, you may or may not have a chance to share more information. Be ready to continue a conversation and to share information about health issues and your services. At the same time, be ready to back off if you need to—don't be too pushy. Be respectful of people's time and interests: they may not have the time at the moment to speak with you. If the person appears to be in a hurry, or if the outreach site is in a difficult setting, keep your message simple and brief, while taking the opportunity to distribute outreach materials if appropriate.

Every outreach setting really *is* unique. Because of this, it is important for you to learn as much as possible about the setting and the community before your first visit. If you are providing outreach in a new setting, you may feel nervous. If the location becomes a site for regular outreach, you will adapt and tailor your approach with time, gaining confidence. You will begin to recognize some of the community members and develop ongoing conversations and relationships.

Depending on the outreach site and the target population, you may develop creative ways to gain access and acceptance into the community you are attempting to reach. For example:

Expand your message and your outreach to *address more generalized needs* of the community. If you are providing outreach to migrant farm workers, brainstorm and network with people at the site to find out what they need. Do they need food, clothing, or school supplies for their children? You may be able to provide some things that are really needed at this location, even if these items have not been explicitly stated as part of your outreach services and goals. Network with other agencies in your city or seek donations of some of the items that are needed at the camp. By meeting some of the basic needs of the target community, you will accomplish several goals at once. Not only will you provide important resources, but you will also build relationships with members of the community so that you can work with them more closely each time you visit their camp.

TRAINING OUTREACH WORKERS AT CITY COLLEGE OF SAN FRANCISCO

At City College of San Francisco, we offer a course on conducting health outreach. During the first month, students are divided up into teams of two, provided with a backpack with HIV prevention materials, and given ten minutes to go out on campus, introduce themselves to someone they do not know, and see if they can initiate a conversation related to HIV issues. When students are preparing to conduct outreach for the first time, they often feel nervous, embarrassed, shy, or worried about whether or not they will be able to initiate a conversation with anyone. Once the students return to the classroom, they analyze their experience and the factors that made it easier or harder to connect with potential clients. As a final assignment, the students design and manage a three-hour campus outreach event that reaches hundreds of students. With repetition, the students gain confidence and skills in approaching potential clients. They learn to relax, have fun, and focus on their successes rather than their disappointments.

Break the ice with humor, games, or fun interactive exercises. At City College of San Francisco, HIV prevention outreach workers have used a variety of participatory activities such as the STI Wheel of Fortune and a Talking Wall. The STI Wheel of Fortune is a large colorful wheel that CHWs set up in a prominent location. They invite people to spin the wheel, which will land on a number that is matched to a question about STIs. As other people gather round to see what is happening, the CHOWs are able to facilitate discussions about topics such as: "What birth control methods also aid in preventing STIs?" Players are provided with prizes whether they win or lose. The Talking Wall is simply a big piece of paper—we have used paper as large as 10 feet high by 15 feet wide—with a series of provocative questions or quotes, and colorful pens also and markers available so that people can add their own comments and questions. Typically, the wall focuses discussion on particular topics or themes, such as the connection between crystal methamphetamine use and HIV. As the wall fills up with anonymous comments and opinions, CHOWs stand by to talk with participants, pass out health materials, and make referrals.

Hold an event in the community you are trying to reach. Work with your outreach team and volunteers to come up with something that will be fun. Make sure that the event allows members of the target population to participate in a way that will energize them so that they will want to get involved. Members of the Queer Youth Action Team (QYAT) in Contra Costa County, California, hosted barbeques with free food that provided lesbian, gay, bisexual, transgender, queer, questioning, and intersex (LGBTQQI) youths with a safe and fun place to socialize. The CHWs were identified by colorful QYAT T-shirts, and they arranged a table with HIV prevention resources for those who were interested. They took a quiet approach to outreach and let the youths choose to initiate conversations about HIV prevention, and most did.

Don't force yourself to do things that make you uncomfortable. If you are having difficulty approaching people you don't know, be aware that this discomfort will subside in time. If you continue to have difficulty, speak with your supervisor or coworkers and listen to their suggestions.

Handling Rejection   When you conduct health outreach, most people will respect your role and your contributions. But not everyone will be interested in what you have to offer, be welcoming, or act polite. Expect and prepare to handle *a lot* of rejection as a CHOW.

Craig Wenzl, CHW, facilitates a "post office" game at a community event to encourage people to approach his outreach table.

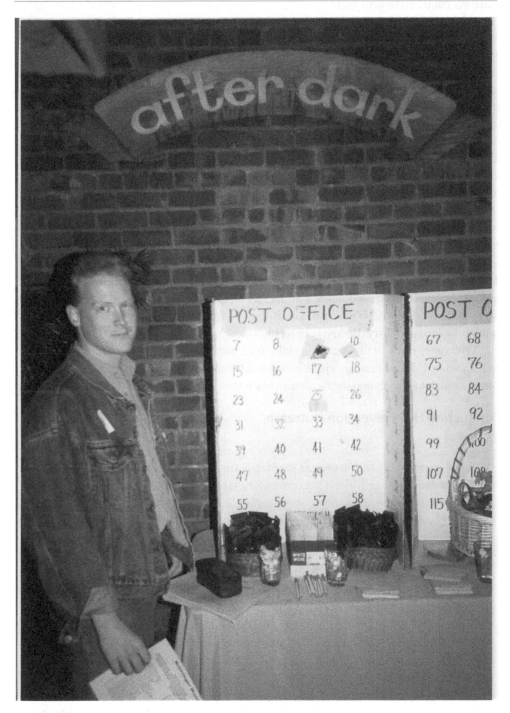

?   *Have you ever encountered a pushy outreach worker or sales representative who didn't take no for an answer?*

?   *Have you ever been followed down the street by someone who wanted to give you a flyer, ask you to sign a petition, or sell you something?*

? *What do you think of these strategies?*

? *How do they make you feel?*

Many people don't like to be approached by strangers, for a variety of reasons. If you continue to bother prospective clients after they have clearly indicated, by their words or actions, that they are not interested in speaking with you, you risk making a strong and lasting negative impression that could hurt future efforts to conduct outreach in the community. If potential clients try to ignore you or avoid you, don't pursue them. If they let you know that they aren't interested (by shaking their head or saying something like "I don't have time" or "I'm not interested"), consider saying something brief and polite—such as "have a nice day"—and move on immediately. Remember that you are likely to return to the same locations again and again, and therefore to encounter the same people in the future: leave a positive and professional impression. At a future visit to this location, you may very well have a chance to interact with the person who could not speak with you today.

Some people will be actively rude. Try not to take it personally. Even if a prospective client is angry or says something vulgar or disrespectful to you (this *will* happen!), don't retaliate in kind. Keep your professionalism and your dignity. When you get a chance, debrief these encounters with a colleague, supervisor, friend, or family member. Vent your feelings in a safe place, and never with the clients and communities you work with. One angry outburst or nasty comment to a prospective client may quickly become news in the community and seriously damage your reputation.

With time, you will find that your skills as an outreach worker become more developed and fine-tuned. Encountering rejection and indifference will aid you in learning to tailor your outreach messages and interactions to reach more people in more effective ways.

Conducting HIV Prevention Outreach

CRAIG WENZL: When I first began working at the Monterey County AIDS Project as a CHOW doing outreach in the gay community, I thought people would be happy to hear about HIV prevention and antibody testing. But I found out right away that this wasn't always true. I was new to the community, so people didn't know me. I had to "prove" myself in order to gain their trust. At first, I was uncomfortable approaching people I didn't know at bars, events, and community gatherings. However, after doing outreach in the community a few times, I began to figure out what did and didn't work. One method that worked well for me was to make sure that I approached and spoke with everyone at an outreach setting. For example, when providing outreach at the After Dark Bar, I started at one end of the busy bar, speaking with each patron with an introductory but nonintrusive message. I would introduce myself and ask if he or she knew about my agency and our programs. I would take the cue from that person to determine how far my interaction with him or her would go at that time. Because I was speaking to everyone, and I was aware that everyone was watching me, I knew that people would be expecting me to approach them. This gave the patrons a chance to prepare. Most people were friendly and welcoming. However, a few were unfriendly and abrupt and let me know that they did not want to be bothered. During my first few visits to the After Dark, I was put off by the reactions of people who appeared to reject me and my message. However—*and here is the key*—many of those same people who initially rejected my message welcomed the opportunity to open up and discuss their personal interest in the topic of HIV/AIDS. I found out that many of the people who had appeared to reject me from the start were doing so because they had very close personal experience with HIV/AIDS. Either they were HIV-positive or living with AIDS, or they had a close family member, partner, or friend who was living with or had passed away from the disease. I learned the importance of being patient and not making any assumptions about prospective clients, especially those who initially rejected my approach.

Recognize and Acknowledge Your Limitations and Mistakes   As a CHW, you will be confronted with questions that you do not know how to answer and situations that you are not sure how to handle. Don't be afraid to acknowledge the limits of your knowledge and skills to clients or coworkers. Rather than try to answer a question when you are not confident in your response, say that you don't know. Choose your own words and say something along the lines of: "I don't know" or "I'm not certain about that" or "I don't want to tell you anything that may not be true. Let me research this question when I get back to the office, and next time I see you, I'll let you know what I have learned." Trust us: You will need these words often!

Many of your clients have suffered from prejudice, discrimination, loss, or abuse. These experiences often influence their interaction with helping professionals, and they may be watching, waiting, and expecting you to be yet another person who lets them down in some way. Inevitably, despite your best efforts and intentions, you will disappoint some clients. For example, you might arrive late for an appointment, run out of food vouchers, forget an important detail that client told you about their life, misinterpret a statement that a client makes, make an incorrect assumption, or say something that triggers previous bad experiences for a client. These are natural, common, and inevitable "mistakes" that we all make at some point in our careers.

As a result of these types of mistakes, some clients will stop working with you and may avoid you and your agency in the future. Others may show their disappointment or anger and say something about your action. We encourage you to view these moments as an opportunity to repair and perhaps deepen the working relationship. A sincere apology often has remarkable power to defuse and transform anger and conflict. It shows that you are a fallible human being who makes mistakes, not someone who thinks that you are better than your client. An apology communicates your commitment, your desire to be supportive, and your intention to treat your clients with the respect they deserve. In many cases, it will actually result in renewed trust for the working relationship and open up dialogue that will assist you get to know your clients in a deeper way.

What words do you use when you apologize or otherwise take responsibility for doing something you wish you hadn't done? Don't apologize simply because someone suggested it to you as a professional technique: whatever you say, *it has to be authentic*.

For example:

> I'm sorry I showed up late. I know your time is valuable, and I want you to know that I will always do my best to get here on time.

Or:

> I apologize. I really didn't express myself very well. I didn't mean to say that I understood what you are going through. What I want to say is that I'd like to learn about your experience and to see how I can best be supportive to you.

We all make mistakes and do things that are hurtful to others. Saying "I'm sorry" to a client does not mean that you knowingly did something wrong. But an apology can aid in repairing a misunderstanding or conflict and provide you and the client with an opportunity to move forward in your work.

? *What are your experiences with and beliefs about apologies?*

? *Are you someone who can apologize easily, or is it difficult for you?*

? *Can you think of a time when you gave or received an apology that aided in strengthening a relationship?*

? *If you have difficulty apologizing, what is it that gets in the way?*

? *What could assist you to learn how to offer a sincere apology to a client?*

YOUR REPUTATION AS AN OUTREACH WORKER

As you conduct health outreach, you will get to know and begin to feel a part of the community in which you are working. People will begin to recognize you and associate you with your work and your agency. Your reputation, both on and off the clock, will follow you wherever you go in the community, and will become one of your most important professional resources. When we asked senior CHOWs how they have built and maintained positive reputations in the communities they serve, they said:

- Don't break confidentiality in any way. This is the quickest way to end your career.
- Don't ever act like you are better than anyone you are working with, talk down to anyone, or criticize anyone behind their back.
- Don't pretend to be something or someone you are not. The community will always see your act and you will lose their respect.
- Don't make things up. If you don't know something, that is okay, just say so.
- Don't spend all of your time speaking with *one* outreach contact. Other people may want to speak with you, and they may feel ignored if you don't give them a chance to interact with you.
- Be careful not to discriminate against any part of the target population you are serving. As an outreach worker, your duty is to provide services and information to *everyone* you interact with—not just the ones you are more comfortable speaking to or the ones you would *rather* approach. Review your own reporting data to make sure that you aren't leaving anyone out—for example, are you serving women as well as men, Latinos as well as African Americans?
- Stay neutral: don't pick sides when the community you are working with is in conflict.
- Take the time to listen to and be kind to everyone you interact with. When you have to cut a conversation short, do so as politely as possible.
- Don't make promises you can't keep. It can damage your reputation if clients feel that you do not keep your word or care enough to follow through with promises.
- Don't flirt: it may be perceived as sexually charged, inappropriate, unprofessional, or unwanted.
- Don't use language that is unfamiliar to the community (such as *epidemiology*): everything you want to say can be communicated using language that is accessible to your audience.
- If you mess up, apologize!

◉   Don't push your own agenda on clients. If you are talking about prostate cancer and the client is telling you he is hungry, listen to him and see if there is anything you can do to help him out. Maybe there is a soup kitchen or food pantry nearby. If you assist clients with their priorities, then they will be ready to listen to yours.

◉   Live by your code of ethics! Don't sleep with clients, do drugs with clients, or give money to clients!

SAFETY ISSUES

Keep in mind that some members of the community may view you with suspicion or fear and treat you as an outsider or intruder. This is one of many reasons that it is so essential to take the time to get to the know the community you will be working in, and to forge respectful relationships with key opinion leaders.

Depending on the type of outreach you are providing, safety may or may not be a major consideration. Safety issues and concerns may include:

◉   Losing sight of your partner
◉   Injuring yourself in dark or dimly lit areas
◉   Witnessing illegal or underground activities such as selling or using drugs
◉   Unintentional involvement in police actions
◉   Witnessing arguments, threats, or violence (such as incidents of domestic violence)
◉   Encountering an angry, aggressive, or threatening person
◉   Experiencing harassment, including sexual harassment
◉   Theft and assault

?   *Can you think of additional safety concerns?*

Your job as a CHW is to provide services to the most vulnerable and at-risk communities, such as homeless and runaway youths, injection drug users, or people living with chronic mental illness. Often society stigmatizes these communities, and others fear them and assume they are dangerous. Sometimes your own prejudices may influence your assessment of safety issues. Try to be aware of the tendency for this to happen and guard against discriminating against clients or communities that have already been harmed in this way. Remember that safety issues are present in any work setting and with clients of all backgrounds.

Chapter Ten discusses safety issues in relation to home visiting and presents safety tips that apply to conducting health outreach as well. Review the safety discussion in that chapter. Here, we present additional tips and issues that are specific to doing outreach.

Work with a partner or outreach team. Keep your teammates within view at all times, and check in with each other regularly. Develop a system to "signal" one another if you need some assistance, whether it be a hand signal or a code phrase ("Hey, Marcos, can you bring me my backpack?"), and come together immediately after the signal is given. Always allow for quick communication with other team members if you or someone else should run into a difficult situation. Listen to your instincts, which will develop over time, and pay attention to them when you feel particularly ill at ease, anxious, or unsafe.

If you find yourself in the midst of a conflict, try to deescalate the situation using conflict resolution skills (Chapter Thirteen). If necessary, ask your team members for assistance. Here is where a code phrase or hand signal can come in handy. If the situation is too intense, however, shout out for assistance. If no other team members respond and the situation is dangerous and immediate, ask for assistance from *anyone* who is nearby and might be able to assist you. If you don't see any hope for calming the situation, *leave*. Document the incident, report it to your supervisor, and debrief it with someone you trust. *Only call the police if it is absolutely required.* Most situations will not require such a drastic measure. You want to avoid bringing the police into a community that has a history of tensions with the law (that is, injection drug or other substance users, sex workers, and so on). You could find yourself losing the trust and respect of this community.

KENT RODRIGUEZ: I always found that doing outreach with at least someone else or in a small group of no more than three people always made it easier to approach people. Safety was not an issue because someone could maintain a lookout at our surroundings while we distributed supplies. *Never go out alone.*

Having some established "safe" words when doing outreach is a good idea. I remember my volunteers, and I had one that was as easy as "let's get coffee." If someone mentioned this at any point during outreach, we all knew that one of us was uncomfortable in the current situation and that we needed to move on.

Do not be afraid to walk away from a situation that makes you feel unsafe.

Make sure to take care of yourself first. This includes debriefing after outreach sessions. Talk to those you are working with about any feelings or thoughts that come up. Allow yourself time to process anything that comes up for you.

TIPS FOR SUCCESSFUL TEAMWORK

We strongly encourage CHOWs to work with a partner or as a part of a team for a variety reasons:

- It is safer to work in a team.
- You can reach a larger number of clients.
- You can provide complementary services (for example, some CHWs can conduct general outreach in a club, and others may provide confidential risk-reduction counseling or screening services in a more private area).
- The more diverse the outreach team, the more choice you offer potential clients. For example, a team with both male and female members provides greater comfort and access to clients who may prefer to speak with one or the other.

Successful teamwork often comes down to good communication. When conducting health outreach with a partner or team, here are a few tips for working together:

- Meet with your team to clarify your goals, objectives, expectations, and the policies and protocols that will guide your work.
- Make time to review and discuss your outreach plan together, including locations, outreach materials, and referrals you will provide.
- Develop a system for responding to safety concerns, including a code that will alert you and your partners to potential danger.
- Ask for and listen to the ideas and opinions of your teammates.
- Be patient with your colleagues.
- Accept and respect the different experiences, cultural perspectives, and opinions of your partners.
- Give your teammates the benefit of the doubt: assume that they have good intentions, even when you may be upset by the consequences of their actions.

- Assert your opinions clearly, calmly, and respectfully.
- Be ready and willing to compromise.
- Learn to accept critical feedback from others without getting defensive. When you make mistakes, apologize.
- Learn to provide critical feedback to others in a way that demonstrates your respect for them. (See the section on critical feedback in Chapter Fifteen.)
- Make time to debrief your work together after every shift. Share your successes and your challenges. Make plans to improve aspects of your teamwork that didn't go as well as you had hoped. Look for and acknowledge the positive contributions of teammates and outcomes of your collaborative efforts.

DEVELOPING AND MANAGING OUTREACH MATERIALS

CHWs use a variety of outreach materials in the course of their work. For example, a CHW conducting outreach to reduce the risks of HIV disease may carry a backpack with materials such as condoms, lubricants, safer sex guidelines, and a list of local resources for testing, counseling, and health care.

Outreach materials may include printed brochures, pamphlets, flyers, posters, and referral cards; health promotion books, booklets, cassettes, CDs, videotapes, or DVDs for distribution, viewing, listening, or display; promotional materials such as key chains, pens, cups, toys, tote bags, and so on that have your agency logo and contact information printed on them; food, clothing, hygiene materials (toothpaste, toothbrush, soap, and so on), or other items that are needed by members of the target community.

Depending on your agency and your program, you will find that some materials work better than others with your target audience. You will want to develop a tailored mix of outreach materials that you can take to different venues or distribute in other ways.

You should plan your collection of materials carefully, based on the demographics and needs of the target population. Trial and error will guide you as you determine what has and hasn't worked in prior visits to that site or to similar sites. Most important, ask the community you are serving what they think about the materials you are using.

MAKING THE MOST OF OUTREACH MATERIALS

A CHW conducting outreach to the homeless always made a point of carrying clean socks in his backpack. Many of his clients slept on the streets and in parks and lacked clean, warm clothes, and they truly appreciated a pair of clean socks. By providing clean socks, he was able to start off a new relationship by offering something valuable to a client. This was often useful in creating an opportunity to start other conversations. For example, if a client pointed to the backpack and asked, "What else do you got in there?" the CHW was able to talk about the full range of services that he could provide.

Keep your outreach materials well organized. Be sure that they are up-to-date and undamaged. For example, make sure that none of the condoms you carry have passed their expiration date. Giving a client outdated or damaged goods is a sure way to damage their trust in you.

Often, CHOWs participate in the development of new outreach materials such as flyers, brochures, or resource guides. When developing any outreach materials, or using those produced by other sources, be sure to pay close attention to the content and the messages being provided. Gather members of the target population and ask for their input and opinions on the materials you are considering developing or distributing. Coordinate focus groups (see Chapter Seventeen) and pilot tests to see what people think about the materials. Collaborate with other agencies who serve the target population to see what they think. If you are purchasing or otherwise acquiring materials produced by another source, make sure that the message is culturally appropriate for your target population(s). Make sure you examine the materials, reading every page of the brochures, watching every minute of the videos, testing out the equipment and promotional materials, and so on. The last thing you want to do is discover that you have been handing out materials that are offensive or inaccurate. Offensive materials are worse than none at all.

CRAIG WENZL: When I started working as a CHOW at the Monterey County AIDS Project, I once made the mistake of handing out materials that hadn't been approved or tested beforehand. There were some materials that had been produced by another agency to target young African American men at risk of contracting HIV/AIDS. I didn't read through the entire collection of materials (a series of brochures)—*bad mistake!* One night when I was facilitating a small group, one of the members—an African American man—took one of the brochures out of his pocket and read it to me. He said it was offensive because it used language that he could not relate to and was clearly targeted to a more urban setting and most likely a more "East Coast" setting. As a group, we examined the materials and agreed that they weren't right for the local African American community. This example illustrates the importance of localizing your materials if you are borrowing from another agency. Be sure to gather members of the target population together and find out what they think about the materials before you distribute them. You might be surprised at what you hear in the discussion.

18.9 DOCUMENTING HEALTH OUTREACH SERVICES

One of the most important tasks of outreach work is the documentation of the services you provide. Documentation of health outreach services has become increasingly important for a variety of reasons:

- Documentation can show what you've accomplished, and if you have met program goals and objectives.
- It provides data that can be used to find additional funding to continue or expand the program.
- It reveals the history of the program and builds a timeline of program development.
- The information gathered can assist your agency and others to develop plans to better promote the health of the community in the future.
- It enables you to be accountable to funders including, in the case of public funding, the general public (taxpayers).

⚙ Documentation makes it possible to evaluate your program. Data is gathered in order to:

 ● Determine who you have and have not reached, and highlight opportunities to reach underserved segments of the community
 ● Better understand the clients and communities served
 ● Refine and improve the quality of services provided
 ● Guard against discriminatory practices, such as the exclusion of certain groups from programs and services
 ● Advocate for the continuation and the expansion of necessary services
 ● Provide evidence that can assist others to develop similar programs and services

? *Can you think of other reasons why documentation is so important?*

Clients, CHOWs, and the agencies they work for sometimes raise concerns about documentation. CHOWS may fear that the information documented may be used to discipline them and could even result in losing their job. Agencies may fear that the information will be used to reduce or eliminate programs and services. Clients and communities may also fear that the data gathered will be used to reduce or eliminate services or to harm them in some other way. This fear is particularly pronounced among communities with the least access to essential health resources, and among those who have experienced a history of discrimination. For example, undocumented immigrants may fear that information will be forwarded to the Immigration and Naturalization Services (INS).

KENT RODRIQUEZ: When I first started doing outreach, I hated all the paperwork I had to do. I felt like all these forms just got in the way of my work, and it just took time away from building relationships in the community or talking to my clients. I didn't really understand what happened after I turned the forms in to my supervisor or how the information would be used.

Depending on your agency, you may be asked to provide a weekly, monthly, quarterly, or annual report. You may have a supervisor who completes some of these reports for the program. Whatever your particular requirements, it is a good idea to keep track of *every* outreach session you complete. Use the outreach tracking forms your agency provides, or talk with your supervisor about creating such a form. In addition to keeping documentation on paper, you may want to use some form of database or a calculating or totaling system to keep track of the numbers and demographics of outreach contacts. This is especially helpful if you provide outreach many times throughout the month or to a large number of different contacts. Also, you will need a simplified method of totaling the number of contacts and other services you provide in order to prepare accurate, detailed reports and to determine if you are reaching program goals.

In order for the documentation to be useful, it should include the following information:

⚙ The date and time when the outreach was provided
⚙ Outreach location(s)
⚙ The names of the outreach worker(s)

- An estimate of the number of people you reached and their demographic profile: Often you will be asked to record demographic information about the identities of the people you serve, such as their sex, ethnicity, age, substance use, sexual orientation, homeless or marginally housed, or health status. You won't always be able to gather this information. Sometimes, you will be asked to make an educated guess about the identities of those to whom you conduct outreach, but be careful not to jump into stereotypes or assumptions. Ask for guidance about how to do this from experienced CHWs and your supervisor.
- The number and type of supplies, materials, brochures, and so on that you distributed
- Other information that is required for your specific program

We don't recommend that you fill out outreach reports as you talk with clients, as it is likely to distract you from focusing on your interaction with them and may harm your relationship (this type of documentation is different from what you will do when you provide case management or client-centered counseling services). However, don't wait too long before you document the services that you provide. Take time during each day to stop and document your work: you won't be able to remember the details later on.

18.10 ETHICS AND HEALTH OUTREACH

Because of the independent nature of their work, CHOWs frequently face ethical challenges, including:

- Requests for food, money, and transportation
- Offers of gifts, sex, and drugs
- Witnessing violence, including incidents of domestic violence
- Maintaining confidentiality when working in public places
- Developing personal relationships with clients, including romantic relationships

For this reason we strongly encourage you to anticipate and prepare to respond to common ethical challenges. Review the section on ethics in Chapter Eight. Talk with more experienced CHOWs to learn how they handle these situations. Be ready to clearly explain your policies to clients—what you can and cannot do, and in some instances, why. For example, be prepared to explain the following to clients:

- Why you cannot give or loan them cash
- Why you cannot accept gifts
- Why you cannot develop personal relationships with them, including romantic or sexual relationships
- Why you need to preserve confidentiality, and the exceptions to this policy (specific types of harm to the client or harm to others)
- That you don't know the answer to a relevant question, but will do your best to find out

To be successful in your career as a CHW, you will need to develop strong interpersonal boundaries that protect both you and your clients. Be prepared to set and maintain your limits and to stand behind them. You will often have to say "no" to clients or otherwise communicate that you cannot provide the services they have asked for. Some clients won't accept the boundaries you attempt to establish and may continue to push for what they want.

For example, a client might say something like: "I haven't had anything to eat in two days! Can't you just give me a little cash to get something to eat this one time? I won't tell anyone about it."

Try not to let yourself get placed in a defensive position, or to spend too much time repeating your ethical obligations and professional policies to clients. Find ways to refocus the conversation on the client's issues and on the services that you *can* offer. Make sure to maintain your professionalism at all times: handling these challenges with grace and compassion often results in renewed trust and the opportunity to do more substantive work with a client. If you are unable to change the focus of the conversation or the client becomes increasingly assertive or aggressive, remember that you can always walk away from the encounter. If you need to do this, however, don't do it in anger. Explain yourself clearly, calmly, and politely.

Some CHWs complain that clients are trying to "manipulate" them. We encourage you to think about this in a different way. It may be helpful to remember that for some clients, what you perceive as manipulation is how they have learned to get the resources they need in order to survive. For some clients, these strategies may be connected to drug and alcohol use. Try not to take a client's behavior personally: it isn't about you. Respect the autonomy of your clients to make their own choices, and remember that you can only control your own words and behavior. Practice the words you will use to end an encounter with a client when you feel the need to walk away. How will you explain this in ways that asserts your own professional boundaries and preserves their dignity?

L<small>EE</small> J<small>ACKSON</small>: I don't lend money to my clients. Sometimes they'll ask me to lend them money and say they'll pay me back double or something like that. I explain what my job is and what my boundaries are. I tell them: "I'm not a loan shark, I'm a health worker. I'm here to get you to your appointments and make sure you're okay and get you back on your feet, and if you need housing we'll help get you housing, but I can't loan you money." Sometimes I have to break it down in a street manner and explain it to them, and they understand because then I ask them, "Do you enjoy me working with you?" If they say, "Yes," I'll say: "If I start breaking the laws, then I will lose my job and then there's a possibility that me and you will have to go to these agencies together because I'll be looking for a job also." So they understand. It's all in the way you explain things.

18.11 SUPERVISION AND SUPPORT

CHOWs often work independently outside of an office, and outreach is not always well understood or appreciated by supervisors. Depending on your agency and your program, supervision may or may not be something you receive regularly.

While we hope that each of you has the opportunity to work with a knowledgeable and supportive supervisor, the truth is that not all supervisors have the skills necessary to provide effective guidance and support to CHWs. Despite this, you have a professional responsibility to do your best to develop and sustain a positive working relationship with your supervisor. Building a positive relationship with your supervisor is essential to doing effective work, preventing stress and burnout, and maximizing your job satisfaction and opportunities for advancement. Ask for regular meetings with your supervisor and take the opportunity to inform them about your accomplishments and the challenges that you face in the field. Remember to turn in documentation of your work in a timely fashion.

When you face an immediate challenge and do not have a supervisor (or another coworker) nearby to consult, rely on what you have learned about ethics, safety, and representing your agency. You will not always know how best to respond to problems that arise in the field. Sometimes, it is better and safer to remove yourself from a situation as soon as possible rather than to try to respond or resolve it in the moment. Check in with your coworkers and teammates to make these difficult decisions together. When this occurs, document what happened and report to your supervisor as soon as possible.

Because CHOWs work in such an independent fashion, sometimes they may feel isolated and wish for more professional support. Other CHOWs will best understand the nature of the challenges that you face and are best equipped to provide meaningful support in terms of how to handle the stresses of the job and to enhance the quality of services that you provide. Try to identify someone who you trust to talk with about the challenges you face on the job. Our recommendation is to seek out a mentor who has years of experience conducting health outreach. This senior CHOW may work at your same agency or with another organization. In many parts of the country and around the world, CHWs have formed local support groups that provide them with an opportunity to meet regularly with peers. These support groups function both as a source of support and of ongoing professional development. For more information about CHOW support groups, please refer to Chapter One, the Web site of the American Association of Community Health Workers (www.aachw.org), or local or state CHW networks.

CHAPTER REVIEW QUESTIONS

To review the concepts and competencies covered in this chapter, we would like you to develop a health outreach plan for a community that you belong to and know well. Please do your best to complete the following worksheet based on what you already know about your community and the information presented in this chapter.

1. Define the community to be served by outreach (demographics, location, and so on). Be as specific as possible.
2. Define the health issue to be addressed by the outreach program.
3. What is the objective of your outreach program (what do you want to accomplish as a result of the outreach services provided)?
4. Who are the key opinion leaders in the community? How will you identify others?

What are three questions that you would like to ask these key opinion leaders?

5. What or where are three venues (places) where your community spends considerable time together and where you can conduct outreach?
6. List three institutions that are respected by the community that you can work with:
7. What outreach level might you use to conduct your outreach?
8. Which types of outreach methods would you select?
9. What types of outreach materials will you bring with you to share with clients?
10. What types of information will you gather to document the outreach services you provide? How might this information be used to improve the quality of your program?

ADDITIONAL RESOURCES

Californians for Pesticide Reform. *Cuando los Pesticidas Invaden su Hogar* ("When Pesticides Invade Your Home"). 2002. Accessed on April 10, 2009: www.migrantphotographyproject.org/Fotonovela1.pdf

The Center for AIDS Prevention Studies at the University of California, San Francisco. Accessed on April 2, 2009: www.caps.ucsf.edu

The Center for AIDS Prevention Studies at the University of California, San Francisco. The Mpowerment Project. Accessed on April 2, 2009: www.caps.ucsf.edu/projects/MPowerment/

Protect the Truth Campaign. 2000. Accessed on April 10, 2009: www.protectthetruth.org/truthcampaign.htm

19

Facilitating Community Health Education Trainings

Jill Tregor

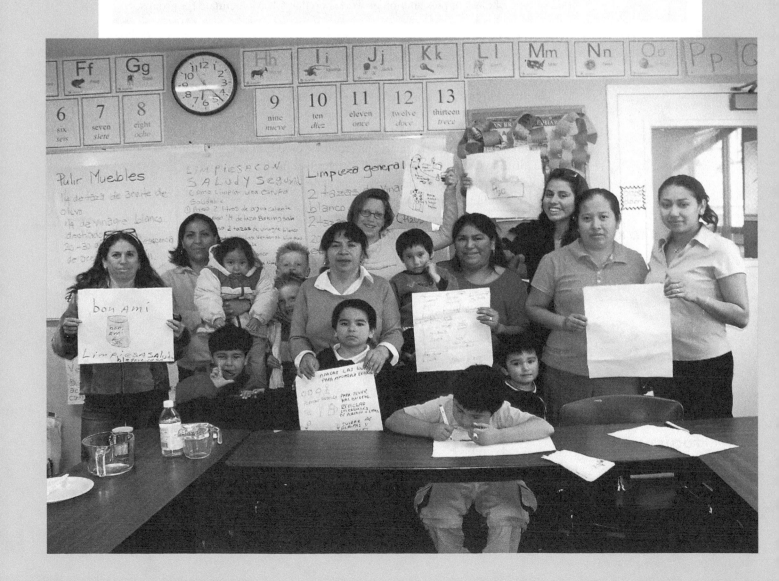

CHW SCENARIO

You receive a call from a staff member at a local nonprofit agency that does violence prevention work. She asks you to facilitate a two-hour training on stress management for a team of CHWs and volunteers who do frontline work in the community. You are knowledgeable about the topic of stress reduction, but haven't facilitated this type of training before.

- ✪ What additional information would assist you to plan for the training?
- ✪ How will you gather this information?
- ✪ How will you plan and prepare for the training?
- ✪ What will your training objectives be?
- ✪ What training methods and exercises will you use?
- ✪ How will you know if the training is successful?

INTRODUCTION

This chapter will address the knowledge and skills for facilitating training or educational presentations to groups. For the purposes of this chapter, we will use the word "training" for any type of class or presentation or workshop that CHWs facilitate for groups.

WHAT YOU WILL LEARN

By studying the information in this chapter, you will be able to:

- ✪ Identify different types of training that CHWs may facilitate
- ✪ Discuss some of the ways that people learn new information and skills
- ✪ Describe and apply approaches to training commonly used by CHWs, including popular education, participatory learning, and problem-based learning
- ✪ Identity and respond to common challenges that facilitators may face
- ✪ Develop a training plan, including goals and learning outcomes
- ✪ Develop a simple evaluation of a training

WORDS TO KNOW

Visual Learners	Kinesthetic Learners	Auditory Learners
Conscientization	Popular Education	Participatory Learning
Problem-Based Learning	Learning Outcome	

19.1 AN OVERVIEW OF TRAINING

As a CHW you may be asked to facilitate or cofacilitate a training. These trainings may vary in many ways including:

FOCUS OR MAIN TOPIC

CHWs facilitate trainings that address a wide range of public health topics including:

- ✪ Chronic illness such as diabetes, depression, and cancer

- ✪ Infectious diseases such as hepatitis, cholera, and HIV
- ✪ Reproductive health topics, including family planning and pregnancy
- ✪ Violence, including domestic violence
- ✪ Healthy relationships, including parenting
- ✪ Environmental health
- ✪ Occupational health
- ✪ Civil rights and human rights
- ✪ Stress management

? *Can you think of other topics that CHWs might address in trainings?*

PURPOSE OR GOAL

The primary purpose or goal of trainings may include:

- ✪ To share and learn new health-related information
- ✪ To promote changes in health-related behaviors
- ✪ To share and learn new skills such as stress management, risk reduction, health outreach, or advocacy skills
- ✪ To promote teamwork and community building
- ✪ To support a community planning or organizing process

? *Can you think of other goals for trainings?*

DURATION

Trainings may last anywhere from thirty minutes to eight hours and may even take place over many days.

NUMBER OF FACILITATORS

Sometimes you will facilitate trainings on your own, and sometimes with a cofacilitator or as part of a training team. When you are starting out, it is helpful to observe other facilitators and to facilitate trainings as a part of a team. This will provide you with opportunities to give and receive critical feedback, and to learn new skills and approaches from trusted colleagues.

AUDIENCE OR PARTICIPANTS

CHWs facilitate trainings for a wide variety of audiences including youths, parents, coworkers, clients, members of a faith community or other group or organization, people diagnosed with chronic illness, and professionals such as teachers, physicians, police, and staff and volunteers of community-based organizations.

? *Can you think of other groups who might participate in trainings?*

LOCATIONS

Trainings take place in a wide variety of locations, including:

- ✪ Schools
- ✪ Clinics or hospitals
- ✪ Churches, mosques, temples, and other religious or faith-based organizations
- ✪ Work sites
- ✪ Housing sites, including public housing and homeless shelters
- ✪ Community-based organizations
- ✪ After-school programs
- ✪ Recreational sites
- ✪ Cultural and arts organizations

?   *Where do trainings take place in your community?*

Facilitating trainings can be intimidating, especially if you feel uncomfortable speaking in front of groups. Most people who lead trainings started out feeling nervous and unsure about what to do. I have been making presentations and conducting trainings for more than twenty years, and I still feel nervous before a training session. The good thing is that being nervous motivates me to do my homework in order to *prepare* for the training. By the end of this chapter, my hope is that you will have the building blocks to develop interesting and engaging trainings and learner-centered activities, and will feel confident that you already have the qualifications necessary to be a great facilitator.

AN EARLY EXPERIENCE AS A TRAINER

My first paid job in the community was with an organization that worked to prevent and respond to hate-motivated violence (when people are threatened or attacked due to their real or perceived ethnicity, religion, sexual orientation, gender, or gender-identity). We were a small organization with a big mission, a limited budget, and not many staff. We received requests for presentations about hate violence from schools and other organizations. Sometimes I had time to learn something in advance about the group I would present to, but more often I showed up to the training without knowing much about the participants.

Because I knew a lot about my topic, I figured I could just tell people about hate violence. But the people in the trainings also knew a lot about the topic because their communities had often been the targets of hate-motivated violence. I didn't think enough about how boring it might be for them if I just stood up at the front of the room and talked for thirty minutes or more, though I knew I did not like it when someone did the same thing to me. Because I didn't always have a training plan, it was also possible (or likely) that I would end a training without covering topics or concerns that the participants most wanted to learn about.

Very quickly, I realized that I needed help and asked for support to learn how to become a better trainer. I talked with my coworkers. I read books and went to workshops. I watched carefully what experienced trainers did. I learned to prepare for every training I do and to tailor that training to fit the needs of the group I am working with. I need to know who they are and what they want to learn.

19.2 UNDERSTANDING HOW PEOPLE LEARN

TYPES OF LEARNERS

Many educational institutions have assumed that people learn by reading and listening to lecturers. In reality, people learn in many different ways, including:

- **Visual learners:** who need to see the material they are learning. They might prefer films, photographs, drawings, or observation. To learn how to facilitate a training, this type of learner may want to watch an experienced trainer in action.
- **Kinesthetic or tactile learners:** who need to interact with the material they are learning, to move around, touch, or practice doing what it is they are trying to learn. To learn how to facilitate a training, this type of learner may want to practice by doing part of a training with an experienced cofacilitator.
- **Auditory learners:** who learn by listening. This learner might enjoy a lecture, a film, or a small or large group discussion. To learn how to facilitate a training, this type of learner may want to listen to a detailed lecture or presentation about training skills.

While some people may be *primarily* one type of learner, all people learn in more than one way. In any training, you will be working with a diverse group that learns in a variety of ways. If you rely on just one teaching method, you will limit the effectiveness of your trainings.

WHAT IS YOUR EXPERIENCE AS A LEARNER?

Think about a training session or class that was *not* effective in facilitating your learning:

- What made it difficult for you to become actively engaged in learning?
- Did the trainer or teacher talk too much?
- Did the training value your experience and knowledge?
- Did the training or class invite your participation?
- What could the trainer or teacher have done to improve the class?

Think about a training or class that was effective in facilitating your learning:

- What did the trainer or teacher do to make you feel comfortable?
- What kind of activities most engaged you?
- What styles of teaching worked best for you?
- How do you know that this training or class was effective for you?

19.3 APPROACHES TO TEACHING AND TRAINING

There are many approaches to facilitating trainings. For the purposes of this chapter, we will emphasize three approaches that are commonly used in the field of public health to actively engage training participants in learning and teaching: popular education, participatory learning, and problem-based learning.

POPULAR EDUCATION

Paulo Freire is considered one of the world's most important thinkers about education. He is widely known in the field of public health as a key theorist and practitioner of popular education. Freire lived and worked in Brazil, where it was illegal to vote unless one was literate (able to read and write), leaving the poor without a voice in elections. Freire worked to address the problem of illiteracy, teaching sugarcane workers how to read in just forty-five days. He initiated a national literacy campaign, which ended when the Brazilian government was overthrown.

> One cannot expect positive results from an educational or political action program which fails to respect the particular view of the world held by the people. Such a program constitutes cultural invasion, good intentions not withstanding.
>
> —Paulo Freire, *Pedagogy of the Oppressed,* 1968/1970.

Freire recognized that unless a learner's own experiences were recognized and valued, truly significant learning could not occur. Education that starts *where people are* has the potential to transform lives. Freire's approach suggested that education that supported people in identifying and analyzing important problems in their lives, and in better understanding how those problems are connected to larger social issues and dynamics, could lead them to develop and implement actions to change and improve their circumstances. Freire called this process **conscientization** or the development of a critical consciousness about social and political realities. He also strongly believed that the true purpose of education should be liberation—the promotion of social justice.

When Freire taught farmworkers how to read, the workers also talked about and analyzed their personal experiences with poverty and injustice. They came to realize that these were not individual problems, but larger problems created by social inequities and oppression. The final step of the popular education process comes when the development of critical consciousness leads to praxis—when the participants use their knowledge to take collective action to promote social justice and the welfare of their community.

Have you ever taken a class in which the teacher lectured the entire time? Freire called this "banking"—a traditional teaching method that treats learners as though they are containers into which information is poured, with the expectation that the learner will be able to repeat back the information exactly as it was told to them. In contrast to this approach, Freire encouraged teachers or trainers to recognize, value, and call forth the experience, the knowledge, and the wisdom of students or participants. **Popular education** supports learners in "speaking their own word," rather than repeating back the language, analysis, and ideas of trainers, or anyone else. To learn more about popular education, review the resources provided at the end of this chapter, including the Paulo Freire Institute.

Popular education is commonly used to guide the work of CHWs. Imagine working with a community who lives near a waste incinerator that produces significant pollution. The community experiences disproportionately high rates of asthma and other health problems. In this context, CHWs might use popular education to support the community in talking about how the incinerator affects the health of their families. As they join together, families are able to connect personal problems to larger community issues, and to analyze the causes of these problems. The group is asked to think about what would improve the welfare of their community and how they could work together to create change. For example, the community may choose to organize and advocate together for policies to reduce their exposure to toxins, such as the closure of the nearby waste incinerator.

SERGIO MATOS: Most education in this country assumes that students know nothing. Popular education is the exact opposite. It holds that people are a fountain of wisdom and knowledge and experience, and they bring all of that life experience and history to education and training. As a CHW, you really need to validate that. We call it liberation education because it provides an opportunity for freedom and critical thinking and organizing for social justice. Liberation education is about the wisdom in the group, not of any one individual.

PARTICIPATORY LEARNING

When we engage people in all aspects of the learning experience, when we presume that a learner is also a teacher, we have begun the process of **participatory learning**. Other ways to describe participatory learning are interactive learning or sharing knowledge. As with popular education, participatory learning views the learner as more than a recipient of information. A participatory learner is involved in identifying what she needs to know, how she would like to learn new information, and in all learning activities. You might say that the learners identify not only what their problems are, but the solutions to these problems as well. This approach to learning eliminates the idea of there being one expert: we are all experts when it comes to figuring out the solutions to our life's problems and challenges. And if we are part of a community working together to identify and solve our problems, then we have much more power to create meaningful changes. To learn more about participatory learning, please refer to the resources at the end of this chapter.

PROBLEM-BASED LEARNING

Another way to engage a community in the learning experience is to organize them into teams that work together to discover solutions to real-life problems. As with the methods described above, **problem-based learning** (PBL) encourages people to think in a critical way. Instead of just memorizing somebody's idea of "the right answer" to a problem, team members talk to and challenge each other to develop their own solutions. Under this model, there are no "right answers" as much as there are a range of possible answers that represent the experience, ideas, and values of the group. One significant benefit of this approach is that the group members get to know each other as individuals and learn how to work together as a team. This creates a sense of community, as well building relationships across differences of class, race, language, and culture.

CHWs use participatory learning, popular education, problem-based learning, and other methods that actively involve community members in the process of learning. These methods respect the experience, knowledge, and wisdom of learners, and support them in using their knowledge to take action that will promote their health and well-being.

How might you apply these approaches to learning as you facilitate a training on stress management for the team of CHWs and volunteers mentioned at the beginning of the chapter?

19.4 DECIDING IF TRAINING IS THE RIGHT STRATEGY

Training is sometimes suggested as the strategy to address most community health issues. But training may or may not be the best way to address the challenge at hand. It may be more effective, for example, to conduct community health outreach, to facilitate a support group, to engage in community planning or to facilitate community organizing and advocacy.

How do you figure out whether training is actually what a group needs? The following questions are designed to guide you in deciding whether or not to conduct training:

- ✪ What does the group want to accomplish?
- ✪ Are there other ways to accomplish these goals?
- ✪ What makes you think that training is the best way to accomplish it?
- ✪ Is there a better way to get the information to people?

In order to answer those questions, you will need to figure out:

- ✪ Who is your audience?
- ✪ Will participation in the training be voluntary or required?
- ✪ Would learning be better in a formal or informal setting?
- ✪ Is the group highly diverse (with different backgrounds, identities, and levels of knowledge about the training issues)?
- ✪ What are the possible barriers between you and your audience? Age, race, language, gender, sexual orientation, national origin, and literacy level are just a few of the walls that may stand between you and the people you are working with.
- ✪ Will the audience be expecting an "expert" as the teacher? What qualifies you to be the one to lead the session?
- ✪ Are you hoping to teach skills or ideas?
- ✪ What is your budget? What will the cost be? Is there a more cost-effective way to have your participants learn the material?

There is no simple formula to determine whether training is the right strategy use. Based on the answers to these questions, use your best judgment to decide whether training is the right approach for the challenge at hand.

19.5 HOW TO PLAN AND PREPARE TRAININGS

How will you prepare for the stress management training that you have been asked to facilitate?

Your first task is to ask questions. You need to know what the supervisor wants, what the CHWs need, and what resources are available for this training.

The following list of general questions does not necessarily have to be answered in any particular order, but we recommend that you find out as much as you can about each one.

1. If you have been asked to conduct this training by someone else, *what are their primary goals*? In the case study presented at the beginning of the chapter, what are the agency's goals for the stress management training? What do they expect CHWs to learn in the two-hour workshop?

2. What do the participants *want to know*? What do the CHWs who will participate in the training most want to know about stress reduction? Do they want to learn specific stress-reduction techniques such as meditation? Do they want to talk about how the stress of their work is affecting them?

3. What do those who will participate in the training *already know*? For example, have the CHWs participated in stress-reduction workshops before? What do they currently do to manage their stress?

CONDUCTING AN ASSESSMENT BEFORE DESIGNING A TRAINING

You will facilitate a better training if you understand what the participants already know and want to learn. If possible, conduct a preassessment to gather this information and prepare for the training. The assessment doesn't need to be complicated or lengthy; it just needs to provide you with some basic information. There a number of options for how to gather the information, each with its own strengths and weaknesses. These options are described in greater detail in Chapter Seventeen and include the following:

Interviewing Stakeholders or Possible Participants   Interviews with potential participants, or another professional who works with the participants, provide useful information for designing a training. Ideally, for the stress management training you have been asked to provide, it would be best to interview the CHWs who will participate in the training. You might be able to visit the agency and talk with them in person, or set up a conference call. Prepare a list of *open-ended questions,* being careful not to take too much time with the people you are interviewing. Decide how many people you are going to interview. One you have conducted a few interviews you can review your notes for common themes.

If you are able to speak with the CHWs who will participate in the stress management training, your questions might include:

- What is your level of interest in attending this training?
- What do you hope to get out of this training?
- What types of stresses are most common in your job?
- What types of training have you already received in stress reduction?
- What do you do now to manage stress?
- What topics do you not need me to cover in detail?
- What kind of trainings do you most enjoy? How do you best learn new information or skills?

?

What other questions would you want to ask?

Administer Surveys   Your agency might use a survey to gather information about future trainings. In general, surveys ask *closed-ended questions.* You need to decide on your goals before you design the survey, and think about the type of answers that people may give to the questions you ask. You can conduct a survey by phone, via the World Wide Web, by distributing paper copies, or with an in-person interview. Survey questions can be of many types, including multiple choice, yes/no, or *interval rating* (such as a Likert Scale, which asks people to rate their feeling or opinion on a 0–10 scale).

Learning to develop a good survey is an art that takes practice. For more information about using surveys, please see Chapter Seventeen and the resources provided at the end of this chapter from the University of Texas at Austin and the National Association of County and City Health Officials.

Conduct a Focus Group   Chapter Seventeen also presents information about focus groups. Briefly, this is an opportunity to bring together six to twelve members of a common group or community to facilitate a discussion about specific topics and record their responses. It is often used as part of a community diagnosis process, to develop new public health programs or educational materials or to evaluate programs, and it may be useful in designing your training as well. Focus groups take a lot of time to prepare for and, depending on the nature of your training, it may be a bigger project than the training itself merits.

FACILITATING A TRAINING ON DOMESTIC VIOLENCE

Recently, I assisted in developing training for people who work in a family court about the issue of domestic violence. The group I was working with felt that court employees did not always know what to do when someone experiencing family violence came to them for assistance. After hearing from the group about what they felt the problem was, the next task was to find out what court employees thought about the issues.

To develop the training, I conducted a preassessment that included a survey of court employees, brief telephone interviews with individual employees, and a focus group discussion. Keep in mind that this assessment was part of a well-funded and ongoing program, so we had the resources and time to conduct a more comprehensive assessment.

When I conducted telephone interviews with court employees, I asked the following questions:

1.   Have you had previous training about domestic violence? If so, who provided the trainings, and when/where were they held?
2.   What were the strengths and weaknesses of those trainings?
3.   What type of information might assist you to do your job better when working with victims of domestic violence?
4.   If you had the opportunity for more domestic violence training, what would you most like to learn?

The questions were designed to give me ideas about possible topics for the training. Question 2 was an opportunity to find out if certain topics or training approaches were either particularly effective or ineffective. Questions 4 and 5 might seem repetitive, but sometimes asking the same question in a slightly different way brings out new information. Even if we had not held focus groups or distributed a survey, these phone calls gave me essential information that assisted to formulate our training agenda.

You will decide how to conduct your assessment based on the amount of time and other resources you have, how easy it will be for you to contact the participants, and what you and your participants are comfortable doing.

ARE YOU THE RIGHT PERSON TO FACILITATE THE TRAINING?

Once you have determined that training is an appropriate strategy to meet the needs of the community or organization, there are still other questions to be answered. Are you the right person to deliver this training? Do you have the expertise and knowledge required? If your answer to that question is "no," you may be able to learn new information and skills that will prepare you to take the lead. Or you may want to identify someone who is more knowledgeable about the topic, and ask that person to facilitate the training or to work with you as cofacilitator. Even if you are highly knowledgeable about the topic, you should still consider whether you are the right person to facilitate the training.

Perhaps the most important issues I consider before deciding to do a training are the potential barriers that may exist between the training participants and me. I don't believe that a facilitator has to resemble the people participating in the training. If I don't share things in common with the group, I want to consider whether our differences are going to get in the way of their learning experience. When I trained public school teachers in the Central Valley of California about the topic of hate-motivated violence, I acknowledged that I was *not* a schoolteacher and that I was not from a rural area myself. My cotrainer grew up just a few miles away from the training site, so while she too had never been a schoolteacher, she was able to assure people that she had some insight into who they were. I shared my areas of expertise and acknowledged that it was different from theirs, and I think this assisted in eliminating a possible source of stress.

Differences of race, class, gender, and age are among the most obvious differences that might exist between you and the people you are hoping to train. Sometimes any or all of those differences might be such significant obstacles that you are not the right person to lead the training. Other times, by acknowledging the differences, by allowing for different points of view during the training, and by doing plenty of homework ahead of time, you can go ahead and act as the trainer. There are no hard and fast rules to follow. Listen to your own gut, and be sure to respect the cultural practices of the group you are working with.

ESTABLISH GOALS AND LEARNING OUTCOMES

Once you have gathered the information you need from stakeholders and potential participants, it is time to establish the goals and learning outcomes or objectives for your training. (For the purpose of this chapter, we will use *learning outcomes* and *objectives* interchangeably.) The feedback you received, whether from a survey, an interview, or a focus group, will be a critical part of determining what these goals and objectives will be.

What is the difference between a goal and a learning outcome? A goal is the broad statement about where we want to go or what we want to accomplish, and is generally an abstract idea. A **learning outcome** should be as specific as possible about what participants will know and know how to do as a result of the training. To learn more about developing goals and objectives, refer to the resources at the end of this chapter from the American Library Association and the Indiana Department of Education.

Here are the goals and two of the learning outcomes we established, after we conducted a preassessment for the training with the court staff mentioned above:

Training Goals

1. To increase awareness of the impact of exposure to domestic violence on victims and their children.
2. To increase the ability to effectively understand and respond to families in crisis.
3. To increase the number of families experiencing domestic violence who are linked to appropriate resources, including legal, mental health, and housing services.

Learning Outcomes

1. For staff who work at the family court to be able to identify at least three symptoms of post-traumatic stress (PTS), and at least one example of how PTS could affect how a victim of domestic violence presents herself at the court.

2. For staff at the court to be able to list at least three new resources they could offer to survivors of domestic violence and their children.

    Good training goals and learning outcomes are realistic and recognize the abilities and desires of your participants. Perhaps most important, it requires you to meet your participants where they are, not where you wish they would be.

    What are the possible goals and learning outcomes for the training on stress reduction that you have been asked to facilitate?

Goals:

Example: To reduce stress for workers and volunteers doing violence prevention work.
    Write down additional goals here:

1. _____

2. _____

Learning Outcomes:

Example: All participants will practice a three-minute breathing exercise designed to reduce stress responses.

Section 1: Introduction to the Training

Objective/ Scope	Key Content	Activity	Materials	Who Is Responsible?
1. To review the purpose and content of the training.	1. Mission, history, and primary tasks of the family court's Domestic Violence Project 2. Review the training agenda, goals, and learning outcomes.	1. Facilitator presents information and invites questions and discussion.	1. Agency brochure; handouts with training agenda, goals, and learning outcomes	1. Jill

Section 3

Dynamics of domestic violence: How families present domestic violence, the relationship between domestic violence and child maltreatment, and roles and considerations for court frontline staff.

Write down additional learning outcomes here:

1. _____

2. _____

CREATE AN OUTLINE FOR YOUR TRAINING

After identifying your goals and learning outcomes, you are ready to develop a detailed outline of what you will do in the training. What information will you cover? What kinds of training methods are you going to use? Be specific about every step and topic you are going to cover. This will assist you in many ways, including allowing you to determine what you really have time to cover.

There are many ways to outline a training plan. Here is an excerpt of the outline format I used for the court training.

19.6 TIPS FOR FACILITATING A PARTICIPATORY TRAINING

You will develop your own approaches and training methods with time and experience. In the meantime, here are some tips I've learned along the way that I hope will be useful to you.

Objective/ Scope	Key Content	Activity	Materials	Who Is Responsible?
1. To understand common signs of post-traumatic stress among victims of domestic violence (DV) and their children.	1. Define post-traumatic stress (PTS) and common trauma responses among victims of DV.	1. Show video about DV. Provide definition of post-traumatic stress and facilitate discussion. Facilitate small-group activity to identify common trauma responses.	1. Video: "The Impact of Domestic Violence on Families." Handout with definition of post-traumatic stress.	1. Tony and Jill

(Continued)

Objective/ Scope	Key Content	Activity	Materials	Who Is Responsible?
		Review the work of small groups with all participants. Highlight common trauma responses. Respond to questions and concerns about trauma responses.	Flip-chart paper and pens for small-group brainstorming. One paper for each small group (of three to four participants) with a different category of trauma response, including: physical, emotional, cognitive (thoughts), spiritual/religious, and behavioral responses.	

PREPARING THE TRAINING

☆ *Ask about the language needs of your participants.* Is there someone who is deaf? If so, make sure they have access to an interpreter and a comfortable place to sit where the participant can clearly see the interpreter and still be part of the group. If the trainers are English speakers, are there participants who speak languages other than English? If you can't afford to pay for interpreters, see if there are community members who are willing to volunteer to play that role. Otherwise, you will need to let people know that the training is not accessible to all.

☆ *Make sure you have a safe, comfortable place for your training* that is accessible to all participants. Will people be able to get there easily by bus, car, or on foot? Will there be seats for everyone? If there are stairs, is there also an elevator for those who are unable to use the stairs?

☆ *Assess child care needs.* If possible, try to arrange for child care, or have a plan for how to handle children if participants bring them. Your participants will appreciate knowing their children are safely occupied so that they can focus on the training. If you can't afford child care (which is probably most of the time), it may be possible to provide some toys and materials for the children to play with.

Now try using the same format to develop a plan for the training you are scheduled to facilitate on stress management.

Section 1: Introduction to the Training

Objective/ Scope	Key Content	Activity	Materials	Who Is Responsible?
1. Example: To provide an overview of the goals and learning outcomes for the training session. 2. Fill this in: What's next? 3.	1. Goals and learning outcomes developed for the session. 2. 3.	1. Presentation and large-group discussion of the goals and learning outcomes. Ask if there are other items people want to cover. 2. 3.	1. Flip-chart paper and pens. Handouts. 2. 3.	1. Your name here! 2. You! 3. You!

- ☼ *Pack up your materials well ahead of time,* including extra pens and paper, plenty of copies of any handouts, newsprint and an easel, markers, tape, and anything else you will be using. Make sure you haven't left anything out. If you plan to show a video or DVD, make sure that the appropriate technology (such as a TV and VCR or laptop and LCD projector) will be available at the training site, or bring what you need with you.
- ☼ *Get to the training location thirty minutes in advance* so that you have plenty of time to set up the room, and to deal with any unexpected problems related to the space.

?

What else would you want to do to prepare for the training session?

FACILITATING THE TRAINING SESSION

Setting the Stage

- ☼ *Introduce yourself and welcome all participants.* Tell them what topics the training will address. Tell them what your goals and learning outcomes are. Review the day's agenda so that they know what to expect. Invite and respond to their questions or concerns. Make sure participants know when breaks will occur, where the restrooms are, and any other logistical information they might need.

✪ *Establish clear ground rules.* Suggest some ground rules to the group and ask them if they would like to add to the list. Sample ground rules include: "No interruptions—let each person finish speaking before you begin," "Turn off cell phones," "Maintain confidentiality—don't share anyone's private or personal information with people outside of the training," and "Offer respect to all of the participants, even if you disagree with them." Ask everyone for their agreement in following the ground rules: this will be helpful if anything happens during the session that creates an unwelcome interruption or disturbance.

✪ *Use icebreakers or opening activities* to assist participants to relax and build trust. This will assist people prepare for the work at hand, and perhaps allow them to meet some or all of the people in the room. There are thousands of great ideas for icebreakers on the World Wide Web (see the resources from the University of Hawaii and the National Park Services at the end of this chapter). Be guided in your choices by how much time you want to spend on this activity. Here is an icebreaker that I have often used:

✪ *The history of your name.* Each participant shares what they know about the history of their first or last name. All sorts of information might be shared: perhaps a family changed their name when they immigrated to the United States, or the name may have a specific historical, cultural, religious, or family meaning. Some participants may know little about the history of their name, and that is all right too.

? **What else would you want to say or do at the beginning of a training?**

Organization and Logistics

✪ *Keep to the training schedule.* You will break trust with the participants if you start late or don't finish on time. Start within ten minutes of when scheduled.

✪ *Schedule breaks during your session,* particularly if you are working for more than an hour. People need time to stretch, use the bathroom, and return phone calls. They will be more capable of giving their full attention to the training if you let them know that they will be able to take care of these needs.

✪ *If possible, provide healthy refreshments for participants.* Fruit, water, fresh vegetables, and dip are good things to provide, and also provide reassurance that you are concerned about the welfare of your participants.

Clarity

✪ *Tie your points together.* Show how one idea leads to the next. Check in regularly with participants to see if they understand what you are saying and doing. Ask them if they have any questions or concerns. Watch for their body language. If you see looks of confusion on their faces, ask if you are communicating clearly enough.

✪ *Build on earlier lessons.* They may be lessons learned at a different time entirely, or lessons learned earlier during the same session. This aids in reinforcing learning.

✪ *Repeat your main points* during the course of the session as a way to emphasize your message. If you do your job well, the participants will begin to take on this role for you.

? **What else would you do to organize the training and to ensure that participants understand the information provided?**

An effective facilitator maintains the interest and attention of participants.

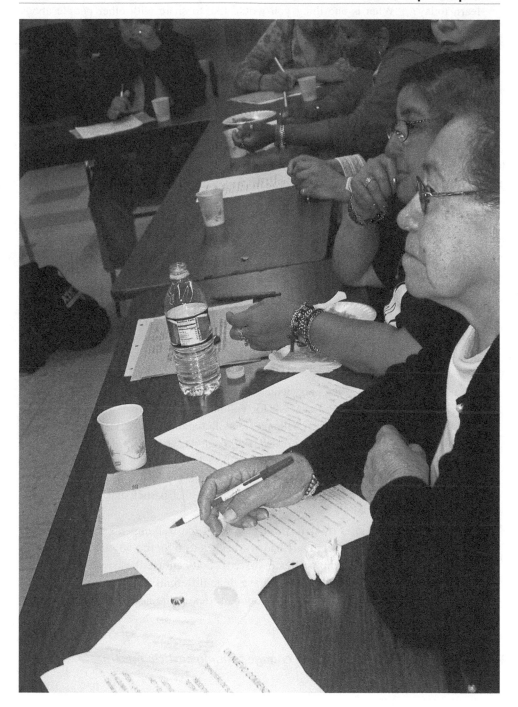

Engaging Participants

☼ *Don't talk too much!* Give people many opportunities to ask questions and to express their own knowledge and expertise.

☼ *Ask questions.* Acknowledge that everyone in the room has knowledge and experience to share. Your role is to facilitate learning, not to be the only source of information. I like to start a training by asking people to introduce themselves and answer a few questions. I might ask, "How long have you worked here?" "What do you hope to learn today?" "What is one thing you would like to share with other people about your experience with this topic?"

○ *Ask participants to work in teams.* There are many methods for getting people into smaller groups including both teams of two and larger groups of three to five. You can ask people to group themselves by twos or threes, "count off," assign people to a group as they enter the workshop (put a symbol on their name tag). When people work in small groups they are more likely to actively participate.

Engage participants in problem-based learning instead of telling them what they need to know. For your stress-reduction workshop, you might assign participants to small teams, and ask each team to develop a proposal for what they and their agency can do differently to reduce stress among frontline workers.

○ *Keep people moving.* Sitting in one place throughout a training often makes it difficult for people to stay alert and to learn effectively. I often ask people to move around the room, meeting in different small groups, or writing down their ideas on large sheets of paper posted on the walls.

○ *Provide games and exercises.* Once people are in small groups, they often enjoy an opportunity to compete in some way with the other groups. Teams might play a version of Jeopardy or another popular game show. Questions to be answered should reflect the material that you want the participants to learn.

○ *Role-play.* This is one of the best ways for participants to practice new skills. Teams can be given a scenario to act out, which they present to the other participants in the workshop or training. Or you can ask for volunteers to participate in a role-play in order to demonstrate a situation, challenge, or skill that the group is learning about.

○ *Have teams teach each other a new skill.* For example, you might give each group a handout about a different stress-reduction method. Each group is given enough time to understand and practice the method, and to make a plan for how to teach it to others. Each group will make a presentation to the other participants about a stress-reduction method.

○ *Use real-world examples as case studies.* When I led trainings about hate crimes, I told stories about the cases that I had worked on as a victim advocate (maintaining the confidentiality of the parties involved). You can use these stories and case studies to ask what participants might have done differently, or even to assist them to learn what *not* to do. You can draw upon stories in the news, historical events, films, or literature.

? *What else would you do to actively engage training participants?*

ROMELIA RODRIGUEZ: I facilitate a lot of trainings in the community, and there is a big difference between being a facilitator and being a teacher. Teachers might want to control the agenda in the workshop, but as a facilitator, someone who understands popular education, I know that the group should control the experience of the training. It's not my job always to be in control or to know the outcomes of the workshop. I need to make space for the group to speak up, to share their experiences and their knowledge. It is harder sometimes for people to give up this control.

But popular education is about sharing power, about being equal with the group, about knowing that the most important knowledge comes from the group. Because the learning that happens is for them, and we hope that it leads to action, and these actions must be carried out by the community.

ENDING YOUR TRAINING

- ✪ *Acknowledge that people may still have questions* and let them know where and how they can continue to learn about the topics addressed in the training. Give people a way to contact you if they don't already have that information.
- ✪ *Make sure you end on time.* Even if you have not been able to cover all your material, you must respect people's time and end when you said that you would.
- ✪ *Make sure that you leave the training space as you found it.* This is particularly important if you are using space that was donated. Make sure your hosts want to invite you back.
- ✪ *Thank everyone for his or her participation.*

PRESENTING STATISTICS IN A TRAINING

In general, we advise you to use statistics and numbers sparingly in the trainings you facilitate. Unless statistics are presented very well, they can be boring and difficult to understand. However, if you have a really punchy, simple statement, like "More women have died this year in St. Louis due to domestic violence than due to cancer," then use it. See Chapter Seventeen for more discussion about this.

? *In Table 19.1, what is the central point that the creators are trying to make? Would you use a table like Table 19.1 in the training you are facilitating?*

? *Do you think most training participants would be able to understand this table?*

? *Can you think of another way that the material could have been presented?*

Now take a look at Figure 19.1.

? *What story is Figure 19.1 telling?*

Table 19.1. Percentage of Respondents Aged ≥18 Years Who Reported a History of Stroke, by Selected Characteristics—Behavioral Risk Factor Surveillance System, United States, 2005.

Characteristic	Total No. of Respondents*	Prevalence of Stroke (%)[†]	(95% CI[§])	Estimated No. of U.S. Residents with a History of Stroke
Age group (yrs)				
18–44	128,328	(0.8)	(0.7–0.9)	852,000
45–64	137,738	(2.7)	(2.5–2.9)	1,926,000
≥65	87,351	(8.1)	(7.7–8.5)	3,036,000
Sex[¶]				
Men	136,201	(2.7)	(2.5–2.8)	2,694,000
Women	219,911	(2.5)	(2.4–2.7)	3,145,000
Race/Ethnicity[¶]				
White, non-Hispanic	279,419	(2.3)	(2.3–2.4)	4,017,000
Black, non-Hispanic	27,925	(4.0)	(3.6–4.5)	772,000
Asian/Pacific Islander	5,974	(1.6)**	(1.0–2.7)	60,000
Hispanic[††]	25,539	(2.6)	(2.1–3.3)	616,000
American Indian/Alaska Native	5,535	(6.0)	(4.5–7.8)	126,000
Multiracial	6,519	(4.6)	(3.7–5.6)	136,000
Education[¶]				
Less than 12 years	38,202	(4.4)	(4.0–4.9)	1,365,000
High school graduate	109,830	(2.6)	(2.5–2.8)	1,863,000
Some college	93,228	(2.7)	(2.5–2.9)	1,474,000
College graduate	113,944	(1.8)	(1.6–1.9)	1,108,000
Total	**356,112**	**(2.6)**	**(2.5–2.7)**	**5,839,000**

*The sums of the sample sizes in each category might not add up to the total number of respondents because of unknown or missing information.

[†]Weighted percentage of respondents who reported a history of stroke.

[§]Confidence interval.

[¶]Weighted percentages are age adjusted to the 2000 U.S. standard population.

**The relative standard error of this estimate is 20%–30% and should be interpreted with caution.

[††]Might be of any race.

Source: Centers for Disease Control and Prevention 2007, p. 471.

Figure 19.1 Assistance for Mentally Ill Homeless Veterans in San Francisco.

➤ No. of beds at the San Francisco V.A. = 101 (1 🛏 = 10 actual beds)

➤ No. of mentally ill homeless veterans in San Francisco = 2200 (1 👤 = 10 mentally ill vets)

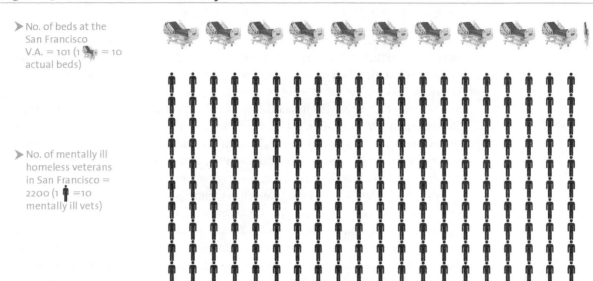

Source: Blecker, 2003.

? *Does it make a different impact on you than Table 19.1?*

? *In what way?*

19.7 RESPONDING TO COMMON CHALLENGES

No matter how well I have planned a training, something unexpected always happens. Mostly, this is a good thing, but sometimes it makes my work more challenging. Recently, one of my cotrainers was over one hour late and I couldn't reach her by phone. I had to decide whether to adjust the agenda and hope she showed up later in the day to do her part, or whether to go ahead and facilitate a section of the training that I didn't feel confident about. I decided to gamble that "Jana" would show up eventually. Sure enough, she showed up, her training segment went extremely well, and I didn't have to be responsible for material that I didn't know very well.

? *What do you think happened during the training at the Vietnamese Youth Center?*

? *If you had the chance to do this training, what would you do differently?*

Following are several other challenges that you are likely to face when you facilitate trainings, and my suggestions for how to handle these situations.

ONE OF MY WORST TRAINING MISTAKES

Mike, a fellow CHW, and I were asked to facilitate a series of trainings about interracial conflict for immigrant teenagers at a Vietnamese youth center. The Vietnamese youths had recently had a series of conflicts with some African American youths. We spent a lot of time trying to think about appropriate ways to work with the group, given that they had life experiences that were enormously different from our own. Mike is Chinese American, I'm Jewish and Caucasian, and neither of us are immigrants. We did not know much about these young people, although we were advised by one of the adult staff members that many of the boys probably wouldn't want to participate in any group activities.

Mike had recently been in a documentary film about the racism experienced by American-born Asian men, and for one of the sessions we decided we would use excerpts from this film as a springboard for discussion. Though there were girls in the group we were working with, we thought that the overall message of the film, about facing racism as Asians in America, would be relevant for the entire group.

Several of the men in the movie cry as they speak about the racism they experienced and the difficulties they faced as Asian men in the United States. Unexpectedly for us, both the boys and the girls started laughing during these scenes. As the minutes passed, the giggling turned into loud laughter. We had thought watching the film would be a moving experience that could promote a deeper conversation about their own experiences as immigrants and Asians, but the youths at the Vietnamese Center didn't feel that they had much in common with the men in the film. After several very long minutes during which we tried to get the youths to talk about the film and their own life experiences, Mike and I realized that we had completely missed the mark.

A PARTICIPANT WHO IS ARGUMENTATIVE OR DOMINATING

At some time, you are likely to encounter a training participant who is argumentative, has something to say about every statement you make, is disrespectful to others, or in some other way makes it difficult to proceed smoothly with the agenda. Each of us has a different tolerance for this type of behavior. It is important to consider, however, how these behaviors may affect the other participants. As a facilitator, it is your responsibility to ensure a productive learning environment for all participants. Once I realize what is going on, I rely on several strategies to try to manage this type of challenge.

First, this is where the ground rules established at the beginning of the training can be very useful. If a person is openly disruptive, it is up to you to remind the individual that everyone agreed to follow the ground rules. If there is a person who is dominating the discussion, I make a point of calling on others to speak. I might even begin to call on people who have not raised their hands or spoken up on their own. I might say, "Let's make sure we hear from everyone today." I have also spoken with disruptive participants one-on-one, during a break. I might say something like: "I see you have a lot to say, and I really appreciate that, but today I need to make sure that everyone gets an opportunity to participate. If you have questions or comments you want to make to me, we can always check in after the training session is over."

This was not the time for a lengthy examination of what had gone wrong. We needed to quickly change direction and find another way to open a door to communication and connection with the participants. We took a short break. I felt overwhelmed and uncertain about what to do next. Thankfully, Mike is both a quick thinker and someone not willing to give up easily. He suggested we ask the group to do a writing exercise. We reconvened, and Mike handed out paper and asked the youths to start writing about their own experiences. We made it through the difficult moment without the youths themselves seeming to be aware that there had been any problem at all. Eventually, we were able to recapture their interest and to get them talking and reflecting about their own lives, the recent conflicts with the other youths, and how they could respond in ways that were positive for both groups.

As trainers, we didn't meet the youths where they were, and the gap between our assumptions and their reality was enormous. Remember what Paulo Freire said: unless a learner's own experiences are recognized and valued, real learning cannot occur.

In retrospect, we could have turned down the request to conduct these trainings, offering referrals to other sources. Alternatively, we might have sought out a cotrainer, perhaps someone from the Vietnamese community, who could have assisted us in developing a curriculum that our participants could better connect with. We might also have asked the staff at the Community Center for the opportunity to meet with some of the youths prior to the training, to learn more from them about what they were interested in and how we might engage them. None of those ideas would be wrong. While Mike and I had spent a lot of time preparing for the trainings, we needed to spend it differently. We were talking to each other, when we needed to be talking to others.

If I have a cotrainer, one of us will take responsibility for keeping their eye on the "room temperature," making sure that disruptions are handled quietly, perhaps even by asking the person to step out into the hallway to talk for a minute, and asking them if they can agree to be present without being disruptive.

In the worst situation I was in, a participant became so disruptive that we stopped the training. One of the cotrainers stepped out into the hallway with the person causing the disruption, and the other trainer stayed inside with the other folks in order to hear from them what they wanted and needed from the situation. Sadly, we ended up asking the disruptive person to leave, because she was unable to make a commitment to peaceful participation. The experience really underscored one basic truth of community health work: no matter how much you plan, the unexpected can, and will, happen. It will be how you respond to the bumps in the road that will determine your success.

WHEN PARTICIPANTS ARE NOT INTERESTED IN THE TRAINING

As with the situation I described earlier about my training mistakes with a group of Vietnamese youths, there are times when your agenda is simply not the right one for the situation or the participants. While there is nothing to stop you from plowing ahead and ignoring the problem, that does nothing to accomplish your goals or those of the participants. In the situation I described, I was fortunate to have a cotrainer who was great at thinking on his feet. The experience also illustrates how valuable it is to have a "Plan B" along with your "Plan A" at all times—alternate methods of delivering your message, or even other topics that could be covered. It is all right to put aside your agenda and to check in with participants about the training. If you learn that the training isn't working well for them, put aside your planned agenda and try using other methods to reach your learning outcomes.

DOING OR SAYING SOMETHING THAT OFFENDS TRAINING PARTICIPANTS

Perhaps my biggest fear is that I am going to say or do something that offends the group I am training, undermining trust and perhaps the opportunity for future partnerships. But I know that despite my best efforts, I will make mistakes, and from time to time—I will unintentionally do something that offends someone. Hopefully, when this occurs, it will be brought to my attention in some way. Ideally, participants will speak up to let me know that they are upset. If I don't learn about the problem, I won't have an opportunity to respond and to restore trust and collaboration. When participants tell me that I have done something that they experienced as offensive, hurtful, or disrespectful, I want to give them my full attention. This is the most important time to be fully present, to listen deeply, and not to respond defensively. I want to understand their experience and point of view so that I can respond in an appropriate manner and prevent similar mistakes in the future. In these moments, I have come to realize that I don't need to explain or defend my actions. What I need to do is to honor the experience of the participants. Even if I didn't intend to be hurtful, I listen, apologize, and try not to repeat the error. When I have done a good and honest job at this, often I have deepened the quality of our relationship by showing that I am a human being who makes mistakes, takes responsibility for them, and expresses my intention to build a respectful professional partnership.

19.8 EVALUATION OF TRAININGS

How are you going to measure what people learned during a training? For most training, you will want to keep your evaluation simple. Determine what you want to know about the training. What information will allow you to do a better job next time? Do you want feedback about your presentation skills? Do you want to know how much people learned? What their favorite part of the session was?

An evaluation can be as simple as asking participants to respond anonymously, in writing, to four questions: What did you think of the training? What did you learn? What else did you want to learn? What would you change about the training? Or it can be a series of questions about each section of the training.

Here is a sample of a brief evaluation for the stress management training mentioned at the beginning of the chapter.

1. Name three things that you learned as a result of today's training.
2. How much has your knowledge of stress management increased as a result of this training?

0	1	2	3	4	5	6	7	8	9	10
Not at all					Neutral					A lot

3. Would you recommend this training to others?

4. What suggestions do you have for how to improve this training?

To learn more about evaluation, review the resources at the American Evaluation Association (www.eval.org).

CHAPTER REVIEW QUESTIONS

PLAN YOUR OWN TRAINING

You have been asked to facilitate a four-hour training on domestic violence for a group of peer educators at a local high school. The peer educators provide information and referrals to other students. You have been working on domestic violence issues for two years and are very knowledgeable about the topic. You also have experience working with youths, but you haven't facilitated a training on domestic violence for that group before. You have four weeks to prepare the training.

1. What steps will you take to plan this training?

2. What do you most want to know in order to prepare for the training? How might you conduct a preassessment to prepare for the training? What questions might you ask?

3. What do you want the participants to come away with at the end of the training? What might be some of your goals and learning outcomes?

4. Explain what Paulo Freire called *conscientization,* or *critical consciousness,* and how this concept could be applied to the training you will facilitate.

5. What training methods will you use? How will you engage different types of learners?

6. Develop a specific training plan for at least two learning outcomes using the format provided in this chapter.

7. How will you evaluate this training?

REFERENCES

Blecker, M. 2003, May. Statement of Michael Blecker, Executive Director of Swords to Plowshares: A Veterans Rights Organization, San Francisco, CA, Before the Committee on Veterans Affairs. U.S. House of Representatives, House Committee on Veterans Affairs. Accessed on November 21, 2005: www.house.gov/va/hearings/schedule108/may03/5-6-03/mblecker.html

Centers for Disease Control and Prevention. 2007. Prevalence of Stroke—United States, 2005. *Morbidity and Mortality Weekly Report* 56 (19): 469–474. Accessed on April 6, 2009: www.cdc.gov/mmwr/PDF/wk/mm5619.pdf

Freire, P. 1968/1970. *Pedagogy of the Oppressed.* Clearwater, FL: H & H Publishing.

ADDITIONAL RESOURCES

American Evaluation Association. Accessed on April 6, 2009: www.eval.org/

American Library Association. Accessed on April 6, 2009: www.ala.org/

Association of College and Research Libraries. Accessed on April 6, 2009: www.ala.org/acrl/

The Buck Institute for Education. 2007. Project Based Learning Handbook. Accessed on April 10, 2009: www.bie.org/pbl/pblhandbook/intro.php#history/

Center for AIDS Prevention Studies. University of California, San Francisco. Good Questions / Better Answers: A Formative Research Handbook for California HIV Prevention Programs. Accessed on April 10, 2009: http://www.caps.ucsf.edu/goodquestions/pdf/Default.html

Indiana Department of Education. Accessed March 2009. How to Write Measurable Goals and Objectives. http://www.doe.state.in.us/sdfsc/pdf/writing-gos.pdf

International Institute for Environment and Development. Sustainable Agriculture Program. 1995. Participatory Learning and Action. What Is Participatory Learning and Action? http://www.iied.org/NR/agbioliv/pla_notes/whatispla.html

National Association of County and City Health Officials. Accessed March 2009. Mobilizing for Action through Planning and Partnerships. Community Themes and Strengths Assessment. http://mapp.naccho.org.

MSP Resource Portal. Participatory Learning and Action (PLA). Accessed March 2009. http://portals.wi.wur.nl/msp/?Participatory_Learning_and_Action_(PLA)

National Park Service. 2002. Community Tool Box. Facilitation Tools. Icebreakers. http://www.nps.gov/phso/rtcatoolbox/fac_icebreakers.htm

Paulo Freire Institute. Accessed March 2009. University of California, Los Angeles. http://www.paulofreireinstitute.org/

University of Hawaii, Honolulu Community College. Accessed March 2009. Break the Ice. http://www.honolulu.hawaii.edu/intranet/committees/FacDevCom/guidebk/teachtip/breakice.htm

The University of Texas at Austin. 2007. Instructional Assessment Resources. http://www.utexas.edu/academic/diia/assessment/iar/how_to/methods/survey.php

Woods, D. R. 1996. *Instructor's Guide for Problem-Based Learning: How to Gain the Most from PBL, 3rd Edition.* Hamilton, Ontario, CAN: McMaster University, Department of Chemical Engineering. http://chemeng.mcmaster.ca/pbl/chap2.pdf

20

Group Facilitation

Philip Colgan • Tim Berthold • Joani Marinoff

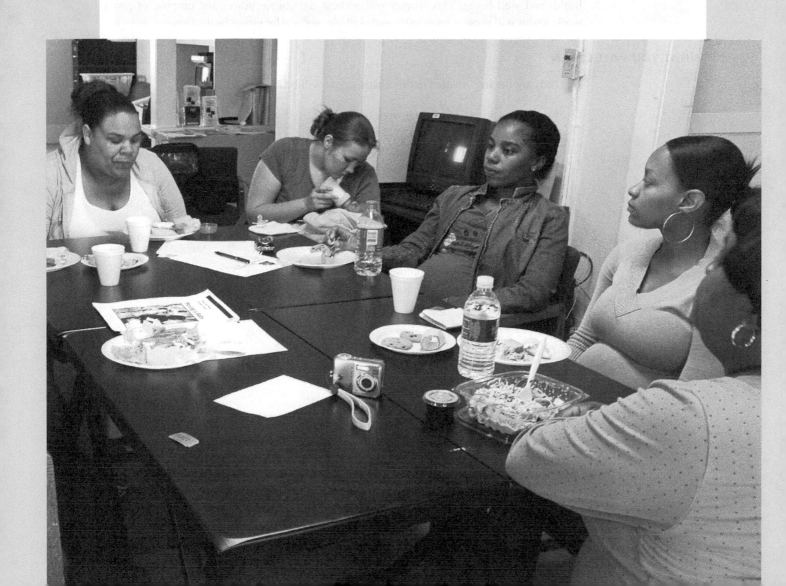

CHW SCENARIO

You have been asked to assist in starting a group in your community for people newly diagnosed with a chronic illness. The purpose of the group is to support participants in better managing and living with their illness, and in preventing further complications.

- ✪ What will your goals be for the group?
- ✪ How will you establish ground rules for the group?
- ✪ What will you do to create a sense of common purpose and community?
- ✪ How will you create a sense of safety necessary for people to talk honestly about their lives?
- ✪ How will you handle disagreements or conflicts in the group?
- ✪ How will you measure the success of the group experience?

INTRODUCTION

CHWs facilitate a variety of groups designed to bring people together to discuss and learn about common concerns and to support each other in taking actions that will enhance their health and well-being. This chapter will address the unique power and purpose of group work, and it will present knowledge and skills for successful group facilitation.

WHAT YOU WILL LEARN

By studying the information in this chapter, you will be able to:

- ✪ Discuss how and why group work is different from working with individual clients
- ✪ Identify and describe different types of groups
- ✪ Describe the unique benefits of group work
- ✪ Explain four key stages of group work and analyze the roles and tasks of facilitators at each stage
- ✪ Analyze how issues of power and authority, including the authority of the group facilitator, influence group dynamics and process
- ✪ Discuss the importance of self-reflection and evaluation to becoming a skilled group facilitator and apply this to your work
- ✪ Identify and respond to common challenges of group work
- ✪ Discuss and apply ethics to group work, including issues of boundaries and confidentiality

WORDS TO KNOW

Self-Disclosure

20.1 THE DYNAMIC NATURE AND PURPOSE OF GROUP WORK

The groups that CHWs and other helping professionals facilitate create a space for people with common experiences or interests to join together and to support one another in experiencing some type of change. Learning from one another in a structured environment, with a trained facilitator, can open new possibilities for people's thinking, feelings, and behavior.

Group work is different from working one-on-one with individual clients because it provides the opportunity for dynamic interaction among several individuals. Group members form working relationships with other participants, and through their interactions they come to understand themselves better. Members improve their communication and other interpersonal skills and take action to make changes in their lives. This makes group work unique: the group itself becomes the agent of change for the participants.

As we will emphasize in this chapter, key roles for facilitators are to create and maintain the necessary safety for group members to be able to participate, and to support the leadership of the participants themselves. When members begin to take responsibility for the group process and relationships, supporting each other to make positive life changes, the facilitator has also supported their empowerment.

If facilitators do not tap into the unique power of group—the dynamic interaction and learning that happens between group members—then it may not be the proper strategy to use.

20.2 TYPES OF GROUPS

? *What type of groups have you participated in?*

? *What motivated you to participate in the group(s)?*

? *What were the benefits for you?*

? *What was your experience like overall?*

There are many different types of groups, including a wide range of therapy groups facilitated by licensed mental health providers such as social workers, counselors, psychologists, or psychiatrists. For the purposes of this textbook, we will focus on the types of groups most commonly facilitated by CHWs, and will refer to them as *educational, social, and support groups.* Different agencies and regions of the United States and the world may refer to these types of groups by different names.

KEY FACTORS AMONG GROUPS

Before we describe the types of groups most commonly facilitated by CHWs, we want to identify additional key possible differences among the groups that CHWs facilitate. These include the following factors:

Group Size Some groups are smaller, others larger, and they may range from three to thirty or more members. Both very small and very large groups pose challenges for participants and facilitators. You may find that groups with approximately six to twelve participants allow for dynamic interaction between members and a diversity of experience and points of view, without being so large that they are difficult to manage.

Open or Closed Groups Some groups are open to anyone who fits the membership criteria on a drop-in basis. For example, Alcoholics Anonymous meetings are public and open to anyone interested in attending. In contrast, closed groups select members in advance, generally through an interview process, and do not accept new members for a stipulated period of time, such as the next time that a new group forms or when there is a need for new participants.

Duration of the Group   Some groups, such as certain educational groups, may meet just once. Other groups may continue to meet for several weeks, months, or even years. Some groups are highly structured, as described below, and may always meet for six or eight or ten weeks, and then start up again with new members. The duration of the groups you facilitate will depend on the agency you work for, the community you work with, the issues the group addresses, and the common purpose that brings the members together.

The Group Focus Issue or Topic   Check online or in the back of your city or county's free paper, if you have one, and you will find a large number of groups addressing a wide variety of topics. CHWs may facilitate groups addressing any number of health-related topics, such as parenting, recovery from drug use, living with disabilities, depression, supporting family members living with different health conditions, sexual assault, domestic violence, surviving the death of a loved one, negotiating healthy relationships, HIV prevention, healthy pregnancy, living with disabilities, diabetes, asthma, or other chronic health conditions: the list of possible topics is almost endless.

? *What issues or topics are the focus of groups that take place in your community?*

? *What topics or issues in your community do you think would benefit from additional groups?*

Purpose of the Group   Some groups are designed to educate participants about a specific health issue such as family planning or hypertension. Other groups aim to support members in changing health-related behaviors, such as smoking, parenting practices, or patterns of drug use. The purpose of other groups is to build self-esteem, community, and a sense of belonging. Most important, facilitators and group members need to have a clear understanding of and a commitment to a common purpose that brings them together.

The reasons people decide to participate in a group include:

- Desire to break isolation and build community
- Desire to learn from others who have had similar experiences
- Desire to talk about experiences, identities, feelings, and ideas that may not be understood or accepted in other settings, including the family
- To learn information and skills to better manage a specific illness
- To learn more about oneself
- To change behaviors and take action to enhance health and well-being

? *Can you think of other reasons why people participate in groups?*

Location   Groups may take place in a variety of settings, including hospitals and clinics, nonprofit agencies, schools, faith-based institutions, local departments of public health, recreational centers and facilities, correctional facilities, community centers, group homes, and housing developments.

Group Structure   Some groups begin with a highly developed structure, purpose, membership criteria, and even an agenda for meetings that are established by the sponsoring program and the facilitators. In others, decisions about the structure of the group are determined by the participants. Educational groups tend to be the most structured. For example, a diabetes education group might always meet once a week for five weeks and have an established purpose and agenda that the facilitator uses to guide each meeting. At the other extreme, social groups are often much more flexible; and the purpose, length, and topics for discussion are determined collaboratively through discussion by the participants and facilitator(s). See the description of a social group for Latino men that follows.

Group Membership Criteria   Membership may be loosely or specifically defined. For example, a group addressing violence in the community may be open to anyone who lives in the community. In contrast, some groups may be open only to people who fit a more specific profile, such as single fathers, Native American youths under the age of eighteen, or African American men living with prostate cancer.

Presence of a Facilitator   Some groups don't have a facilitator. For example, a Lesbian, Gay, Bisexual, Transgender student group might function without an outside facilitator. Other groups may have one or more facilitators.

Number of Facilitators   Sometimes you will facilitate groups on your own and on other occasions with a cofacilitator. Educational groups are more likely to be facilitated by just one CHW. We recommend cofacilitation as the best model for support groups. As part of your training, we hope that you will have the opportunity to work with an experienced cofacilitator. Later on in your career, you may have the opportunity to aid in training a new group facilitator.

Role of Facilitators   In most groups, facilitators have a strongly defined leadership role. As we will discuss in this chapter, the facilitator is responsible for creating a safe environment that encourages participation and dialogue, for assisting to prevent and resolve conflicts, and for modeling how to provide meaningful support. In other groups, such as the social groups that we will discuss in this chapter, the leadership role of the facilitator is less pronounced. In that case, the facilitator's key role is to support the leadership and empowerment of group members, who make most or all of the key decisions about membership, purpose, ground rules, and the topics addressed during group meetings.

Regardless of the level of formality and structure of the group, and the authority of the facilitator, CHWs should always be guided by client and community-centered practices designed to enhance the capacity and leadership of group members themselves.

For the purposes of this chapter, we will emphasize three different types of groups that CHWs commonly facilitate: educational, support, and social groups.

EDUCATIONAL GROUPS

Educational groups bring people together who are seeking to learn new information about a well-identified health topic. For example, an educational group may focus on the prevention of conditions such as HIV disease. Other groups provide people newly diagnosed with a health condition, such as asthma, lupus, or hepatitis C, with information about the condition, how to manage it, and how to prevent progression of the disease. The groups typically focus on enhancing health-related knowledge and skills, and provide an opportunity for people to share questions, concerns, feelings, and knowledge that they have gained through their own experience.

In general, educational groups are time limited. Once the basic health information has been covered, the group ends. Some groups might meet just once, and others might meet four or five times, depending on the nature of the health issues. Educational groups might be held in a variety of locations, including a clinic or hospital, schools, and community-based and faith-based organizations. Educational groups are commonly facilitated by one CHW, but may be cofacilitated. The emphasis is on providing health information that will assist participants to enhance their wellness.

? *Can you think of other examples of educational groups that are offered in your community?*

? *Who facilitates these groups?*

? *What issues do they address?*

SUPPORT GROUPS

Support groups may or may not have a facilitator. They provide a place for people who share a common experience, concern, or goal to meet and talk together, and to provide each other with support for improving their health or life circumstances. These groups are widely used for people who have survived difficult experiences (such as rape or the death of a family member), face stigma and discrimination based on their identity or behavior (such as for Latino immigrants, transgender women, or people who have been incarcerated in prison), share risks for a specific health condition (such as HIV, hepatitis C, or risk from smoking tobacco), or are living with a disease or health condition (such as breast cancer, alcoholism, or depression). Alcoholics Anonymous is a well-known example of a support group. Rape crisis centers and domestic violence agencies across the country also commonly facilitate support groups for survivors. Increasingly, clinics, hospitals, and health plans are also providing support groups for patients living with a specific health risk or disease such as asthma or diabetes. The emphasis is on the emotional support that peers can provide.

? *Can you think of other examples of support groups that are offered in your community?*

? *Who facilitates these groups?*

? *What issues do they address?*

SOCIAL GROUPS

Support groups are not familiar to or appropriate for all communities. Some people feel that support groups are a culturally specific model, that they emphasize problems or challenges, and that they are based on therapy groups. For these reasons and others, some communities prefer to form and facilitate social groups. Social groups tend to be less formal than support groups and are generally characterized by greater autonomy of the group members. For example, participants often take responsibility for determining what the group will address, membership criteria, ground rules, and when and how the group will meet. A key role of facilitators is to support the leadership of the members, to assist in fostering a sense of community, to step in when needed, and to resolve conflicts or address issues that the members themselves may not be prepared or willing or able to address. The emphasis is empowerment and community building.

A SOCIAL GROUP FOR LATINO MEN

A local health department, concerned about the increase of HIV infections among Latino men who have sex with men (MSM), asked a community-based agency to start support groups for this population. When the agency conducted interviews with this community, they found little interest in attending traditional support groups. However, the men did report a sense of isolation and the lack of meeting spaces in their home county. Instead, they visited urban areas outside of the county to meet other men. The men were very interested in creating meeting spaces and a stronger sense of community nearer to home. Based on this formative research, agency staff initiated a social group that met for dinner on a weekday evening. Eventually, the men decided to cook dinner together, using the agency's large kitchen on a night when they could use it with privacy. Together, the participants determined when and where they would meet, what they would talk about, and decided to keep the group open to new members. While the CHW who facilitated the social group informed participants that his primary job was to work on HIV-prevention issues, he didn't push any particular agenda for discussion. As the men began to build relationships with each other and to establish a basis for trust, they began to talk about a range of issues including coming out, family and community acceptance, dating, sex, healthy relationships, drug use, and HIV and other STIs (sexually transmitted infections). Over the course of a year, participants reported increased comfort with their sexual orientation, a deeper sense of belonging to a community, and increased commitment to and confidence in their ability to negotiate safer sex.

20.3 THE UNIQUE BENEFITS OF GROUP WORK

?

Reflect on your experiences participating in different types of groups.
What was it about the group that was helpful to you?

Participating in group work is different in many ways from the services that individuals receive. Dr. Irvin Yalom identified several factors that make group work unique, based on his years of work as a mental health clinician. He identified twelve therapeutic factors that people who participated in groups reported as being particularly helpful to them (Yalom, 1995.) While Dr. Yalom comes from a clinical perspective, the factors that he identified hold true for the types of groups facilitated by CHWs. These twelve factors are as follows:

1. INSTILLATION OF (OR BUILDING) HOPE

Hope is a strong motivator and is one primary reason people give for beginning a process of change.

2. UNIVERSALITY (OR BUILDING A DEEP CONNECTION WITH OTHERS)

Universality refers to the human experience of finding that one is not alone. While each person's problems may be unique, connecting with others who have experienced similar events, circumstances, and emotions can be a powerful experience, particularly for people who have survived traumatic experiences or whose identity or behaviors are stigmatized by the larger society. Finding commonality with others assists to quiet self-doubts that may arise when one feels isolated and alone with a difficult experience. For example, the rape crisis movement created safe spaces for survivors of rape to meet together and provide each other with meaningful support, breaking silences and isolation.

3. ALTRUISM (OR TRUE GENEROSITY TO OTHERS)

Altruism refers to acts of unselfish giving to others. Research has shown that in interpersonal relationships where individuals find a high degree of satisfaction, they sometimes act for the benefit of the other without expectation of return. In social or support groups, participants develop a connection that fosters generosity and unselfish giving to other members. The experience of providing meaningful support to others in need can also boost the self-esteem of those who offer support.

4. CORRECTIVE RECAPITULATION OF THE PRIMARY FAMILY GROUP (OR HEALING FROM BAD FAMILY EXPERIENCES, AND LEARNING NEW WAYS OF BUILDING HEALTHY RELATIONSHIPS)

Essentially, this means that group participants may have the opportunity to replay the tape of earlier experiences with family and to learn emotional responses that are more productive and supportive of good health. For example, if one was the victim of trauma in childhood, one can now develop the skills to put a stop to abuse in adulthood.

5. DEVELOPMENT OF SOCIALIZING SKILLS

Group participation provides a rich opportunity to improve interpersonal skills such as listening more deeply to the experience of others, expressing feelings, handling conflict, negotiating safe and meaningful relationships, or promoting health and wellness. Participants receive feedback and support from their peers in practicing behaviors that reinforce their health and that of their families and communities.

6. IMITATIVE BEHAVIOR (OR THE INFLUENCE OF ROLE MODELS)

In groups, people observe others making choices that they might like to incorporate into their own lives. By observing the behavior of others, participants learn different ways of communicating and living. This is the same process by which younger children learn from observing their older brothers and sisters. For example, participants might learn from one another new ways to manage anger, reduce stress, or cook traditional foods that are lower in calories.

7. INTERPERSONAL LEARNING (OR LEARNING FROM INTERACTIONS WITH OTHERS)

Interpersonal learning means that we learn more about how our own behavior affects and is perceived by others, as well as how to create meaningful connections and offer support. The advantage of the group experience, in this regard, is that participants don't have to guess at the impact of their actions. Under skilled leadership, the group can explicitly assist the members to understand themselves in an interpersonal context and can develop and enhance the skills essential to creating and maintaining healthy relationships with others. For example, participants might learn new ways to respond to differences of opinion, to receive feedback from others, and to take responsibility for actions that are harmful or hurtful to others.

8. GROUP COHESIVENESS (OR CREATING COMMUNITY AND EXPERIENCING A SENSE OF BELONGING)

This may be the most powerful factor of all. Group cohesiveness refers to the feeling of belonging to a group of people you admire and want to be a part of. When the group is working well, participants may experience a sense of deep connection and commitment.

9. CATHARSIS (OR THE EXPRESSION OF STRONG EMOTION)

Catharsis is the experience of having expressed strong and often difficult emotions in a way that feels healthy, productive, and healing. Catharsis requires a safe environment that supports not only the expression of experiences and emotion, but also the opportunity to reflect on the meaning of these emotions. For example, survivors of sexual assault may express emotions that are difficult for them to share anywhere else. Through expressing these emotions, survivors may begin to better understand how assault has affected their lives and their individual paths to recovery.

10. IMPARTING INFORMATION (OR SHARING INFORMATION WITH OTHERS)

Group participants share information with each other, including information about what they do to promote their own health and well-being. Because group members share a common connection and experience, the information they share with each other is often highly relevant. Hearing information from someone you know and respect is generally much more powerful than reading about it in a book or brochure. For example, people living with HIV disease might share information about how they navigate the health care system to get the care they need or what they do to manage stress or depression.

11. EXISTENTIAL FACTORS (OR LIFE CHOICES AND MEANING)

It has been said that group work recapitulates (or repeats) key aspects of life. The behavior of members in the group, including positive experiences of handling conflict and building connections with others, can motivate participants to make similar choices elsewhere in their lives.

12. SELF-UNDERSTANDING

In many cases, people who participate in groups gain new insights and knowledge about themselves, the way they interact with others, and the feelings and thoughts that may unconsciously influence their behavior. This is often associated with increased acceptance of themselves and enhanced self-esteem.

These twelve factors have been identified as key opportunities and benefits from participating in groups.

? *Have you ever experienced or benefited from participating in a group in any of the twelve ways described above?*

? *Can you think of other factors that contribute to the power and benefit of group participation?*

20.4 GROUP FUNCTIONS AND PROCESS

The group itself—through the power of its cohesion or togetherness—influences people to try new ways of thinking, feeling, and behaving. While every experience is unique, groups often go through common processes. By understanding these common processes, you can be prepared for the sorts of things that might come up in the group you are facilitating. The following section is adapted from the American Group Psychotherapy Association (American Group Psychotherapy Association, 2007).

THE GROUP AS A SOCIAL SYSTEM

It is helpful to think of a group as its own culture, with its own rules, roles, boundaries, and values.

Rules   Members establish group rules with the assistance of facilitators. Rules cover expectations about everything from being on time, when and how much to talk, respecting different experiences and opinions, to practicing nonviolence in all interpersonal interactions. They are similar to the ground rules that govern our participation in classes or trainings and at work.

Roles   Group members will likely find a role to perform within the larger circle of group treatment. The facilitator's role is clear: to assist the group to achieve and maintain cohesion. Finding one's role is frequently the task of early group membership. People report greater calm and less anxiety once they establish what they can expect of others. Facilitators can aid in acknowledging and appreciating the role that each participant plays in the life of the group.

Boundaries   Boundaries are enforced by rules, and they assist in making a group physically and emotionally safe to explore new challenges and new choices. Boundaries overlap with the ground rules discussed above. They include maintaining the confidentiality of participants, and professional relationships between participants and facilitators. The boundaries that will guide group work must be developed at the beginning of a new group in order for members to feel comfortable participating.

Values   Groups universally come to value openness, honesty, and respect in interpersonal communication. They also value interpersonal safety, including confidentiality, and creating opportunities for participants to learn, grow, and change. Groups may wish to articulate shared values and to revisit them during times of conflict.

BENEFICIAL AND HARMFUL GROUP PROCESSES

Group processes may be beneficial or harmful (or neither).

Beneficial Processes   Beneficial processes include the following:

Conflict management and resolution: For some participants, the group may offer an opportunity to experience a healthy resolution of conflicts. With skilled leadership and facilitation, group members can experience conflict as a natural and inevitable part of life. They learn strategies for managing conflict that lead to greater understanding of themselves and others.

Contagion: Contagion refers to the spread of attitudes or behaviors from one member to the group. It can be either harmful or beneficial. It may be harmful to the group process when, for example, it undermines the willingness to address difficult issues, or it reinforces discriminatory treatment of group members or other behaviors that may be harmful to participants. At its best, contagion represents the spread of positive attitudes and behaviors to others, such as an attitude and feeling of hope, or a desire to listen and support one another.

Cohesion: As identified above as a key benefit of group participation, cohesion is a sense of belonging to a community. It motivates members to achieve positive growth and change. A cohesive group often feels that: "We are growing and changing in positive directions together, and we are all important members and contributors to this process!"

Harmful Processes   Harmful group processes work to defeat the primary task of the group and include the following:

Subgrouping: When part of the group splits off and forms a subgroup, the cohesion of the group as a whole is threatened. Subgrouping, or splitting, can occur when individual members' differences are not resolved and become a source of division. At its worst, subgrouping results in discrimination against certain members based on real or perceived differences in experience, identity, values, or beliefs. The group may ignore, isolate, insult, or fail to provide support or validation to these members.

Absence: An individual member's lack of ability to be physically and psychologically present due to any number of personal reasons. Carefully screening participants in advance about their ability to be physically, emotionally, and intellectually present can prevent this.

Avoidance: When the group is unable or unwilling to approach important topics, including issues or conflicts that arise among members, the group can become ineffective and lifeless. Avoidance can include an individual member's psychological defenses as well as the group's defenses as a whole.

It is the responsibility of the group facilitator to address and minimize the harmful factors identified above, and to maximize those factors that are beneficial.

20.5 THE ROLE OF GROUP FACILITATORS

For the group to be effective in its work, the facilitator must be adequately prepared for the intellectual, emotional, and behavioral challenges that group members will bring and create. A comprehensive study of leadership functions identified four key functions of group facilitators (Lieberman, Yalom, and Miles, 1973). They are as follows:

EXECUTIVE FUNCTION

Executive functions are those that manage the rules and boundaries of the group, assisting to create and preserve safety and to prevent and resolve discriminatory treatment. They include resolution of conflicts, time and space management, as well as other administrative tasks that keep the group on task. The facilitator monitors each member's participation and acts to create opportunities for those who have been silent to be able to speak, and for those who have spoken a lot to listen more.

CARING

Caring refers to the group facilitator's ability to convey to each group member individually, and to the group as a whole, that their well-being matters. This is done in many ways, including listening attentively to the contributions of each group participant, respecting the experience and perspective of each participant, asking members if they would like to speak, and acknowledging the positive contributions of each member.

SUPPORT FOR THE EXPRESSION OF EMOTION

The group facilitator sets the tone for the group and supports and affirms the expression of feelings, personal value statements, and personal attitudes.

MEANING ATTRIBUTION

The group facilitator effectively assists the group as a whole, as well as the individual members, to understand themselves more deeply and thoroughly. The group facilitator does this by inviting individuals and the group to talk about the significance and meaning of their participation and experience. For example, a facilitator might ask questions such as: "There aren't any public places for gay and bisexual Latino men to meet here, and many of you have spoken about being hesitant to come out in your families and churches. How do you think that affects you?" "What do you think it would be like to be able to come out and to be fully accepted by your families and communities?" "What role does this group play in your life?" "Last week, we touched on some powerful topics. Did anything take place during group that had particular meaning for you?" These questions are also designed to provide opportunities to the group to talk about issues that have particular significance and meaning in their lives.

The success of group work is also enhanced by the ability of the facilitator to do the following:

Show Up   The effective group facilitator is personally, emotionally, and intellectually present to assist the group to create and maintain a safe environment for personal exploration. Facilitators need to learn to let go of their own agendas and emotions and to concentrate on the participation of group members.

Pay Attention   The effective group facilitator pays close attention to all the communications of the group as a whole as well as the individual members so that people feel heard and cared for.

Tell the Truth   The effective group facilitator is able to see and comment on both potentially harmful and beneficial group dynamics including, as referenced above, dynamics of subgrouping, avoidance, and conflict. The facilitator keeps the focus on telling the truth about what is taking place during the group.

Let Go of the Outcome   The effective group facilitator trusts that the individual members will do their best to learn from the group. Letting go of the outcome expresses your deep faith in the capacity of group members to be responsible for what they get out of the group.

GUIDING PARTICIPANTS INTO THE LEARNING ZONE

Figure 20.1 is used to represent a central task of the facilitator.

Figure 20.1 Learning Zones.

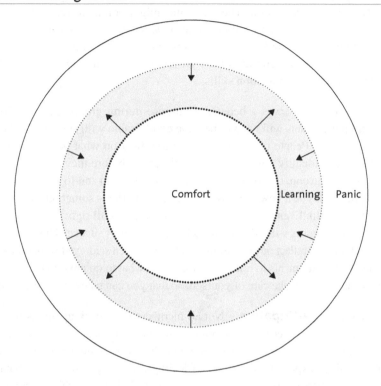

The three concentric circles represent three different "zones" of group work. These are the comfort zone, the learning zone, and the panic zone. Groups often like to stay in the *comfort zone* because it is easy and familiar and does not challenge them to reveal personal information or to otherwise take risks that can inspire learning and change.

In the *learning zone,* participants interact with each other in an honest way, disclosing their own life experiences, feelings, and opinions. They learn from one another and about themselves. The learning zone implies taking risks by opening up and participating in ways that may not always be familiar or comfortable.

A group is in the *panic zone* when interactions are characterized by persistent conflict, and when one or more members become so emotional (fearful, humiliated, or angry, for example) that the group can no longer interact in a safe and productive way, diminishing trust.

A successful facilitator will try to guide the group away from both the comfort and the panic zones, and to stay close to the learning zone in which interactions are dynamic, imply risk, and result in meaningful learning and motivation for positive action.

FACILITATION TECHNIQUES

The following techniques are used to fulfill the basic role and functions of group facilitators:

Naming   "Naming" means to acknowledge a dynamic that is happening in the group such as prolonged silence, tension, anxiety, fear, or conflict. These dynamics may be neutral (silence), positive (enthusiasm, support for a group member, a deep common connection, humor, silence), or negative (such as discrimination against certain group members). The idea is to name or to ask the group to name what is happening in order to interrupt potentially harmful behavior, and to provoke reflection and learning about the nature of the group dynamic or interaction. The facilitator might comment on what is happening ("So, it seems like people aren't talking right now. What is coming up for you?"). The facilitator could ask the group to name what is happening ("What is going on in the group right now?"). This is an opportunity for the group to analyze their interactions, increasing their knowledge and communication skills.

Silence   Silence often serves a beneficial purpose during group sessions. Sometimes, facilitators and participants will need to become comfortable with silence, instead of rushing to say something. People often require time to reflect on what has been said or what has occurred, and to identify their feelings and thoughts, before they speak. When silence arises naturally in a group, try to sit back and just let it be for ten to twenty seconds. See what will happen. Maybe a new idea will come up, or perhaps somebody who hasn't participated will speak up. Even if nothing new happens, that is all right.

Sometimes facilitators will ask the group for a moment of silence. This can be useful to give people a chance to reflect on something that has just been said. And sometimes, the facilitator may need a few moments to reflect and figure out what to do next. Asking for silence in these moments is a way to take care of yourself, so that you can take care of the group.

Guiding Inclusive Participation   Not all members will speak up and actively participate in group discussions. Yet it is important for the group to hear all voices and to benefit from the input of all members. A key role of the facilitator is to support all members in talking and sharing their experiences, ideas, and feelings, and to guard against dynamics that are dominated by a minority of speakers (see Common Challenges, which follows).

Mapping the Conversation   A technique that can be helpful for understanding group interactions is to map the conversation. Start by drawing a representation of the group, as in Figure 20.2, that shows where each group participant sits. During the group conversation, draw in:

- ✪ Solid directional arrows to indicate when one member speaks directly to another
- ✪ Dotted lines to indicate a statement made to the entire group

It is easiest to do this when there are two facilitators, and one can focus on mapping the conversation. After the group session ends, analyze the map you have created to identity patterns of communication. Who is speaking most often? Who is not speaking as much or at all? How often are comments being made to the entire group? Your analysis can assist you to redirect the flow of conversation to increase the participation of all members and prevent just a few members from dominating the discussion.

?   *What does the map provided above tell you about participation in the group?*

Triangulation   Triangulation is the act of preventing group interactions from being dominated by prolonged conversation between one group member and the facilitator. Your role as group leader is to facilitate interaction and dialogue among *all* group members. (See Figure 20.3.) Imagine, for example, that you ask an open-ended question to the group, and Peter answers. Instead of responding to Peter, you might ask the group as a whole, or another member, what they think about what Peter just said. Triangulation fosters inclusive participation and supports all members to benefit equally from the unique power of group dynamics.

Figure 20.2 Mapping the Conversation.

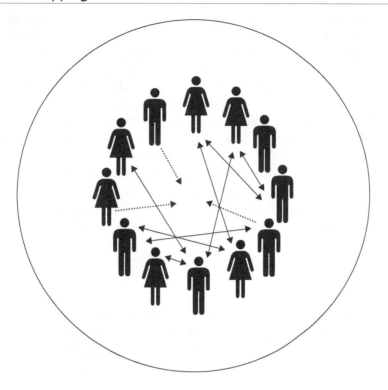

Figure 20.3 Triangulation.

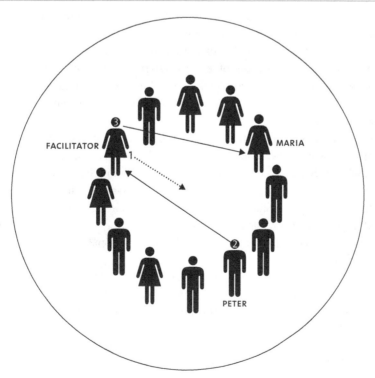

PREVENTING DISCRIMINATORY TREATMENT

In societies characterized by bias, prejudice, and discrimination, group members are likely to act these out. Intentionally or unintentionally, participants may sometimes act in ways that exclude, confront, shame, or punish people who are perceived as belonging to groups that historically face discriminatory treatment such as women, gay or lesbian people, and communities of color. For members who are the targets of this behavior, the group experience may repeat the very traumatic experiences that negatively impact their health. For this reason, groups often define membership criteria in ways that are designed to create a safer environment for members from a common community, such as Latino men who have sex with men or Native American women.

Nothing can damage the life, value, reputation, and success of a group as powerfully as uninterrupted prejudice or discriminatory treatment of certain participants. As a facilitator, one of the most important roles is to carefully monitor the group and to quickly intervene to restore respect, equity, and safety if you observe discriminatory treatment.

COFACILITATION OF GROUPS

Sometimes CHWs will facilitate groups on their own and sometimes with a cofacilitator. While each model poses slightly different challenges, in both circumstances you are responsible for ensuring the physical and emotional safety of participants and successful group interactions that provide members with information and support designed to promote their health.

We encourage CHWs who are facilitating groups for the first time to seek out opportunities to cofacilitate with an experienced colleague. Through working together, you will be able to observe, practice, and learn essential skills and techniques.

When working with a cofacilitator, you will want to meet in advance to plan how you will work together to create and sustain a positive group process. Take this opportunity to clarify your goals for the group, how you will establish membership criteria and ground rules, and your approach to ensuring group safety and responding to conflicts. The more that you and your cofacilitator are on the same page, the more effective the group process will be. The success of groups suffers significantly when cofacilitators are unable to work together in a collegial, respectful, and coordinated fashion. During your planning, talk about how you wish to handle differences of opinion that may arise between the two of you.

Be sure to check in with each other between each group sessions, to debrief what occurred in the last session, and to make plans for the next. This is the time to raise concerns about individual members, the group process, and cofacilitation. It is also an opportunity for you to talk about any personal issues or challenges that have come up as a consequence of facilitating the group. For example, you might have a strong reaction to a particular event that occurred in group that is related to your own life experience. Talking about this openly and honestly with your cofacilitator can ensure that your personal issues don't unduly influence the group process.

If you are unable to productively work through challenges or disagreements between you and your cofacilitator, make an appointment as soon as possible to talk with a supervisor and ask for guidance and support for moving forward in a productive fashion. This is your ethical obligation to the group. You must always put their interests and welfare above your own and address your own challenges, no matter how difficult, in order to keep your ethical commitment to the group and its members.

THE POWER AND AUTHORITY OF FACILITATORS

Regardless of the level of formality and structure of the group, CHWs should always be guided by client and community-centered practice designed to enhance the leadership of group members. Facilitators also need to acknowledge the power of their authority as group leaders. Group participants will give power to the facilitator even if the facilitator doesn't want it. For example, participants will often wait for the facilitator to set the agenda, to respond to a comment, to offer support to a member, or to intervene in the early stages of a potential conflict. A skilled facilitator works in ways that encourage participants to demonstrate their own leadership in these moments. Because group members may defer to the authority of the group facilitator, it is particularly important that facilitators don't bring their own issues, concerns, and experiences into the group or otherwise make the group about themselves.

COMMUNITY AND PARTICIPANT EMPOWERMENT

Perhaps the most important measure of the success of a group is the extent to which it fosters the participation and empowerment of its members. While group facilitators must be strong leaders in order to ensure nondiscrimination and safety for all members, the transformative power of the group process to promote life changes must come from the participants themselves. As a facilitator, you will support group members, to the extent possible, to establish ground rules, to identify common values and goals, to develop skills in providing meaningful support to each other, and in honoring differences and resolving conflict. When this occurs, participants emerge from the group process more competent and capable of employing these same skills in other relationships and areas of their lives. A truly healthy and effective group may not require much participation, intervention, or direction for the group facilitator: members learn how to keep the group process on track and to support each member in gaining the confidence to make significant life changes.

Strong group facilitation skills are often embodied by a quiet but firm leadership style that becomes more prominent when events occur that could be harmful to members, and stays in the background when participants are engaged in dynamic and supportive discussion. As always, be aware of your tendencies to dominate the life of the group and to unconsciously undermine the autonomy and leadership of participants.

HOW PERSONAL ISSUES MAY DIMINISH EFFECTIVE GROUP FACILITATION

Our own experiences, feelings, opinions, culture, and values sometimes get in the way of providing culturally sensitive and client-centered services (you may hear this phenomenon referred to as "counter-transference" by those who work in mental health settings). The most effective group facilitators are those who recognize that their own issues may be triggered (become active) and are prepared to take action to minimize the potential damage to the group.

Because group work is dynamic and requires the development of relationships between group members, issues related to our own relationships are likely to be triggered. These may include unresolved issues in our family of origin, current relationships and family, or our prior experience participating in different types of groups. For example, if your role in your family of origin was to be silent when conflicts developed, you may feel uncomfortable about speaking up or addressing conflicts, even if that is part of your role as group facilitator.

Signs that the facilitator's own issues may be getting in the way of the work include:

- ✪ Finding it difficult to listen to what others are saying
- ✪ Strong emotional reactions to what occurs in group
- ✪ A tendency to avoid particular topics, dynamics, or group members
- ✪ Making assumptions about the experience, values, emotions, or ideas of others
- ✪ Negative reactions, thoughts, or feelings about certain group members
- ✪ Paying less attention to some group members than others
- ✪ Strong opinions or judgments about the behaviors or beliefs of clients
- ✪ A strong desire to share personal information

? *Can you think of other signs that a CHW's own issues might be getting in the way of their ability to work effectively with clients?*

? *Can you identify personal issues (we all have them!) that might get in the way of your work?*

A good group facilitator is *not* one who has it all together and who has worked through and resolved all personal issues that could possibly interfere with their ability to provide effective services: this isn't an attainable goal. The key is to recognize what personal issues may be triggered, to do what you can ahead of time to address these issues, and to seek out consultation when your issues are triggered.

All CHWs, regardless of whether or not they facilitate groups, have an ethical duty to develop self-awareness and to identify personal issues that could get in the way of their work. This challenge is also addressed in Chapters One, Seven, and Eight.

To reflect on whether or not personal issues may be getting in the way of your work, think about what you say and do during group work. When you speak, are you doing so for the benefit of the group, or to fulfill a personal need? If you find that you have a thought that you are compelled to share, it may be about yourself rather than the group or individual group members. If you find that the motivations are more personal than professional (the feeling that I *must* share my point of view), try not to speak until you have a chance to reflect on and to understand what is influencing you. Chances are it is you, not them, who wants to hear your story.

As always, we strongly encourage you to reflect on and talk about these personal issues with others. This may be a colleague, your cofacilitator, a counselor, or a trusted friend. The most important thing is not to avoid these insights, but to investigate and strive to understand them. Remember that you need to do this not only for yourself, but also out of concern for the welfare of group members and other clients. If you are facilitating a group, you should receive regular supervision. Some of the many things to explore during your supervision are personal issues that are being triggered by group work and how you are handling them.

? *What resources do you have to reflect on personal issues that may get in the way of your work with groups and other clients?*

? *Who can you talk to about these issues?*

GUIDELINES FOR SELF-DISCLOSURE

Self-disclosure means that a CHW or other helping professional shares personal information about themselves with clients. As a rule, we encourage facilitators not to disclose personal information about themselves to the group. Self-disclosure can sometimes change the dynamic of the group to focus on the experiences, needs, and ideas of the facilitator rather than of those in the group. This risk is particularly significant because of the unique power and authority of group facilitators. If you consider disclosing personal information to the group, we suggest the following guidelines:

1. Have a clear purpose for self-disclosure that is clearly in the best interest of the group. If you are motivated to disclose information for a personal reason, don't!
2. Be brief. You may reveal a fact about yourself. You don't need to get into all the details and should not take up time and space discussing the issues.
3. Be specific. For example, the facilitator of a group for people living with HIV disease may disclose that they are also living with HIV disease (we are not making a value judgment about the wisdom of disclosing such information). But they should not go on to explain how they were infected, how many T cells they have, or what kinds of medications they take. This is likely to unduly influence the focus, direction, or safety of the group.

We strongly encourage you to talk with coworkers and your supervisor about the issue of self-disclosure before you consider doing it. Ask them to share their beliefs and practices in relation to self-disclosure.

? *What are your personal beliefs and guidelines about self-disclosure?*

? *Would you ever disclose personal information to a client?*

? *If so, what information might you share, when, and why?*

20.6 THE STAGES OF GROUP WORK

Various authors have described a predictable sequence of stages that represent the development of emotional and physical safety necessary for a well-run, high-functioning group. Knowing about these common stages may assist you to identify how your own group is progressing and to manage challenges that arise. Bruce Tuckman's memorable names for these stages are Forming, Storming, Norming, Performing, and Adjourning (Tuckman, 1965). Marianne Schneider Corey and Gerald Corey (2006) describe the stages as the following:

THE INITIAL STAGE (FORMING)

At the beginning of a new group, members may be somewhat hesitant to participate and may have concerns about whether the group facilitators are competent, whether the group offers a format that will be useful to them, if they will be accepted and come to belong, and more. Participants may be on their best behavior and be cautious about sharing their life experiences, challenges, and doubts. In the beginning stages, people are searching for structure and safety that will support them in taking risks and sharing more intimate and difficult information.

Bruce Tuckman called this the *Forming Stage.* The group forms around its tasks and boundaries. Participants decide what they want to accomplish, how to define membership, and what the ground rules are that will allow them to function well together. There is a high sense of individuality at this stage.

The membership functions in the initial stage are to begin to participate by sharing relatively safe personal information, telling stories about life experiences, cooperating to set rules for the group for attendance and confidentiality, and establishing expectations of each other and the facilitator(s).

The early stages of a group are about building connection and trust.

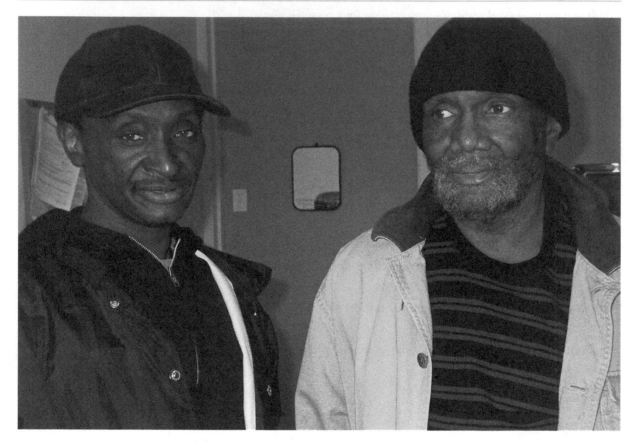

FACILITATING A SUPPORT GROUP FOR MIDDLE-SCHOOL YOUTHS

When I was starting my career in public health, I facilitated a support group for seventh and eighth graders at a middle school. The school counselor referred students to the group whom she considered to be "at risk" (this included students struggling with academic, family, and personal issues). The group met for eight weeks in a confidential space and provided participants with a hot lunch. I was initially surprised that youths would be willing to participate in such a group, and was inspired by their ability to cocreate a supportive group experience that addressed real issues associated with adolescence.

The Work of Facilitators in the Initial Stage In the first stages, the facilitator's task is to establish physical and emotional safety by assisting the group to identify common goals, expectations, and ground rules that will guide their participation. Overall, your goal in the initial stage of group work is to assist the group in creating an atmosphere of safety.

You will assist the group to anticipate differences in terms of their experiences, opinions, beliefs, and values. This is important to do at the beginning of new groups, as is framing conflict as a natural, inevitable, and often productive aspect of life and group work. You can also assist the group to establish agreements about the way they will handle disagreements and conflicts, and you should emphasize that a key part of the group's role is to ensure that conflicts don't spiral out of control in way that is harmful to individual members and the group itself. To read more about conflict resolution concepts and skills, please refer to Chapter Thirteen.

As facilitator you direct the flow of communication, encouraging but not pushing all members to participate and ensuring that no individual group member dominates the discussion or pushes an agenda that does not resonate and is not supported by the group as a whole.

A strategy for assisting the group to establish safety is to assist members to recognize the similarities they share with others. In the beginning, encourage each group member to speak, and assist them to identify experiences, ideas, feelings, and values that they share in common. It is important that each person identify at least one other person in the group who appears to share some point of view, experience, or value system.

Any similarity between members, however superficial, opens the door for personal sharing. This is one reason why the membership of groups is often structured around common identities and experiences. For example, groups might be established for Cambodian women living with breast cancer, Latino parents with a child who is developmentally disabled, or men diagnosed with high blood pressure. Active participation in the group is one predictor of a positive outcome, so getting people to join with others right from the beginning is important. You can do this by asking everyone to share their name and something about themselves. Ask everyone to share one expectation that they have about participating in the group.

Be sure to reinforce any behavior that is for the good of the group. If someone arrives breathless and says, "I worked really hard to be here on time!" respond with positive affirmation about the effort and reinforce how important it is to use the full time allotted for the group. Be generous and explicit with your praise. When a participant first takes a risk to share something personal, thank them for this contribution. When one participant offers support to another, point out that this is the kind of support that is important to provide in the group.

During the first session, I asked each student to introduce themselves and to share one hope that they had for the group. At the very least, everyone introduced themselves to each other (this was a large middle school, and not everyone knew each other's name). Occasionally, someone expressed a hope ("I really hope this group can be different and everyone can really try to respect where everyone is coming from.") that resonated powerfully with other members and sparked an initial discussion.

From there, we set up expectations and ground rules designed to make the group a safe and productive place to be. As facilitator, I introduced certain ground rules, such as privacy (confidentiality), and asked participants to talk about why it is important to them. Confidentiality was a big concern for the youths, as many had experienced

(Continued)

hurtful rumors, or had a friend or family member break a promise to keep something private. The group would then identify other ground rules to guide participation, such as the importance of accepting different experiences and points of view, and of respecting the participation of all members, including not using put-downs (making negative comments about other group members). Not only did this result in a set of ground rules and expectations to guide the group process, it also provided members with a first experience of working together with a common purpose.

Together the youths brainstormed and prioritized a list of topics to be addressed during group. Students never had difficulty identifying issues for conversation, and worked well together to prioritize the lists. When it was difficult for the group to decide which topics to select, the participants voted to select the issues they most wanted to talk about: the topics with most votes formed the agenda for the next six weeks. The agenda selected by the participants generally included topics

THE TRANSITION STAGE (STORMING AND NORMING)

In the transition stage, members begin to talk more directly about the issues that motivated them to participate in the group. People work to establish trust by telling the truth or talking honestly about their lives.

Some participants may resist hearing the truths of others, or acknowledging certain aspects of their own experience and behavior, particularly those that may imply making changes. This is a rich and productive stage in the life of the group when issues and challenges are identified.

Tuckman called this the *Storming Phase,* when conflicts may emerge and people with apparently different agendas seem to struggle for attention. The necessary group task is to develop tolerance and patience for the process of becoming a group with a common purpose.

The membership functions in the transition stage are to learn to manage themselves and each other in ways that move toward the positive and affirm participation. In many cases this means that group members will begin to identify and name their fears out loud, including fears of revealing certain aspects of their life experience and identity, of being rejected or accepted by the group, of intimacy or getting to close to others in the group. The other main task in this stage is to learn how to listen; to accept, validate, and support other participants; and most important, to accept and respect people with different experiences, identities, and points of view.

FACILITATING A SUPPORT GROUP FOR MIDDLE-SCHOOL YOUTHS (*Continued*)

Middle school (seventh, eighth, or ninth grade) is often a difficult time for students. Not only are the students going through adolescence, but the school environment is often characterized by popular and unpopular groups, bullying, teasing, and discrimination. It is only natural that participants bring some of these dynamics to group. A key part of my job was to watch for and to quickly respond to early expressions of conflict. For example, one group member might roll their eyes as another was talking, such as depression and suicide, family conflict, divorce, dating and sexual involvement, immigration and discrimination (a significant percentage of students in the school and in the support group were immigrants), alcohol and drug use, peer pressure, and gang involvement.

During the first session, I made a point of encouraging each member to participate. For example, I might turn to a member and say: "Julio, is there anything you would like to add to the ground rules?" I also tried to model ways of affirming their participation by making a comment such as: "Thanks, Julio, I agree that it is really important that just one person talk at a time if we are going to be able to work well as a group." Or "You did a really great job working together to come up with this list of expectations for the group." How you express support and affirmations must be authentic and true to who you are.

—Tim Berthold

The leadership functions of this stage are to assist the group resolve their ambivalence toward becoming a group. The ambivalence of this stage may be marked by behavior that is confusing to a beginning group facilitator. But, to the experienced group facilitator, the necessary emergence of the ambivalence—"I want to change and I don't want to change"—signals that people are becoming emotionally more involved in the group, and a group identity is beginning to emerge.

The Work of Facilitators in the Transition Phase   The group facilitator's job at this stage is to assist the participants see that conflicts and differences can be resolved. As a facilitator, you will need to become comfortable witnessing and responding to anger and conflict. You will need to develop skills in assisting members to reflect on their experiences and their participation in the group and to demonstrate empathy for each other's point of view.

Tuckman called this the *Norming Phase,* where individuals settle down, become a group, and create new norms for emotional and social interaction. Members are committed to the group and find that they can trust each other even if they disagree.

A key role for the group facilitator is to assist each member to be viewed as valuable to the group. You do this by using your active listening skills to support participants in identifying, validating, and striving to understand different points of view. The end of this stage is marked by group members having a solid sense of safety within the group—a sense of belonging by choice and by inclusion.

turn to whisper to another participant, or make a disrespectful comment, such as: "That's nothing new coming from you," or "Yeah, but you're always depressed anyway: look at how you dress!" While the form of put-down would always vary, I made sure to respond right away. I also kept in mind that, while I was watching for conflict to emerge, group members were watching me to see if and how I would respond, and if I would keep my promise to enforce the group's ground rules.

In general, I would first direct my comments to the entire group, reminding them about our common purpose and ground rules, and emphasizing that all group

(Continued)

members deserve and require their respect. This was often enough to stop the negative behavior.

If, however, an individual or individuals continued to tease or otherwise disrespect other members of the group, I would gently confront them by saying something like: "K., I want you to be a part of the group, and I really need for you follow the ground rules." I would also make time to address my concerns to K. privately, after group, explicitly describing the behavior that I had observed and why I found it harmful. I would always try to do this in the most respectful and supportive way, encouraging the participant to rejoin the group and to make positive contributions. Occasionally, I would ask the student to provide the target of their behavior with an apology and let them decide when and how to do so.

If I judged the behavior to be more harmful, I would have immediately interrupted the group and removed the participant who had put down another member. Depending on the nature of what they did, they might not be invited to return. Acting in a prompt and effective method to remove a serious threat to the welfare of the group is important to preserving its integrity and your leadership (I facilitated five or six groups at the middle school, and never reached a point where a member had to be asked to leave).

Perhaps most important, I want to ensure that when a group member shares something that seems highly personal, emotional, or difficult, they are met with

THE WORK STAGE (PERFORMING)

The most in-depth work takes place at this stage. The individual members and the group as a whole commit themselves to the deeper work of understanding the issues that trouble or challenge them, and identifying what they can do to address these problems. For example, this is the stage when the Latino men's group talked about the people they had lost to the HIV epidemic; about not being accepted by their families; about their desire for community, healthy relationships, and love; and what they can do to create healthier and more satisfying lives.

Tuckman called this the *Performing Phase,* when the group is functioning best, offering members opportunities for self-expression and personal growth within the functioning of the group as a whole.

In some groups, this is the stage in which members examine behaviors that are harmful to their own health or that of others. They move beyond health information to consider making changes in behavior. The deep work comes with understanding the full impact of thoughts, feelings, and behaviors in one's own life as well as on others. It is through sharing these experiences and insights in the group and creating connections with other members that participants gain the motivation and commitment to changing and growing in other relationships and areas of their lives. Group members provide support to each other in making changes, and report on their progress in future sessions.

THE WORK OF GROUP FACILITATOR IN THE WORK PHASE

The facilitator's function at this stage is to assist members to access and express their emotions and thoughts in the here and now, and to reflect on the meaning of their experiences. As always, the group facilitator works to maintain the emotional cohesion of the group respect and support. Ideally, there are several participants in the group who do this naturally and well. As group facilitator, I also tried to model this. For example, during a discussion about depression, a student said that his older brother had killed himself three years before. While he was clearly emotional, he also continued to talk about what had happened. We listened and, when he stopped, I acknowledged what a significant loss the death of a family member is, and asked him if he wanted to talk about how the death of his brother had affected him. Generally, other group members will follow this lead and rise to the occasion, offering condolences and listening to whatever else the participant cares to say. If something occurred that might be harmful in the moment, I would intervene and say something like: "H. just shared something really important with us. That isn't easy to do. The purpose of this group is to be able to talk about the real things that happen in our lives, to listen to each other, and to provide support." If I were concerned about the individual participant who took a risk to share something personal, I would check in with them as soon as the group ended, in a private space.

In general, the young people were naturally good at providing support to each other in these moments. I would make sure to acknowledge and reinforce this. For example, I might say something like: "I was impressed today with how supportive you were when S. was talking about his brother. That is what this group is all about."

—Tim Berthold

Effective groups support participants in making positive changes in their lives.

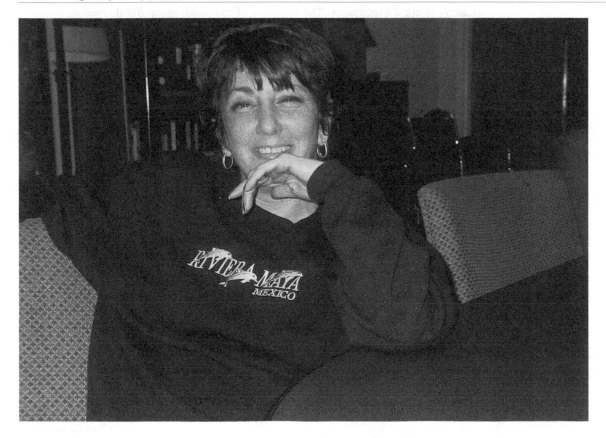

by addressing any behavior that may be harmful and is not adequately addressed by the members themselves. Facilitators also ask the group to focus on actions that they can take, including changes in behavior that will promote their health and well-being and that of others.

Essentially you will work to assist the group members to understand and respond to each other in supportive and positive ways. You continue to solve problems created by misunderstandings, and you continue to assist group members to see each other's points of view. You steer the conversation toward topics that are beneficial for the participants' growth and away from conversations that reinforce unhelpful behavior. The effective group facilitator continues to assist individual group members understand how their behavior in group affects other people. The facilitator assists individuals in understanding how they can try out new knowledge and skills with people they trust—the other group members.

In this stage of the group process, the facilitator does not need to speak or step into discussions unless there is a good reason. Good facilitation includes being able to trust group members to stay on track with their discussions, interactions, and values, and understanding that the leadership of group members is critical to the ultimate success of the process.

FACILITATING A SUPPORT GROUP FOR MIDDLE-SCHOOL YOUTHS (*Continued*)

During this stage, I monitored participation and tried to provide opportunities for all members to talk. For example, I might turn to a member who has mostly been silent and say: "E., I'm wondering if you have anything to say about this topic."

An important part of my role as facilitator was to guide members to reflect on the meaning of their experiences. The members of the youth group did this naturally, as talking about what matters is a common part of adolescence. For example, when the youth group was talking about the issue of depression, which was a common experience, I might ask something like: "So how does being depressed influence your life?" (or "How does depression affect your life at home or your performance at school?" or "Does being depressed change the way you think or feel about yourself?"). If we had done our work well up to this point, the group would have created an environment in which the participants wanted to share their experiences, feelings, and ideas.

By this stage, group members were generally skilled at supporting each other in identifying possible actions to improve their lives. Occasionally, as a facilitator, I might ask something like: "What do you think would be helpful for you to do about this situation?" In addition, I watched for members who, out of an effort to be supportive, might try to give advice or otherwise tell another participant what to do. In such a circumstance, I might say something like: "That sounds like a great suggestion, but we need to keep in mind that everyone is unique. Is this something that you might be interested in?"

While in some ways working with youths can be more challenging than working with adults, in other ways the very nature of adolescence supported the middle-school students in talking about real issues in a real way. A guiding principle for every group I facilitated was some version of "keeping it real." This meant that group members could drop the false front they sometimes showed to parents, teachers, and each other, and talk about common challenges, like depression, in a very direct way. They were also able to identify realistic steps that might encourage them to make positive changes rather than suggestions that were out of reach for most people.

— Tim Berthold

Be aware of your tendencies to impose your own agenda on the group. If you are working with a cofacilitator, discuss these issues to ensure, to the best of your ability, that the work of the group is guided by the interests, experiences, emotions, and values of the members rather than the facilitators. Any actions that members decide to take to promote their health must be their own, in order to maximize the chance that they will follow through in making those changes.

THE FINAL STAGE (ADJOURNING)

The final stage of group work consolidates what people have done and allows them to say "good-bye" in a healthy fashion. Tuckman calls this the *Adjourning Phase.* Participants confront the realization that the group—like other aspects of life—may end before they are ready. Simultaneously, members report that they incorporate what they have learned in group into their lives.

Membership issues at this stage include expressing feelings about any chances passed up or missed in the group and other losses, as well as risks taken in group and positive changes made. Ambivalence returns as people are both ready and not ready for the experience to end. For those who have had a satisfying experience, saying good-bye provides yet another opportunity to be in the here and now with emotions, thoughts, and new behaviors. For those who wish for more, the experience of closure provides a way to acknowledge the limitations of self, others, and relationships. Most people experience a little of each.

The Work of Facilitators in the Final Stage   Leadership functions at the final stage are, as before, to guide members to experience and express their thoughts and feelings as they

FACILITATING A SUPPORT GROUP FOR MIDDLE-SCHOOL YOUTHS (*Continued*)

Each time I facilitated the support group at the middle school, I was struck by how difficult it was for participants to say good-bye.

One activity that I have used to end a class or group takes just a few minutes. It requires an eight- to ten-foot length of colored ribbon, one for each participant. The group stands in a circle, and one participant begins the activity by sharing something that they appreciate about the contributions that another participant made to the group and hands them the other end of their colored ribbon. This member in turn selects another, acknowledges something positive about their participation in the group, and hands them the other end of a second piece of colored ribbon. At the end of this brief activity, all group members have been acknowledged and appreciated by others, and a web of ribbon has been created that visually represents the interconnections among all group members.

With the middle-school students, I also asked each member to share something meaningful that they learned from the group, something they plan to do to promote their own health, and one resource they can realistically turn to when they face life challenges. Typically, students mentioned their parents, best friends, sports teammates, respected teachers, and the school counselors.

It was typical for group members to stay late after the last group, talking further with each other, with the facilitator, and with the school counselor (who was invited, with permission from members, to attend the last session).

— *Tim Berthold*

confront the ending of the group. It is also time to revisit and reinforce the commitments that participants have made to making changes that will enhance their health and wellness.

It is not unusual for people to have a tough time saying good-bye to an experience that has become valuable. A key role is to support members in saying good-bye to the group and affirming the connections they have made, the knowledge and skills they have gained, and the changes they intend to make.

? *What do you do to say good-bye to a group when it ends?*

? *What sorts of activities would you choose to facilitate?*

Rᴀᴍᴏɴᴀ Bᴇɴꜱᴏɴ: I facilitate a couple of different groups for women at the Black Infant Health Program. One way I measure my success is when women who were in a group before come back to speak to a new group. They might share what they went through and what they learned, because they want to give back and help other women. And they might tell me: "I'm in school now. I'm working for my GED or my Associate's Degree." One lady said, "Can I get a referral to a therapist?" And that's success to me because they are still working to change their life, and not ashamed to reach out and ask for help.

20.7 COMMON CHALLENGES OF GROUP FACILITATION

The "client" in group work is both the individual participant and the group itself. The group is the agent of change, and maintaining an environment that *supports group learning* is the responsibility of the facilitator. Some of the common challenges to facilitating a successful group include the following:

THE CULTURE OF INDIVIDUALITY

The United States places great emphasis on the individual, often at the expense of the group or community. The society often celebrates the right of individuals to go their own way, and to oppose the will of the group. These cultural values and messages sometimes make it difficult for people to work collaboratively in a group setting. They may feel restricted by the group process and start to rebel by asserting their unique needs.

Unconscious Issues   Group work is affected by unconscious and unspoken issues that group members bring with them, such as unresolved experiences with their families or other groups. These issues may be acted out in any number of ways including blaming, criticizing, denial, trying to please others, or attempting to control the dynamic and focus of the group.

Unclear Intention of the Group   Group members are often unclear, and sometimes suspicious, about the intentions of the group. What is it trying to accomplish? What are its values? Is it right for me? Will the group accept me? These doubts can undermine safety and participation.

Other Challenges

- Members who do not actively participate
- Members who dominate discussions
- Put-downs, insults, threats, or attacks on any member of the group
- Prejudice, cultural bias, or discriminatory treatment targeting any group member related to their identity or perceived identity
- Development of subgroups or cliques
- Persistent negativity from individuals or the group: Sometimes groups get stuck focusing on what isn't working well in their lives. It is important for members to be able to talk honestly about the challenges they face. But it is also important for them to talk about and to support each other in taking positive actions that will improve the quality of their lives.
- Members bringing private issues between themselves into the group: Sometimes group members have preexisting relationships as friends, family, or coworkers, and sometimes new personal relationships are established by members outside of the group. Sometimes conflicts within these relationships are brought into the group. The group is not the proper place to raise or resolve these issues, and this situation may place other participants in the very awkward or harmful position of being asked to take sides, to provide critical feedback, or to aid in resolving the conflict. None of this is appropriate, and group facilitators must be prepared to set a firm boundary.
- A participant who is under the influence of drugs or alcohol: Ground rules should include not coming to group after drinking alcohol or using drugs. This can change the behavior of a group member and may contribute to many of the other challenges identified here. If you suspect that someone has been using, pull them aside and privately address your concerns. Focus on any conduct that may not be in line with your ground rules. Ask the participant not to return to that group session. If the behavior continues in future sessions, you may need to ask the member to leave the group permanently.
- Breaking confidentiality: This is one of the most powerful ways of harming or destroying safety and trust in a group. Facilitators can prevent this by strongly reinforcing the ground rules that require members to maintain the privacy of all members. If confidentiality is broken, it must be addressed immediately and decisively. In some circumstances, it may result in expelling any member who has broken the confidentiality of any other member.

? *Have you experienced these challenges as either a group participant or facilitator?*

? *Can you think of other common challenges that you might face as a group facilitator?*

- Lack of support for group members in moments of vulnerability: People sometimes participate in group to talk about intimate and challenging issues that they are not comfortable or able to discuss elsewhere. Participants understandably have a strong expectation that if they share personal information in the group (such as HIV status, sexual assault, or sexual orientation), it will be received with respect. If this does not occur, it may also harm the ability of the group to establish or maintain trust and safety and to continue working productively together. Group facilitators should model how to provide respect and support to participants who share intimate information, and intervene to restore respect if it is not provided in these moments.

✪ Other situations of conflict: Please refer to Chapter Thirteen for more information about handling conflict. We encourage you to anticipate conflict as an inevitable part of the group process and to discuss it with the group up front, developing mutual ground rules to guide the way you will respond in the moment of conflict. We encourage you to share some of the information addressed in Chapter Thirteen, including concepts such as shifting from certainty to curiosity, from blame to contribution, and disentangling intentions from impact.

✪ Crisis situations: These may include reports or threats of violence or other physical harm to self or others, including the disclosure of suicidal thoughts or plans. When such situations arise, they immediately become your number one priority. You may have to interrupt the group (or ask a cofacilitator to continue) as you meet with the individual or individuals involved, and you may be required to report this information to legal authorities. When a group member experiences crisis, it also affects the group and should be addressed with all participants. The focus here should be on the impact on the group, and personal information about the member undergoing a crisis must be kept confidential. Whenever a crisis emerges, be sure to report it to your supervisor and to debrief it with your cofacilitator.

✪ Resistance to "keeping it real": Sometimes group members will try to keep conversations on a more superficial level, avoiding the issues that brought them to the group in the first place.

Expect to face some of these challenges, and more, when you facilitate groups. Briefly, we wish to highlight classic mistakes that facilitators sometimes make, and share a few tips designed to enhance the quality and effectiveness of your work with groups.

CLASSIC MISTAKES THAT FACILITATORS MAY MAKE

✪ *Avoidance (or doing nothing):* For a variety of reasons, including a lack of comfort with anger or conflict, facilitators sometimes fail to act when events take place that may be harmful to group members. Members must be able to trust that facilitators will take action swiftly and effectively to stop harmful dynamics such as insults or discriminatory treatment. If facilitators fail to do this, they are modeling avoidance, may send the message that the problematic behavior is acceptable, and may quickly undermine the integrity and effectiveness of the group process. While handling conflict is difficult, it is an ethical obligation. When facilitators don't step in to resolve a conflict that members themselves are unable to prevent, they are putting their own self-interest and needs above those of the group members.

✪ *Dominating the group process:* Facilitators sometimes forget that the group exists for the benefit of the members, not themselves. When facilitators dominate the group process, they undermine opportunities for participants to express themselves and to claim their own leadership potential.

✪ *Failing to demonstrate and model empathy and support:* Participants need to know that facilitators care about them, want to learn about their life experiences, and will support them in taking positive steps to promote their health. Responding with empathy and compassion when members share something personal and difficult about their lives also provides participants with a model for how to do this.

✪ *Imposing personal values or opinions on the group:* It is common for the personal issues of helping professionals to unconsciously influence our work with clients and groups. Unfortunately, when we impose our own values or opinions (about faith, relationships, love, sex, treatment options, behavior change, politics, and so forth), we undermine the autonomy of participants. Effective group facilitation requires being able to get out of our own way; to leave our own experiences, feelings, and ideas outside of the meeting space; and to listen, encourage, and support group members in expressing their own values, doubts, emotions, and opinions.

✪ *Disagreements or conflicts between cofacilitators during group sessions:* Cofacilitators may disagree about a range of issues. This is natural. However, when these disagreements are shared with the group, or result in a conflict that influences the ability of facilitators to work cooperatively together, it undermines the integrity, quality, and effectiveness of the group process.

? **Have you faced or witnessed other challenges to effective group work?**

? **Which of these challenges do you think will be most difficult for you to address?**

SUGGESTIONS FOR GROUP FACILITATORS

✪ *Screen potential group members:* We recommend, if appropriate, conducting brief interviews to screen potential group participants. This is an opportunity for you to explain the focus of the group to potential members. It is also an opportunity for the prospective member to determine whether or not they are interested in participating in the group. During the interview, try to assess whether the prospective member is ready to make positive contributions to the group process. When people are unable to make use of the group as a learning environment, it is unethical to include them in the group where their behavior may be a threat to the integrity of the work of others.

✪ *Regular meetings for cofacilitators:* As described above, meet with your cofacilitator to plan the group, and check in after every group meeting to debrief what happened, to identify potential challenges and areas of disagreement, and to come up with a coordinated plan of action for the next group meeting.

✪ *Regular meetings with supervisors:* CHWs who facilitate groups should have regular meetings with a supervisor who can provide guidance regarding the work and support for personal issues or challenges that may arise as a consequence of facilitating group work.

✪ *Participate in professional development opportunities:* Seek out opportunities to enhance your skills. Identify skills that you would like to enhance, such as resolving conflict, cofacilitation, or self-care. Talk with your supervisor to see if there are opportunities to attend local workshops or trainings. Consider enrolling in a class at your local college or university.

✪ *Self-care:* Facilitating groups is deeply rewarding work. As you have learned in this chapter, it is also often challenging. Make time to do the things that assist you to relieve stress and prevent burnout. Refer to Chapter Fourteen.

? **What other suggestions would you share with a colleague who was preparing to facilitate their first group?**

20.8 ETHICS AND GROUP FACILITATION

The foundation of ethical practice for facilitating groups is the same as for individual practice as outlined in Chapter Eight. Everything that CHWs do should be designed to put the best interests of the client first (in this case, the group and its members). The difference between group work and individual work is that the client is, for ethical decision making, both the group and the individual.

Some ethical issues are relatively easy to understand, such as preventing discrimination, physical violence, or threats of violence. Other ethical issues are more complex, such as the boundaries of confidentiality. The ethical duty of the CHW is clear: clients' rights to confidentiality are the same as with any individual counseling relationship. What is said to the CHW is held in the strictest confidence with only a few exceptions (see Chapter Eight). But what about the boundaries of confidentiality within an agency? Should you, as a group facilitator, be allowed to share client information with other agency workers? Are you obligated to divulge information you think would benefit the client in work with another agency professional? The answers become complex when agencies don't have explicit guidelines about intra-agency policies and when those policies aren't made explicit to clients.

What about confidentiality between group members? What can a group member expect from the group with respect to privacy? In fact, the group member can only expect what one would expect from any human interaction. There is no law to prevent others—nonprofessionals, that is—from talking to people who are not in the group, or talking to other group members outside of group time. The best that can be hoped for is that group members pledge to each other that what is said in group stays in group. This is a mutual promise made by group members, but it does not carry the weight of law.

The group facilitator should make the limits of confidentiality clear to group members as they join the group. This is best done by facilitating a discussion among group members about privacy. The group facilitator can guide the group toward the mutual promise of confidentiality and be ready to intervene should the promise be broken. It is best to get the group to come to a consensus about their pledge to each other, with the understanding that everyone in the group will work to enforce that rule.

Finally, every group facilitator and cofacilitator should meet regularly with a supervisor. This is your opportunity to raise ethical concerns and other challenges and to receive direction and support from a trained professional in how best to respond to these issues. If you are ever confused about how to handle a potential problem in group, seek guidance as soon as possible from your supervisor.

CHAPTER REVIEW QUESTIONS

DESIGN YOUR OWN GROUP

Develop your own model for a social or support group that you would facilitate. Please develop a realistic model based on the information in this chapter. Choose a community to serve, and health issues to address, that you are already familiar with.

1. Describe the community that will participate in the group:

2. What health issue or concern does the group have in common?

3. What are the membership criteria for the group?

4. Describe the structure for the group:
    - Where will you meet and how often?
    - How many times will the group meet?
    - Will the group be open or closed?
    - How will you start and end each group session?
    - What ground rules will guide the work of the group? How will these be established?

5. What will some of the primary goals for the group be?
6. What will you do to promote participation of all group members?

7. How will you work to promote the leadership of group members?
8. How will you know if you have been successful in facilitating this group? What outcomes will group members achieve?

REFERENCES

American Group Psychotherapy Association. 2007. Practice Guidelines for Group Psychotherapy: A Cross-Theoretical Guide to Developing and Leading Psychotherapy Groups. Accessed on April 10, 2009: www.agpa.org/guidelines/index.html

Lieberman, M. A., Yalom, I. D., Miles, M. B. 1973. *Encounter Groups: First Facts*. New York: Basic Books.

Schneider Corey, M., and Corey, G. 2006. *Groups: Process and Practice* (7th Ed.). Belmont, CA: Brooks/Cole.

Tuckman, B. 1965. Developmental Sequences in Small Groups. *Psychological Bulletin* 63: 384–399.

Yalom, I. 1995. *Theory and Practice of Group Psychotherapy*. New York: Basic Books.

ADDITIONAL RESOURCES

Rosenberg, P. R. 1984. Support Groups: A Special Therapeutic Entity. *Small Group Research* 15(2): 173–186.

21

Using the Arts to Promote Community Health

Tim Berthold

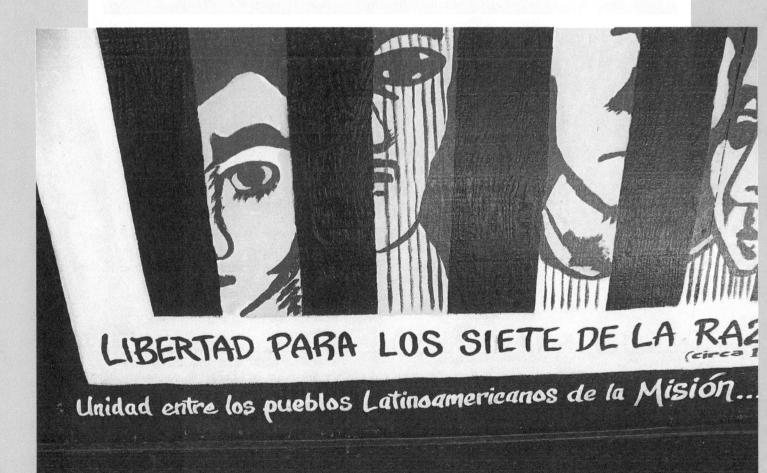

In 1939, Billie Holiday sang "Strange Fruit" to raise awareness of the lynchings (death by hanging) of African-Americans in the United States. This song is based on a poem published in 1937 by Abel Meeropol (National Public Radio, 2003).

> Southern trees bear a strange fruit,
> Blood on the leaves and blood at the root,
> Black bodies swinging in the Southern breeze,
> Strange fruit hanging from the poplar trees.
>
> Pastoral scene of the gallant South,
> The bulging eyes and the twisted mouth,
> Scent of magnolias, sweet and fresh,
> Then the sudden smell of burning flesh!
>
> Here is a fruit for the crows to pluck,
> For the rain to gather, for the wind to suck,
> For the sun to rot, for the trees to drop,
> Here is a strange and bitter crop.
> —Abel Meeropol

"We Shall Overcome," a gospel song written in 1900 by Charles Tindley, became a source of inspiration and hope for the civil rights movements of the 1950s and '60s (National Public Radio, 2005).

> We shall overcome
> We shall overcome
> We shall overcome some day
> Chorus: Oh, deep in my heart
>   I do believe
>   We shall overcome, some day
> We shall all be free
> We shall all be free
> We shall all be free, some day
> —Charles Tindley

These songs are examples of how art can inspire and promote social justice: "Throughout American history, songs have cried out against inequality, poverty and war, and in support of workers, civil and human rights" (National Public Radio, 2003).

INTRODUCTION

This chapter will describe how and why the arts are used to promote community health and will highlight five community health projects that incorporate the arts.

WHAT YOU WILL LEARN

By studying the information in this chapter, you will be able to:

- ⚙ Explain how various art forms are used to promote community health and provide several examples

- Discuss why the arts are effective resources for promoting community health
- Discuss the role that CHWs may play in projects that use art to promote community health
- Begin to plan a community art project

21.1 ART FORMS USED TO PROMOTE COMMUNITY HEALTH

The arts are commonly used to provoke thought, emotion, dialogue, and action about a wide range of topics. The arts often address public health issues such as child abuse, domestic violence, lynching and other hate-motivated violence, cancer, AIDS, homelessness, civil rights, and the Tuskegee Syphilis Trials. All creative and performing arts may be used to promote community health, including:

- Music
- Theater
- Radio, television, video, and film
- Dance
- Poetry
- Fine arts (drawing and painting), including murals
- Photography, including photo novella and Photovoice projects
- Cartoons, comics, and graphic novels
- Other art forms

? *Have you seen or heard art works—murals, plays, music, comics—that address public health topics?*

? *Have you recently seen a television show, film, billboard, or advertisement related to a health issue?*

In this chapter, we will highlight five projects that used art to promote community health, including a Photovoice project, a digital story project, a postcard campaign, a popular theater project, and a drumming project.

21.2 WHY THE ARTS ARE USED TO PROMOTE HEALTH

The arts are powerful resources for promoting community health for many reasons, including the following:

- The arts engage people's creativity, imagination, and humor, resources that in turn motivate learning and action.
- The expression "a picture is worth a thousand words" speaks to the ability of visual arts to convey complex information in a brief and compelling way.
- The arts can document or depict challenging life issues in a way that deeply moves people. Photography and documentary film, for example, provided Americans with images

of the civil rights movement, the Vietnam and Iraq wars, and the HIV/AIDS epidemic that motivated resistance, protest, and changes in public policy.

A classic example is Pablo Picasso's painting *Guernica*. It depicts the bombing of the city of Guernica, Spain, by the Nazis on April 26, 1937, during the Spanish Civil War. It is estimated that the bombing killed from 250 to 1,600 people, with many more injured. Picasso said: "In the panel on which I am working, which I shall call Guernica, and in all my recent works of art, I clearly express my abhorrence of the military caste which has sunk Spain in an ocean of pain and death" (Public Broadcasting Service, 1999). To view Guernica, go to: www.pbs.org/treasuresoftheworld/a_nav/guernica_nav/main_guerfrm.html

✪ The arts engage audiences emotionally and provide opportunities to express strong emotion (including sorrow, despair, fear, terror, humiliation, anger, and rage) that can inspire learning and action.

✪ The arts can support the expression people's most important hopes and dreams, including dreams of health, peace, and justice.

✪ The arts provide people with opportunities to express common experiences, feelings, and ideas and can motivate community building, organizing, and action, such as the use of protest music and songs to inspire the actions of the civil rights movement in the United States.

✪ The arts sometimes provide a "safer" opportunity for communities to express contradictory, radical, marginal, or emotionally laden ideas. This is particularly true for communities experiencing discrimination and state-sponsored violence.

✪ The arts are effective at engaging different types of learners, including visual (people who learn through seeing), auditory (people who learn through listening), and kinesthetic learners (people who learn through moving, doing, and touching).

✪ Specific art forms may be culturally appropriate or significant to a particular community, and may already be used to communicate important concepts.

✪ The arts are accessible to most communities, often more accessible than other mediums used for health promotion (such as written materials or traditional health education presentations). Some clients and communities have limited literacy and may not be able to read written health education materials.

✪ Arts projects can be based on the creative and artistic talents of the community.

✪ The arts provide opportunities for communities to participate actively in their creation. For example, they may create and act in plays or skits, or design or paint on a mural. Participation often fosters learning, collaboration with others, and a sense of investment in the issues being addressed.

? *Can you think of other reasons why the arts may be used to promote community health?*

? *What are your favorite art forms?*

? *Do you have a favorite artist (musician, poet, writer, or painter)?*

? *What is it about the type of art or the artist that attracts you?*

? *Have you ever been particularly engaged, provoked, or motivated by a work of art, whether it was music, a mural, a poem, or a photograph?*

? *What thoughts or feelings were generated by the work of art?*

21.3 EXAMPLES OF COMMUNITY HEALTH PROJECTS THAT INCORPORATE THE ARTS

"My daughter, Gina Marie Muniz, failed to receive proper medical care for cervical cancer while in prison at the Central California Women's Facility. She died on November 27, 2000, at the age of 27, two days after being given compassionate release."—Grace Ortega

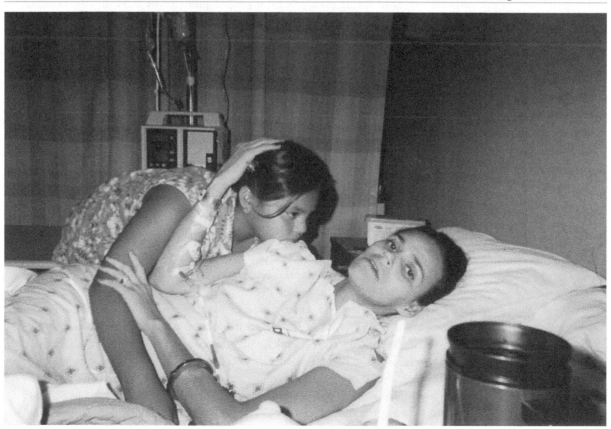

PHOTOVOICE PROJECT

Invisible Punishment: Photovoice Challenges the Prison System

Legal Services for Prisoners with Children (LSPC), a San Francisco–based human rights organization that advocates for the rights of incarcerated people and their families, invited people most affected by the prison system to use cameras to document the impact of incarceration on their lives and the lives of their communities. The project used Photovoice, a community-based participatory research method developed by Caroline Wang, which engages communities in taking, displaying, and analyzing photographs that depict important aspects of their lives. LSPC worked with three different groups to tell their stories through photography: formerly incarcerated women from A New Way of Life, a supportive housing program in South Central Los Angeles; students from Oasis High School in Oakland; and members of the Family Advocacy Network, a group of family members who support their incarcerated loved ones.

In the *Invisible Punishment* project, the process was as important as the product. Project facilitators emphasized the importance of people sharing and speaking from their own experience, seeing connections among their individual situations, creating a way to relate their situations to root causes, and developing solutions and strategies for change. After a brief technical training and a discussion of the ethics and responsibilities of taking photographs of people, participants went into the community, took photos of people or situations that had particular meaning to them, and then brought their strongest photos to a group discussion in which people analyzed the story behind the image.

These photographs were put together to form an exhibit entitled *Invisible Punishment*. The exhibit questioned the "tough on crime" attitudes and the "War on Drugs" that have led the United States to have the highest per-capita incarceration rate in the world. It shed light on the connections between prisons and cycles

A POSTCARD CAMPAIGN

Advocating for Health Care Services for Immigrants

The Community Voices Project in Oakland, California, was funded by the W. K. Kellogg Foundation to expand health care services at the local level, and give underserved communities a greater "voice" within the national debate on health care access. The project is a collaboration of two community clinics, Asian Health Services and La Clínica de la Raza, and the Alameda Health Consortium, a policy advocacy organization that works with Alameda County community clinics to expand services to the poor and underserved. Through Community Voices, the three organizations worked to increase health care services to all Alameda County residents, regardless of their immigration status, by educating policymakers, health care advocates, and community members about the issues that impact the uninsured and underserved. The project addressed a range of health issues including oral health, mental health, local health coverage expansion, language access, and expansion of the CHW model of care.

of abuse, addiction, poverty, and homelessness, and raised questions about the ways that incarceration diminishes the health and well-being of entire communities.

These discussions served to build community capacity to relate to a larger social and political environment. In the words of one project participant, "I like seeing my community through my sisters' eyes." The director of A New Way of Life summed it up this way:

> I had been searching for a way to broaden the vision and perspective about social conditions in South L.A. When the women saw their photos and began to describe what they saw in their photos I knew Photovoice was the educational tool I had been searching for. The Photovoice sessions produced an opportunity for formerly incarcerated women to think about the environment and how it impacts their lives. We came together every week in harmony to discuss our photos, looking at the problems and possible solutions. Photovoice has expanded our minds and changed our focus as to what we can do as individuals in a community that has complicated social problems.

Invisible Punishment was first brought to the community through an opening reception at the Watts Labor Community Labor Action Committee; its Northern California opening in Oakland drew an enthusiastic crowd of 150 people. Over time, the exhibit was used to "speak truth to power," as participants found creative ways to use their images to influence policymakers to listen to their vision of what is needed. By using the photos to demonstrate their ideas at town hall meetings on the rights of formerly incarcerated people, community members challenged policymakers to rethink failed approaches and create policies to decrease our society's dependence on incarceration as the primary solution to public safety. In addition to being shown at conferences and community meetings, the images from *Invisible Punishment* were also incorporated into two different art exhibits that traveled around the United States and in Europe as part of grassroots organizing against the prison industrial complex.

Source: Project description by Donna Willmott, Legal Services for Prisoners with Children, 2009. (www.prisonerswithchildren.org)

In 2004, cuts to the California state budget decreased services to the poor, and anti-immigrant sentiments pushed more community members into the shadow of our society. Community Voices decided to do a postcard campaign to highlight the contributions of immigrants to society and to educate policymakers about the importance of maintaining preventive care for all communities. The postcards were used not just as advocacy and educational tools, but also as a means to engage community members in civic participation.

To create the postcards, project staff worked with local community clinics, social services agencies, and a photographer to highlight the experiences of immigrant families and communities. Ten different postcards were created; each included a personal story and a message that stressed the importance of preserving and increasing health care access to immigrants and other underserved communities. By making ten different postcards, the project was able to convey the diversity and richness of the various immigrant cultures, as well as put many faces and voices to their advocacy efforts.

(*Continued*)

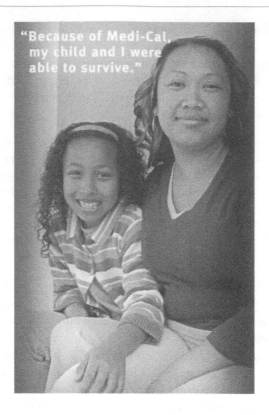

?

What do you think about the way this campaign used photo-graphs, stories, and postcards?

POPULAR THEATER

*Youth Theater Project, The Pittsburg Pre-School
Coordinating Council*

The modern tradition known as popular theater is connected to the popular education movement developed by theorists and activists like Paulo Freire (1992), discussed in greater detail in Chapters Seventeen, Nineteen, and Twenty-Two. Both popular education and popular theater seek to engage communities in a creative and educational process that supports them to express their own realities, their own vision, and ideas for social change. Both are rooted in a strong commitment to social justice.

Traditional theater is usually performed in formal settings and on stages for audiences who can afford to pay to see the work. Popular theater is usually performed in community-based settings such as market places, churches, union halls, and parks, often for free. The productions address a range of public health and social justice issues such as human rights, AIDS, or gun violence. Popular theater often seeks to

The project printed more than ten thousand postcards and distributed them throughout California at conferences and meetings. The postcards were used by CHWs to engage community members in discussing their health care access issues, to educate community members about the democratic process, and to highlight their role in educating policymakers to expand health care services in their local community.

Community members signed the postcards at street health fairs, Immigrant Day at the state capitol, local conferences, and through the local outreach efforts of CHWs. Within two years, almost five thousand postcards were signed and delivered to legislative representatives and the governor. The signed postcards were delivered by community members who traveled with CHWs during Immigrant Day—a day when advocates for immigrants from throughout the state gather at the state capitol to visit and educate policymakers about their issues and concerns. For many of the community members, Immigrant Day was their first time visiting the state capitol and speaking to lawmakers.

By using the postcards, CHWs were able to engage their communities in dialogue about the importance of civic participation and advocacy. They also used the postcards as a tool to organize and enable community members (many of whom were non–English speakers) to have the courage to visit legislators and tell their stories firsthand. While we have a long way to go before our public policies effectively promote the health and welfare of all immigrant groups, this project supported CHWs and community members in developing the skills they need to continue to advocate for social justice.

Source: Project description by Darouny Somsanith, Alameda Health Consortium, 2009.

? *Have you ever participated in a grassroots advocacy campaign like the one described above?*

dissolve the artificial wall or divide between actors and audience and often creates opportunities for audience participation. Audiences may provide direction or participate in the play or skits, or may be asked to engage in dialogue with the actors after the performance. The goal is always to reflect the audience's reality, to engage them in reflection and the contemplation of action. An example is El Teatro Campesino, the cultural wing of the United Farm Workers, which performed *actos* (skits) on flat-bed trucks in the fields of California's Central Valley during the campaigns for workers' rights in the mid-1960s.

The Pittsburg Pre-School Coordinating Council (PPSCC) is a nonprofit agency serving low-income communities in Pittsburg, California. While it began as a pre-school, the agency developed other programs and services over the years in response to local needs, including senior housing; outreach, education, and counseling; and case management services addressing a range of public health issues. These community health programs are managed by a large team of CHWs selected from the local community and provided with extensive training.

(Continued)

Since the early 1980s, the CHWs at the PPSCC had been providing HIV prevention outreach and education services, including programs designed to reach school-aged youths. By the mid-1990s, local youths had received a lot of information about HIV/AIDS from the media, social marketing campaigns, and through educational presentations mandated by California law. As a result, youths were often jaded (they felt they already knew it all) and difficult to engage in HIV-prevention efforts. At the same time, youths were continuing to engage in behaviors that increased their risks for HIV infection. CHWs at the pre-school wanted to develop fresh approaches to educating and supporting youths to reduce their risks for the transmission of HIV and other STIs.

Together, they developed a new program that recruited and trained local youths to serve as Volunteer Peer Educators (VPEs). The youths were trained by CHWs to provide basic health information about HIV and other sexually transmitted infections (STIs), and worked as a team to develop and perform a series of short skits about HIV disease that were inspired by their own realities. The skits dramatized the situations and factors that increased risks for HIV transmission, as well as the consequences of living with HIV disease. The popular theater group took care not to condescend to their audiences, to reinforce fear-based messages about AIDS, or to stigmatize particular behaviors or identities. For example, the skits took special care not to reinforce hurtful stereotypes about women, lesbian, gay, or transgender youths, or people living with HIV disease. The skits did not provide simplistic

? *Have you ever seen or participated in a popular theater production?*

DIGITAL STORY TELLING

Silence Speaks in South Africa: Digital Storytelling to End Gender-Based Violence and Prevent HIV/AIDS

Academic research and our own experiences make it clear that long-term healing from violence is supported by creating opportunities for survivors to tell their stories. Six years ago, with partnership from the Center for Digital Storytelling in Berkeley, California, I founded *Silence Speaks*. The project supports survivors and witnesses of violence in sharing their own stories through short videos and presenting these videos in training, community organizing, and policy advocacy settings. This article provides an overview of digital storytelling and explores the process of doing *Silence Speaks*, with South Africans working to prevent gender-based violence.

WHAT IS DIGITAL STORYTELLING?

The digital storytelling method, initiated in the early 1990s at the Center for Digital Storytelling, brings small groups of people together in workshops to make short answers to complex challenges, such as the pressure to be sexually active, and often posed questions to the audiences and invited them to share their own ideas, beliefs, and experiences. One skit featured a young woman who is being pressured to have unprotected sex with her boyfriend. She does not want to have unprotected sex, but she is worried about losing the relationship. Rather than providing the audience with an ending to the skit, the actors stopped to talk with the audience about the young woman's situation, what she might be feeling, what choices she may make, and why. Together, the actors and the audience developed one or more endings for the skit, and the actors performed them.

The skits were performed in English and Spanish in a wide variety of settings including schools, churches, youth-serving agencies and programs, and community centers. Volunteer Peer Educators were trained to facilitate discussions and to answer questions following their performances. One measure of the success of the project was the extent to which audience members asked questions and actively engaged in dialogue. Audience members often remained behind after performances or scheduled follow-up appointments with CHWs to talk further about their own risks and concerns, about their own HIV status and that of families and friends, and to participate in confidential HIV antibody test counseling. This project featured the participation and leadership of local youths and was developed, managed, and evaluated by CHWs.

Source: Project description by Tim Berthold, City College of San Francisco, 2009.

? *Are there groups in your community who use popular theater to raise awareness of public health issues?*

(usually two to three minutes in length), first-person digital videos. Over the course of three to four days, participants share aspects of their own life experiences in a group story circle; write and record voiceover narration that becomes the foundation of their stories; and select photos, artwork, and short video clips to use in illustrating the pieces. Next, participants are guided through hands-on computer tutorials that cover the basics of digital editing and allow them, with facilitator assistance, to piece together their materials into finished videos, or "digital stories." An important moment of the workshop comes at the end, when participants' work is screened and celebrated by all.

TAKING DIGITAL STORYTELLING TO SOUTH AFRICA TO SUPPORT AN END TO VIOLENCE

The Men As Partners Network (MAP) began in South Africa in 1998 (Engender Health, 2008). The many organizations involved in the Network have joined together to address the relationship between rigid gender roles, domestic and sexual violence, and HIV and AIDS in South Africa. The Network calls on men and women to take

(Continued)

a stand against violence, reduce their risk-taking behaviors, and play an activist role in preventing the spread and impact of the epidemic. As MAP spokesperson Dean Peacock explains, "To bring about change at all levels of society, the Network conducts street outreach, holds workshops, engages in community education and mobilization activities, and advocates for policy change."

Given that *Silence Speaks* highlights the voices of people rarely depicted with any degree of sensitivity in mainstream media, it felt right to take our work to South Africa in 2005. The MAP Network had sponsored many creative arts projects, including community murals, street theater, and photo essays, so the digital storytelling sessions were a logical next step in the Network's understanding of art and media as tools for social change. The project reflected the MAP Network's deepening commitment to healing (from the trauma of abuse and HIV stigma) through action—in this case, by providing its supporters with the chance to share their stories. The workshops also had a clear purpose: these stories would go up on the Web and be shown throughout the country in trainings and at community events. As is our practice in *Silence Speaks*, we were careful to make this known in advance to potential participants. We also talked at length at the beginning of the two workshops about the implications of personal disclosure to broad audiences.

We held two *Silence Speaks* workshops with staff and volunteers from MAP, one in Cape Town and one in Johannesburg. In the Cape Town workshop, Juliana Davids was the first to make the leap into the unknown. As she started telling a story about rape within her family when she was growing up, the memory and pain brought tears. With gentle support, fellow students and I asked questions, encouraged clarification, and inspired Juliana to find even better words to describe the core of what creates her foundation today, as a mature young woman. "It seems you are searching for liberation from what happened to you," one friend commented. Juliana's eyes lit up. That was the concept she was looking for, her own key to unlocking herself and her story.

Later, as we reviewed her script, Juliana assured me that she was comfortable using photos of herself and sharing her story with thousands of people. She made it clear that she wanted the piece to inspire viewers to examine their own histories and cultivate a new sense of urgency about the need to take action against HIV and violence. This is the story she told:

> I started working at Pollsmoor prison about three years ago, educating men about the importance of being tested for HIV. The day I was sexually harassed by an inmate, I realized I was still imprisoned by my own past. By my stepfather, who physically

? *What kinds of music do you listen to, and when?*

? *How does music influence your mood?*

and emotionally abused my mom for thirteen years, and who sexually abused me. Sleepless nights, being tired at school the next day, out of fear that if I slept he would come and force himself on me. He only stopped when I got my period. . . .

It didn't stop for the other girls in my family. When I was fifteen, my eleven-year-old cousin was raped and strangled to death by a male family friend on a local sports field. I began to believe all men are monsters, dangerous, potential rapists—and that they use their physical powers to get what they want.

The day after harassing me, the same prisoner apologized in front of an entire group of inmates. I thought it was brave of him, and I forgave him. But when I went home that night, I realized my stepdad would probably never apologize. He was going on with his life and seemed happy. I was not. I knew that unless I could let go of my bitterness and fear of him, I wouldn't be at peace.

So I made the choice to forgive him for taking away my innocence. After that, I made the decision to free other men and women by working with college students. They're trapped by their own attitudes about gender-based violence, relationships, and HIV/AIDS. I help them realize they can make different choices—their own choices.

The best thing is, I started to trust men. I determine how I feel and how I react to those feelings. Back when I was a kid, I didn't have that choice. But now I do.

Juliana's hope that her story would be seen far and wide was gratified in a way none of us had expected. Just weeks after we finished the workshops, the MAP stories were shown in the South African Parliament. A lengthy discussion ensued among the elected officials present about the links between violence against women and HIV, and the government proceeded to pledge a large amount of funding to the broader MAP Network, for their community organizing and policy change work.

In the two years since the digital storytelling workshops, Juliana and the MAP Network have shared the stories at trainings for youths and adults throughout South Africa. With careful facilitation, they discuss the messages carried by the stories and encourage viewers to examine their own histories and see how their experiences reflect larger cultural, societal, and political messages about violence. Through these trainings, and by screening the stories on the Web and at community speak-out events, they are giving rise to a new sense of urgency and commitment among South Africans, to take action against HIV and violence.

For more information about Silence Speaks, please visit us online at www.silencespeaks.org. To see Juliana's story and the other MAP stories online, visit www.engenderhealth.org/our-work/gender/digital-stories-south-africa.php.

To view more stories online go to: www.storycenter.org/stories.

Source: Project description by Amy Hill, community projects director, Center for Digital Storytelling, 2009. (www.storycenter.org)

? *What role does it play in your life?*

? *Have you ever participated in community health or social justice projects that used music in some way?*

DRUMMING AND HEALTH

Drumming Circulos at Instituto Familiar de la Raza, San Francisco, California

Music is an important part of every culture. People use music to promote health on a daily basis, often without being conscious of it. We listen to music to feel more energized, relaxed, inspired, reflective, or romantic. Music and rhythm surround us and are manifested as heartbeats, the way we walk and talk, the sounds of the tides of the ocean, of birds, and the wind. Our bodies, brain, heart, and sprit respond to music and rhythm; we are all susceptible to its influence.

For thousands of years, communities throughout the world have used drumming and music to promote community, cultural identity, and health. In the United States, the use of drumming to promote health is gaining recognition and momentum. The American Music Therapy Association (AMTA, 2009) has actively promoted the use of music as a healing modality or approach. Researchers have also started to investigate the health effects of drumming and music, and their findings affirm ancient wisdom: music promotes our well-being.

Many groups use drumming and other types of music to promote community health. One of these is Instituto Familiar de la Raza (IFR), a behavioral health clinic located in the Mission District of San Francisco, California. For the past ten years, IFR has offered drumming groups tailored to meet the health needs of youths, families, CHWs, clinicians, and the community at large. These healing groups are offered on a weekly basis to youths and families, on a monthly basis for the Mission Community Response Network, a group of CHWs and clinicians, and every three months or as needed to the community at large.

The community drumming groups, or *circulos,* promote education, social support, community dialogue, and organizing efforts. These healing circles are also used to provide an outlet for community members to heal from experiences of trauma, violence, injury, loss, grief, stress, burnout, and psychological rehabilitation. Participating in drumming groups can promote self-care, spiritual development, membership in a community, cultural awareness, and well-being.

Over 650 youths have participated in drumming circles over the past ten years at IFR, including groups for young men ages eleven to seventeen, and groups facilitated in both English and Spanish. Participants are recruited by conducting outreach to schools, community health agencies, and youth-serving programs. Drumming circles are held at IFR on Thursdays after school. I facilitate the group and am an experienced musician, drummer, and therapist. I teach the youths how to drum, and together they talk about the history and meaning of drumming in their communities and cultures and how drumming can promote physical, mental, and spiritual health and strength. As the group becomes more comfortable with drumming and

Are there groups in your community that use drumming or other forms of music to promote health and wellness?

each other, I engage them in discussions about the challenges and stresses they face in life, including the risks for dropping out of school, gang involvement, street violence, drug use, and other health issues. The young men talk about strategies that can empower them and promote their health and wellness along with that of their families and communities.

Over the course of many weeks, the young men develop more advanced drumming skills and talk about the lives they want to create for themselves, their families, and their communities. Because drumming captures the attention of young participants, the group has made it easy to provide health education and teach youths about the impact of substance abuse, sexually transmitted illnesses, nutrition, exercise, and self-care. Participants have also been able to learn about general mental health issues and how to manage and cope with stress.

The drumming group has proved to be an effective model for reaching young men who need community support, as it offers a physical and developmentally appropriate means of expression. Most youths mention that the drumming circle offers them a sense of community and a way to reconnect with their heritage and healing practices that speak to their cultural traditions. They have mentioned that the spiritual and health education components elevate their level of consciousness and prepare them to deal with some of the hardships of life.

Occasionally, the young men perform at local community and cultural events and share the experience of drumming with other youths. The drummers report that performing gives them a sense of purpose and pride. They mention feeling empowered and good about themselves, as well as a sense of keeping their culture alive. Participants have also reported positive changes in levels of anxiety; feeling good, relaxed, tranquil, and at peace; and a sense of increased confidence, self-esteem, energy, appetite, group cohesiveness, and community. Other positive outcomes have been increased awareness of the importance of culture, increased academic functioning, and decreased distress. Some youths have also pursued advanced training in music and have been accepted in the local school of the arts, colleges, and universities.

Participating in a drumming group is accessible to anyone because it does not require previous experience with music or drums. If you have access to a drum and a place where you can drum without being concerned about disturbing anyone, sit comfortably, take a deep breath, and drum away.

We do recommend that drumming groups who seek to do in-depth work around chronic and severe health issues should be facilitated by people who are experienced and skilled musicians, group facilitators, and health or mental health providers, like CHWs. The facilitator must be prepared to respond immediately to health-related issues that arise in the group.

Source: Project description by Sal Núñez, faculty, City College of San Francisco Health Education Department, and musician, 2009.

21.4 THE ROLE OF CHWs

CHWs play many roles in programs that use the arts to promote health. They may collaborate with artists to produce the art, and then share it with communities, facilitating learning and action. They also support communities in creating and producing their own art. As a CHW, your role will depend many factors, including your experience, skill, and comfort level with artistic projects. As always, the best projects are characterized by leadership from the community in all phases of development, production, and evaluation. To the extent that you can facilitate and support the community's leadership, the more effective the project will be.

At the same time, we encourage CHWS to participate in the creative process of producing the art (mural, theater work) that will be used to promote the community's health. Sometimes CHWs stand on the sidelines, worried that they don't have artistic talent, or that their participation may undermine the autonomy of the community. However, this may be perceived as being "standoffish." In general, we encourage you to participate as fully as possible, and as a member of the team, in the work that communities do, whether it is digging a latrine or painting a mural.

Finally, try to keep in mind that perceptions about the "quality" of artwork are subjective and ultimately not as important as the process of community empowerment. You don't need to be a professional artist to paint a mural or a professional actor to take part in a skit. What you need most is a sense of commitment, some creativity, a sense of play and humor, and a great deal of humility.

?   *Have any of the examples provided in this chapter inspired you?*

?   *Which example or examples, and why?*

?   *Have you ever participated in any type of an arts project?*

?   *Do you have experience and skill with any particular forms of art?*

CHAPTER REVIEW

Please develop your own proposal for a community health program using art. Use the examples above, and your own experience and skills, as sources of inspiration.

Write down the following elements of your plan:

1. Define and describe the community you will work with:
2. Identify the health issue or issues that your project will address:
3. What health outcomes will the project hope to achieve?
4. Describe the form of art that the project will use:
5. What materials will you need?
6. Describe how you will use art in your project:
7. Explain why you will use art as a resource in this project:
8. Describe the role of the community in your project. How will they participate?
9. What will your role be?
10. How will you know if the project has been successful?

REFERENCES

The American Music Therapy Association (AMTA). Accessed on April 6, 2009: http://www.musictherapy.org

EngenderHealth and Men as Partners. 2008. Accessed on April 6, 2009: http://www.engenderhealth.org/our-countries/africa/south-africa.php

EngenderHealth. Juliana's Story. Accessed on April 6, 2009: http://www.engenderhealth.org/our-work/gender/digital-stories-south-africa.php

Freire, P. 1992. *Pedagogy of the Oppressed*. New York: Continuum.

Legal Services for Prisoners with Children. Accessed on April 6, 2009: http://www.prisonerswithchildren.org/

National Public Radio. 2003. Strange Fruit. Accessed on April 6, 2009: http://www.pbs.org/independentlens/strangefruit/film.html

National Public Radio. 2005. Get Up, Stand Up: The Story of Pop and Protest. We Shall Overcome. Accessed on April 6, 2009: http://www.pbs.org/wnet/getupstandup/music_overcome1.html

Public Broadcasting Service. 1999. Treasures of the World. Guernica: Testimony of War. Accessed on April 6, 2009: http://www.pbs.org/treasuresoftheworld/a_nav/guernica_nav/main_guerfrm.html

ADDITIONAL RESOURCES

Bates, R. 1996. Popular Theater: A Useful Process for Adult Educators. *Adult Education Quarterly* 46: 224–236. Accessed on April 6, 2009: http://aeq.sagepub.com/cgi/content/abstract/46/4/224

The Bay Area Popular Theater Project. Accessed on April 6, 2009: http://www.rasmo.net/poptheaterframe.html

Burgess, J. 2006. Hearing Ordinary Voices: Cultural Studies, Vernacular Creativity and Digital Storytelling. *Continuum: Journal of Media and Cultural Studies* 20: 201–214.

The Center for Digital Storytelling. Accessed on April 6, 2009: http://www.storycenter.org

Diallo, Y., and Hall Mitchell. 1989. *The Healing Drum: African Wisdom Teachings*. Vermont: Destiny Books.

Drum Circle Facilitators Guild. Accessed on April 6, 2009: http://www.dcfg.net/dcfg06/home.html

Friedman, R. L. 2000. *The Healing Power of the Drum*. Reno, NV: White Cliffs Media.

Healthy Drumming Institute. Accessed on April 6, 2009: http://www.healthydrumming.org/.

Instituto Familiar de la Raza. Accessed on April 6, 2009: http://www.ifrsf.org

Lambert, J. 2002. *Digital Storytelling: Capturing Lives, Creating Community*. Berkeley, CA: Digital Diner Press.

Ochs, E., and Capps, L. 1996. Narrating the Self. *Annual Review of Anthropology* 25: 19–43.

The Popular Education News. Accessed on April 6, 2009: http://www.popednews.org/.

Rappaport, J. 1995. Empowerment Meets Narrative: Listening to Stories and Creating Settings. *American Journal of Community Psychology* 23: 795–807.

USA Drum Circle Finder Directory. Accessed on April 6, 2009: http://www.drumcircles.net/circlelist.html.

22

Community Organizing and Advocacy

Alma Avila-Esparza

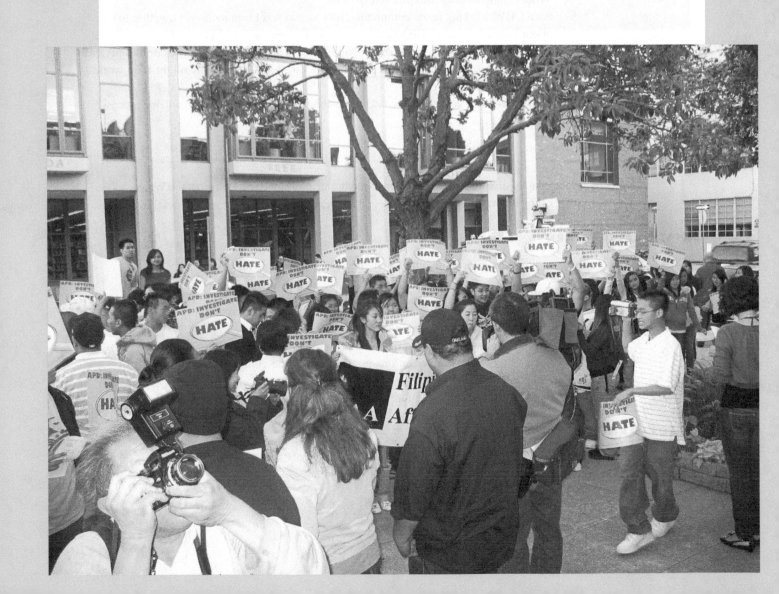

CHW SCENARIO

A local community is deeply concerned about increasing handgun violence. This predominantly low-income Latino and African American community includes a large number of public housing units and faces a wide range of other health concerns, including high rates of asthma and diabetes. The neighborhood has a city-funded health center, schools, parks, and several churches, temples, and nonprofit agencies that provide social services. Community members have a long history of participating in social movements, including civil rights movements. Recently, a young mother and her infant were killed by stray bullets during a drive-by shooting. Over six hundred community members attended the memorial service. The community wants to find a way to prevent further shootings and deaths. They want to reclaim their community and make it a safer place to live and raise their families.

Based on the situation described above:

- What are the community's primary concerns?
- What other challenges does the community face?
- What resources does the community have?
- As a CHW working in the community, how would you bring members together to talk about their concerns and to identify strategies to promote social change?
- How could community organizing promote the health and safety of the community?
- What possible actions might the community take? What solutions might they work toward?
- As a CHW, what are your roles and responsibilities in the community organizing process?

INTRODUCTION

This chapter provides an introduction to the basic knowledge and skills that CHWs use when supporting communities in organizing and advocating for social change and social justice.

WHAT YOU WILL LEARN

By studying the information in this chapter, you will be able to:

- Define and discuss community organizing
- Discuss at least two ways that contemporary models of community organizing are different from models used in the past
- Explain the five steps of the Community Action Model (CAM)
- Discuss the CHW's roles and responsibilities in the community organizing process, and put them into practice
- Apply the Community Action Model to issues facing the communities you work with

WORDS TO KNOW

Media Advocacy

22.1 WHY ORGANIZE?

We all want to live in healthy communities. Yet many communities lack access to the basic resources necessary for health such as clean water and air, safety, housing, food, education, employment, health care, and civil rights. They face a wide range of other public health problems such as high rates of infant mortality, heart disease, HIV/AIDS, drug use, incarceration, or homelessness. They may live close to an oil refinery or waste incinerator. It is to face these challenges that communities come together and organize for social change. They want a better life for themselves and their children.

Because CHWs have a special relationship with communities, they are often ideally situated to facilitate community organizing efforts. CHWs are also skilled at connecting community members to information and resources that can assist them to find solutions to their identified problems or concerns.

A LITTLE HISTORY

The concept of community organizing is not new. Throughout history, people excluded from power and decision making have come together and organized to assert their needs. Examples include:

- Labor movements organized to demand safe working conditions, the right to organize, limits to working hours, and a living wage.
- The feminist movement organized to demand the right to vote and other civil rights protections for women and girls.
- The civil rights movement allowed communities of color to gain new rights and access to essential resources.
- Disabled communities organized for civil rights protections to pass the Americans with Disabilities Act.
- Cesar Chavez and the United Farm Workers (UFW) won rights for better working conditions and treatment for California farm workers.
- The Queer Youth Action Team (QYAT)—as described in Chapter Sixteen—organized queer youths and their allies to successfully advocate for protections against discrimination in local high schools.
- In Bolivia, communities organized and fought off the efforts of Bechtel, a large transnational corporation, to regain control over water resources.

? *Can you think of other examples of successful community organizing campaigns and movements from the United States or elsewhere in the world?*

? *What about the history of communities that you belong to?*

? *Have these communities organized to advocate for social change in the past?*

? *Are they currently organizing?*

? *Have you or your family and close friends participated in any of these efforts?*

The term *community organizing* was first used in the 1800s by U.S. social workers to describe their efforts to coordinate services for newly arrived immigrants and the poor

(Garvin and Cox, 1995). While community organizing has aided in starting national movements and resulted in major changes in policy and social conditions (the right to vote, the 1964 Civil Rights Act), it often begins at the local level when a group of people come together to talk about a common problem or vision. The history of community organizing shows that communities do have the power to challenge and change social and political situations that have a negative impact on their health.

DEFINING THE COMMUNITY

Which communities participate in community organizing efforts? There are many ways to define communities. Communities share something important in common. They may live in the same neighborhood or region. They may share a common gender, gender identity, sexual orientation, ethnicity, religion, cultural identity, nationality, immigration status, disability, health condition, profession, political affiliation, values, or other identity or interest. Communities may organize locally or within a region, county, nation, or even internationally. As discussed above, some of the communities who have organized for social change in the United States include women, communities of color, the disabled, and farm workers.

There are many formal definitions for community. Early leaders in the field of community organizing have defined "community" as "a group of people living in the same defined area, sharing the same basic values, organization, and interests" (Rifkins and others, 1988).

Other definitions include: "An informally organized social entity, which is characterized by a sense of identity" (White, 1982).

What is most important is that the members of the community identify for themselves what they share in common, rather than having their identity defined by anyone else.

? *How do you define community?*

? *What communities do you belong to?*

? *What communities have you worked with?*

22.3   WHAT IS COMMUNITY ORGANIZING?

Community organizing is a process by which people, usually a group of people who have been denied resources and participation in the decision-making process, work together to create social change that results in meaningful improvements such as access to new resources and rights or improved health and living conditions. Community organizing identifies and supports leadership from within the community and increases their capacity to work together and take effective action for social change. In this way, the balance of power and resources shifts toward the community.

PHUONG AN DOAN BILLINGS: Every year there is an Immigrant Day in Sacramento [the state capitol of California]. Many different immigrant groups and communities go. My agency, Asian Health Services, participates. They rent some buses and take those who want to go up to Sacramento. We go to express our opinion, and there is always a big demonstration. This is advocacy. Immigrant communities still face so much prejudice. We need more respect for our histories and cultures and contributions to California and the United States.

WHY IS COMMUNITY ORGANIZING SO IMPORTANT?

Community organizing is important for many reasons. It is one of most effective strategies for creating lasting social changes that will improve the lives and health status of large groups of people. For example, community organizing efforts significantly expanded the rights of disabled people for access to basic resources such as transportation, education, housing, and employment. Community organizing by groups like ACT UP and the AIDS Treatment Action Group have significantly expanded the rights of people living with HIV disease and their access to medical treatments and social resources such as housing. At its best, community organizing also honors the resources, wisdom, and leadership of local communities and leaves them with a greater capacity to take action on their own to tackle other problems and create other types of meaningful social change in the future.

POPULAR EDUCATION—A RESOURCE FOR COMMUNITY ORGANIZING

Popular education and the work of Paulo Freire were introduced in Chapters Seventeen and Nineteen. Popular education is often used in the field of public health to guide the work of CHWs and to support community organizing efforts.

Freire was a Brazilian educator who believed that education should lead to liberation or freedom from oppression and the creation of social justice. Popular education is the process by which people come together to talk about their social conditions, to analyze the factors that harm their communities, and to take collective action to change these conditions. As people begin to talk about their lives, their values and hopes, and the factors that harm their health and limit the future of their children, they develop a new awareness of the world and their own potential. Freire referred to this process as "conscientization" or the development of critical consciousness.

The process of conscientization must be carried out and defined by the community. Freire wrote about the importance of local communities speaking "their word" or using their own language and concepts to identify and analyze social conditions.

Based on his experience, Freire believed that community action or organizing should first address the issues that the community cares most deeply about. These deep feelings are a key resource for bringing and keeping community members together and motivating them to continue to take action in the face of significant obstacles and challenges.

Popular education, like community organizing, may be initiated and facilitated from outside the community. But the role of outsiders is to facilitate the leadership and decision making of community members rather than to claim such power for themselves. Any process that undermines the leadership, autonomy, and empowerment of the community is not consistent with the principles of popular education.

By posing questions, the facilitator supports community members in analyzing their social reality and in developing a plan of action to advocate for meaningful change (such as improved working conditions, civil rights protections from discrimination, access to clean drinking water, or affordable health care). These questions provide community members with a way to speak their own word and to express their identity:

- What are the factors, problems, and institutions that harm the health and well-being of the community?
- What are the community's leading concerns or priorities?
- What are the common values and visions or goals for social change and a better future?
- What are the key community resources, including knowledge, wisdom, skills, accomplishments, institutions, relationships, and leadership?

✪   What actions can the community take to reach their goals?

✪   Who are the key allies who may support the community in advocating for social change?

22.4 MODELS OF PRACTICE

There are many different models for community organizing, and these models have changed over time.

EARLY APPROACHES

Early approaches to community organizing, such as those developed by Rothman and Tropman (1987) and Alinsky (1971), were need-based and emphasized the important role that outside experts play in providing communities with leadership and assistance.

Rothman's model featured the role of outside experts who worked with the community to build its identity, to identify their needs by conducting research, and to propose solutions to these needs or problems. Outside experts also aided in linking communities with existing direct services, such as food programs or housing. This model was need-based or focused on what the community needed or lacked. It focused on reaching a common agreement to get the community what it needed.

Alinsky's model of social change focused on challenging the existing power relations that contribute to the inequalities facing poor communities. While it moves away from having outsiders do most of the work for the community, it still assumes that a disadvantaged group needs to be organized from the outside in order to successfully advocate for increased resources. Alinsky's social action model focused on:

✪   Addressing issues that a majority of the community would support, such as ending gun violence or supporting affordable housing policies

✪   Challenging the imbalance of power and privilege between the disadvantaged and the larger community

✪   Assisting to increase the problem-solving ability of the community with the advice of an expert

✪   Goals of social justice, democracy, and the redistribution of power, resources, and decision making

CONTEMPORARY MODELS OF COMMUNITY ORGANIZING

More recent models of community organizing have emphasized an empowerment approach in which the community learns to assume leadership for itself rather than relying on outside experts. These models also include a strength-based or asset-based approach that focuses not only on what communities lack and need, but also on the resources they already have. For example, the process of *community building* (CB) emphasizes the positive resources a community has to offer, including its people as community leaders. These newer models draw on ideas of community development, which emphasize self-help and collaboration within existing power structures. Other examples include:

✪   *Community capacity building,* which refers to the ability to develop and sustain strong relationships to work together in order to identify problems and goals, make group decisions, and take action. This is accomplished by having members of a community share skills, talents, knowledge, and experiences (Mattessich and Monsey, 1997).

✪ *Collaborative partnerships,* which entail building alliances with people and institutions who share your values and goals. For example, an effort to improve the quality of education in local schools might involve establishing a collaborative partnership among students, parents, teachers, school officials, faith-based and other community based organizations, and local businesses. Because these partnerships bring people together from all parts of the community, they can build on a diversity of strengths and resources to increase the chances of success.

As Wallerstein (1992) writes: "The empowerment process at the heart of community organizing promotes participation of people, organizations, and communities toward the goal of increased individual and community control, political efficacy, improved quality of community life, and social justice."

Today's community organizing seeks to accomplish four things:

1. To increase community participation and ownership
2. To build the capacity of the community through leadership and understanding
3. To address the imbalance of power and shift power and local resources back to the community
4. To build a stable power base through coalition building to ensure sustainable social actions

A WORD ABOUT MEDIA ADVOCACY

Media advocacy is often important to the success of a community organizing campaign. It is the strategic use of any form of media—newspapers, radio, television, the World Wide Web, advertisements, billboards, and so on—to publicize and raise awareness about the problems that a community is facing and their goals for social change.

The media is an efficient way to communicate with a large audience. The media can be used to:

✪ *Inform* the public about the causes and consequences of a specific issue
✪ *Recast* these problems as social concerns that affect everyone, not just a distant group
✪ *Encourage* community members and their leaders to find out more about the problems and to get involved in solving those problems
✪ *Promote* agencies and services within your community that address the identified problems

Media advocacy can assist community organizing efforts by:

✪ *Changing* the way key decision makers and the general public look at community issues or problems
✪ *Creating* a reliable, consistent stream of publicity or media focus for your community's issues and activities
✪ *Offering possible explanations* of how these problems could and should be solved
✪ *Motivating* community members and policymakers to get involved

Working with the media becomes easier with training and experience. One step that community members and leaders may wish to take is to seek out local opportunities to learn or enhance media advocacy skills.

Chapter Sixteen described the work of the Queer Youth Action Team (QYAT), a group of youths who successfully advocated for new policies to protect lesbian, gay, bisexual, and transgender youths from discrimination in local schools. The youths did extensive media advocacy, and their work was featured by local and statewide newspapers, radio, and television. The coverage by the media served to change the nature of the debate about student rights and to convince local policymakers to work with the QYAT.

22.5 THE COMMUNITY ACTION MODEL

The Community Action Model (CAM) is an approach to community organizing developed by the Tobacco Free Project of the San Francisco Department of Public Health (Tobacco Free Project). The CAM (Figure 22.1) is deeply influenced by the theories of Paulo Freire and popular education. It features a five-step process designed to assist community members to further develop their capacity to advocate for social justice by creating changes in social policies.

The goals of the CAM are:

1. *Environmental or social change:* To move away from projects that focus only on changing individual lifestyles and behaviors in order to focus on mobilizing community members and agencies to change environmental factors that promote economic, political, and health inequalities.

Figure 22.1 The Community Action Model: Creating Change by Building Community Capacity.

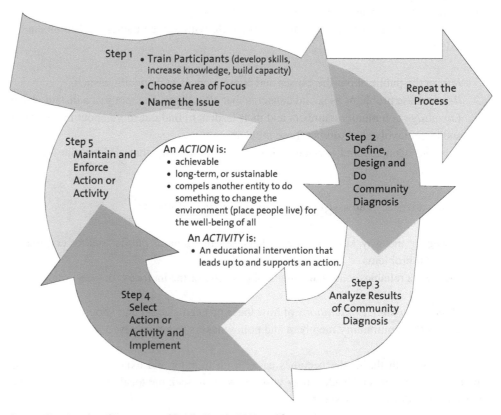

Source: San Francisco Department of Public Health, 2009, p. 16.

2. *Empowerment and community leadership:* Through asset-based action research, the CAM provides a framework for community members to acquire the skills and resources to investigate the health of the place where they live and to plan, implement, and evaluate actions that change the environment to promote and improve health.

Fundamental to implementing the CAM is the *action* or proposed solution that communities work toward. The selected action should meet three criteria:

1. It must be achievable, meaning that you must be able to complete it within the near future (such as year or two rather than twenty or fifty years).
2. It must be long lasting or sustainable, meaning that after your project goes away, the actions or the changes achieved will continue.
3. It must compel another entity (person or organization) to do something to change the environment (the place where people live) for the well-being of all. It must benefit a large number of people or a community rather than just one individual.

THE FIVE STEPS OF THE CAM

Below is a summary of the five steps of the CAM, including a list of activities that may take place at each step.

Step 1: Identify the Problem   Members of a community come together to address key problems or concerns. They invite other members of their community to join them. They discuss the problem or concern and what they would like to change as a result of working together.

Step 1 activities may include:

- ⊛ Conducting outreach to involve more community members (flyers, meetings, emails, and so on)
- ⊛ Meeting at diverse settings (private homes, community centers, faith-based organizations, and so forth) to share information, concerns, and hopes
- ⊛ Facilitating group discussions about the concerns that people care most about
- ⊛ Identify and prioritize leading concerns or problems
- ⊛ Begin to conduct research to learn more about the issues or concerns identified

Step 2: Assess the Problem/Community Diagnosis   Community diagnosis was described in Chapter Seventeen. It is a process of gathering information to better understand the causes and consequences of an issue or problem that the community has identified, such as handgun violence, homelessness, or breast cancer. This process takes time and cannot be rushed. It is important for the community to look deeply at the root causes of their concerns, and to discuss and analyze these together. The community diagnosis is vital to the success of the CAM: it provides information that will guide the actions and strategies that the community will take to advocate for social change. This is a step that communities may best be able to take with the support or facilitation of a CHW or other experienced public health provider or community organizer.

Step 2 activities may include:

- ⊛ Interviewing key opinion leaders in the community
- ⊛ Conducting surveys or facilitating focus groups with community members
- ⊛ Making sure that important groups in the community were not left out of the community diagnosis process
- ⊛ Conducting research to find existing data about the issue at hand, such as study the rates of handgun violence or breast cancer

By meeting together, communities can identify the root causes of the problems they face.

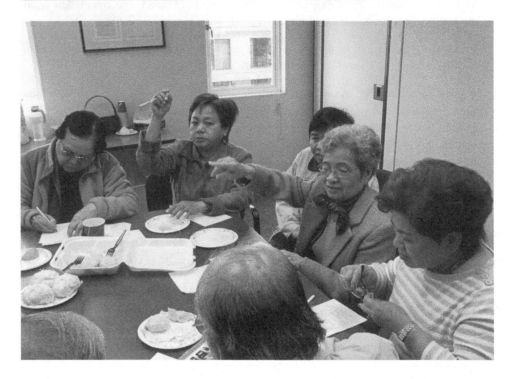

- ⊛ Conducting community-mapping activities
- ⊛ Researching existing records, laws, and policies
- ⊛ Looking for examples of actions that other communities have taken to address similar concerns or problems
- ⊛ Identifying policymaking institutions and individuals
- ⊛ Identifying potential allies and opponents (people who may support or stand in the way of efforts to create social change)

Chapter Seventeen gives more detail and explanation about how to conduct the community diagnosis.

Step 3: Analyze Findings   The next step is for the community to meet together to analyze the information that they gathered during the community diagnosis. Again, this is often a step in which the community can benefit from the support of CHWs or other experienced facilitators. Community members will learn how to read and make sense of different types of data, including survey data or epidemiological data from a local health department. Together the community will decide what the information gathered tells them about the problem at hand and what questions remain.

Step 3 activities may include:

- ⊛ Tallying numbers from a survey
- ⊛ Discussing the information learned from interviews with key opinion leaders
- ⊛ Reviewing reports from focus-group discussions
- ⊛ Reviewing data from existing studies, including public health studies, and arranging this data in ways that make it most accessible, understandable, and useful for the community (such as pie charts, graphs, and picture collages)

✪ Summarizing the findings or information gathered from all sources
✪ Deciding together what the information says about the causes and consequences of the problem or concern, and identifying issues that still may not be clear or well understood
✪ Identifying any outstanding needs to gather more information
✪ Converting this information into visual resources such as graphs, tables, or facts sheets

Step 4: Identify and Implement an Advocacy Action   In this step, community members identify and discuss a list of potential actions to address their identified issue or concern. These actions will include policies that they may want to change. They will analyze these potential actions to see whether they meet the three criteria of the CAM. Together they will analyze the possible choices they identified and select one or more actions that will assist them to create meaningful change and promote the well-being of the community as a whole. Advocates will develop a detailed action plan, including a list of all activities to be undertaken and timelines for completing these activities, and support the community in implementing this plan.

Step 4 activities may include:

A.   *Develop the action plan:*
  ● Coming up with a list or menu of possible actions
  ● Proposing a model policy around the issue or concern identified
  ● Developing a timeline for accomplishing tasks
  ● Identifying and meeting with stakeholders and decision makers
  ● Developing one to three activities to support your proposed policy and raise awareness, such as a health fair, community forum, media advocacy (see below), or presentations to schools or community groups
B.   *Implement the action plan.* The following activities are the building blocks to support the proposed action:
  ● Meeting with stakeholders and policymakers
  ● Getting media coverage of your work and your proposal for policy change
  ● Mobilizing the community to write letters, make calls to policymakers, or participate in public demonstrations
  ● Mobilizing the community to testify before policymakers such as the city council, housing authority, or health commission
  ● Celebrating your hard work and accomplishments

Step 5: Maintain Actions and Results   This step focuses on continuing the activities detailed in the action plan to ensure that the efforts accomplished will be maintained over the long term and enforced by the appropriate bodies.

Step 5 activities may include:

✪ Continuing to meet with policymakers and groups that enforce public policies
✪ Gathering new data to see if the situation or problem has changed
✪ Setting up groups to monitor outcomes such as PTA groups, neighborhood watch groups, and so on
✪ Continuing to do media advocacy to keep the public informed about community organizing efforts
✪ Continuing to raise money to support your advocacy work

The San Francisco Department of Public Health has developed resources to guide community groups in implementing the CAM, including a facilitator's guide. These resources are available online at: www.sfdph.org/dph/comupg/oprograms/CHPP/CAM/default.asp.

THE CAM IN ACTION: THE GOOD NEIGHBOR PROGRAM

Since 1995, the San Francisco Tobacco Free Project, a program of the Department of Public Health, has provided funding to community-based organizations to implement the CAM. The following example illustrates how one project used the model to organize around food security or the extent to which an individual, family, or community has access to regular and sufficient quantities of healthy food to eat.

Food security was identified as a concern by residents of the Bayview Hunters Point Neighborhood in San Francisco. This largely low-income community is home to many public-housing projects, but lacks supermarkets and other places for the community to shop for healthy foods, including fresh fruits and vegetables. Most residents shop at corner liquor stores that sell mostly alcohol, tobacco, and processed foods with poor nutritional content. The only other available food outlets in the community are fast-food restaurants. Not surprisingly, the community experiences high rates of diabetes, hypertension, and other chronic conditions.

Literacy for Environmental Justice (LEJ), an urban environmental education and youth empowerment organization, received funding to implement the CAM in the Bayview neighborhood (www.lejyouth.org). Their goal was to increase food security and improve the health of local residents.

STEP 1: IDENTIFY THE PROBLEM

This is an example of a community organizing project that was funded to address a problem that had already been identified as a priority by community residents. To begin the project, staff from LEJ recruited youth advocates from the neighborhood high school. The advocates were trained on a variety of issues including health, food security, diversity, the legislative process, and public speaking. As a result, the young people came to understand how the lack of high-quality fresh food contributes to increasing rates of chronic disease and premature death in their community. Together, they decided to focus their work on increasing local access to healthy and affordable food and reducing the availability of processed foods and products such as tobacco.

STEP 2: COMMUNITY DIAGNOSIS

The youth advocates conducted a community diagnosis that included a review of existing research and information gathered by previous projects and the local health department. They mapped the community to identify food sources, interviewed local merchants, and created diagrams of the products available in local stores. They conducted interviews with residents and community agencies to learn where they shop for food products and what they buy. They researched policies around tobacco and alcohol and identified policymakers and local leaders who might have an interest in assisting them to reach their goal. Please refer to Chapter 17 to view the survey and map developed by the LEJ youth advocates.

STEP 3: ANALYZE FINDINGS

When they came together to review and analyze the information they had gathered, the youth advocates found out that most residents shopped in corner liquor stores and ate fast food. To reach a supermarket, they had to take two buses and travel to another neighborhood. The products most available in local stores were tobacco, alcohol, and junk food, especially Kraft and Nabisco products made by tobacco subsidiary companies. Some local merchants said that they were interested in offering healthier choices, but didn't have the economic means to buy refrigeration units or to establish contracts with companies selling healthier foods. The youth advocates then used this information to create diagrams, charts, tables, and maps illustrating the problem of access to healthy food in the community. This information was used to paint a picture of the problem and to work to educate the policymakers.

STEP 4: IDENTIFY AND IMPLEMENT AN ADVOCACY ACTION

Based on their findings, LEJ and the youth advocates developed the concept of the Good Neighbor Program (see Figure 22.2). They decided to assist local merchants to sell healthier food and educate the community about the dangers of tobacco, processed food, and fast food, including foods sold by big tobacco companies. They met with local food cooperatives that produce and sell locally grown produce and other healthy foods and established an agreement for them to make their products available to interested stores in the Bayview. They also created posters and stickers to promote what they called the Good Neighbor (GN) Program to provide access to healthy food.

LEJ and the youth advocates conducted media advocacy by writing an article that was published by the local community newspaper, *The Bay View*. They were also successful in getting coverage about their work on local television and radio.

The youth advocates wrote a model policy to promote the Good Neighbor Program and presented it to their district representative on the San Francisco Board of Supervisors (or City Council) and other local policymakers. The City of San Francisco agreed to provide free refrigeration and training to merchants willing to participate in the Good Neighbor Program. They convinced two community agencies and the school district to adopt a policy not to buy Kraft and Nabisco products. A local merchant signed on to become the pilot store for the Good Neighbor Program, selling locally grown produce.

Their work fulfills the three criteria for CAM actions: it was sustainable, achievable, and successful in compelling an entity, in this case a corner store and the city of San Francisco, to change something for the better of the whole community.

STEP 5: MAINTAIN ACTIONS AND RESULTS

Advocates from LEJ and other members of the Bayview Community continue to promote the Good Neighbor idea and monitor and provide assistance to any interested merchants who want to become a Good Neighbor store. Not only did this community organizing project improve food security, it also trained and empowered local youths to become effective advocates for social change. To learn more about the work of LEJ and the Good Neighbor campaign, please go to www.lejyouth.org/programs/food.html.

Figure 22.2 The CAM in Action: The Good Neighbor Program.

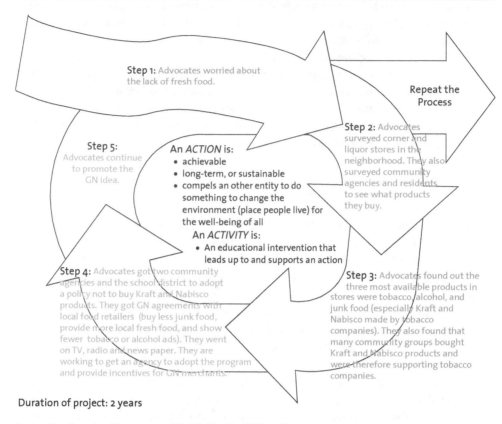

Step 1: Advocates worried about the lack of fresh food.

Repeat the Process

Step 2: Advocates surveyed corner and liquor stores in the neighborhood. They also surveyed community agencies and residents to see what products they buy.

Step 5: Advocates continue to promote the GN idea.

An *ACTION* is:
- achievable
- long-term, or sustainable
- compels an other entity to do something to change the environment (place people live) for the well-being of all

An *ACTIVITY* is:
- An educational intervention that leads up to and supports an action

Step 4: Advocates got two community agencies and the school district to adopt a policy not to buy Kraft and Nabisco products. They got GN agreements with local food retailers (buy less junk food, provide more local fresh food, and show fewer tobacco or alcohol ads). They went on TV, radio and news paper. They are working to get an agency to adopt the program and provide incentives for GN merchants.

Step 3: Advocates found out the three most available products in stores were tobacco, alcohol, and junk food (especially Kraft and Nabisco made by tobacco companies). They also found that many community groups bought Kraft and Nabisco products and were therefore supporting tobacco companies.

Duration of project: 2 years

Source: San Francisco Department of Public Health, 2009, p. 22.

22.6 THE ROLE OF CHWs

Have you ever worked with others to plan a meeting, party, or a family reunion? Have you ever spoken to a group of people about a problem that concerned you? Have you ever spoken out on behalf of a friend or relative? If you have, then chances are you already have experience and skills that are relevant to the task of community organizing.

CHWs have many qualities and skills to support community organizing, including:

- A commitment to social justice
- The ability to develop and maintain trusting relationships with diverse clients and communities
- The ability to listen to the concerns, experiences, and ideas of others with compassion and without judgment
- Information about resources that may be beneficial to the community
- Group facilitation and teamwork skills
- Cultural humility and respect for the experience, wisdom, and skills of others
- Flexibility and the ability to adapt to changing circumstances
- A client- and community-centered approach to their work and a commitment to supporting the self-determination of individuals and communities

? *What other qualities and skills do you and other CHWs have that may be helpful to community organizing efforts?*

Community organizing may take place with or without the participation of a CHW, and the CHW may or may not belong to the community in question. Regardless of whether you are a member of the community, we hope you keep the following suggestions in mind.

When participating in community organizing efforts, we hope that CHWs *will not:*

✪ *Assume that they know or understand the problems that most affect the community.* Only by listening to the community can you come to understand these problems.

✪ *Be the leader.* The role of the CHW is to facilitate the leadership of others rather than to assume it themselves.

✪ *Decide who participates.* All members of the affected community should be invited to take a place at the table and to contribute their knowledge and skills to the community organizing effort.

✪ *Prioritize tasks and activities or make key decisions.* The community must decide which issues or problems to work on and what actions they will take.

✪ *Do all the work.* Remember that your role is to assist people to acquire new skills so that they can take ownership of their own community organizing efforts.

We hope that CHWs *will:*

✪ *Listen to the community.* Your most important job is to listen deeply to the concerns, ideas, aspirations, fears, and accomplishments of the community. You can facilitate this by creating opportunities for people to meet together, and by asking simple open-ended questions that encourage people to speak up and share their knowledge.

✪ *Learn local history.* Take time to learn about the history of the community, including past community organizing efforts and accomplishments, and any previous attempts to address the same problem or concern.

✪ *Recruit and honor the participation of diverse members of the community.* Drawing upon your existing connections in the community, reach out and invite all members to participate.

✪ *Provide training to community members.* You may have a role to play in supporting community members in enhancing their skills in areas such as group facilitation, planning, conducting a community diagnosis, or media advocacy. As always, you need to take direction from the community about which areas, if any, they would like to learn more about. You may provide the training yourself, or identify others who can facilitate workshops for the community.

✪ *Mentor key people.* Often CHWs play a key role in mentoring community participants and leaders, assisting them to learn new skills and to gain confidence in their own ability to contribute to and to lead a community organizing effort.

✪ *Aid in facilitating the critical thinking process.* CHWs often support the development of critical consciousness by facilitating meetings and posing open-ended questions designed to provide community members with an opportunity to "speak their word" and arrive at a deeper understanding of the problems they face. As people begin to gain a common understanding of the problems affecting their communities, they will come up with possible actions and strategies to address these problems.

✪ *Assist the community to build on their strengths.* By supporting community members in conducting a community diagnosis, you can help them to identify existing resources (experience, knowledge, skills, institutions, and leaders).

✪ *Facilitate the implementation process.* Once an action plan has been developed, CHWs can help the community to implement it. Again, you may facilitate group discussions or mentor others to facilitate this process. The community will have a lot of decisions to make: What activities will we undertake? Who will do which activities?

How much money do we need? How will we raise these funds? Whom do we need to reach to participate in our efforts? What potential allies do we need to talk with? What additional training and resources do we need? How much money will be needed? How can we raise these funds?

? *What else do you hope that CHWs who participate in community organizing efforts will and will not do?*

SUPPORTING COMMUNITY MEMBERS TO IMPLEMENT THEIR PLAN

RAMONA BENSON: Some of the clients at the Black Infant Health Program decided they wanted to get involved in policy decisions about welfare. They were upset about how the state government [California] was gonna change the program. They decided to go to Sacramento [the state capitol] to testify to legislators. We helped them decide what they wanted to say, and if they wanted to write it down in advance. We met and talked, and they practiced what they were gonna say—and not say. That was a fun meeting because everyone was supporting each other to speak out. I provided a few tips and suggestions here and there, but mostly they helped each other figure it out. We got these big buses and went up to Sacramento. We provided lunch and encouragement. But the ladies decided who would speak first and what they were gonna say. I think everyone felt good about raising their voices that day. And I hope it made it easier for them to speak out the next time they face a problem.

THE COMMUNITY BUILDER'S TOOL KIT

We have adapted the following list from *A Community Builder's Tool Kit: 15 Tools for Creating Healthy, Productive Interracial/Multicultural Communities* (1998), developed by the Institute for Democratic Renewal and the Claremont Graduate University (www.race-democracy.org/publications.htm). The *Tool Kit* is a resource to guide the work of CHWs and other activists participating in community organizing efforts.

1. Plan with people, not for them. Start by listening to local residents and involve them from the start.
2. Goals will better allow you to see the big picture. There must be clarity or purpose among the group before you can go forward and this should be identified in two to three sentences.
3. Strategies will assist to get you there. Once needs and capacities have been identified (sometimes referred to as asset mapping), it is easier to see what needs to be done and to plan for those steps.
4. Identify leaders. Leadership is about assisting a community empower itself. Every community has leaders, whether they are formal or informal; all they need is someone who can help bring them together. This group will have great influence in the decision-making process.
5. Assist the community in drawing strength from multicultural identities. We can all learn from each other and have something unique to contribute that helps to strengthen the group.
6. Bridge the language barrier. For people to be included in the conversation, they must be able to understand and be understood. CHWs can help to ensure that these needs can be met before any gathering of the group.

7. Safety comes first. Ensure that meetings are a safe place for people to come together, including space and ground rules. Don't forget about your own safety.

8. Assist with the research. Work with community leaders to access information that only an agency may have access to. Whether this is statistical information or knowledge of key decision makers, the community will need this information to come up with a strategic plan.

9. The planning process. You may be able to tap into your own agencies to help a community identify and plan out the steps they wish to take. A detailed, step-by-step approach will best serve to guide the group, although adjustments and refinements will happen along the way.

10. Stay grounded in the community. Issues may change and other priorities may arise, so stay informed to share information.

11. Build partnerships. Gain allies or friends by being an ally yourself. Participate in community meetings or advisory boards so that you can help each other. There is power in numbers (agencies and people).

12. Cultivate the media. Television, newspapers, and the Internet influence people's thinking about public issues and about the causes of problems and possible solutions. Professional relationships with reporters and editors can better get the fair media coverage you may need.

13. Be committed; it's a long road. Positive social change does not come quickly, but focus on the game plan, and long-term planning to move you forward.

14. Take care of yourself. CHWs often consider their communities before considering their own health. Remember that if you are not healthy, you cannot assist your community. Knowing when to let go and setting boundaries will keep you healthy and involved.

22.7 CAM IN THE CLASSROOM

We teach the Community Action Model to students enrolled in the CHW Certificate Program at City College of San Francisco. We also ask them to participate in a modified CAM, selecting and researching an issue and taking an action to advocate for social change.

During the semester, students complete a modified version of the CAM: they research and learn about a specific public health issue; they analyze the information they gather; and they research existing policies that affect their selected health topic and identify key policymakers. Finally, they write a letter to a relevant policymaker and propose or support a policy change to promote the health of the affected community.

At the beginning of their training, CHW students are asked to identify their greatest health concerns for their own communities. Later in the semester, students are assigned to work in groups. Each group selects one of the health concerns identified earlier to address using the CAM.

Students are provided with the following knowledge and skills related to the CAM:

- Overview of the CAM and its applications
- Basic research skills including a library workshop
- Basic information on how to develop and conduct a survey and a key informant interview
- How to develop a basic fact sheet—with proper citations—summarizing key information about the selected health issue or concern. (Citations are the way you refer people to the sources of your information. Citations in this book are included in parentheses after we quote or use information from another sources. Complete information about

these resources—author, title, publisher, publication or Web site, place, and the date published—are provided at the end of each chapter.)

- ✪ Teamwork skills
- ✪ How to develop a work plan to guide their group work
- ✪ The legislative and policy process at the local and state levels
- ✪ How to influence the public policy process, and how to write a letter to a decision or policymaker

A FAMILY ANYWHERE PROJECT

One of the public health issues identified by CHW-certificate students at the beginning of the semester was the devastating impact that high rates of incarceration have on their communities. In class, students learned that the United States has the highest rate of incarceration in the world. Several students shared that they had family members who were or had been incarcerated for significant periods of time.

One small group decided to conduct further research about incarceration and health (Figure 22.3).

Figure 22.3 The CAM in Action: A Family Anywhere Project.

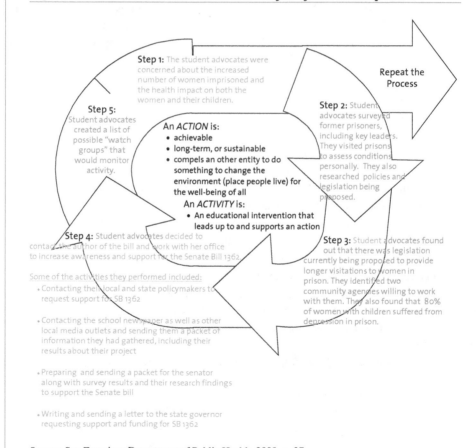

Source: San Francisco Department of Public Health, 2009, p. 27.

✪ How to assemble a poster board illustrating their project and providing policy recommendations

The example that follows, "A Family Anywhere Project," represents the work of one group of CHW students.

STEP 1: CHOOSE AN AREA OF FOCUS

Students conducted research and learned about the increasing number of mothers who are incarcerated, and the health impact on the women and their families. Incarcerated women in California often have little or no contact with their children due to the remote locations of correctional facilities, limited family resources, and limited visiting hours. For women especially, separation from their children can lead to mental health issues and difficulty reentering their communities and reuniting with families upon release.

Step 1 activities included:

✪ Sharing personal knowledge and experience related to the health impacts of incarceration
✪ Discussing goals and objectives for the project and the group
✪ Developing group rules and agreements about work responsibilities
✪ Setting a schedule for meetings and a timeline for completing the CAM project

STEP 2: COMMUNITY DIAGNOSIS

The students conducted various types of research to learn more about the extent and nature of the problem and the consequences for incarcerated women and their families. This included archival research of existing studies and current policies and laws regarding family visitation. Students identified key policymakers and community-based organizations representing the needs of incarcerated people and their families, including Legal Services for Prisoners with Children (LSPC).

Step 2 activities included:

✪ A survey of CCSF students and San Francisco residents to determine their level of knowledge and interest in the selected topic
✪ Interviewing formerly incarcerated women—including students at CCSF— to learn more about their experiences and the impact on their health and families
✪ Interviewing staff at LSPC and other agencies representing the needs of incarcerated women
✪ Attending meetings of local coalitions representing the interests of incarcerated and formerly incarcerated communities
✪ Researching through the Internet current bills, laws, or policies around parental visiting, as well as current policies for lifers and nonviolent offenders
✪ Visiting a local prison to learn more about living conditions and family visitation

(Continued)

STEP 3: ANALYZE RESULTS

The students analyzed the information they gathered and summarized their findings. They found that:

- Nearly 80 percent of female inmates are mothers.
- Seventy percent of women have one or more children under eighteen years of age.
- Women in prison suffer severe depression as a result of being cut off from their children.
- Prison visiting rooms lacked privacy and weren't conducive to family visitation.
- A majority of children whose mothers are imprisoned feel isolated and responsible for their mother's absence, and often do poorly in school.
- Current California law does not permit life-term inmates access to family visits.
- There was a bill before the California legislature (SB 366) that would improve visiting conditions between parents in state prisons and their children.
- Based on the people surveyed, most people feel children need contact with their mothers, regardless if they are incarcerated.

Step 3 activities included:

- Tallying and summarizing survey results.
- Converting numbers into easier-to-read graphics such as pie charts and bar graphs.
- Developing a fact sheet on their findings with the appropriate citations.
- Developing a poster board about the project for use in presentations.
- Conducting presentations to the class and to several community agencies.

STEP 4: IDENTIFY AND IMPLEMENT AN ADVOCACY ACTION

Based on their analysis, the students decided to focus on expanding access and contact between incarcerated mothers and their children, including the right to overnight family visits. They also agreed to support Senate Bill (SB) 366.

Step 4 activities included:

- Contacting the office of the legislator sponsoring SB 366 to ask if and how they could assist to raise awareness and support for this legislation.

CHAPTER REVIEW QUESTIONS

1. Review the scenarios presented at the beginning of this chapter about the community facing increasing handgun violence. Based on the information provided, answer the following questions:
   - What are the primary concerns of the community?
   - What other challenges does the community face?
   - What resources does the community have?
   - As a CHW working in the community, how would you bring members together to talk about their concerns and to identify strategies to promote social change? Specifically, what would you do?
   - What type of community diagnosis might the community undertake to gather more information about the nature, causes, and consequences of their identified concern? What type of key decision and policymakers might

✪ Sending a summary of information gathered, and the fact sheet they prepared, to the office of the legislator sponsoring SB 366.

✪ Contacting legislative representatives to request their support for SB 366 and policy changes that would expand visitation rights for incarcerated women.

✪ Contacting the school newspaper, as well as other media outlets, and sending them a fact sheet on the issue and SB 366.

✪ Writing and sending a letter to the state governor requesting support and funding for the bill.

STEP 5: MAINTAIN ACTIONS AND RESULTS

Because implementing CAM in the classroom has limitations, and students are not able to work on an issue for more than two semesters, the focus is on planting the seed for policy recommendations, rather than following a campaign all the way through to policy implementation. In this case, students spoke with legislators and other activists to learn how the proposed policy would be implemented and monitored over time.

Step 5 activities included:

✪ Researching agencies and coalitions willing to continue monitoring the progress of the bill.

✪ Preparing and sending a packet of information on the project, including a list of possible volunteers.

Each student had the opportunity to present their project to the class and send a letter to a decision maker. The skills they acquired assisted them to take ownership of the solutions and empowered them to take more active leadership roles.

SB 366 was not passed into law in California. Efforts continue, however, to expand the rights of incarcerated people to family visitation. To read more about these and other efforts to advocate on behalf of incarcerated people and their families, including the rights of pregnant women, please go to the Web site of Legal Services for Prisoners with Children (www.prisonerswithchildren.org). You will also find links to other agencies and resources on their Web site.

be able to influence the issue of concern to the community?

● What challenges might the community face in analyzing the information they gather? How might a CHW facilitate this process?

● What types of goals might the community develop? What types of actions or activities might they engage in? What types of policy changes might the community advocate for?

● How might the community work to maintain their organizing efforts? How could they monitor the results of their work and any changes created?

● As a CHW, what role could you take in this community organizing process?

2. Now think about *your* community. Think about a community you belong to and answer the following questions:

● What health issues does the community face? Which issues are you most concerned about? Which issue would you select to be the focus of a community organizing effort?

● What factors contribute to this problem or otherwise harm the community? What needs to change?

- What information do you want to gather to better understand the causes and consequences of this problem? How will you gather this information?
- Who are the key decision makers or policymakers with the ability to influence or change the issue you want to work on?
- What are some of the key resources in this community? Who are some of the key opinion leaders you would ask to participate in a community organizing effort?

- What goal (or goals) might you select to work toward? Does it meet the three criteria of the CAM model?
- What type of actions and activities would better allow you to reach this goal?
- How will you know if your community organizing efforts are successful?

3. Now you try:
   - Use the information you have collected from the questions above and plug them into the CAM. What does this reveal and what else would you still need to research or do?

REFERENCES

Alinsky, S. D. 1971. *Rules for Radicals: A Pragmatic Primer for Realistic Radicals*. New York: Random House.

Garvin, C. D., and Cox, F. M. 1995. A History of Community Organizing Since the Civil War with Special Reference to Oppressed Communities. In J. Rothman, J. L. Erlich, and J. E. Tropman, Eds., *Strategies of Community Intervention: Macro Practice* (5th ed.). Itasca, : F. E. Peacock.

Institute for Democratic Renewal. 1998. School of Politics and Economics. Claremont Graduate University. A Community Builders Tool Kit. Accessed on April 11, 2009: www.race-democracy.org/publications.htm

Legal Services for Prisoners with Children. Accessed on April 11, 2009: www.prisonerswithchildren.org

Mattessich, P., and Monsey, B. 1997. *Community Building: What Makes It Work; A Review of Factors Influencing Successful Community Building*. St. Paul, MN: Amherst H. Wilder Foundation.

Rifkin, S. B., Muller, F., and Bichmann, M. 1988. Primary Healthcare: On Measuring Participation. *Social Science and Medicine* 26: 931–940.

Rothman, J., and Tropman, J. E. 1987. *Models of Community Organization and Macro Practice Perspective: Their Mixing and Phasing*. In F. M. Cox, J. L. Erlich, J. Rothman, and J. E. Tropman, Eds., *Strategies of Community Organization: Macro Practice* (pp. 3–26). Itasca, IL: F. E. Peacock.

San Francisco Department of Public Health. Community Health Promotion and Prevention: Community Action Model. Accessed on April 11, 2009: www.sfdph.org/dph/comupg/oprograms/CHPP/CAM/default.asp

Wallerstein, N. 1992. Powerlessness, Empowerment, and Health: Implications for Health Promotion Programs. *American Journal of Health Promotion* 6: 197–205.

White. 1982. Cited in W. R. Brieger, *Definitions of Community*. Baltimore, MD: John Hopkins Bloomberg School of Public Health, 2006. Accessed on April 11, 2009: http://ocw.jhsph.edu/courses/SocialBehavioralFoundations/PDFs/Lecture10.pdf

ADDITIONAL RESOURCES

Administration on Aging. Department of Health and Human Services. Accessed on April 11, 2009: www.aoa.gov/press/more/Media_Advocacy/Media_Advocacy.aspx

Bobo, K. A., Max, S., and Kendall, J. 2001. *Organizing for Social Change: Midwest Academy Manual for Activists* (3rd ed.). Washington, DC: Seven Locks Press.

Freire, P. 1973. *Education for Critical Consciousness*. New York: Seabury Press.

Paulo Freire Institute. University of California, Los Angeles. Accessed on April 11, 2009: www.paulofreireinstitute.org/

Heaney, T. 1995. Issues in Freirian Pedagogy. Accessed on April 11, 2009: www3.nl.edu/academics/cas/ace/resources/documents/FreireIssues.cfm

Himmelman, A. 1992. Communities Working Collaboratively for Change. Unpublished paper. Minneapolis, MN: Himmelmann Consulting Group.

Lavery, S. H., Smith, M. L., Avila-Esparza, A., Hrushow, A., Moore, M., and Reed, D. F. 2005. The Community Action Model: A Community-Driven Model Designed to Address Disparities in Health. *American Journal of Public Health* 95: 611–616.

Literacy for Environmental Justice. Accessed on April 11, 2009: www.lejyouthy.org

McKenzie, J. F., Neiger, B. L., and Smeltzer, J. L. 2005. *Planning, Implementing, and Evaluating Health Promotion Programs: A Primer* (4th ed.). San Francisco: Benjamin Cummings.

The Midwest Academy. Accessed on April 11, 2009: www.midwestacademy.com

Minkler, M., and Wallerstein, N. 1997. Improving Health Through Community Organization and Community Building: A Health Education Perspective. In M. Minkler, Ed., *Community Organizing and Community Building for Health* (pp. 30–52). New Brunswick, NJ: Rutgers University Press.

GLOSSARY

Active listening   Communication skills used to demonstrate that you are listening closely and accurately to others, to improve the quality of communication and professional and personal relationships. Also used in conflict resolution.

Advocacy   The act of speaking up or speaking out in support of a client, community, or policy change.

Advocate (noun)   Someone who speaks up on behalf of someone else or in support of a change; frequently, in support of changing a law or policy.

Advocate (verb)   To speak out in favor of a client, community, or policy change.

Ambivalence   Having thoughts or actions in contradiction with each other.

At risk   Individuals or communities who have a greater chance of developing a specific illness, disability, or other health condition.

Auditory learners   People who learn primarily by listening.

Body language   Nonverbal communication through facial expressions and how people move, position, or hold their body.

Boundary crossing   When a CHW or other service provider crosses or breaks professional or ethical guidelines and is at risk of causing harm to the client, the community, themselves, or their agency.

Burnout   The point a person reaches when the demands made over an extended period of time are too great for the resources the person possesses. Burnout has been described as a physical, emotional, psychological, and spiritual phenomenon—an experience of personal fatigue, alienation, and failure—or a progressive loss of idealism and energy. A common risk for people working in the helping professions.

Capacity building   Strengthening the knowledge, skills, and confidence of individuals or communities.

Caseload   The number of clients that a service provider is working with at the same time. For example, some providers work with no more than 25 clients at a time; others may serve 50 or more.

Child mortality   The number of children who die before the age of five, out of every one hundred thousand live births.

Chronic disease or health conditions   Illness or other health conditions that are ongoing or last for at least three months and often for a long period of time. Chronic conditions often have no cure, but may be treated or managed to improve the quality of life. Examples include cancer, diabetes, asthma, hypertension, depression, and heart disease.

Closed-ended questions   Questions that can be answered with a few words, like *yes* or *no*. They are used when you want to focus the conversation and gather specific information.

Code switching   Recognizing and following the rules of conduct of a different culture, institution, or profession in order to be successful in that environment.

Competencies   For the purposes of this book, competencies are the knowledge and skills that CHWs and other people need to perform a job well or to provide high-quality services.

Compliance   For the purposes of this book, compliance refers to following a prescribed set of treatments, standards, or policies. Treatment compliance or adherence refers to whether or not clients accurately follow prescribed treatments including diet and the use of medicines.

Confidentiality   The policy of not sharing private information about clients, including the client's identity (name or Social Security number), with others, unless the client provides written consent. There are important exceptions: If a client discloses information about harm or the threat of harm to themselves or others, the CHW may have an ethical and legal obligation to report this to a third party, such as their supervisor or law enforcement agencies.

Conscientization and critical consciousness   The process of developing a new awareness of the social, economic, and political factors that influence our social condition, health, and well-being. A first step in popular education that leads to taking collective action for social change and social justice.

Copayments   The out-of-pocket expenses that patients pay to cover part of the costs for insurance premiums or a share of costs for receiving services at a clinic or hospital, or for medications.

Corrective feedback   Feedback usually provided to a coworker that indicates desired changes in behavior, by explaining what didn't work, went badly, or needs improvement.

Credentialing   Requires people to prove that they have completed a program of education or training and mastered essential knowledge and skills before they begin to work in a particular occupation (such as a teaching credential or CHW certificate).

Crisis intervention   Working with a client who is in crisis to prevent further harm or trauma and to assist them in accessing resources that will facilitate their safety and recovery.

Cross-cultural   Working in more than one cultural context or with people from more than one cultural identity or background.

Curriculum   A set of classes, and their content and materials, for a particular course or field of study.

Deductible   A fee that a patient must pay annually before the health insurance company will cover additional costs of health care. For example, some patients will have to pay a deductible of $500 to $1,000 or more for hospitalization, with the insurance company paying for additional costs.

Demography   The study of human populations, their composition, structure, and change.

Demographic information   Information or data about an individual or population including, for example, their age, income, educational level, ethnicity, employment status, and so forth.

Dual/multiple relationships   When a CHW or other helping professional has another type of relationship or connection with someone who is also a client. For example, a client may be a former coworker, a neighbor, a friend of a family member, or a member of your church, synagogue, or mosque.

Ecological models of health   These models are used to show the broad range of factors that influence human health, including individual behavior and biology, relationships, the place where people live and work, and social, economic, and political policies.

Environmental justice   Refers to organizing and advocacy efforts to redress environmental racism (see below) and to equalize and diminish the risks of exposure to environmental toxins and other risks among all communities.

Environmental racism   Increased exposure to environmental toxins and other hazards for communities of color, racial discrimination in the enforcement of environmental rules and regulations, or the exclusion of minority groups from public and private boards, commissions, and regulatory bodies.

Epidemiology   The study of the distribution and causes of disease, disability, or death in populations.

Ethics   A set of principles that provide guidance for professionals regarding "right conduct," or what to do when faced with a challenge or dilemma. Designed to prevent abuse, discrimination, or other harm to clients, customers, or patients.

External resources   Resources that lie outside of ourselves and that support our health and well-being, such as friends, family, safe housing, employment, health insurance, and so on.

Food security   Food security implies that people have regular access to enough food so that they won't face hunger.

Gender identity   A person's own sense of identification as male or female, both, or neither.

Grassroots organizing   Grassroots organizing efforts and campaigns are those characterized by the participation and leadership of the communities who have the most to gain or lose from the outcome of the organizing effort.

Gross domestic product (GDP)   The total value of all goods and services produced by a nation in a given period of time, typically within a year. *GDP per capita* is GDP divided by the size of the population, often used to estimate the relative prosperity of a nation.

Harm-reduction/risk-reduction counseling   An approach that does not expect clients to eliminate risky behaviors altogether, and supports them in making any small or incremental changes designed to reduce harms, such as the risk of HIV infection.

Health inequalities   Unequal and unfair rates of illness and death between different populations often based on income, wealth, location, ethnicity, or immigration status.

Homophobia   Prejudice and discrimination against homosexuals (people who have romantic or sexual relationships with members of the same sex).

Infant mortality   The number of infants who die before the age of one, out of one thousand live births. One of most commonly used statistics to evaluate the health of a nation or population.

Infectious diseases   Diseases that are caused by pathogens (disease-causing agents) such as bacteria or viruses and that may be transmitted from person to person. Examples include the flu, cholera, tuberculosis, HIV, malaria, and syphilis.

Informed consent   The obligation to provide clients with information they need in order to make a sound decision about whether or not to participate in a program or service. Usually obtained in writing. Minor children or otherwise dependent clients may require the consent of a parent or guardian.

Interdisciplinary   Incorporates and builds upon more than one academic discipline or field of study.

Internal resources   Strengths that lie within each of us, such as our knowledge, skills, personality, values, beliefs, and accomplishments.

Key opinion leaders   The natural leaders found in all communities, not necessarily holding formal positions of authority. People in a community who are trusted and whom others turn to for information and guidance.

Kinesthetic learners   People who often learn best by doing or through a "hands-on" approach.

Leading Questions   Questions that are designed to lead to or result in a specific answer or response.

Learning outcomes   What participants or students will know, and know how to do, at the end of a training, class, or course of study.

LGBTQQI   Lesbian, Gay, Bisexual, Transgender, Queer, Questioning, and Intersex. An umbrella term that is sometimes used to refer to a large group of communities who have sexual orientations other than heterosexual and diverse gender identities. Please note that transgender and intersex people and communities sometimes object to being included in this broad category.

Life expectancy   An estimate of the number of years that people who belong to a specific population will live at birth or after a given age.

Maternal mortality   The number of women who die as a result of pregnancy or childbirth, out of one hundred thousand births.

Media advocacy   The strategic use of any type of media (radio, television, newspapers, and so on) to help advance an organization's objectives or goals.

Mediation   A process of dispute resolution in which one or more impartial third parties intervenes in a conflict, with the consent of the participants, and assists them in negotiating a resolution.

Morbidity   Illness or disease.

Mortality   Death.

Needs assessment   A process of conducting research to find out what a community or other population lacks or needs.

Open-ended question   Invites a client or other person to respond with more than a "yes or no" answer. It encourages people to talk and may facilitate dialogue.

Participatory learning   When students or other learners are actively engaged in the learning experience.

Popular education   A system of education based on the writings of Brazilian educator Paolo Freire that helps people to identify social and political problems and develop solutions for social justice based on their own life experience and wisdom.

Population   A group of people with common characteristics that may be based on one or more factors such as geography, nationality, age, sex, ethnicity, occupation, illness, or disability.

Post-traumatic stress (PTS)   A type of stress response that may occur when people are exposed to war, torture, child abuse, sexual assault, incarceration, natural disasters, and other traumatic experiences characterized by intense fear, loss of control, and helplessness.

Premiums   The amount that we are charged to purchase health insurance. Premiums are usually paid monthly by an individual, a family, or an employer.

Prevalence   The percentage of a population with a certain illness or risk. For example, the prevalence of HIV among adults in the United States is approximately 1 percent (1 in 100), while it is approximately 20 percent (20 in 100) in Zimbabwe.

Problem-based learning   Students or participants learn by working together and applying knowledge and skills to solving reality-based problems.

Professional boundaries   Limitations or guidelines that a professional establishes within relationships, including relationships with clients. These boundaries guide professionals in maintaining an ethical relationship with clients that seeks to do no harm.

Professional development   Learning new or enhancing existing professional skills.

Qualitative data   In research and in public health evaluation, information that is gathered directly from people that is subjective and not easily summed up by numbers (as opposed to quantitative methods).

Quantitative data   In research and in public health, information that can be measured through counting and numbers, such as the number of clients served or the percentage or prevalence of an illness in a population.

Relapse   Returning to unhealthy behaviors after reducing or eliminating them.

Resilience   The ability to survive and recover well from stress, crisis, trauma, or a series of negative events.

Résumé   A formal document listing your work experience, skills and education.

Safety net   Hospitals, clinics, and community health centers that provide health care to the poor and the uninsured.

Scope of practice   The tasks and services that a professional is qualified to provide on the job.

Secondary or vicarious trauma   The effect on helping professionals of working closely with survivors of traumatic events including war, rape, and child abuse. In these circumstances, helping professionals may themselves begin to experience symptoms of post-traumatic stress.

Secondary or vicarious resilience   When helping professionals working closely with survivors of traumatic events are positively affected and inspired by the resilience, healing, and recovery of those they work with.

Self-disclosure   Revealing personal information to others, such as when CHWs or other service providers share personal information with clients.

Sexual orientation   Refers to whether or not people are romantically and sexually attracted to people of the same or opposite sex, or both (homosexual, heterosexual, bisexual).

Social determinants of health   The economic, social, and political policies and dynamics that influence whether or not populations have access to basic resources and rights and their health status.

Social justice   Promoting human rights and equal access to essential resources within a society including education, housing, food, employment, safety, and health care.

Social marketing   Applying the same methods that businesses use—including the use of radio, television, and other media—to sell products in order to promote specific health outcomes such as breast cancer screening, HIV antibody testing, or healthy eating.

Stakeholder   Anyone who has an interest in the outcome of a decision (usually a policy change).

Stress   Stress is defined as the way we respond to and are affected by events or situations that place a demand on our internal and external resources.

Stressor   The event or circumstance that places demands upon our internal and external resources.

Structural discrimination   When discrimination against a group of people (based on sex, gender identity, ethnicity, sexual orientation, religion, nationality, immigration status, disability status, or other criteria) is supported by private or government policies and practices.

Structural racism   When inequities based on race or ethnicity are built into the key systems of a society, such as the educational, legal, employment, housing, and health care systems.

Supportive feedback   Reinforces the current behavior of coworkers by identifying what they are doing well or right.

Transphobia   Prejudice or discrimination against transgender or gender-variant people.

Treatment Adherence or Compliance   Supporting clients or patients to understand and be able to follow treatment guidelines such as the proper use of medications.

Universal health care   A government policy or set of policies that guarantees access to health care to everyone.

Venue   Place. Used to describe places where a community spends significant time or where outreach or events take place.

Visual learners   People who generally learn through the ability to see the material that they are learning.

NAME INDEX

SUBJECT INDEX

Anxiety, 300, 354

AOL, 431

Apartheid, 75

APHA. *See* American Public Health Association

Apologizing: to clients, 249, 303, 441; for conflict resolution, 329

Applications, job, 363

Appropriations Committee, 128

Arguing, 474–475, 509

Arizona, 40

Arts: benefits of, 515–517; examples of projects incorporating, 517–527; forms of, 515; role of CHWs in, 527–528

Asian Health Services, 19–20, 126, 429, 430, 518, 534

Asian Pacific Environmental Network, 75–76

Asian people: ethnic identity of, 141; examples of outreach to, 429; health inequalities of, 70; interpreters for, 126; number of CHWs who are, 6; number of, served by CHWs, 6; population changes regarding, 138; professional boundaries of, 170

Assessment writing, 285

Association for Conflict Resolution, 335

Assumptions: about clients, 249, 256, 474–475; about conflicts, 324–325

At risk populations, 50

Audience, for training: assessing interest of, 461; challenges of, 474–476; description of, 455; engaging, 468–471

Auditory learners, 457

Australia, 99

Authentic apologies, 441–442

Avoidance behaviors, 320, 489, 508

B

Bangladesh, 8

Banking, 458

Bankruptcy, 132

Banks, 92

Behavior change: in client-centered care, 189, 193; common mistakes in facilitating, 183–189; as counseling outcome, 225; developing a plan for, 226–230;

factors that influence, 180–183; group facilitation for, 502, 504–505; implicit theories about, 193–194; need for, 179; personal assessment of, 180; resistance to, 244–245; scale to assess, 242–244; theory of, 232–234; types of behaviors to undergo, 179. *See also* Counseling, client-centered

Behavior responses, to stress, 343

Behavior, risky, 191–192

Bias, 15, 404–405

Bill, 128–131

Birth weights, 74, 81–82

Black Infant Health Program, 30, 81, 82, 434, 506

Black Panther Party, 29

Blame: of clients, 186–188; for conflicts, 325, 326

Blood poisoning. *See* Septicemia

Body language: during client interviews, 205, 206; definition of, 206; home visit safety and, 302; in workplace communication, 370–371

Bolivia, 92, 533

Boston, City of, 34

Boundary crossing, 168–169

Brandeis University, 29, 32, 257

Brazil, 105

Bread for the World, 97

Breathing technique, 354, 355

Bretton Woods Project, 93, 97

Bubble charts, 229–230

Buddhism, 103

Budgets, 96

Bureau of Primary Health Care, 37

Burnout: aggravating factors for, 344; assessment of, 346–350; definition of, 344; possible outcomes of, 345

Business cards, 216, 280

C

Calendars, 376

California, 40, 121, 138

California Budget Project, 121

California Healthcare Foundation, 115, 117

California Newsreel, 74, 78, 79

California Pan Ethnic Health Network, 112

Californians for Pesticide Reform, 432

CalWORKS, 77

CAM. See Community Action Model

Canada, 93, 132, 231

Cancer, 48

Capacity building: AACHW code of ethics regarding, 165; CHWs' core competencies in, 14; CHWs' personal qualities and, 14; CHWs' role in, 12, 152; community partnerships for, 63; cultural humility and, 152; definition of, 33; models of, 536–537, 538–544; training for, 33–36

CAPS. *See* Center for AIDS Prevention Studies

Carbon dioxide, 98, 102

Cardiovascular health, 6, 353

Care plans, 260, 270*f*, 285

Caring, conveying, 489–490

Case conferences, 285–286, 378

Case management: advocacy in, 276; assessments in, 264–266, 273; challenges of, 259, 277–278; CHWs' responsibilities in, 261–262; CHWs' work time and, 7; clients' responsibilities in, 261; communication in, 263, 275; confidentiality in, 271, 283; definition of, 257–258; documentation of, 272–273, 282–285; elements of, 260; function of, 257; goal setting in, 266–267, 275; during home visits, 306; identifying resources in, 259, 278–281; maintaining client contact in, 275; plan for, 260, 263–274; for prevention of illness, 258; priority setting in, 267–268; professional boundaries in, 275, 277–278; referrals from, 281–282, 282; resource identification in, 278–281; scope of practice of, 259, 260–261; self-care during, 278; stages of, 262–263; teamwork for, 260–261; termination of, 274; time management of, 282; timing of guidance during, 275–276

Case studies, 470